CONCEPTS IN ONCOLOGY THERAPEUTICS

Made possible through a grant from Amgen

SECOND EDITION

CONCEPTS IN
ONCOLOGY THERAPEUTICS

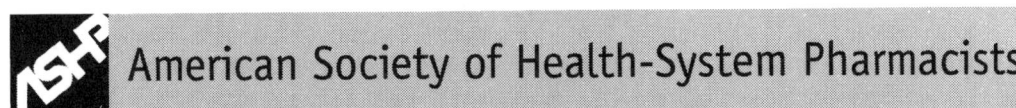
American Society of Health-System Pharmacists

SECOND EDITION

Editors

REBECCA S. FINLEY, Pharm.D., M.S.
Chair and Associate Professor
Department of Pharmacy Practice and Pharmacy Administration
Philadelphia College of Pharmacy
Philadelphia, Pennsylvania

CAROL BALMER, Pharm.D.
Associate Professor
University of Colorado School of Pharmacy
Denver, Colorado

Any correspondence regarding this publication should be sent to the publisher, American Society of Health-System Pharmacists®, 7272 Wisconsin Avenue, Bethesda, MD 20814, attn: Jane S. Ricciuti, Pharmacist Editor/Project Manager, Special Publishing. Produced in conjunction with the ASHP Publications Production Center (Technical Editor/Production Manager: Bruce Hawkins; Production Assistants: Nancy L. Kelih and Michelle M. Noble). Cover and Page Design: Hector L. Coronado

The information presented herein reflects the opinions of the contributors and reviewers. It should not be interpreted as an official policy of ASHP or as an endorsement of any product.

> **Drug information and its applications are constantly evolving because of ongoing research and clinical experience, and it is often subject to professional judgment and interpretation by the practitioner and the uniqueness of a clinical situation. The authors and ASHP have made every effort to ensure the accuracy and completeness of the information presented in this book. However, the reader is advised that the publisher, authors, contributors, editors, and reviewers cannot be responsible for the continued currency of the information, for any errors or omissions, and/or for any consequences arising from the use of the information in the clinical setting.**

©1998, American Society of Health-System Pharmacists, Inc. All rights reserved.

No part of this publication may be reproduced or transmitted in any form or by any means, electronic or mechanical, including photocopying, microfilming, and recording, or by any information storage and retrieval system, without written permission from the American Society of Health-System Pharmacists.

ASHP® is a trademark of the American Society of Health-System Pharmacists, Inc.; registered in the U.S. Patent and Trademark Office.

ISBN: 1-879907-78-X

Contents

List of Tables v
List of Figures ix
Preface xiii
Reviewers xv

Chapter 1—Overview of Cancer 1
  by Rebecca S. Finley

Chapter 2—Principles of Cancer Treatment 15
  by Carol Balmer and Rebecca S. Finley

Chapter 3—The Pharmacology of Cytotoxic Chemotherapy I 33
  by Rebecca S. Finley

Chapter 4—The Pharmacology of Cytotoxic Chemotherapy II 51
  by Rebecca S. Finley

Chapter 5—Pharmacology of Immunotherapies 67
  by Carol Balmer

Chapter 6—Optimizing Chemotherapy Outcomes 81
  by Rebecca S. Finley and Carol Balmer

Chapter 7—Systemic Toxicity 99
  by Carol Balmer and Rebecca S. Finley

Chapter 8—Major Organ Toxicity 121
  by Carol Balmer and Heidi Mabay

Chapter 9—Gastrointestinal Complications of Cancer Chemotherapy 147
  by Amy Valley

Chapter 10—Administration of Cancer Chemotherapy 173
  by Rebecca S. Finley

Chapter 11—Management of Lung and Colorectal Cancers 197
  by Jane Pruemer

Chapter 12—Management of Breast and Prostate Cancers 211
  by Carol Balmer and Marianne Irani

Chapter 13—Management of Hematological Malignancies 231
  by Andrea Iannucci

Chapter 14—Bone Marrow Transplantation 251
  by Laura E. Wiggins

Chapter 15—Infectious Complications 269
  by James A. Trovato and Rebecca S. Finley

Chapter 16—Pain Management 289
  by David S. Johnson

Chapter 17—Psychosocial and Palliative Care **309**
  by Rowena N. Schwartz
Chapter 18—Nutritional Support **323**
  by Cynthia L. LaCivita and Jeannine Schreiber
Chapter 19—Oncological Complications **341**
  by Cynthia L. LaCivita
Chapter 20—Pharmacy Practice Issues in Oncology **357**
  by Rebecca S. Finley and Carol Balmer

Appendixes **391**
  The Mammalian Cell Cycle 391
  Common Toxicity Criteria 394
  Karnofsky Performance Status Scale 397
Answers to Self-Study Questions **399**
Glossary **411**
Index **417**

List of Tables

1-1.	Types of Genetic Mutations	3
1-2.	Examples of Genes Associated with Human Cancer	3
1-3.	Types of Proteins Involved with Malignant Characteristics	3
1-4.	Characteristics of Benign and Malignant Tumors	4
1-5.	Proposed Etiologic Factors Associated with Carcinogenic Risk in Humans	5
1-6.	Tumor Nomenclature for Common Malignant Neoplasms	7
1-7.	Recommendations for Early Detection of Cancer	8
1-8.	Examples of Paraneoplastic Syndromes Associated with Some Malignant Cancers	9
1-9.	Clinically Useful Tumor Markers	9
2-1.	Goals of Cancer Therapy	19
2-2.	Toxicities Associated with Radiation Treatment	21
2-3.	Responsiveness of Specific Tumors to Chemotherapy and Hormonal Therapy	23
2-4.	Examples of Nononcological Uses of Chemotherapy and Immunotherapy Drugs	23
2-5.	Examples of Regional or Localized Administration of Chemotherapy	24
2-6.	Guidelines for Use of Adjuvant Chemotherapy	29
3-1.	Alkylating Agents in Clinical Use in the United States	38
3-2.	Toxicities Associated with Alkylating Agents	38
3-3.	Antitumor Antibiotics in Clinical Use in the United States	42
3-4.	Toxicities Associated with Antitumor Antibiotics	44
4-1.	Antimetabolite Cytotoxic Drugs in Clinical Use in the United States	52
4-2.	General Guidelines for Modification of Leucovorin Dosage Following High-Dose Methotrexate in High-Risk Patients	54
4-3.	Toxicities Associated with Antimetabolite Cytotoxics	54
4-4.	Plant Alkaloids Used as Anticancer Drugs	58
5-1.	Guidelines for Withholding IL-2 Therapy	74
5-2.	Examples of FDA-Approved Cancer Detection Agents	75
5-3.	Alternative Cancer Therapies	77
6-1.	Breast Cancer: 10-Year Survival Related to Size of Primary Tumor and Lymph Node Involvement	83
6-2.	Mechanisms of Tumor Cell Resistance to Antineoplastic Drugs	85
6-3.	Examples of Antineoplastic Drugs Cross-Resistant via the P-Glycoprotein–Mediated Multidrug Resistance Mechanism	85
6-4.	Advantages and Disadvantages of Combination Chemotherapy	89
6-5.	Potential Toxicities of the CAP Regimen	89
6-6.	An Alternating Regimen Compared with a Hybrid Combination	90
6-7.	MOPP Chemotherapy Regimen Dose Adjustment Guideline	93
6-8.	Recommended Dose Adjustments of Cytotoxics for Organ Dysfunction	95
6-9.	Steps in Selection of a Chemotherapy Regimen	95

7-1.	FDA-Approved Indications for Clinical Use of G-CSF and GM-CSF	102
7-2.	Summary of ASCO Recommendations for Use of Hematopoietic CSFs	103
7-3.	Common Causes of Thrombocytopenia in Cancer Patients	104
7-4.	Nonmyelosuppressive Hematological Toxicity of Chemotherapy Agents	105
7-5.	Potential Causes of Skin Reactions in Patients with Cancer	107
7-6.	Cytotoxic Drugs That May Cause Alopecia	110
7-7.	Recommended Premedication Regimens for Paclitaxel and Docetaxel	110
7-8.	Anticancer Drugs That Cause Hypersensitivity Reactions	111
7-9.	Comparison of Secondary AML Induced by Alkylating Agents and by Type II Topoisomerase Inhibitors	112
7-10.	Relative Risk of Secondary Malignancies After Hodgkin's Disease Treatment	113
7-11.	Fertility Effects of Individual Chemotherapy Agents	114
8-1.	Antineoplastic Drugs That Are Only Occasionally Implicated in Hepatic Damage or That Have Infrequent Clinical Use	132
8-2.	Antineoplastic Agents Associated with Pulmonary Toxicity	134
8-3.	Selected Cytotoxic Agents Associated with Neurological Toxicity	136
9-1.	Gastrointestinal Toxicity Grading System	148
9-2.	Relative Emetogenic Potential of Antineoplastic Agents	151
9-3.	General Principles of Antiemetic Therapy	152
9-4.	Comparison of Antiemetic Agents	154
9-5.	Commonly Used Chemotherapy Regimens and Suggested Antiemetic Regimens	158
9-6.	Oral Mouth Care Protocols	160
10-1.	Orally Administered Cytotoxic Drugs	175
10-2.	Locally Reactive Cytotoxic Drugs and Suggested Interventions	176
10-3.	Potential Complications of Central Venous Catheters	179
10-4.	Thrombolytic Therapy for Occluded Venous Access Devices	182
10-5.	Features and Specifications of Ambulatory Infusion Devices	183
10-6.	Anticancer Drugs Administered by IM or SC Injection	184
	Appendix 10-A—Recommended Vesicant and Irritant Administration Procedures to Minimize Risk of Extravasation	192
	Appendix 10-B—Suggested Procedures for Minimizing Toxic Effects of Vesicant Extravasation	193
	Appendix 10-C—Intraperitoneal Catheter Care and Recommendations for Drug Administration	194
11-1.	Comparison of NSCLC and SCLC	199
11-2.	Common Signs and Symptoms of Lung Cancer	199
11-3.	TNM Staging System Definitions for Lung Cancer	199
11-4.	Chemotherapy Agents with Activity Against NSCLC	201
11-5.	Combination Chemotherapy Regimens for NSCLC	201
11-6.	Chemotherapy Agents with Activity Against SCLC	202
11.7.	Combination Chemotherapy Regimens for SCLC	202
11-8.	American Cancer Society Guidelines to Reduce Risk of Colorectal Cancer	203
11-9.	American Joint Committee on Cancer (AJCC) Classification of Colon and Rectal Cancer	205
11-10.	AJCC Staging of Colorectal Cancer	205

11-11.	Adjuvant Therapy for Patients with Stage III Colon Cancer	205
11-12.	Regimens Established as Superior to Fluorouracil Alone in Advanced Colorectal Cancer	206
12-1.	Summary of Environmental Risk Factors for Breast Cancer	213
12-2.	Stage Grouping for Breast Cancer	215
12-3.	Chemotherapy Regimens Used in the Adjuvant Therapy of Breast Cancer	216
12-4.	Relationship Between Estrogen and Progesterone Receptor Status of Breast Tumor and the Patient's Objective Response to Endocrine Therapy	217
12-5.	General Criteria to Select Patients for Endocrine Manipulations or Chemotherapy for Management of Metastatic Breast Cancer	218
12-6.	Guide to Interpretation of Prostate-Specific Antigen Values	221
12-7.	Risk of Death and Cure Rates by Stage of Prostate Cancer	222
12-8.	Hormonal Interventions for Management of Advanced Prostate Cancer	224
12-9.	Representative Chemotherapy Regimens for Management of Patients with HRPC	226
13-1.	Classification and Epidemiology of Leukemias	233
13-2.	FAB Classification of AML	234
13-3.	Differentiating Between AML and ALL	235
13-4.	FAB Classification of ALL	237
13-5.	Immunologic Classification of ALL	237
13-6.	Commonly Used Chemotherapy Regimens for Remission Induction in ALL	238
13-7.	Rai Staging System for CLL	241
13-8.	Comparison of Hodgkin's Disease and Non-Hodgkin's Lymphoma	243
13-9.	Ann Arbor Staging Classification for Lymphomas	244
13-10.	Working Formulation for Classification of Non-Hodgkin's Lymphoma	245
13-11.	Combination Chemotherapy Regimens in Treatment of Hodgkin's Disease	245
13-12.	Combination Chemotherapy in Non-Hodgkin's Lymphoma	246
14-1.	Types of Bone Marrow Transplantation (BMT)	252
14-2.	Applications of BMT in the Treatment of Cancer	254
14-3.	Clinical Staging of GVHD According to Organ Involvement	257
14-4.	Clinical Grading of GVHD Severity	257
14-5.	Examples of GVHD Prophylaxis Regimens	258
14-6.	Side Effects Associated with GVHD Prophylaxis	258
14-7.	Organ Involvement in Chronic GVHD	260
14-8.	Common Infections Following BMT	261
15-1.	Defects in Host Defense Mechanisms in Patients with Cancer	270
15-2.	Predominant Pathogens Associated with Infections in Cancer Patients	271
15-3.	Examples of Antibiotic Regimens Used as Empiric Therapy for Fever in Granulocytopenic Patients	273
15-4.	Suggested Amphotericin B Regimens for Immunocompromised Cancer Patients	277
15-5.	Prophylactic Oral Antibiotic Regimens Used in Granulocytopenic Cancer Patients	280
16-1.	Barriers to Cancer Pain Management	291
16-2.	Etiologies of Pain in Cancer Patients	292
16-3.	Adjuvant Analgesic Drugs for Cancer Pain	296
16-4.	Nonsteroidal Anti-inflammatory Drugs (NSAIDs)	298

16-5.	Comparison of Opioid Analgesics	300
16-6.	Nerve-Blocking Agents	305
17-1.	Factors Contributing to Patient Distress	310
17-2.	Adult Dosages for Antidepressant Medications	313
17-3.	Symptoms and Signs of Anxiety	314
17-4.	Etiology of Confusion in the Patient with Cancer	315
17-5.	Potential Causes of Dyspnea in Advanced Cancer	317
18-1.	Mechanical and Physical Problems That Contribute to Inadequate Enteral Intake	325
18-2.	Comparison of Metabolic Parameters in Starved, Injured, and Cancer Patients	328
18-3.	Harris-Benedict Equation for Estimating Basal Energy Expenditure (BEE) in Kilocalories	329
18-4.	Factors for Adjusting BEE for Activity and Injury	330
18-5.	Nutritional Supplements for the Cancer Patient	332
18-6.	Specialty Enteral Nutrition Immune-Enhancing Formulas	335
18-7.	Promising Cancer Chemoprotective Agents in Phase I Clinical Trials and Preclinical Toxicology Testing	337
19-1.	Diseases and Drugs Associated with Hypercalcemia	343
19-2.	Organ System Effects of Hypercalcemia	344
19-3.	Causes of Back Pain	348
19-4.	Therapies Contributing to Electrolyte Abnormalities with Tumor Lysis	351
19-5.	Sclerosing Agents	353
20-1.	Indirect Methods of Assessing Occupational Exposure to Hazardous Drugs During Routine Manipulations	359
20-2.	Important Steps and Techniques in Preparing and Administering Hazardous Drugs	362
20-3.	Examples of Abbreviations That Increase the Risk of Chemotherapy Errors	365
20-4.	Printed Sources of Drug Information for Anticancer Drugs and Related Therapies	370
20-5.	On-line Sources of Drug Information for Anticancer Drugs and Related Therapies	371
20-6.	Other Sources of Drug Information for Anticancer Drugs and Related Therapies	371
20-7.	Information Sources for Alternative Cancer Therapies	372
	Appendix 20-A—ASHP Technical Assistance Bulletin on Handling Cytotoxic and Hazardous Drugs	374

List of Figures

1-1.	Estimated new cancer cases and deaths by sex for all sites, United States, 1997	10
1-2.	Age-adjusted cancer death rates of females and males by site, United States, 1930–93	11
2-1.	The growth history of cancer	16
2-2.	Representation of the relationships among the rate of cell production, the rate of cell loss, and the tumor size	17
2-3.	Gompertzian tumor growth curve	17
2-4.	Pathogenesis of cancer metastases	18
2-5.	Selected anticancer drugs developed since 1940	22
2-6.	Measurement of objective solid tumor response	25
2-7.	Survival curves	26
2-8.	Hypothetical representation of potential benefit from adjuvant systemic therapy in patients with primary breast cancer	28
3-1.	Organization of DNA	35
3-2.	Simplified pathways of DNA and RNA synthesis	35
3-3.	Interaction of topoisomerase II with DNA and the mechanism by which some drugs interact with the enzyme–DNA complex to cause double-strand breaks in DNA	36
3-4.	Cell cycle specificity of anticancer drugs	37
3-5.	The process of alkylation	39
3-6.	Structures of bifunctional alkylating agents	39
3-7.	Structures of cisplatin and carboplatin	41
3-8.	Structures of anthracycline drugs and the related anthracenedione compound mitoxantrone	43
3-9.	Structure of bleomycin	45
4-1.	Structures of folic acid and its analogue, methotrexate	53
4-2.	Utilization of reduced folates in the synthesis of DNA and the inhibitory effect of methotrexate	53
4-3.	Serum methotrexate concentrations that identify patients at high risk for severe toxicity	53
4-4.	Structures of cytarabine, fludarabine, and gemcitabine	55
4-5.	Metabolic activation of fluorouracil	56
4-6.	Structures of docetaxel and paclitaxel	59
5-1.	Immune system response to an antigen	69
5-2.	How recombinant DNA is made	70
5-3.	Using hybridoma technology to make monoclonal antibodies	71
5-4.	Interferon antitumor mechanisms	72
5-5.	Antitumor mechanism of interleukin 2	73
5-6.	Concept of immunoconjugates, illustrated using an immunotoxin example	75
6-1.	Effects of chemotherapy on tumor growth and regression	83

6-2.	A single cell transformed by a neoplastic event undergoes clonal expansion	84
6-3.	Response continuum of tumors to combination chemotherapy regimens	87
6-4.	Theoretical points of blockade of metabolic pathways by drugs	87
6-5.	Biomodulation of fluorouracil action by leucovorin	88
6-6.	Body surface area of children	91
6-7.	Body surface area of adults	92
6-8.	Algorithm of treatment decisions in early-stage breast cancer	96
7-1.	Blood cell development	100
7-2.	Patterns of chemotherapy myelosuppression	102
8-1.	Risk of congestive heart failure (CHF) with cumulative doxorubicin doses	123
8-2.	Anatomy of the renal tubules	127
8-3.	Example of cisplatin hydration regimen for outpatient administration in patients without cardiovascular compromise	128
8-4.	High-dose Ara-C (HDAC) dose modification algorithm	137
9-1.	Pathways and neurotransmitter receptors in chemotherapy-induced nausea and vomiting	149
9-2.	Mechanisms of action of antiemetic agents in chemotherapy-induced nausea and vomiting	155
9-3.	Physiology of GI mucosa	159
10-1.	Small vein needle with Luer-Lok adapter	177
10-2.	Tunneled central venous catheter, such as a Hickman or Broviac catheter	180
10-3.	Single-lumen Groshong or slit-tip catheter	180
10-4.	Implantable vascular access port	181
10-5.	Diagrammatic view of subcutaneous reservoir and pump device with an intraventricular catheter	185
10-6.	Theoretical aspect of intra-arterial infusion of drugs	187
10-7.	Schematic diagram of isolated limb perfusion with heart-lung machine	188
11-1.	New International Staging System for lung cancer (the "TNM staging system")	200
11-2.	Actuarial survival curves for different stages of non-small cell lung cancer	203
11-3.	Anatomy of the colon and rectum	204
12-1.	Anatomy of the female breast	212
12-2.	Five-year disease-free survival versus the number of pathologically positive axillary lymph nodes in breast cancer patients	214
12-3.	Kaplan-Meier plot of relapse-free survival and overall survival in premenopausal patients in the first Milan study of adjuvant cyclophosphamide + methotrexate + fluorouracil (CMF) therapy	215
12-4.	Male anatomy of the pelvis and transverse section through the midportion of the prostate gland	219
12-5.	Gleason grading system	220
12-6.	Modified Whitmore-Jewett or American Urologic Association (AUA) staging system for prostate cancer	221
12-7.	Hormonal regulation of the prostate gland	223
13-1.	Normal hematopoiesis and differentiation in the bone marrow	232

15-1.	Relationship between risk of infection and absolute neutrophil count	270
16-1.	Continuing pain management in patients with cancer	293
16-2.	Pain intensity scales	294
16-3.	The World Health Organization three-step analgesic ladder	297
18-1.	Normal function of the gastrointestinal system, with sites of nutrient absorption	326
20-1.	Example of a chemotherapy order sheet	366
20-2.	Example of a chemotherapy checklist	367
20-3.	Example of appropriate chemotherapy labeling	368
A-1.	The cell cycle	391
A-2.	Mitosis (cell division)	392

Preface

Much of cancer therapy involves the use of drugs—whether those drugs are administered as chemotherapy or for patient support in managing infection, pain, nausea, or nutrition. Also, many cancer patients receive multiple drugs. Therefore, it is important that pharmacists working with oncology patients understand how the drugs work and why they are used.

Concepts in Oncology Therapeutics, now in its second edition, is designed for practicing pharmacists, postgraduate trainees (e.g., residents and fellows), and for pharmacy students to be used as an introduction to the field of oncology. All chapters have undergone extensive revision, and material has been updated to reflect current information. Information on the treatment of breast, colon, lung, and prostate cancers is included. Relevant terminology is defined in the glossary, and the index provides easy reference.

Oncology therapeutics is subject to rapid changes as new drugs are approved, new therapies developed, and new practice standards created. Keeping abreast of these constant changes requires both practice and diligent reading of related current literature.

November 1998

Reviewers

ASHP gratefully acknowledges the following individuals, who donated their expertise in reviewing chapters for this publication:

Anthony M. Abang, Pharm.D.

Mary Pat Anderson

Richard L. Barron, M.S.

Susan Berg

Diane M. Caravone

Robert B. Catalano, Pharm.D.

Judy L. Chase

Terri Graves Davidson, Pharm.D., F.A.S.H.P.

Priscilla Amos Dollard, Pharm.D.

Sarah E. Donegan, Pharm.D.

Denise M. Erkkila

Richard Gannon, Pharm.D.

Barry R. Goldspiel, Pharm.D., F.A.S.H.P.

Susan Goodin, Pharm.D.

R. Elizabeth Gregory, Pharm.D.

Lea Ann Hansen, Pharm.D.

R. Donald Harvey, Pharm.D.

Mark T. Holdsworth, Pharm.D., B.C.P.S.

Lisa M. Holle, Pharm.D.

Philip E. Johnson, M.S., F.A.S.H.P.

Reginald S. King, Pharm.D.

Kim C. Larkins, Pharm.D.

Melvin E. Liter, M.S., Pharm.D., F.A.S.H.P.

J. Kelly Martin, Jr.

Jeanine McCune, Pharm.D.

Helen M. McFarland, Pharm.D.

Christopher P. Murphy, Pharm.D.

M. Jane Nolte

Cynthia L. Osowski, Pharm.D.

James Partyka, Pharm.D., B.C.P.S.

Nomita H. Patel, Pharm.D.

Janelle B. Perkins, Pharm.D., B.C.P.S.

Jean M. Scholtz, Pharm.D.

Terrence L. Schwinghammer, Pharm.D.

Steven P. Smith, Pharm.D., B.C.P.S.

Scott Soefje, Pharm.D.

Nancy L. Sommers, Pharm.D.

Suzanne M. Walton, Pharm.D.

Gary C. Yee, Pharm.D., F.C.C.P.

Chapter 1 | Overview of Cancer

Rebecca S. Finley, Pharm.D., M.S.
Chair and Associate Professor
Department of Pharmacy Practice and Pharmacy Administration
Philadelphia College of Pharmacy
Philadelphia, Pennsylvania

Characteristics of Cancer 2
Malignant Transformation 2
    Oncogenes and Proto-oncogenes 2
    Tumor Suppressor Genes 3
    Protein Products of Genetic Alterations 3
    Tumor Cell Proliferation 3
Benign Tumors 4
Etiology of Cancer 4
    Environment 4
    Lifestyle 4
        Diet 5
    Drug Therapy 6
    Heredity 6
    Links to Other Diseases 6
    Viruses 6
Tumor Nomenclature 6
Cancer Diagnosis 7
    Cancer Screening 8
    Diagnosis in Symptomatic Individuals 8
Cancer Statistics 9
Summary 10
References 10
Self-Study Questions 12

Optimal outcomes for patients with cancer result from the collaboration of many health care professionals. An understanding of the characteristics of malignant diseases is fundamental to comprehending the principles and practices of cancer management. Pharmacists need this information to be able to improve the care of patients with malignant diseases.

After completing this chapter, the reader should be able to:

1. Discuss the differences between normal and malignant cells and describe how oncogenes, proto-oncogenes, and tumor suppressor genes are involved in the development of a malignancy.
2. Describe the differences between benign and malignant tumors and discuss the principles of tumor nomenclature.
3. List common carcinogens and the tumors they are associated with.
4. Discuss trends in cancer statistics and the screening initiatives that are recommended to detect cancers in asymptomatic individuals.

The chapter begins with a discussion of the nature of cancer, including its causes, characteristics, and methods of proliferation. The introduction to cancer terminology that follows is limited to those terms used to describe some common malignant tumors. Finally, there is a brief overview of cancer diagnosis, the impact of screening or early detection initiatives, and current trends in cancer statistics.

CHARACTERISTICS OF CANCER

Cancer is a group of diseases characterized by uncontrolled growth or division of cells that are genetically dysfunctional. Normal cells proliferate only until there are enough cells to maintain the physiological needs of the body or until the tissue or structure is complete; then, feedback mechanisms inhibit further replication of that particular cell line. Cancer cells lack this growth control mechanism. Malignant cells have the ability to invade tissues surrounding them (loss of contact inhibition) and spread throughout the body (metastasize), destroying distant tissues and organs. If the process is not halted, these malignant characteristics ultimately cause death. There is compelling evidence that cancers arise from the transformation of a single cell and are therefore monoclonal.

Most normal cells are differentiated—that is, they have developed specific morphology and function. Cancer cells have lost these differentiated characteristics and are not capable of the physiological functions of their mature tissue of origin. For example, normal granulocytes migrate to the site of infection and phagocytize microorganisms, whereas leukemic cells cannot accomplish either function. In addition, cancer cells may exhibit several other differences from normal, healthy cells, including changes in the cellular membrane, different protein and enzyme content, and chromosomal abnormalities—all of which may influence the cells' sensitivity to chemotherapy and radiation. Cancer cells also exhibit changes in cellular fibers and filaments, which give them a different shape or appearance from normal cells.

MALIGNANT TRANSFORMATION

Cancer is a disorder that occurs at the cellular level. All cellular functions, both normal and malignant, are controlled by proteins encoded by DNA organized into genes (see Appendix I for a review of DNA, RNA, and protein synthesis). Protein production involves several steps, each dependent on essential enzymes, which are also encoded by DNA and regulated by other proteins. Most of the steps in this very complex process can be affected, eventually leading to alterations in the amount or structure of a protein, which in turn alter cellular function. The most enduring hypothesis about the origin of cancer is that genetic alterations result in the unregulated proliferation of cells. Although many cellular functions can be affected by a disturbance or alteration (mutation) of one gene, a malignant transformation is believed to require two or more mutations in the same cell. Thus, carcinogenesis results from an accumulation of changes in an assortment of genes.[1] Advances in the understanding of cellular and molecular biology over the past decade have further elucidated malignant transformation at the cellular level. This understanding has opened new avenues of research in cancer prevention and treatment.

Oncogenes and Proto-oncogenes

Theories conceived as long ago as the late 1960s postulated that cells of vertebrates contain information for producing RNA viruses.[2] The DNA that encodes for viral information includes portions responsible for malignant transformation; these portions have been termed viral oncogenes. Subsequent research revealed that all tissues contain DNA sequences homologous to the viral oncogenes. These normal cellular sequences are called proto-oncogenes.[3] Proto-oncogenes are present in all cells and are passed on from generation to generation. Under normal, well-controlled conditions, the proto-oncogenes may be expressed, apparently playing a role in the growth and development of the organism, or they may be inactive. However, certain factors (e.g., irradiation or chemical exposure) can cause partial or complete activation or alteration of these oncogenes by mutations. Genetic changes referred to as mutations may include point mutations, deletions, insertions, translocations, and amplification (Table 1-1). Such genetic alterations may result in malignant transformation. However, activated oncogenes have not been detected in the majority of human tumors,[4] and it is clear that other genetic events must also influence carcinogenesis.

Table 1-1. Types of Genetic Mutations

Point mutations	Change of one base pair in the genetic material may lead to a single amino acid substitution in a critical portion of the protein.
Deletions	Removal of one or more base pairs may result in loss of expression (production) of a protein.
Insertions	Addition of one or more base pairs may result in altered expression (production) of a protein.
Translocations	All or part of a gene recombines with other genes, which may result in altered expression of a protein.
Amplifications	Increase in the amount of DNA from a specific region of a chromosome, which may result in altered expression of a protein.

Table 1-2. Examples of Genes Associated with Human Cancer

Type of Genes	Type of Cancer
Oncogenes/Proto-oncogenes	
N-myc	Neuroblastoma
c-myc	Breast
erb-B	Breast, cervical, head and neck
ras	Acute myelogenous leukemia
ABL	Chronic myelogenous leukemia
RASK	Lung, ovarian, and bladder
Tumor Suppressor Genes	
p53	Breast
BRCA1	Breast
BRCA2	Breast
WT1	Wilms' tumor
RB	Retinoblastoma

SOURCE: references 1–6.

Tumor Suppressor Genes

Inactivation of genes that inhibit cellular growth or proliferation under normal conditions also appears to facilitate tumor growth. Mutations that result in the inactivation of these tumor suppressor genes are frequently observed in malignant transformation and tumor progression.[5,6] Some of the most well-characterized tumor suppressor genes are the retinoblastoma susceptibility (RB), the p53, and the BRCA1 genes. Table 1-2 lists some of the genes known to be commonly associated with carcinogenesis. Interestingly, it does not appear that tumor suppression is the primary function of these genes in their unaltered form. Instead, tumor suppression is probably an indirect consequence of more general functions in normal cellular growth and differentiation. In some cases, mutations or alterations of these genes may be hereditary; in other cases, they are sporadic. When the mutations occur in the germ line, the cancer could be inherited like other genetic traits. When they occur in a single somatic cell, the cancer should be sporadic. However, multiple cases of a sporadic cancer may occur in the same family because of mutations caused by environmental or dietary factors that the family shares. Mutations in proto-oncogenes appear to be restricted to somatic cells.[1]

Protein Products of Genetic Alterations

Like their normal counterparts, mutated genes direct the production of various proteins (Table 1-3) that constitute the biochemical pathways. However, structural alterations or overexpression of such proteins is common in the transformed cell. These qualitative and quantitative changes in protein production are likely to be responsible for many of the characteristics of the malignant cell, such as uncontrolled cellular growth or loss of contact inhibition, and they may also affect the cells' sensitivity to chemotherapy or radiation.

Tumor Cell Proliferation

Once a cell has been transformed, it may proliferate slowly or rapidly to form a clone. Because human tumors appear to arise from one stem cell, they are considered monoclonal. Once a clone of tumor cells is established, the immune system may recognize the clone as being foreign and eliminate it, or the tumor cells may possess receptors for hormones or growth factors that may stimulate their growth. Cancer cells are much more prone to genetic mishaps than normal cells. During the time in which a single transformed cell proliferates into a clinically detectable tumor (about a billion cells), many mutations take place, resulting in a mass of heterogeneous cells. (See also chapters 2 and 5.) This means that the subpopulations of cells within a single tumor mass may have very different biochemical and morphological characteristics. This heterogeneity ex-

Table 1-3. Types of Proteins Involved with Malignant Characteristics

Growth factors
Growth factor receptors
Membrane-associated binding proteins
Cytoplasmic kinases
Nuclear proteins and transcription factors

Table 1-4. Characteristics of Benign and Malignant Tumors

Characteristics	Benign Tumors	Malignant Tumors
Potential to metastasize	No	Yes, may invade surrounding tissues or spread to distant sites via the blood or lymph or both
Encapsulated	Yes	No
Morphologically typical of tissue of origin	Yes	No
Rate of growth	Slow	Unpredictable and unrestrained
Recurrence after surgical removal	Rare	Common

plains why some cells in a tumor may be sensitive to the lethal effects of a particular chemotherapy agent or radiation therapy and others may not.

BENIGN TUMORS

The terms *malignancy*, *neoplasm*, and *tumor* are often used as synonyms for cancer; however, tumors may be either benign or malignant. Benign means nonmalignant, which may suggest that benign tumors are harmless. In many cases they are, but benign tumors, though they lack most of the other harmful characteristics of cancer, may be characterized by uncontrolled cellular division, which can lead to death if the tumor continues to grow in a vital tissue and interrupts normal function. Characteristics that distinguish benign and malignant tumors are shown in Table 1-4.

ETIOLOGY OF CANCER

Over the years there has been a great deal of emphasis on cancer prevention. Prevention is often difficult, however, because the exact cause or causes of most cancers are not understood. Most of the known and suspected causes of cancer are related to either environmental exposure or heredity. Some of the environmental factors are most commonly associated with lifestyle. Exposure to other causes is more likely to be associated with the workplace or, in some situations, the therapeutic use of some drugs.

Environment

It is believed that environmental factors probably contribute to a significant proportion of human malignancies.[7,8] The first environmental cause of cancer was recognized more than 200 years ago, when it was observed that chimney sweeps had a high incidence of scrotal cancer.[9] Several more contemporary occupational exposures have now been implicated in the etiology of various cancers. For example, lung cancer is more prevalent among those who mine or work with asbestos,[10] chromate, or uranium, especially if they are also cigarette smokers[11,12]; workers in the aniline dye industry have an increased risk of bladder cancer.[13] The association between asbestos exposure and mesothelioma is also well established. Benzene exposure has been associated with acute leukemia.[14] Other potential carcinogens are listed in Table 1-5.

Lifestyle

Lifestyle-related factors that have been most strongly implicated as carcinogenic risks include cigarette smoking, alcohol ingestion, sun exposure, and diet. A strong association between cigarette smoking and lung cancer has been recognized for over 40 years.[15] It is estimated that >80% of all lung cancers in the United States are related to smoking.[11,16] Because lung cancer is the leading cause of cancer deaths in the U.S. adult population, strong antismoking campaigns have been advocated by the federal government, the American Cancer Society, and health care organizations. Many epidemiologic studies have also concluded that the risk of lung cancer is significantly increased in the nonsmoking spouses of smokers.[17] This effect is referred to as passive smoking and has been the driving force behind strict no-smoking policies and laws in the workplace and in public sites.

Radiation exposure (both accidental and therapeutic) has been linked to several types of malignant diseases. This link has been most striking in the survivors of the atomic bomb explosions at Hiroshima and Nagasaki, who subsequently had an increased incidence of cancers, particularly leukemias and breast cancer.[18,19] Thyroid cancer is also more common in individuals who received irradiation to the neck as children.

Radon, a natural gas that emanates from the ground, decays to a short-lived radioactive form inside buildings and attaches to aerosol particles. These particles are then deposited in the tracheobronchial tree. It is feared that high radon levels in the home can increase the risk of lung cancer, and some estimates suggest that 40,000–50,000 cases of lung cancer per year are at least partially related to radon exposure.[20,21] The Environmental Protection Agency recommends that if

Table 1-5. Proposed Etiologic Factors Associated with Carcinogenic Risk in Humans

Carcinogenic Risk Factor	Associated Neoplasm(s)	Degree of Evidence
Environmental		
Ionizing radiation	Leukemia, breast, thyroid	Sufficient
Ultraviolet radiation	Skin, melanoma	Sufficient
Viruses	Leukemia, lymphoma, nasopharyngeal	Limited
Radon	Lung	Sufficient
Occupational		
Asbestos	Lung, mesothelioma	Sufficient
Aniline dye	Bladder	Sufficient
Benzene	Leukemia	Sufficient
Vinyl chloride	Liver	Sufficient
Chromium	Lung	Sufficient
Nickel	Lung, nasal sinus	Sufficient
Cadmium	Lung	Limited
Lifestyle		
Alcohol	Esophagus, liver, stomach, oropharynx, larynx	Sufficient
	Breast	Limited
Tobacco	Lung, mouth, pharynx, larynx, esophagus, bladder, lip	Sufficient
Aflatoxin (food contaminant produced by *Aspergillus flavus*)	Liver	Sufficient
Dietary factors	Colon, breast, endometrium, gall bladder	Sufficient
Reproductive history		
Late first pregnancy	Breast	Sufficient
Zero or low parity	Ovary	Sufficient
Sexual promiscuity	Cervix, uterus	Sufficient
Medical drugs		
Tamoxifen	Endometrium	Sufficient
Diethylstilbestrol	Vaginal in offspring	Sufficient
Estrogens	Endometrium	Limited
Alkylating agents	Leukemia, bladder	Sufficient
Azathioprine	Lymphoma	Sufficient
Chloramphenicol	Leukemia	Limited

SOURCE: references 7–31. Sufficient, causal relation established; limited, causal interpretation credible but not firmly established.

the annual average radon level in the home exceeds 4 pCi/L of air, corrective measures should be taken.[22]

Diet

Diet has also been implicated in the risk of several cancers, particularly colon cancer. Animal experiments have also shown that dietary variables, such as the intake of fat, calories, and several micronutrients, influence carcinogenesis. It has been postulated that the reduction in roughage and bulk in the diet of Western cultures (resulting from widespread availability of refrigeration and processed foods) has led to the increased rate of colon cancer observed during this century. High-fiber foods produce much more bulk of waste, which moves through the intestine faster and produces large, soft stools that are easy to excrete. Low-fiber foods have the reverse effect, resulting in the formation of potential carcinogens in the large bowel by the action of certain bacteria on bile salts. Thus, with low-residue diets, carcinogens take longer to pass through and expose the lining of the large bowel for longer periods of time. Although animal studies have been widely publicized, there is little evidence to substantiate a link between various food additives (e.g., saccharin or nitrate preservatives) and human cancer.[23]

Dietary fats, especially unsaturated fatty acids, also appear to act as cancer-promoting agents. An association between fat intake and the risk of breast cancer has been postulated. The per capita consumption of fat correlates with both the incidence of breast cancer and its mortality, although the actual relationship is far from conclusive.[24] A metanalysis of 12 studies that included over 10,000 women found a positive correlation between fat intake and breast cancer for postmenopausal women.[25] However, a large prospective study of nurses in the United States published in 1987 revealed no relationship between the development of breast cancer and fat consumption.[26] Also, other studies of vegetarian groups and those with minimal animal fat consumption have not confirmed lower breast cancer risk. Because of the obvious difficulty of quantitating fat intake over long periods of time (i.e., decades) and the limited range of difference among the fat intake of various populations of study subjects, it is unlikely the epidemiologic studies will ever be unequivocally convincing regarding the link between fat intake and breast cancer.[24]

Causal relations have been suggested between the ingestion of alcohol and the development of esophageal, liver, gastric, oropharynx, breast, and larynx neoplasms; however, in many cases, the development occurs in association with another known carcinogen.

Drug Therapy

Higher than expected incidences of certain malignancies have been reported after therapy with some drugs. For example, the risk of leukemia increases after therapy with an alkylating agent, such as mechlorethamine (with or without radiation therapy), for the treatment of Hodgkin's disease, and bladder cancer has been associated with cyclophosphamide therapy. In other circumstances, the incidence of cancer, particularly lymphomas, has increased following long-term therapy with immunosuppressive agents (e.g., azathioprine).[27] Estrogen use in postmenopausal women and tamoxifen in women with a history of breast cancer have each been associated with an increased risk of endometrial carcinoma.[13,28,29] Both oral contraceptives and contemporary postmenopausal hormone replacement therapy have sometimes been linked to an increased risk of breast cancer. Most experts feel that the reduced doses of estrogens used today are not associated with a significant increase in risk.[30,31]

Heredity

Genetic factors probably play an important role in the familial tendencies toward some common malignancies, such as breast, stomach, and colon cancer. Evidence supporting the role of genetic factors in cancers also comes from animal breeding experiments that led to the development of animal families with a high incidence of cancer. Breast cancer is one of the best examples of a malignancy for which a genetic predisposition influences clinical practice. The incidence of breast cancer increases substantially when one or more first-degree female relatives of a woman (mother, sister, or daughter) have had breast cancer.[32] It is now recognized that mutations of the tumor suppressor gene *BRCA1* are largely responsible for this familial risk.[33] Women with mutations of the *BRCA1* gene also have an increased risk of ovarian cancer. Identification of this gene has led to considerable ethical debate regarding whether women from high-risk families should undergo genetic screening and counseling.[34] Much of the debate centers around whether acknowledgment of the gene would have to be made available to potential employers or insurers. Although aggressive early detection programs are routinely advocated for these high-risk women, some individuals have advocated a more extreme prevention technique—prophylactic mastectomy.

Links to Other Diseases

Because cancer has been linked to genetic damage, it is not surprising that there is a higher incidence of cancer in individuals with diseases that have associated altered chromosomes or the inherent inability to repair DNA.[1] Examples of such conditions include xeroderma pigmentosum, Fanconi's anemia, Bloom's syndrome, and ataxia telangiectasia (Louis-Bar syndrome).

Viruses

Viruses have been linked causally to several cancers in animals and have been reported to account for one in seven human cancers worldwide.[35] Some of the first viral associations with human cancers included the observations that the Epstein-Barr virus was present in a high percentage of African children with Burkitt's lymphoma[36] and in association with nasopharyngeal carcinoma.[37] Infection of cells with specific viruses is believed to lead to genetic mutations that ultimately contribute to the malignant transformation. The hepatitis B virus and human papillomavirus have been linked to hepatocellular carcinoma and cervical cancer, respectively.[35] Human T-cell leukemia virus type 1 (HTLV-1), a retrovirus, is associated with adult T-cell leukemia. Although several cancers are clearly related to infection with the human immunodeficiency virus (HIV), it is not clear whether the virus is directly responsible or the resulting immunodeficiency leaves cells more susceptible to other viruses.

TUMOR NOMENCLATURE

Tumors are classified according to their tissue of origin (Table 1-6). When a malignancy is diagnosed, it is important to know the tissue in which it originated, because various histological types respond differently to therapy and prognosis varies significantly.

Epithelial tissue covers or lines all body surfaces, both inside and outside the body. It includes the skin and the mucosal lining of the entire gastrointestinal tract and the bronchial tree, the inner lining of the peritoneum, and other mucosal tissues. Its major function is to protect the body's vital organs. The term carcinoma is reserved for malignant tumors that arise from epithelial cells (Table 1-6).

Connective tissue is the most abundant and widely dis-

Table 1-6. Tumor Nomenclature for Common Malignant Neoplasms

Tissue of Origin	Malignant Tumor
Epithelial	
Glands or ducts	Adenocarcinomas
Respiratory tract	Bronchogenic carcinomas (e.g., small cell, large cell carcinomas)
Renal	Renal adenocarcinoma (hypernephroma)
Liver	Hepatocellular carcinoma (hepatoma)
Bile duct	Cholangiocarcinoma
Urinary tract	Transitional cell, squamous cell, and papillary carcinomas
Testicular	Seminoma, embryonal carcinoma
Skin	Squamous cell, epidermoid, and basal cell carcinomas
Neuroectoderm	Melanoma
Connective	
Fibrous tissue	Fibrosarcoma
Fatty tissue	Liposarcoma
Cartilage	Chondrosarcoma
Bone	Osteogenic sarcoma, Ewing's tumor
Blood vessels	Angiosarcoma, endothelioma, Kaposi's sarcoma
Lymph vessels	Lymphangiosarcoma
Synovia	Synovial sarcoma
Mesothelium (lining of body cavities)	Mesothelioma
Blood cells	Leukemias
Lymph tissue	Lymphomas, including Hodgkin's disease, lymphocytic leukemia, multiple myeloma
Nerve	
Glial	Glioma
Meninges	Meningeal sarcoma
Peripheral nerve	Neuroblastoma
Retina	Retinoblastoma
Adrenal medulla	Pheochromocytoma
Nerve sheath	Schwannoma (neurofibroma)

tributed of all tissues. It is found throughout the body and includes the bones, cartilage, muscle, blood, lymphatics, and vascular tissue. It connects, supports, and protects other tissues. Most malignant tumors of connective tissues are called sarcomas. There are two exceptions: malignancies affecting the lymphatic system are called lymphomas, and cancers involving the blood cells are called leukemias.

Nerve tissue is found in the brain, spinal cord, and accompanying nerves. Functions of the nervous system tissue include movement and coordination of all bodily functions. Tumors of the nervous system are named according to the cell from which they arise. For example, a brain tumor arising from a glial cell is called a glioma, and one arising from an astrocyte is called an astrocytoma.

CANCER DIAGNOSIS

Cancers may be diagnosed in persons who (1) develop symptoms and seek medical attention, (2) are asymptomatic and take part in screening efforts, or (3) seek medical attention for unrelated problems or have routine physical examinations that coincidentally reveal the cancer.

Cancer Screening

Unfortunately, the most common types of cancer (lung, prostate, breast, colorectal, and ovarian cancers), as well as many of the less common malignancies, cannot be cured if they are detected when the disease has already advanced (i.e., a large tumor or metastatic disease is present). The individual's only chance of cure, therefore, is detection when the cancer is localized. However, when many of these cancers are still localized they produce almost no symptoms. Screening initiatives may use physical examinations, laboratory tests, or radiological studies to detect disease in asymptomatic individuals.

The optimum criteria for widespread screening initiatives in either general or high-risk populations are that the tests should be:

- sensitive (distinguish true positives) and specific (distinguish true negatives) enough to lead to a decrease in morbidity and mortality associated with the target cancer;
- acceptable to the target population (e.g., not excessively painful or inconvenient);
- low risk; and
- economically justifiable to society.

Organizations and expert panels have, over the years, offered recommendations regarding screening tests that meet these criteria. Currently, these include early detection strategies for breast, cervical, testicular, skin, colorectal, and prostate cancers (Table 1-7). Although numerous investigators have evaluated strategies for early detection of lung cancer, programs such as chest X-rays and sputum cytology at regular intervals have not had an impact on the death rates of this major cancer killer. As shown by the controversy surrounding screening mammography in women aged 40–49 years that was highly publicized during 1996 and 1997, the expert panels are not always consistent with their recommendations, and sometimes public emotion and political pressures play a role in determining recommendations.

Diagnosis in Symptomatic Individuals

Cancers may produce signs and symptoms by invading, obstructing, or displacing other normal tissues at the site of the primary tumor or at sites of regional or metastatic spread. For example, a patient with lung cancer may develop a cough, chest pain, and hemoptysis related to the primary lung tumor, or hepatic dysfunction secondary to metastatic involvement in the

Table 1-7. Recommendations for Early Detection of Cancer

Cancer/Test	American Cancer Society	National Cancer Institute	U.S. Preventative Services Task Force
Breast			
Self-exam	Age ≥20, monthly	Not recommended	Not recommended
Clinician exam	Age 20–40, every 3 yr Age ≥40, annually	Age 20–40, every 3 yr Age ≥40, annually	Age ≥40, annually High risk, annually from age 35
Mammography	Age ≥40, annually	Age ≥40, annually	Age ≥50, annually
Prostate			
Digital rectal	Age ≥40, annually	Age ≥40, annually	Not recommended
Prostate-specific antigen	Age ≥50, annually	Not recommended	Not recommended
Colorectal			
Stool guaiac	Age ≥50, annually	Age ≥50, annually	Not recommended
Sigmoidoscopy	Age ≥50, every 3–5 yr	Age ≥50, every 3–5 yr	Not recommended
Cervical			
Pelvic exam	Age 20–40, every 1–3 yr; Age >40, annually	Annually	Not recommended
Pap smear	At age 18 if sexually active, annually for 3 yr, then less frequently if normal	At age 18 if sexually active, annually for 3 yr, then less frequently if normal	When sexually active, every 1–3 yr
Testicular			
Self-exam	Not recommended	Periodic	Not recommended unless high risk
Skin	Not recommended	Part of regular physical exam	High risk

SOURCE: adapted from Bloom JR. Early detection of cancer. Psychologic and social dimensions. *Cancer* 1994;74:1464–73.

Table 1-8. Examples of Paraneoplastic Syndromes Associated with Some Malignant Cancers

Syndrome	Cancer
(Addison's disease) Chronic adrenocortical insufficiency	Adrenal, lymphomas
Autoimmune hemolytic anemia	Chronic lymphocytic leukemia, lymphomas, ovary
Cushing's syndrome	Lung, thyroid, testes, adrenal
Dermatomyositis and polymyositis	Lung, stomach, ovary
Disseminated intravascular coagulation	Acute promyelocytic leukemia, lung, prostate, pancreas
Hypercalcemia (not associated with bone metastases)	Lung
Myasthenic syndrome (MS or Lambert-Eaton syndrome)	Small cell lung, stomach, ovary
Sensory neuropathies	Lung
Sweet's disease	Hematological malignancies and various carcinomas
Syndrome of inappropriate secretion of antidiuretic hormone (SIADH)	Lung
Thrombophlebitis	Lung, breast, ovary, prostate

liver, or both. Tumors can also produce signs and symptoms at a distance from the tumor and its metastases. These effects are referred to as paraneoplastic syndromes or remote effects of the malignancy. Some paraneoplastic syndromes are listed in Table 1-8. They are believed to be the result of biologically or immunologically active substances that are secreted by the tumor. Some patients may also develop constitutional or generalized symptoms associated with their malignancy, including anorexia, weight loss, fatigue, and fever.

Many tests are used to diagnose malignancies, but ultimately a sample of the suspicious tissue must be obtained for pathological confirmation. X-rays and computed tomography (CT) and magnetic resonance imaging (MRI) scans are commonly used to locate and assess the size of tumor masses. The results of these tests help determine the prognosis and selection of the most appropriate treatment. Tests may also be repeated periodically during therapy to assess the response to treatment. Radionucleotide scans may be used to look for additional tumor involvement. Blood chemistries and organ function tests are valuable in assessing the amount of functional impairment caused by tumor invasion. Several substances have been identified that may be found in abnormal concentrations in the presence of a neoplasm. They are secreted or associated with particular tumor types and are referred to as tumor markers. Examples of some clinically useful tumor markers are given in Table 1-9.[38] In some cases, identification of a tumor marker in conjunction with other clinical findings is diagnostic for the presence of a tumor. These substances are also widely used in assessing response to therapy, because as the tumor diminishes, the level of the tumor marker in the blood should decrease correspondingly.

CANCER STATISTICS

The American Cancer Society estimated that in 1997 approximately 1,382,400 new cases of invasive cancer would be diagnosed. It is also predicted that about 30% of the U.S. population now living will eventually have some type of cancer. Cancer may strike at any age. It kills more children 3–14 years of age than any other disease, and it strikes more frequently with increasing age. From 1930 until 1989 there was a steady overall rise in the age-adjusted death rate due to cancer; however, since then the mortality rates have trended downward. The major cause of the steady increase over 60 years was tobacco use and lung cancer. Except for that form of cancer, age-adjusted cancer death rates for other major sites leveled off and in some cases declined because of

Table 1-9. Clinically Useful Tumor Markers

Marker	Associated Cancers
α-Fetoprotein (AFP)	Liver, testes
Carcinoembryonic antigen (CEA)	Colon, lung, breast
Human chorionic gonadotropin (HCG)	Trophoblastic tumors, germ cell tumors of testes
Calcitonin	Medullary cancer of thyroid
Prostatic acid phosphatase (PAP)	Prostate
Cancer antigen 125 (CA-125)	Ovary
Immunoglobulins	Multiple myeloma

SOURCE: adapted with permission from reference 38.

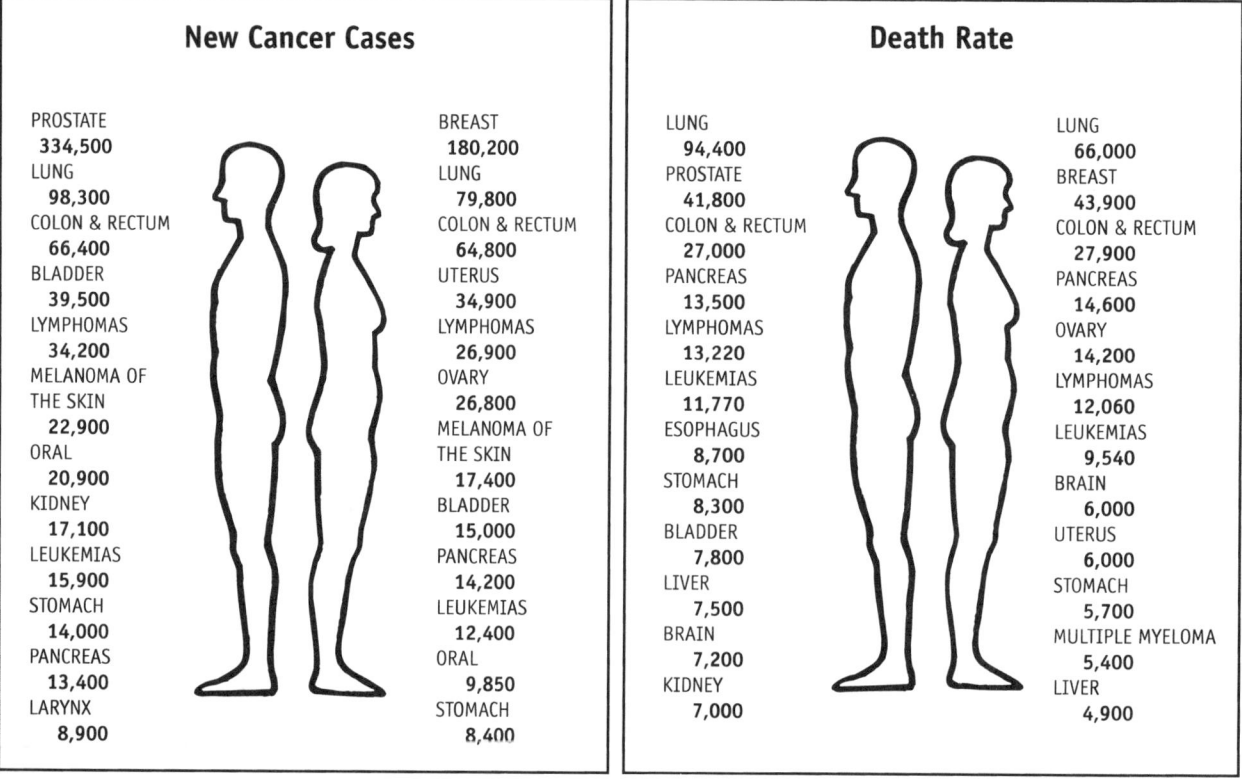

Figure 1-1. Estimated new cancer cases and deaths by sex for all sites, United States, 1997. Excludes basal and squamous cell skin cancers and in situ carcinomas except bladder.

SOURCE: adapted with permission from American Cancer Society web page, Nov. 1997. Copyright 1997, American Cancer Society, Inc.

improved early detection, treatment strategies, and access to care. Recent data further suggest that this downward trend will continue at an accelerated rate. This trend is due, at least in part, to reduced tobacco use by male smokers and the subsequent reduction in mortality from lung cancer over the past 25 years.[16,39] Figures 1-1 and 1-2 illustrate the most common types of cancer among American adults and the leading types of cancer death, respectively. Today, about 4 of every 10 patients who are diagnosed with cancer will be alive 5 years after diagnosis. Major emphasis on identifying and avoiding carcinogenic factors (smoking, high-fat and low-fiber diets, and excessive sunlight exposure), coupled with initiatives aimed at the early detection of major cancers (breast, colorectal, prostate, and skin), are targeted at reducing these death rates. If you would like to learn more about these factors, contact your local office of the American Cancer Society.

transformation proposes that cancers arise from a single stem cell that has been genetically altered. Altered proto-oncogenes and tumor suppressor genes contribute to this malignant transformation.

Patients with cancer are usually diagnosed in one of three ways: from complaints of symptoms, from screening or physical exams, and from complaints of unrelated symptoms. Many tests are used for detecting tumors. Tumor markers are substances in the blood that can be used to monitor a tumor's presence.

Well over a million new patients were diagnosed with cancer in 1997 in the United States. Environmental, lifestyle, and hereditary factors contribute to the overall rise in cancer-related deaths. Many types of cancer-related deaths have decreased over the last several decades as a result of changing lifestyles, public education efforts, and better detection methods.

SUMMARY

Not all cancers are the same. Malignant tumors are classified by their tissue of origin, which is important to know when deciding which therapy to give. Malignant cells may invade neighboring tissue or travel to another site in the body. Tumors may also recur after therapy. The theory of malignant

REFERENCES

1. Squire J, Phillips RA. Genetic basis of cancer. In: Tannock IF, Hill RP, editors. *The Basic Science of Oncology.* 2nd ed. New York: McGraw-Hill; 1992. p. 41–60.
2. Huebner RJ, Todaro GJ. Oncogenes of RNA tumor viruses as determinants of cancer. *Proc Natl Acad Sci USA* 1969;64:1087–94.
3. Minden MD, Pawson AJ. Oncogenes. In: Tannock IF, Hill

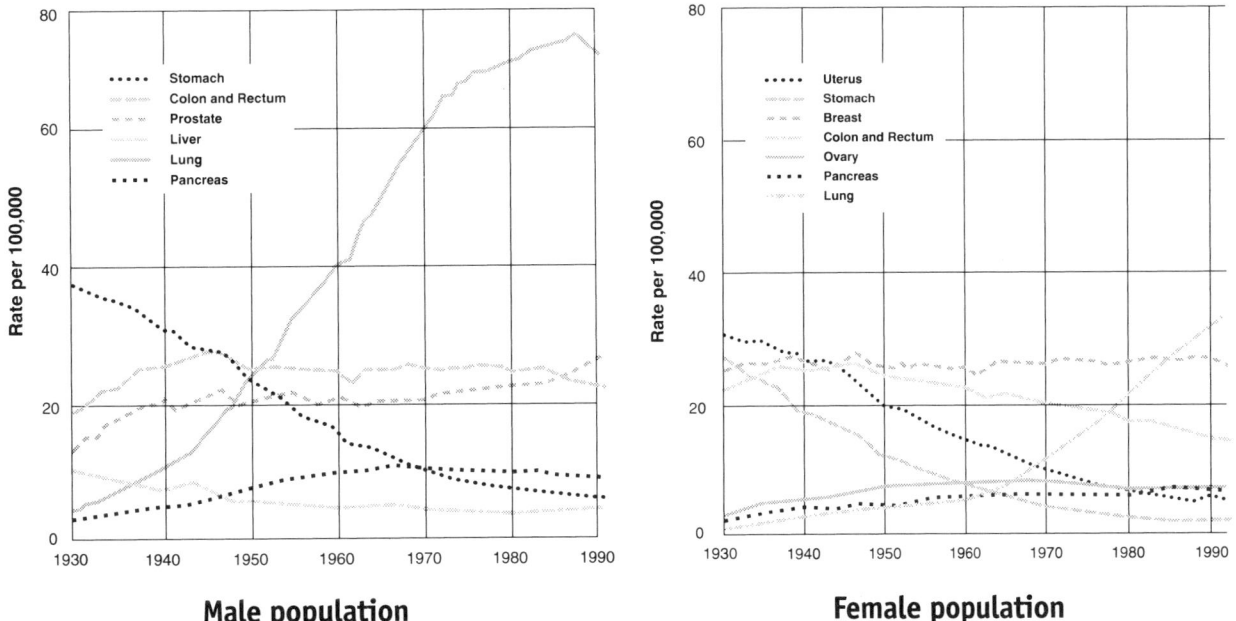

Figure 1-2. Age-adjusted cancer death rates of females and males by site, United States 1930–1993. Uterine cancer death rates are for cervix and corpus combined. Rates are per 100,000 and are age-adjusted to the 1970 U.S. standard population.

SOURCES: adapted with permission from American Cancer Society web page, Nov. 1997. Copyright 1997, American Cancer Society, Inc. Data from Vital Statistics of the United States, 1993.

RP, editors. *The Basic Science of Oncology.* 2nd ed. New York: McGraw-Hill; 1992. p. 61–87.

4. Bishop JM. The molecular genetics of cancer. *Science* 1987;235:305–11.
5. Hollingsworth RE, Lee WH. Tumor suppressor genes: new prospects for cancer research. *J Natl Cancer Inst* 1991;83:91–6.
6. Sager R. Tumor suppressor genes: the puzzle and the promise. *Science* 1989;246:1406–12.
7. Pitot HC. The natural history of neoplastic development: the relation of experimental models to human cancer. *Cancer* 1982;49:1206–11.
8. Yuspa SH, Shields PG. Etiology of cancer: chemical factors. In: DeVita VT, Hellman S, Rosenberg SA, editors. *Cancer: Principles and Practice of Oncology.* 5th ed. Philadelphia, PA: JB Lippincott; 1996. p. 185–202.
9. Pott P. *Chirurgical Observations Relative to the Cataract, the Polypus of the Nose, the Cancer of the Scrotum, the Different Kinds of Ruptures, and the Mortification of the Toes and Feet.* London: Hawkes, Clarke and Collins; 1775.
10. Nicholson WJ. Cancer following occupational exposure to asbestos and vinyl chloride. *Cancer* 1977;39:1792–1801.
11. Doll R, Peto R. The causes of cancer: quantitative estimates of avoidable risks of cancer in the United States today. *J Natl Cancer Inst* 1981;66:1191–308.
12. Selikoff IJ, Chung J, Hammond EC. Asbestos exposure, smoking and neoplasm. *JAMA* 1968;204:106–12.
13. Trichopoulos D, Petridou E, Lipworth L, et al. Epidemiology of cancer. In: DeVita VT, Hellman S, Rosenberg SA, editors. *Cancer: Principles and Practice of Oncology.* 5th ed. Philadelphia, PA: JB Lippincott; 1996. p. 213–57.
14. Rinsky RA, Young RJ, Smith AB. Leukemia in benzene workers. *Am J Ind Med* 1981;2:217–45.
15. Hammond EC, Horn D. Smoking and death rates—report on forty-four months of follow-up of 187,783 men. *JAMA* 1958;166:1294–308.
16. Cunningham MP. Giving life to numbers. *CA Cancer J Clin* 1997;47:5–6.
17. U.S. Environmental Protection Agency [EPA]. Respiratory effects of passive smoking: lung cancer and other disorders. Publication No. (EPA) 600/6-90/006. Washington, DC: Government Printing Office,1993.
18. McGregor DH, Land CE, Choi K, et al. Breast cancer incidence among atomic bomb survivors, Hiroshima and Nagasaki. *J Natl Cancer Inst* 1977;59:799–811.
19. Bizzozero OJ, Johnson KG, Ciocco A. Leukemia in Hiroshima and Nagasaki. *N Engl J Med* 1966;274:1095–101.
20. Lubin JH, Boice JD. Lung cancer risk from residential radon: meta-analysis of eight epidemiologic studies. *J Natl Cancer Instit* 1997;89:49–57.
21. Rosco R, Steenland K, Haplerin W, et al. Lung cancer mortality among nonsmoking uranium miners exposed to radon daughters. *JAMA* 1989;262:629–33.
22. Hall EJ. Etiology of cancer: physical factors. In: DeVita VT, Hellman S, Rosenberg SA, editors. *Cancer: Principles and Practice of Oncology.* 5th ed. Philadelphia, PA: JB Lippincott; 1996. p. 203–18.
23. Boyd NF. Epidemiology of cancer. In: Tannock IF, Hill RP, editors. *The Basic Science of Oncology.* 2nd ed. New York: McGraw-Hill; 1992. p. 7–22.
24. Harris J, Morrow M, Norton L. Malignant tumors of the breast. In: DeVita VT, Hellman S, Rosenberg SA, editor. *Cancer: Principles and Practice of Oncology.* 5th ed. Philadelphia, PA: JB Lippincott; 1996. p. 1557–616.
25. Howe GR, Hirohata T, Hislop TG, et al. Dietary factors and

risk of breast cancer: combined analysis of 12 case-control studies. *J Natl Cancer Inst* 1990;82:561.
26. Willet W, Stampfer M, Colditz G. Dietary fat and risk of breast cancer. *N Engl J Med* 1987;316:22.
27. Hoover R, Fraumeni JF. Drug-induced cancer. *Cancer* 1981;47: 1071–80.
28. Fisher B, Costanino JP, Redmond CK, et al. Endometrial cancer in tamoxifen-treated breast cancer patients: findings from the National Surgical Adjuvant Breast and Bowel Project (NSABP) B-14. *J Natl Cancer Inst* 1994;86:527–37.
29. Rutqvist LE, Johansson H, Signomklao T, et al. Adjuvant tamoxifen therapy for early stage breast cancer and second primary malignancies. *J Natl Cancer Inst* 1995;87:645–51.
30. Issacs CJD, Swain S. Hormone replacement therapy. *Hematol Oncol Clin North Am* 1994;8:179–95.
31. Prentice RL, Thomas DB. On the epidemiology of oral contraceptives and disease. *Adv Cancer Res* 1987;49:285–91.
32. Anderson DE. A genetic study of human breast cancer. *J Natl Cancer Inst* 1972;48:1029–34.
33. Easton DF, Bishop DT, Ford D, et al. Genetic linkage analysis in familial breast and ovarian cancer—results from 214 families. *Am J Hum Genet* 1993;52:678–701.
34. Biesecker BB, Boehnke M, Calzone K, et al. Genetic counseling for families with inherited susceptibility to breast and ovarian cancer. *JAMA* 1993;269:1970.
35. Proeschla EM, Wong-Staal F. Etiology of cancer: viruses. In: DeVita VT, Hellman S, Rosenberg SA, editors. *Cancer: Principles and Practice of Oncology*. 5th ed. Philadelphia, PA: JB Lippincott; 1996. p. 153–184.
36. Reedman BM, Klein G. Cellular localization of an Epstein-Barr virus (EBV)-associated complement fixing antigen in producer and nonproducer lymphoblastoid cell lines. *Int J Cancer* 1973;11:499–520.
37. Ho JHC. An epidemiologic and clinical study of nasopharyngeal carcinoma. *Int J Radiat Oncol Biol Phys* 1978;4:183–98.
38. Virji MA, Mercer DW, Heberman RB. Tumor markers in cancer diagnosis and prognosis. *CA Cancer J Clin* 1988;38:105–26.
39. Cole P, Rodu B. Declining cancer mortality in the United States. *Cancer* 1996;78:2045–8.

SELF-STUDY QUESTIONS

1. Describe the differences between the proliferation of normal cells and malignant cells.

2. Give examples of morphological and physiological differences between normal and malignant cells. Describe the impact that these differences may have on response to chemotherapy.

3. A malignant transformation is believed to require:
   a. viral DNA
   b. two or more genetic mutations in the same cell
   c. inactivation of tumor suppressor genes
   d. only b and c
   e. all of the above

4. *BRCA1* and *p53* are examples of _____.

5. Even though cells within a tumor mass are believed to be _____, they are _____.
   a. polyclonal, homogeneous
   b. polyclonal, heterogeneous
   c. monoclonal, homogeneous
   d. monoclonal, heterogeneous

6. The terms malignancy, tumor, and cancer are all synonymous.
   a. true
   b. false

7. Benign tumors may cause pain and symptoms; however, they are far less likely to cause death because _____.

8. List at least four lifestyle factors that are believed to increase the risk of cancer.

9. The Environmental Protection Agency recommends that if the annual average radon level in the home exceeds _____ of air, corrective measure should be taken.
   a. 4 pCi/L
   b. 40 pCi/L
   c. 400 pCi/L
   d. 4000 pCi/L

10. List at least six cancers that have been associated with tobacco exposure.

11. Hereditary mutations of *BRCA1* are associated with an increased risk of _____ and _____ cancers.

12. List at least three viruses that have been linked to human cancers and discuss how they are believed to influence the development of cancer.

13. _____, _____, and _____ are tumors that arise from connective tissues.

14. According to the American Cancer Society, what types of cancer screening procedures should a 45-year-old woman undergo during her annual physical examination?

15. A 55-year-old man is undergoing his first physical examination in over 10 years. According to the American Cancer Society, what types of cancer screening should he receive?

16. Discuss the desirable criteria for cancer screening initiatives.

17. Carcinoembryonic antigen (CEA) is a clinically useful tumor marker for _____, _____, and _____ cancers.

18. _____ cancer is the most common cause of cancer deaths in the United States.

19. About _____ of the U.S. population now living will eventually develop some type of cancer.

    a. 10%
    b. 30%
    c. 50%
    d. 60%

Chapter 2

Principles of Cancer Treatment

Carol Balmer, Pharm.D.
Associate Professor
University of Colorado School of Pharmacy
Denver, Colorado

Rebecca S. Finley, Pharm.D., M.S.
Chair and Associate Professor
Department of Pharmacy Practice and
  Pharmacy Administration
Philadelphia College of Pharmacy
Philadelphia, Pennsylvania

Tumor Growth Kinetics	16
Goals of Cancer Treatment	19
Modalities of Cancer Treatment	19
Surgery	19
Radiation Therapy	20
Chemotherapy	21
Endocrine Therapy	22
Biological Therapy	24
Evaluation of Response	25
Duration of Survival	25
Response Rate	26
Duration of Response	27
Toxicities Associated with Treatment	27
Impact on Quality of Life	27
Adjuvant Therapy	27
Summary	29
References	29
Self-Study Questions	30

Once the diagnosis of cancer has been made, the question of how to treat the patient must be answered. Many tumor- and patient-specific factors must be considered in the decision-making process for an individual patient. These specific factors will be addressed in detail in chapter 6. But some are important basic concepts fundamental to the decision-making process: how tumors grow and spread; how the goals of treatment are established and how they vary based on stage of the disease; how success or failure of treatment is evaluated; how choices are made among the four main types of cancer treatment: surgery, radiation, chemotherapy, and biological therapy; and why chemotherapy is sometimes given to patients who have no signs or symptoms of cancer.

This chapter will discuss the basic principles of cancer growth and treatment. Although treatment with drugs is the main focus of the pharmacist in the management of cancer patients, it is important to recognize the advantages and limitations of surgery and radiation therapy as well, and to understand how drug therapy may supplement, complement, or replace other modalities of cancer treatment. Chemotherapy has many roles in the overall management of cancer patients. These will be discussed, as well as methods for evaluating both desirable and undesirable responses to cancer drug therapies. Upcoming chapters will build on this knowledge base to describe how this understanding leads to the establishment of principles by which cytotoxic drugs are selected for use, dosages and schedules of administration are chosen, and combinations of chemotherapy agents are established.

After completing this chapter, the reader should be able to:

1. Define the terms that describe the growth of tumors (such as doubling time, growth fraction, Gompertzian growth curve, and metastases) and explain why tumors may be clinically undetectable for much of their life span.
2. Describe three goals of cancer treatment and give examples of situations in which each of these goals would be an appropriate choice.
3. Describe the roles of the four major methods used in treating cancer, including the advantages and disadvantages of each modality.
4. Compare hormonal therapy with traditional chemotherapy, outlining advantages and limitations of each.
5. Identify and define four categories of response to cancer therapy and describe the measures of outcome commonly used in oncology clinical trials.
6. Discuss the rationale, advantages, and disadvantages of adjuvant anticancer therapy.

TUMOR GROWTH KINETICS

Understanding how tumors grow is essential to understanding how they are treated. As explained in chapter 1, clinically detectable cancers are believed to develop from a single cell that has undergone malignant change. One cell divides to become two, two cells become four, and so on. The time it

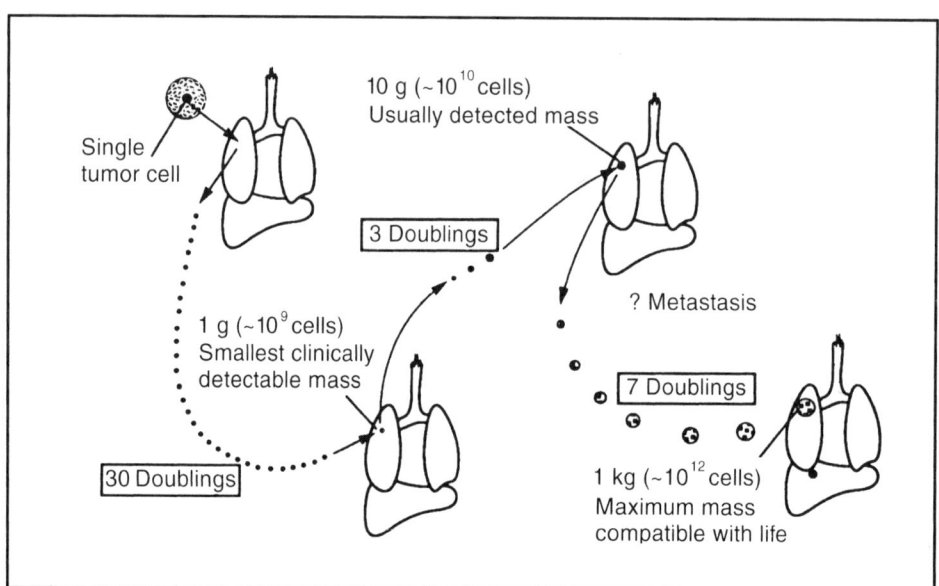

Figure 2-1. The growth history of cancer. A human solid tumor must undergo about 30–33 doublings in volume from a single cell before it achieves a detectable size of 1–10 g. Metastases may have been established prior to detection of the primary tumor. Only a few further doublings of volume lead to a tumor whose size is incompatible with life.

SOURCE: reprinted with permission from Tannock IF. Cell proliferation. In: Tannock IF, Hill RP, editors. *The Basic Science of Oncology.* 2nd ed. New York: McGraw-Hill; 1992. p. 142.

takes a tumor mass to double in size is called the doubling time. Wide variability exists in the doubling times for various cancers, but the doubling times of solid tumors are usually longer than those of hematological malignancies. The doubling time for most solid tumors averages about 2–3 months, although the range extends from 1 month to several years. Breast cancer cells, for example, have an average doubling time of 100 days, or about 3 months. In contrast, Burkitt's lymphoma, one of the most rapidly growing hematological malignancies, may demonstrate a doubling time as short as a day. There is wide variation in growth rate, even among tumors of the same type.[1,2]

A tumor mass usually cannot be detected by either physical examination or radiological studies until it is at least 1 cm in diameter, about the size of a small marble. Tumors of deep internal organs, such as the colon, are likely to escape detection until they are much larger, because a mass this size can be easily hidden in the large abdominal cavity of most adults. A 1-cm mass weighs about 1 g and contains approximately 1 billion (1×10^9) cells. To put this in a human perspective, 1 billion is more than the combined total population of North America, Latin America, and the Caribbean Islands.[3] It requires about 30 doublings in cell number for a tumor to grow from 1 cell to 1 billion cells (Figure 2-1).

This process takes roughly 5–8 years at the average rate of growth of most solid tumors. It only takes 10 additional doublings for this 1-g mass to reach 1 kg (approximately 1×10^{12} cells). A total tumor mass of 1–2 kg is considered lethal.[1] Thus, a tumor is clinically undetectable for much of its life span but may appear to progress rapidly once it has been diagnosed.

Actual tumor growth within the body (net tumor growth) depends on the rate of cell death as well as the rate of cell division within a tumor mass (Figure 2-2). The Gompertzian growth curve (Figure 2-3) demonstrates the theoretical pattern of tumor growth.[1,4]

Benjamin Gompertz was an English insurance actuary who described the mathematical relationship between age and expected death in humans. A very similar relationship holds true for the growth of tumor masses. Tumor growth may be slow very early in the tumor's development, since the tumor cells may have to overcome immunologic defense mechanisms of the host. After an initial lag period, overall growth is rapid during the early period of growth. The curve is steep, which means that a large portion of the tumor cells are actively dividing and the rate of cell death is low. This phase of rapid

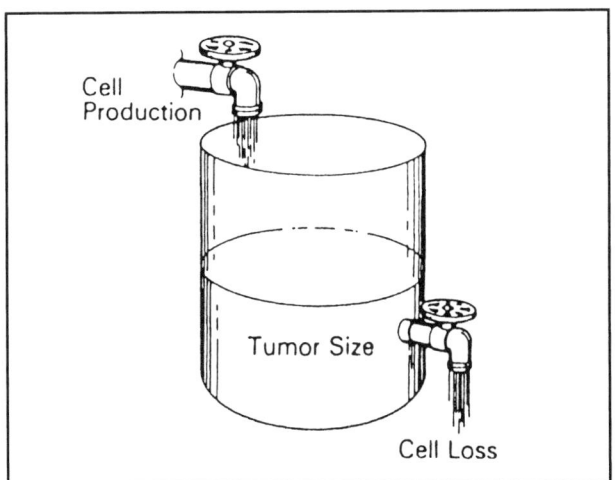

Figure 2-2. Representation of the relationships among the rate of cell production (water inflow), the rate of cell loss (water outflow), and the tumor size (water level in the tank). If water flows rapidly into the tank (high rate of cell production) and water flows out just as rapidly (high rate of cell loss), the water level in the tank will not change (stable tumor) although the overall rate of flow of water is high (high rate of cell turnover). If a trickling inflow is balanced by a trickling outflow, again the water level will not change; in this case the turnover rate is low. If the rate of inflow exceeds the rate of outflow, then the water level will rise progressively (tumor growth).

SOURCE: reprinted with permission from Shackney SE. Tumor growth, cell cycle kinetics, and cancer treatment. In: Calabresi P, Schein PS, editors. *Medical Oncology: Basic Principles and Clinical Management of Cancer*. 2nd ed. New York: McGraw-Hill; 1993. p. 44.

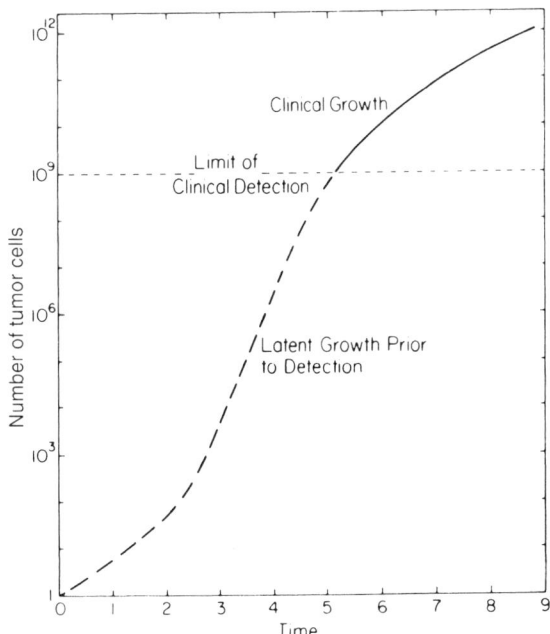

Figure 2-3. Gompertzian tumor growth curve. Hypothetical growth curve for a human tumor, showing the long latent period prior to detection. Tumors may show an early lag phase, followed by rapid growth and the progressive slowing of growth as the tumor reaches large size.

SOURCE: reprinted with permission from Tannock IF. Cell proliferation. In: Tannock IF, Hill RP, editors. *The Basic Science of Oncology*. 2nd ed. New York: McGraw-Hill; 1992. p. 143.

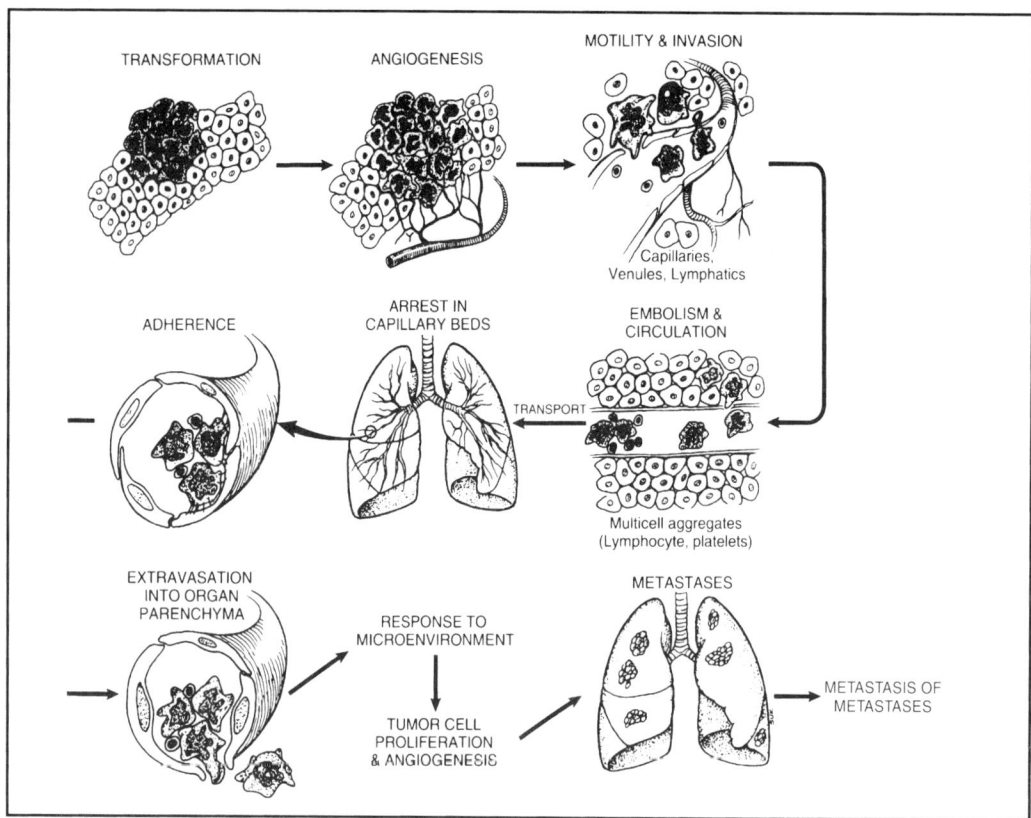

Figure 2-4. Pathogenesis of cancer metastases. To produce metastases, tumor cells must detach from the primary tumor, invade through the wall of the blood vessels or lymph channels that supply nutrients to the tumor mass to enter the circulation, and survive in the circulation to eventually come to rest in the capillary bed of another organ. There the tumor cells adhere to the lining of the vessels and invade through the vessel wall to gain entrance into the tissue of the organ itself. The cells respond there to a variety of growth factors in the organ's microenvironment, proliferate, induce the growth of new blood and lymph vessels, and evade host defenses to establish a new satellite or metastasis of the primary tumor.

SOURCE: reprinted with permission from Fidler IJ. Molecular biology of cancer: invasion and metastasis. In: DeVita VT Jr, Hellman S, Rosenberg SA, editors. *Cancer: Principles and Practice of Oncology*. 5th ed. Philadelphia, PA: Lippincott-Raven; 1997. p. 136.

growth is called exponential growth. The percentage of actively dividing cells is called the growth fraction. The growth fraction decreases as the tumor mass increases in size, and the doubling time increases in length. A larger tumor mass has a greater percentage of nondividing and dying cells and therefore grows more slowly because of restrictions of space, nutrient availability, and blood supply to the tumor mass. Some tumor cells die as a result of these restrictions. Others are destroyed by the body's immune system. Thus, the Gompertzian curve begins to plateau.

The Gompertzian growth curve has important implications for the treatment of cancers with chemotherapy. In general, chemotherapy is most successful in killing tumor cells when the total number of tumor cells (the tumor burden) is low and when the growth fraction is high. These two conditions occur together in the early part of the growth curve and are an important reason for screening programs for early detection of cancers. (The factors that determine the effectiveness of cancer chemotherapy will be discussed more thoroughly in chapter 6).

Treatment of cancer depends not just on the patterns of tumor growth but also on its spread. Metastasis is the spread of cancer cells from the primary tumor, or site of origin, to distant sites. It is a term that is generally used to refer to solid tumors but not to hematological malignancies. The concept of tumor spread is not relevant to cancer of the blood-forming organs (leukemia) because the cancerous blood cells begin circulating throughout the blood stream very early in the course of those diseases.

There are two main pathways of metastasis: through the blood and through the lymphatic system. Metastasis is a complex, multistep process (Figure 2-4). Cells from the transformed cancerous mass invade the small blood vessels and lymphatic channels that feed the tumor. They survive and circulate in the blood or lymph vessels, eventually adhering to the vessel wall; then they invade through the wall into the organ supplied by that vessel. There the cells multiply, inducing new vessel formation to feed the new tumor mass, and become established satellites, or metastases.[5-7]

Metastasis may begin very early in the life of a tumor, and the rate of metastasis often increases with time. It is common for cancers to spread from the original or primary site, even before they are large enough to be clinically evident. About 30% of patients will have detectable metastatic disease (metastatic tumor masses ≥1 cm in diameter at the time of diagnosis). Another 30% of cancer patients will have microscopic cancer metastases that are too small to be detected by current methods. The proof that these deposits exist is that these patients eventually experience cancer recurrence, even when the primary tumor has been completely removed or destroyed.[5-7]

Not all of the cells shed from a tumor result in metastatic lesions. The situation is often compared to that of seed with soil. The shed cancer cells, or "seeds," must first find the appropriate "soil," an environment suitable for the cell's growth. Different cancers have different growth requirements, which result in characteristic patterns of metastasis for specific types of cancer.[6] For example, colorectal cancers metastasize most commonly to the liver, and prostate cancers spread to bones. The liver, lungs, lymph nodes, bones, brain, skin, and adrenal glands are the most common metastatic sites for solid tumors. It is relatively unusual for tumors to spread to the gastrointestinal tract, heart, reproductive organs, kidney, bladder, or sensory organs.[7] Efforts to interfere with the process of metastasis are an important current focus of anticancer research.

GOALS OF CANCER TREATMENT

The primary goal of cancer treatment is to cure patients—to render them clinically and pathologically free of disease and return their life expectancy to that of healthy individuals of the same age and sex. However, currently available treatments do not offer cures for all patients. When cure is not an option, the best alternate goal of therapy is to prolong survival while maintaining the patient's functional status and quality of life.

The third goal of cancer therapy is to relieve symptoms, such as pain, for patients in whom the likelihood of cure or prolonged survival is very low. The practice of administering therapy to relieve symptoms is referred to as palliative therapy.[8,9]

A fourth goal is sometimes included to account for experimental use of cancer drugs in phase I trials. Although study medications are always given to patients with therapeutic intent (that is, with the hope that they will benefit the patient), the main purpose of these studies is to determine safe doses of new cancer drugs in humans.[9]

Many factors are considered in determining treatment goals for an individual patient: the type of cancer, its stage of growth, the age and medical condition of the patient, social and economic factors, and the patient's or family members' wishes. It is important that the patient and health care professionals understand and agree on the goals of treatment. These goals, to a large extent, determine the acceptable balance of toxicity and benefit that is appropriate for a particular patient. This is outlined in Table 2-1.

MODALITIES OF CANCER TREATMENT

Once the goals of treatment have been established, the method or combination of methods to achieve those goals must be selected. Surgery, radiation therapy, chemotherapy, and immunotherapy are the major modalities used to treat cancer. The type and extent of tumor involvement—as well as the treatment goals, performance status, age, and concomitant diseases of the patient—determine the most appropriate type of therapy. Many patients receive two or more of these therapies for treatment of their cancer.

Surgery

Surgery is the oldest cancer treatment. For many years it was the only method that could produce cures, and it still provides the best chance of cure for most patients with solid tumors. Also the most invasive treatment method, it requires that patients be able to withstand the physical challenges of the surgi-

Table 2-1. Goals of Cancer Therapy

	Cure	Extend Life	Palliate Symptoms	Phase I (research study to determine safety of new drug)
Tolerance of acute side effects	High	Moderate	Low	Expected
Special concerns	Delayed and late side effects	Value of added time	Symptom control	Finding correct dose
Challenges in patient selection and management	Avoid treating those who are already cured	Treat when added time outweighs side effects	Treat when *not* treating leads to lower quality of life	Respond ethically to patient's perception of intent

SOURCE: adapted from reference 9.

cal procedure. In America, surgery was first used in 1809 to treat a cancer that was not on the surface of the body. A frontier surgeon, Ephraim MacDowell, removed an ovarian tumor weighing 22 pounds from a woman who survived the surgery and lived for another 30 years after the operation. The success of the operation is particularly remarkable because general anesthesia was not introduced until 1846 and the idea of aseptic surgical technique was nearly a century away.[10]

Surgery can be a curative therapy when solid tumors are confined to one anatomical site or region (localized disease). It is most commonly used to treat the primary or original cancer, but it is also sometimes used to remove isolated metastatic masses, such as brain metastases in malignant melanoma patients or pulmonary metastases in patients with osteosarcoma. Surgical techniques may also be needed to make other methods of treatment possible. Indwelling intravenous catheters or ports, implanted infusion pumps, intraperitoneal or hepatic artery catheters, chest tubes, or central nervous system drug reservoirs (Ommaya reservoirs) are all examples of surgical procedures used to provide access for chemotherapy delivery (see chapter 10).

Surgery also plays a major role in other aspects of cancer management, including diagnosis, staging, relief of symptoms, reconstruction, and prevention. The role of surgery in cancer diagnosis lies in acquiring tissue for histological diagnosis. Biopsy of the suspected tumor may be done by aspirating cells, by taking a small core of tissue from the tumor with a needle, or by surgically removing either part or all of the tumor. Surgical procedures are also used to determine the extent of tumor involvement in some types of cancer, such as ovarian carcinoma.

Surgical procedures are sometimes necessary to treat complications caused by a tumor, such as hemorrhage, perforation, bowel obstruction, or spinal cord compression. Occasionally, surgery may be performed to debulk (reduce the size of) the tumor even though the entire tumor cannot be resected. Debulking procedures are used primarily to relieve pain or other symptoms or to increase the effectiveness of radiation or chemotherapy that may be more effective on smaller tumors. Surgical removal of a source of hormones, a form of hormonal therapy, is often used to treat tumors whose growth depends on those hormones. The most common examples of this kind of surgery are removal of the testes in men with prostate cancer and removal of the ovaries in women with breast cancer. Surgery also aids in rehabilitating cancer patients after therapy. The ability to reconstruct anatomical defects can substantially improve function, cosmetic appearance, and quality of life. Surgery plays a significant role in cancer prevention by permitting removal of precancerous lesions, such as abnormal moles or colon polyps.[10,11]

Radiation Therapy

Radiation therapy is the destruction of cancer cells by ionizing radiation. It is a component of treatment for half to two thirds of all patients with cancer.[12] The radiation is usually generated by machines outside of the patient (external beam radiation). Most external beam radiation is produced by linear accelerators, in which high-energy electrons bombard a target and produce high-energy photons called X-rays. This is the source of the abbreviation "XRT" commonly used for radiation therapy. Less frequently, radiation sources are placed close to the body surface or within a body cavity (brachytherapy). Sometimes, radiation sources are implanted into or around the cancerous tissue, a process called interstitial brachytherapy.[13]

Radiation therapy doses are measured by the amount of energy absorbed by the radiated tissue. This energy was formerly measured in rads but is now measured in grays (Gy) or centigrays (cGy). One gray equals 100 rads; one centigray equals one rad. Radiation doses are determined both by the sensitivity of the cancer type and of the normal body tissue being irradiated. Some examples of typical doses are 60 Gy (6000 cGy or rads) to brain tissue and 50 Gy (5000 cGy or rads) to breast tissue. Radiation therapy is usually administered in small doses over several weeks rather than in one large dose. This process, called fractionating the dose, permits the administration of levels of radiation sufficient to kill tumor cells while allowing normal surrounding tissue to recover from damage.[12,13]

The energy given off by radiation therapy results in the formation of highly reactive free radical compounds. These radicals cause double-strand breaks in DNA, which interfere with the cells' ability to reproduce. Cancer cells are more likely to be dividing than normal cells and are therefore usually more sensitive to the destructive effects of radiation.

As the dose of radiation increases, more cells are destroyed. Depending on the radiosensitivity of the tumor cells, a dose can sometimes be achieved that completely eradicates the tumor. However, normal cells and tissues are also damaged by radiation, since the beam can never be directed only at the tumor. The most sensitive tissues of the body are those that undergo continuous cell renewal, such as the skin, hair, gastrointestinal mucosa, bone marrow, reproductive tissues, and sweat glands. Damage to these tissues is usually seen rapidly. In slowly growing tissues, such as the lungs, the effects of radiation are seen much later. Radiation can result in fibrosis and edema of affected tissues, and it can sometimes lead to necrosis, or tissue death.[12–14]

Since body tissues have different tolerances to radiation, the ability to produce a cure with radiation therapy depends on the capacity of the normal tissues surrounding the tumor to withstand the toxic effects. If the normal tissues are very sensitive to radiation effects, the range of radiation doses used to treat the tumor may be limited. Table 2-2 shows toxicities associated with radiation treatment. The more severe toxicities are much less common now than in the past, because of the greater specificity of today's radiation therapy delivery techniques.[12]

Radiation therapy can cure some tumors, but others

Table 2-2. Toxicities Associated with Radiation Treatment

Potentially severe or fatal radiation injury	
Bone marrow	Pancytopenia, aplasia
Liver	Hepatitis
Stomach	Ulcer, hemorrhage
Intestine	Ulcer, perforation
Rectum	Stricture, ulcer
Brain, spinal cord	Infarct, necrosis
Lung	Acute and chronic pneumonitis
Fetus	Death
Potentially mild or moderately severe radiation injury	
Scalp	Alopecia (may be permanent)
Upper abdomen	Nausea, vomiting
Skin	Pigmentation changes, burns
Head and neck	Mucositis
Breast	No development (child); atrophy (adult)
Testes, ovaries	Sterilization
Prostate	Proctitis, cystitis, impotence

SOURCE: adapted from reference 12, p. 29.

are relatively resistant. Radiocurability depends on the size and location of the tumor, the type of tumor, and the tumor's radiosensitivity. Like surgery, curative radiation therapy is generally limited to localized tumors. Total body irradiation is sometimes used to prepare patients for bone marrow transplantation, but it is highly toxic. When surgery and radiation therapy have similar ability to cure the patient, the choice of treatment methods is often determined by the general medical condition of the patient. For example, a cancerous prostate will usually be surgically removed from patients who are healthy enough to withstand that major surgical procedure, but it would be treated with radiation in more frail patients. Radiation therapy also may permit destruction of a tumor mass with less damage than surgery would cause to the structure, function, and cosmetic appearance of normal tissues.[12-14]

Radiation may also be used as a supplement to surgery to destroy cancerous cells that may remain after a tumor has been removed surgically. In breast cancer, when a patient selects excision of the cancerous lump (lumpectomy) rather than removal of all of the breast (mastectomy), the remaining breast tissue is irradiated to reduce the chance of local recurrence or new cancers in that breast.

Radiation therapy is often used palliatively when the cancer cannot be cured. The most common use of palliative radiation therapy is to relieve pain caused by skeletal bone metastases. This treatment is usually administered by external beam radiation directed at the painful bone lesion or lesions. The radioisotope strontium-89 is available for management of cancerous bone pain, especially in situations in which multiple painful sites make external beam radiation impractical.

Strontium-89 is a bone-seeking radioisotope that accumulates in sites of high bone turnover, such as cancer lesions, and emits low doses of radiation to that spot as the strontium-89 decays over several months.[15] Radiation is also used to prevent symptoms, such as seizures, associated with brain metastases, and to treat or prevent complications of cancer, such as spinal cord compression caused by growth of tumors on the spine or respiratory compromise from obstruction or external compression of a bronchus with tumor.[14]

Chemotherapy

The word *chemotherapy* was originally coined to describe treatment with antimicrobial compounds. However, today it is almost synonymous with drug therapy used to treat patients with cancer. The term most traditionally refers to use of conventional cytotoxic drugs but also includes hormonal or endocrine drug therapy. The era of modern chemotherapy began in the early 1940s when Goodman and Gilman first administered nitrogen mustard to patients with lymphoma. Nitrogen mustard was developed as a war gas rather than as a medicine. Its precursor, sulfur mustard, was used on battlefields during World War I. The toxic effects observed on the lymphatic system of mustard gas victims led to clinical trials of similar compounds in patients with lymphoma.[16,17] Now there are >50 conventional cytotoxic agents available in the United States and >15 hormonal agents for cancer treatment. Some of these agents are listed in Figure 2-5.

Chemotherapy has a limited role in the primary treatment of localized cancer, since only a few solid tumors are sensitive enough to chemotherapy to be cured with drug therapy alone. These cancers are outlined in Table 2-3.

Surgery and radiation therapy are generally much more effective than drug therapy in treating localized tumors, but these modalities are of limited value in treating disseminated cancers. Chemotherapy becomes the main treatment method in these cancers, because drug therapy can go almost anywhere in the body. Disseminated or systemic cancer includes several clinical situations[8,17,18]:

- Cancers that, by their nature, are considered widespread from the time of diagnosis. This includes most hematological malignancies, such as leukemias, and many lymphomas. Chemotherapy is used as the primary treatment method in these cancers and is given with the intent of curing the patient or prolonging survival.
- Cancers with clinically evident metastatic spread. Chemotherapy is only very rarely curative in treatment of metastatic solid tumors. It is administered with the goal of prolonging life or palliating symptoms. Tumors in which chemotherapy is recognized to prolong life are listed in Table 2-3.
- Cancers that, although they appear to be localized, may have developed clinically undetectable micro-

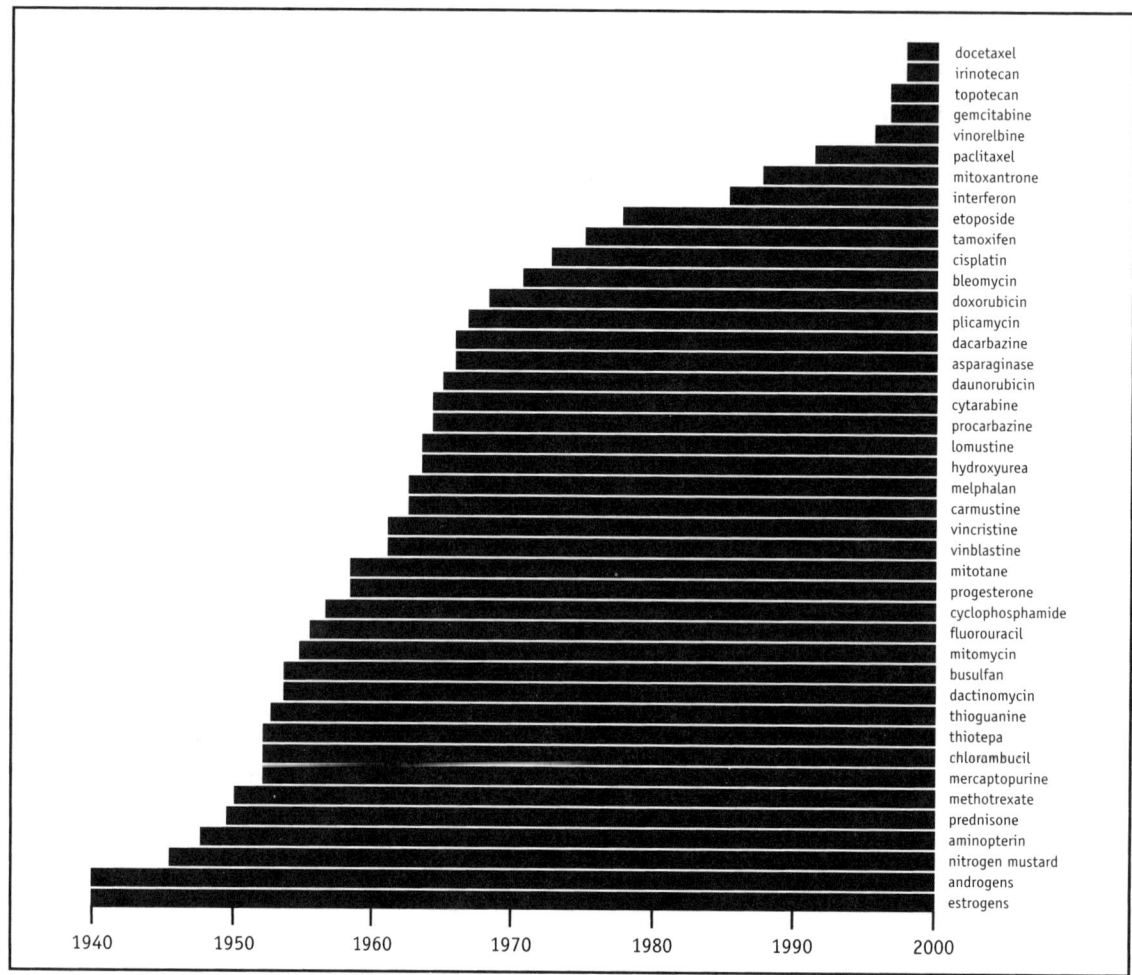

Figure 2-5. Selected anticancer drugs developed since 1940

metastases. Systemic therapy is given in an attempt to eradicate these micrometastases and increase the cure rate following surgery or radiation therapy. This is called adjuvant therapy and is discussed later in this chapter.

Although the special strength of chemotherapy is that it can reach widely disseminated cancers, two areas of the body are exceptions to this. The central nervous system and testes are two areas where most chemotherapy drugs do not penetrate well. These can act as sanctuary sites for tumor cells—sites where tumor cells are protected from the effects of circulating chemotherapy drugs.

Chemotherapy may also be administered in other clinical situations.[17] It may be administered to make other methods of cancer treatment more effective, such as when chemotherapy is administered to debulk a tumor so the surgical removal is less extensive. Some chemotherapy agents (e.g., fluorouracil, doxorubicin, and cisplatin) can increase the effects of radiation therapy. Called radiosensitizers, they are given before or during radiation therapy. Anticancer drugs, especially hormonal agents, are occasionally given to prevent cancer. Large national studies are under way to evaluate the efficacy of estrogen receptor antagonists in preventing breast cancer in women at high risk for developing that disease. Sometimes chemotherapy drugs are also administered for noncancerous conditions—most commonly, to take advantage of their immunosuppressive effects. Examples of nononcological uses of chemotherapy drugs are given in Table 2-4.

Although the major advantage of chemotherapy over surgery or radiation is its ability to reach most cells in the body, sometimes cancer drug therapy is purposefully administered to limited areas, to treat localized disease. Some examples of regional administration are given in Table 2-5. Unusual routes of administration for chemotherapy drugs are discussed in chapter 10.

Endocrine Therapy

Endocrine or hormonal therapy is a special subset of chemotherapy. Like traditional antineoplastic agents, hormonal agents are administered systemically and can therefore be used as adjuvant therapy and to treat disseminated cancers. Endocrine therapy is an alternative to traditional antineoplastics

Table 2-3. Responsiveness of Specific Tumors to Chemotherapy and Hormonal Therapy

Chemotherapy-induced cures possible
- Choriocarcinoma
- Neuroblastoma
- Acute leukemias
- Testicular cancer
- Hodgkin's disease
- Wilms' tumor
- Ewing's sarcoma
- Small-cell lung cancer
- Embryonal rhabdomyosarcoma
- Intermediate-grade lymphomas
- Lymphoblastic lymphoma
- Burkitt's lymphoma

Adjuvant or neoadjuvant chemotherapy-induced cures possible
- Breast cancer
- Colorectal cancer
- Osteogenic sarcoma
- Soft tissue sarcoma
- Head and neck cancer

Tumors that are responsive in advanced stages but are not yet curable
- Bladder cancer
- Breast cancer
- Cervical and endometrial cancers
- Prostate cancer
- Multiple myeloma
- Low-grade lymphomas
- Head and neck cancer
- Glioblastoma multiforme
- Soft tissue sarcoma
- Gastric cancer
- Colorectal cancer
- Chronic leukemias

Tumors that are poorly responsive in advanced stages to chemotherapy
- Osteogenic sarcoma
- Pancreatic cancer
- Renal cell carcinoma
- Thyroid cancer
- Non-small cell lung cancer
- Melanoma

SOURCE: adapted from references 16 and 18.

for systemic treatment of tumors that derive from tissues whose growth and function are normally controlled by endogenously secreted hormones. These tumors may regress if the hormones that normally "feed" their growth are withdrawn or antagonized. Because hormonal effects are receptor mediated, hormonal cancer therapies produce little effect on cells that do not bear hormone receptors. This relative specificity makes endocrine therapy the least toxic systemic anticancer treatment; it seldom results in myelosuppression, alopecia, or major organ toxicity. Fortunately, the most common cancers in males and females, prostate and breast cancers, derive from hormonally regulated tissue and are usually hormone dependent. Levels of gonadal hormones—estrogens, progestins, and androgens—can be manipulated to produce anticancer effects in patients with these cancers.[18,19]

Some hormonal agents appear to have anticancer ef-

Table 2-4. Examples of Nononcological Uses of Chemotherapy and Immunotherapy Drugs

Body System	Drug	Disorder
Musculoskeletal	Methotrexate	Rheumatoid arthritis
Reproductive	Methotrexate	Ectopic pregnancy
Dermatological	Fluorouracil (topical) Bleomycin Methotrexate Interferon alfa	Actinic keratosis Plantar warts Psoriasis Venereal warts
Renal	Cyclophosphamide	Lupus nephritis
Gastrointestinal	Mercaptopurine Methotrexate	Inflammatory bowel disease
Pulmonary	Methotrexate	Asthma
Hematological	Vincristine	Idiopathic thrombocytopenia

Table 2-5. Examples of Regional or Localized Administration of Chemotherapy

Body Region	Cancer Type	Type of Administration
Leg or arm	Melanoma	Isolated limb perfusion
Abdomen	Ovarian cancer	Intraperitoneal ("belly bath")
Central nervous system	Leukemia, lymphoma, breast, lung, others (meningeal involvement)	Intrathecal or intraventricular
Skin lesions	Skin (squamous, basal)	Topical
Liver	Hepatoma; liver metastases	Hepatic artery infusions
Pleura	Lymphoma, breast, others (malignant pleural effusions)	Pleural instillations
Bladder	Superficial bladder cancer	Bladder instillation

fects independent of their effects as hormones. The antiestrogen tamoxifen, for example, interferes with a variety of growth factors. This may be the basis of tamoxifen's clinical use in malignant melanomas and hepatomas, cancers that arise from tissues not considered hormonally dependent.[20] Diethylstilbestrol (DES), an estrogen formerly used to manage advanced prostate and breast cancers, interferes with apoptosis (programmed cell death) in hormonally independent prostate cancer cells in culture.[21]

Adrenal hormones, though less widely used as anticancer agents than gonadal hormones, play important roles in managing hematological malignancies and in supportive care of patients with cancer. Corticosteroids are lymphocytotoxic, making them especially useful for treating malignancies in which lymph tissues are involved, such as lymphocytic leukemias, lymphomas, and multiple myeloma, a plasma cell malignancy of B-lymphocyte origin. In addition to corticosteroids, the adrenal glands also produce small amounts of gonadal hormones, so manipulation of adrenal hormones may also be used to treat breast and prostate cancers.[22]

Biological Therapy

Surgery, radiation, and chemotherapy are sophisticated methods of cancer treatment, but many cancer patients still are not cured by any of these three modalities. Surgery and radiation therapy are limited to treatment of localized disease. And although cytotoxic chemotherapy can be administered systemically to attack tumor cells throughout the body, intolerable toxicity to normal cells may limit the use of cytotoxic agents to doses inadequate to destroy all tumor cells. Endocrine therapies are less toxic, but they are used to treat only a few hormonally responsive tumors.

Because of these limitations, the possibility that the body's own immune system might be exploited to destroy cancerous cells has been under intense investigation for the last two decades. The immune system has traditionally been considered as a defense against disease-causing bacteria and viruses, but it is now well recognized as an effective antitumor defense as well. It is thought that malignant cells occasionally arise in healthy bodies as a result of mutations, but not all of these malignant cells give rise to clinically evident cancers. There are also rare but well-documented cases of spontaneous regression in some patients with metastatic cancers, particularly renal cell cancer and malignant melanoma. Apparently, an intact immune system can identify cells as malignant and destroy them. And, in contrast to the relatively indiscriminate effects of cytotoxic agents, the immune system can distinguish between tumor cells and normal body tissues.[23,24]

Biological therapy, also known as biotherapy, immunotherapy, or biological response modification, includes all anticancer treatment approaches that attempt to influence the patient's own immune response to the tumor. In its broadest definition, biological therapy is any therapeutic alteration in the relationship between the patient and the tumor (except direct killing of the tumor) that improves the ability of the patient to reject the tumor.[23] By this interpretation, biological therapy can include treatments to help the bone marrow recover from chemotherapy. For the purposes of this chapter, however, biological therapy will mean the use of immune system therapies, such as interferons, interleukins, tumor vaccines, and antibody and gene therapies, to treat cancers (see chapter 5).

Chemotherapy and immunotherapy are the most important cancer treatment modalities for pharmacists. Much of this book is devoted to detailed discussion of the safe and effective use of anticancer drug therapies. The next sections of this chapter will address how the responses to chemotherapy and immune therapy are evaluated and the special situation of adjuvant drug therapy for cancer. Other chapters will discuss pharmacology of the drugs and biologicals used in cancer therapy, factors that determine therapeutic outcomes of chemotherapy, toxicities, therapeutic uses of chemotherapy drugs in specific cancers and bone marrow transplantation, safe administration techniques, and practice issues with these agents.

EVALUATION OF RESPONSE

The question of whether or not a particular drug or biological treatment is effective must be answered in both the general and the individual sense. In other words, is the therapy effective in the treatment of a specific cancer type and, if so, is it also effective for the individual patient? Several objective classifications are used to categorize a particular patient's response to chemotherapy or biological therapy.[8,17,18] Although definitions may vary slightly from one institution or research group to another, the following categories of response are widely used:

- Complete response or remission (CR): the complete disappearance of all clinical evidence of the tumor for at least 1 month. This definition also commonly includes the return to normal performance status, referring to the patient's physical level of function.
- Partial response (PR): ≥50% decrease of measurable tumor, with no new areas of cancer and no evidence of tumor progression. The size of tumors is usually measured as the sum of the products of two perpendicular diameters of all measurable lesions (Figure 2-6).
- Disease progression (treatment failure): increase of measurable tumor by >25%, appearance of new lesions, or tumor-induced death.
- Stable disease: measurable tumor that does not meet the criteria for CR, PR, or disease progression. The tumor mass does not increase or decrease in size by >25%.

These categories are used to assess the response of a single patient. The overall efficacy of a drug or regimen administered to a group of patients, such as those enrolled in a clinical trial, may be summarized and evaluated in a variety of ways. To compare the outcome of one trial with another, or with a specific patient, it is necessary to understand what evaluation methods were used. The measures of comparison most commonly used are:

- Duration of survival,
- Response rate: the percentage of patients who demonstrate an objective response (the sum of CRs and PRs),
- Duration of response,
- Toxicities associated with treatment, and
- Impact on quality of life.

Duration of Survival

Duration of survival is the time a patient or group of patients lives after a specific event. Duration of survival may be measured in days, weeks, months, or years. Because the duration of survival may be calculated and presented in several different ways, comparisons between trials can be difficult and confusing. An apparent improvement in the duration of survival resulting from one therapy versus another may be more attributable to the method of calculation than to the actual treatment. For example, duration of survival in one report may be measured from the date of diagnosis of the disease, whereas in another it may be measured from the date of initial therapy or the date on which a response to therapy was documented.

Most oncology trials report the median survival rate, defined as the time from diagnosis, treatment, or documented

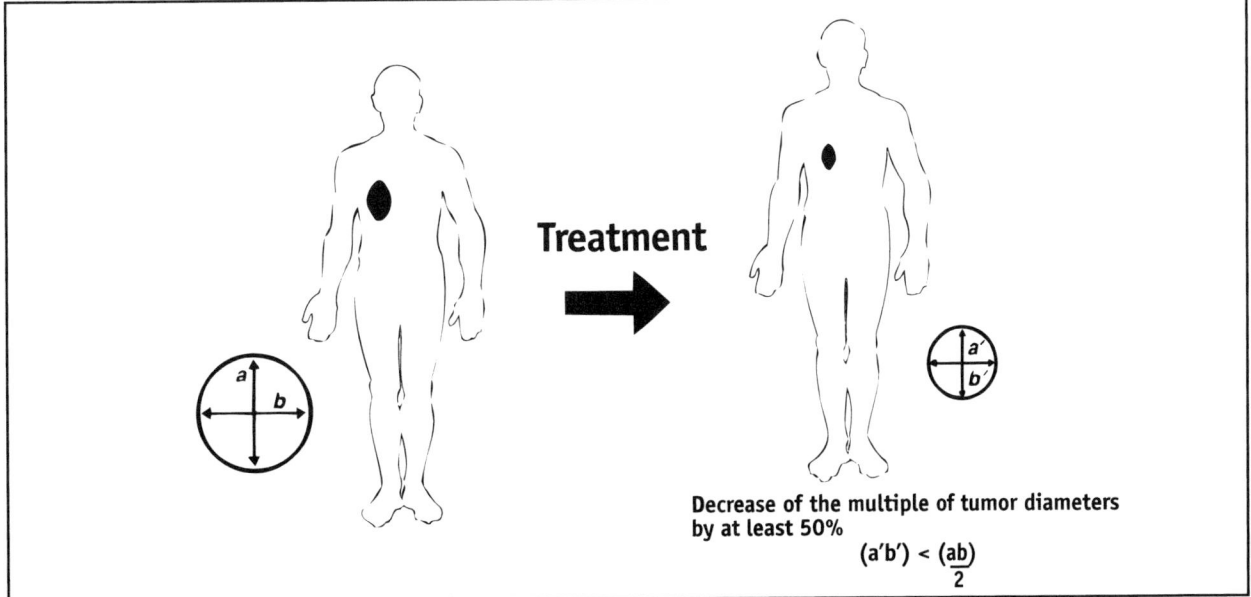

Figure 2-6. Measurement of objective solid tumor response
SOURCE: reprinted with permission from Rhone-Poulenc Rorer Oncology.

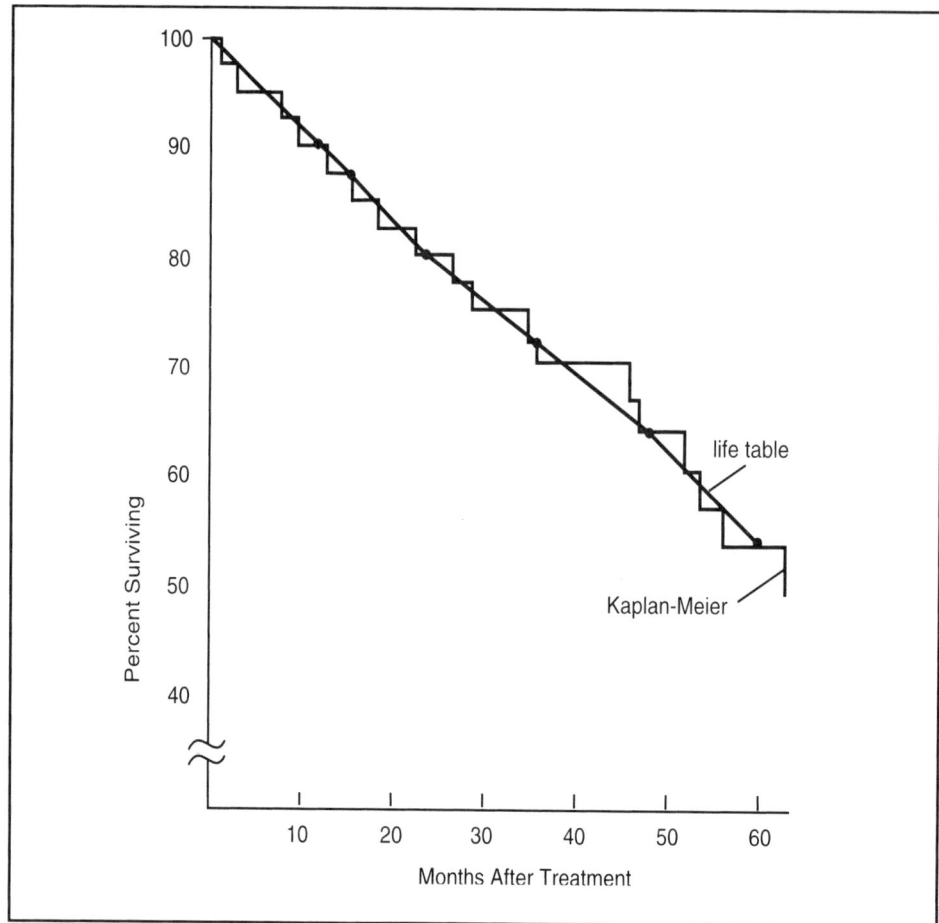

Figure 2-7. Survival curves. The smooth line represents the proportion of patients who remain alive at any time in follow-up of a specified patient population. This is called a life-table survival curve. The "stepped" line is a Kaplan-Meier survival curve, which permits calculation of the proportion of patients surviving to each point in time that a death occurs. Each patient's death is represented by another step in the curve.

SOURCE: reprinted with permission from American Joint Committee on Cancer. *Manual for Staging of Cancer*. 4th ed. Beahrs OH, Henson DE, Hutter RVP, et al., editors. Philadelphia, PA: JB Lippincott; 1992. p. 22.

response until the time when 50% of patients have died and 50% are still alive. This measure is a better indicator of survival than the average (or mean) survival because it is not skewed by patients whose survival was either very short or very long compared with other patients receiving the same therapy. Because the median survival cannot be calculated until 50% of patients have died, other measurements must be used until that criterion has been met. Improvement in actual survival is the most stringent and demanding evaluation criteria for a new pharmacologic agent or treatment.[25] Duration of survival is often represented graphically by curves (Figure 2-7).

Clinical trials may also report an observed survival rate—the percentage of patients alive at the end of a specified interval of observation. For example, a report may state that 65% of patients were alive 2 years after therapy. It would be difficult to compare this report with one that reported different median durations of survival, such as 3 or 5 years. Because relapse of disease may precede death by many months or years, disease-free survival can be calculated earlier than overall or actual survival and is considered a weaker measure for evaluation of an agent or treatment.

Survival may also be reported as the median duration of disease-free survival for patients who achieve a CR to therapy. This indicates the time from documentation of CR until the disease recurs or the patient dies without evidence of the disease.

Response Rate

The response rate reflects the percentage of patients who had documented tumor regression following therapy. The CR rate is the percentage of patients who have had complete tumor regression. The overall response rate, also called the objective response rate (RR), is the sum of CRs and PRs divided by the total number of evaluable patients. The CR rate is far more important than the PR rate in evaluation of chemotherapy agents because only patients with a CR have the potential for cure, and they are usually the only patients who have significantly prolonged survival. However, when a new therapy demonstrates a high PR rate, it is an indicator that there may be merit in the new therapy and further research is warranted.

A clinical CR indicates that total tumor regression was documented by clinical parameters, such as physical examination or radiological studies. In contrast, a pathological CR is documented by biopsy and microscopic examination of previous tumor areas in addition to clinical documentation. In some cancers, such as ovarian cancer, microscopic evidence of disease often is found after therapy, even though no clinical evidence (masses on examination, computed tomography scan, etc.) remains. Therefore, pathological documentation of CR is used in ovarian cancer and some other tumors to determine whether the patient should receive further therapy.

Duration of Response

The duration of response is the time from the first documentation of response to the recurrence or progression of the tumor. For patients who achieve a CR, duration of response is equivalent to the duration of disease-free or relapse-free survival. For a clinical trial, duration of response is usually reported as a median value for all patients who achieve a response. This measurement is important because it is an indicator of the durability of the effectiveness of the therapy. For a therapy to produce a meaningful prolongation in survival, it must produce a durable (lasting) response.[25] In fact, prolongation of survival is usually demonstrated only when >50% of the patients achieve durable CRs.

Toxicities Associated with Treatment

Toxic effects of cancer chemotherapy and complications associated with surgery or radiation therapy often are serious and may limit the amount of treatment that a patient can receive. For this reason, it is important that clinical trials summarize the toxicities experienced secondary to the therapy. Definitions and rating scales of toxicities should be specified in the report so that toxic effects can be assessed. To state that a specific proportion of patients experienced stomatitis after therapy, for example, could mean that those patients had a few oral lesions, that they had serious tissue damage leading to life-threatening infections, that they had damage severe enough to require parenteral nutrition support, or all three. Specifying the degree of toxicity in a standardized way gives reliable measures of toxicity. Therefore, many institutions use standardized rating scales, such as the Common Toxicity Criteria grading system developed by the National Cancer Institute (see Appendix II). Toxicities associated with chemotherapy are described in chapters 7, 8, and 9.

Patients who are debilitated by their tumors or other concomitant diseases are more likely to experience serious toxicities. In these patients, the benefit-to-risk ratio is less favorable than it is in otherwise healthy patients. In clinical trials, it is necessary to provide information about the baseline performance (physical) status of patients so that toxicities may be compared among patients who have similar relative risks. The Karnofsky scale (see Appendix III) is the most widely used rating system for performance status.

Scales to assess performance status have also been developed by the Eastern Cooperative Oncology Group (ECOG). Cooperative groups are organizations of cancer research institutions who pool their resources to develop and carry out oncology research studies. The ECOG performance status scale is a simpler scale than the Karnofsky scale. Patients are rated as fully ambulatory without compromise of their activities (ECOG performance status of zero) to being in bed 100% of the time and unable to care for themselves (ECOG performance status of 4).

Impact on Quality of Life

New cancer treatments are increasingly being judged by the overall impact of treatment on patients' quality of life as well as by clinical efficacy. This is particularly true for cancers for which cure is unlikely. When the best possible outcomes of treatment are prolongation of life or palliation of symptoms, it is essential to consider what trade-offs are necessary to achieve those goals. For example, a toxic treatment that increases the duration of survival by 2 months but requires prolonged hospitalization or has debilitating side effects may or may not be judged by patients as a fair trade-off. An evaluation of the impact of a new treatment on quality of life is now required by the Food and Drug Administration as part of the new drug approval process. This impact is most commonly evaluated by the use of patient survey instruments completed before, during, and after the treatment.[26] Some examples of commonly used instruments are the FLIC (Functional Living Index—Cancer), and Q-TWiST (Quality-Adjusted Time Without Symptoms and Toxicity). The Q-TWiST method makes treatment comparisons by penalizing treatments that have negative quality-of-life effects, such as toxicity, and rewarding those that increase survival and have other positive quality-of-life effects.[9]

ADJUVANT THERAPY

Evaluation methods such as CR, PR, and duration of response work well for assessment of patients with metastatic and measurable disease, but there is one common use of chemotherapy and biological therapy that is much harder to evaluate because there is, by definition, no evidence of disease at the time the treatment is given. This type of therapy is called adjuvant therapy.[8,17]

In the past, it was believed that cancers began in one particular organ and spread from that site only by direct extension, cell by cell, going first into the regional lymph nodes nearest the primary tumor. These lymph nodes were thought to act as barriers to further cancer spread. According to this theory, it was only in advanced-stage disease that tumor cells spread throughout the body via the blood or lymphatic fluids. Unfortunately, this view was false. Cancer cells can be shed from the original tumor mass at any time and may circulate throughout the body very early in the course of the disease, even before malignant cells are detectable in regional lymph nodes. More than one fourth of breast cancer patients with pathologically negative lymph nodes at the time of mastectomy or lumpectomy, for example, have recurrence of breast cancer sometime during their lives. Often the recurrence is in a site other than breast tissue, such as the bones, liver, or lungs. Clearly, some clinically undetectable or micrometastatic breast cancer cells remained in the bodies of these patients after surgery. Thus, early "localized" cancer is often already a systemic disease at the time of diagnosis.

Adjuvant therapy is administration of systemic therapy to eradicate any residual micrometastases and prevent them from growing into clinically evident disease. It is called adjuvant (or adjunctive) therapy because it is a form of treatment that helps another type of treatment. Traditionally, adjuvant therapy refers to systemically administered therapy with cytotoxic drugs, hormones, or biological agents after the primary solid tumor mass has been eliminated with surgery or radiation therapy.[27]

Adjuvant therapy can also be administered after the primary disease has been eliminated with antineoplastic drugs. An example of this is the treatment of patients with acute leukemias. Once clinically evident disease has been eliminated with aggressive chemotherapy, additional chemotherapy courses are given to eliminate residual disease. Postremission therapy in leukemia may include intensification, consolidation, and maintenance therapies.[28] These therapies are described in detail in chapter 13.

Neoadjuvant therapy, a less conventional form of adjuvant therapy, does not strictly fit the definition of adjuvant chemotherapy. Systemic treatment with antineoplastic drugs or hormones is given before surgery to debulk the tumor, reducing the extent and disfigurement of surgery. Drug therapy administered in this situation serves a dual purpose because it may also eradicate micrometastases. Neoadjuvant chemotherapy, which is also called preoperative or primary chemotherapy, is particularly useful for head and neck cancers and the bone cancer osteogenic sarcoma.[29] Hormonal therapy may be used neoadjuvantly for management of locally advanced prostate cancer. Cancers that can be cured with chemotherapy in the adjuvant or neoadjuvant setting are listed in Table 2-3.

Determining which patients should receive adjuvant chemotherapy treatment is a major dilemma. By definition, patients do not show any clinical evidence of residual cancer following surgery or radiation therapy. Patients whose cancers have a high statistical chance of recurrence should be selected. Although some of these patients may already be cured, others will only be cured by the addition of adjuvant therapy (Figure 2-8).[30] Unfortunately, it is not yet possible to accurately distinguish cured patients from those who harbor micrometastases that will eventually cause cancer recurrences.

There are many tests or factors that can be used to assess an individual's risk of cancer recurrence, however. In breast cancer patients, for example, premenopausal patients who have positive lymph nodes and negative hormone receptors in their tumor sample have a very high risk of recurrence. Although such prognostic factors give hints of how a patient's cancer may act in the future, none are 100% accurate. Cancer may recur even in patients with excellent prognostic factors. Recurrent cancer usually means metastatic disease, which is, with rare exceptions, incurable. Therefore, patients are asked to consent to the risks and costs of adjuvant treatment to decrease their statistical odds of cancer recurrence without knowing whether they actually have residual disease. The unusual situation of making cancer treatment decisions based on

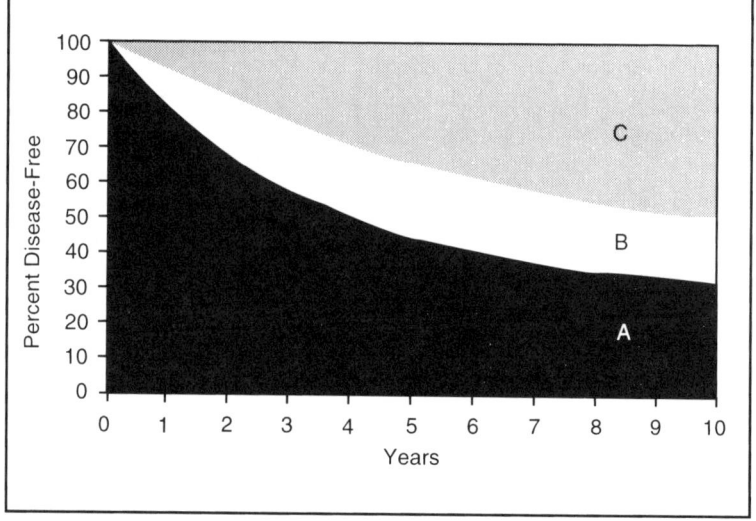

Figure 2-8. Hypothetical representation of potential benefit from adjuvant systemic therapy in patients with primary breast cancer. *A:* patients cured after local/regional therapy. *B:* patients with residual micrometastases after local/regional therapy whose tumor cells are responsive to the adjuvant therapy used (and who may therefore be cured by addition of adjuvant therapy). *C:* patients with resistant residual micrometastases after local/regional therapy (who will not be cured even with adjuvant therapy).

SOURCE: reprinted with permission from Hortobagyi GN, Buzdar AU. Current status of adjuvant systemic therapy for primary breast cancer: progress and controversy. *CA Cancer J Clin* 1995;45:201.

statistical risk rather than clinically evident and assessable disease also makes it impossible to determine, for a given patient, whether they were cured by the primary therapy or by the adjuvant chemotherapy.

The risks of adjuvant therapy are not risks to be taken lightly. Aggressive adjuvant therapy with cytotoxic drugs, hormones, or biologicals produces all the unpleasant side effects and risks of these agents when they are given for known metastatic cancer. Financial costs of therapy may also be high, both in terms of drugs and medical resources and in loss of the patient's productive time from job and family responsibilities.[31] Development of less toxic agents and improved methods of patient selection may decrease the risks of adjuvant therapy, but it is likely to remain a very serious undertaking for patients and physicians alike.

The risks of adjuvant therapy would be easier to justify if undergoing this therapy was a guarantee that the cancer would not recur. Unfortunately, that is not the case for any adjuvant therapy used today. In general, these therapies delay the time to recurrence of cancer and decrease but do not eliminate the risk of recurrence. The strongest adjuvant therapies improve overall survival as well as disease-free survival and increase the number of patients ultimately cured of their cancer. This is illustrated using the example of adjuvant chemotherapy or hormonal therapy for breast cancer in Figure 2-8. The improvements in disease-free survival and overall survival that are accomplished with adjuvant therapy provide the justification for subjecting large groups of patients to the risks of these treatments.[30] The role of adjuvant chemotherapy is also well established for osteogenic sarcoma (a bone cancer) and for patients with lymph-node-positive colon cancer.[32] The biological agent interferon alfa-2b is approved by the Food and Drug Administration for adjuvant treatment of patients with a high risk of recurrence following surgical management of malignant melanoma.[33]

The failures of adjuvant therapy probably occur because of the biological nature of cancers. Even microscopic tumor masses are not composed of identical cells. Most cancers are genetically unstable (have high mutation rates). Mutational changes that occur during cell division may make the offspring resistant to some or all of the agents that are used in adjuvant therapy. (See the discussion on tumor heterogeneity in chapter 6.) If even one cell remains after therapy, it is possible for that cell to eventually multiply into a lethal tumor mass.[34,35] This is one of the reasons why adjuvant therapy is best begun as soon after treatment of the primary tumor as possible, when the tumor burden is smallest. Early treatment decreases the likelihood that resistant cell lines have developed and increases the chance that chemotherapy can destroy all of them and result in a true cure of the patient's cancer. Smaller tumor masses also tend to have higher growth fractions, making them more susceptible to the cytotoxic effects of chemotherapy drugs, which are most effective against actively dividing cells.[8,36] Some general guidelines for administering adjuvant therapy are outlined in Table 2-6.

Table 2-6. Guidelines for Use of Adjuvant Chemotherapy

Stage patients for probability of recurrence

Evaluate benefits and risks of treatment

Use drugs that are effective against advanced forms of that cancer

Begin as soon as possible after surgery or radiation therapy

Give combinations of drugs with different mechanisms of action

Give maximum tolerated doses of drugs as frequently as possible

Discontinue after maximum benefit has been obtained

SOURCE: adapted from reference 27.

SUMMARY

The treatment of cancer includes four treatment modalities: surgery, radiation, chemotherapy (which includes endocrine treatment), and immunotherapy. Surgery and radiation are limited by their local nature. Chemotherapy is administered systemically, and it is used for cancers that are disseminated either because of the nature of the cancer (e.g., leukemias) or because of metastases. Immunotherapy attempts to bolster the patient's immune response to the "foreign" presence of cancer cells. Some patients are treated with only one modality, but most often a combination of therapies is used to achieve the primary goal of cancer treatment—curing the patient. Adjuvant therapy, which attempts to destroy clinically undetectable micrometastases, is a special subset of cancer treatment with intent to cure. The secondary goal of cancer treatment is to prolong survival when a cure is not possible. If neither the primary nor the secondary goal is achievable, palliative therapy can be employed to relieve symptoms and improve the quality of the patient's life.

There are four commonly used criteria for evaluating cancer treatment outcomes. An individual patient is said to have a complete response, partial response, disease progression, or stable disease. The measures of comparison for results of oncology trials are duration of survival, response rate, duration of response, toxicities associated with treatment, and impact on quality of life.

REFERENCES

1. Tannock IF. Cell proliferation. In: *The Basic Science of Oncology*. 2nd ed. Tannock IF, Hill RP, editors. New York: McGraw-Hill; 1992. p. 154–77.
2. Buick RN. Cellular basis of chemotherapy. In: Dorr RT, Von Hoff DD, editors. *Cancer Chemotherapy Handbook*. 2nd ed. Norwalk, CT: Appleton & Lange; 1994. p. 3–14.
3. Famighetti R, editor. *World Almanac 1994*. New York: Funk and Wagnalls; 1993. p. 828.

4. Shackney SE. Tumor growth, cell cycle kinetics, and cancer treatment. In: Calabresi P, Schein PS, editors. *Medical Oncology: Basic Principles and Clinical Management of Cancer.* 2nd ed. New York: McGraw-Hill; 1993. p. 43–60.
5. Fidler IJ. Molecular cell biology of cancer: invasion and metastasis. In: DeVita VT Jr, Hellman S, Rosenberg SA, editors. *Cancer: Principles and Practice of Oncology.* 5th ed. Philadelphia, PA: Lippincott-Raven; 1997. p. 135–52.
6. Hill RP. Metastasis. In: *The Basic Science of Oncology.* Tannock IF, Hill RP, editors. New York: Pergamon; 1987. p. 160–75.
7. Beitz J, Calabresi P. Biology and patterns of metastases. In: Calabresi P, Schein PS, editors. *Medical Oncology: Basic Principles and Clinical Management of Cancer.* 2nd ed. New York: McGraw-Hill; 1993. p. 61–76.
8. Pratt WB. Choice of drugs for cancer chemotherapy. In: Pratt WB, Ruddon RW, Ensminger WD, et al., editors. *The Anticancer Drugs.* 2nd ed. New York: Oxford Univ Pr; 1994. p. 235–46.
9. Cella DF. Measuring quality of life in palliative care. *Semin Oncol* 1995;22(*Suppl* 3):73–81.
10. Rosenberg SA. Principles of cancer management: surgical oncology. In: DeVita VT Jr, Hellman S, Rosenberg SA, editors. *Cancer: Principles and Practice of Oncology.* 5th ed. Philadelphia, PA: Lippincott-Raven; 1997. p. 295–306.
11. Markman M. Surgery for support and palliation in patients with malignant disease. *Semin Oncol* 1995;22 (*Suppl* 3).91–4.
12. Parker RG, Withers HR. Principles of radiation oncology. In: Haskell CM, editor. *Cancer Treatment.* 4th ed. Philadelphia, PA: WB Saunders; 1995. p. 23–31.
13. Ciezki J, Macklis RM. The palliative role of radiotherapy in the management of the cancer patient. *Semin Oncol* 1995; 22:(*Suppl* 3):82–90.
14. Coleman CN, Howes AE. Overall principles of cancer management: radiation therapy. In: Osteen RT, Cady B, Rosenthal PE, editors. *Cancer Manual.* 8th ed. Boston, MA: American Cancer Society; 1990. p. 85–98.
15. Robinson RG, Preston DF, Schiefelbein M, et al. Strontium 89 therapy for palliation of pain due to osseous metastases. *JAMA* 1995;274:420–4.
16. Pratt WB. Some milestones in the development of cancer chemotherapy. In: Pratt WB, Ruddon RW, Ensminger WD, et al., editors. *The Anticancer Drugs.* 2nd ed. New York: Oxford Univ Pr; 1994. p. 17–25.
17. DeVita VT Jr. Principles of cancer management: chemotherapy. In: DeVita VT Jr, Hellman S, Rosenberg SA, editors. *Cancer: Principles and Practice of Oncology.* 5th ed. Philadelphia, PA: Lippincott-Raven; 1997. p. 333–47.
18. Haskell CM. Principles of cancer chemotherapy. In: Haskell CM, editor. *Cancer Treatment.* 4th ed. Philadelphia, PA: WB Saunders; 1995. p. 31–57.
19. Swain SM. Endocrine therapies of cancer. In: Chabner BA, Longo DL, editors. *Cancer Chemotherapy and Biotherapy: Principles and Practice.* 2nd ed. Philadelphia, PA: Lippincott-Raven; 1996. p. 59–108.
20. McClay EF, McClay MET. Tamoxifen: is it useful in the treatment of patients with metastatic melanoma? *J Clin Oncol* 1994;12:617–26.
21. Robertson CN, Robertson KM, Padilla GM, et al. Induction of apoptosis by diethylstilbestrol in hormone-insensitive prostate cancer cells. *J Natl Cancer Inst* 1996;88:908–17.
22. Schwartzman RA, Cidlowski JA. Corticosteroids. In: Holland JF, Frei E III, Bast RC Jr, et al., editors. *Cancer Medicine.* 4th ed. Baltimore, MD: Williams & Wilkins; 1997. p. 1087–102.
23. Quan WD Jr, Mitchell MS. Principles of biologic therapy. In: Haskell CM, editor. *Cancer Treatment.* 4th ed. Philadelphia, PA: WB Saunders; 1995. p. 57–69.
24. Rosenberg SA. Principles of cancer management: biologic therapy. In: DeVita VT Jr, Hellman S, Rosenberg SA, editors. *Cancer: Principles and Practice of Oncology.* 5th ed. Philadelphia, PA: Lippincott-Raven; 1997. p. 349–73.
25. American Joint Committee on Cancer. *Manual for Staging of Cancer.* 4th ed. Beahrs OH, Henson DE, Hutter RVP, et al., editors. Philadelphia, PA: JB Lippincott; 1992. p. 11–23.
26. Beitz J, Gnecco C, Justice R. Quality of life endpoints in cancer clinical trials: the U.S. Food and Drug Administration perspective [monograph]. *J Natl Cancer Inst* 1996;20:7–9.
27. Wittes RE. Adjuvant chemotherapy—clinical trials and laboratory models. *Cancer Treat Rep* 1986;70:87–103.
28. Mayer RJ, Davis RB, Schiffer CA, et al. Intensive postremission chemotherapy in adults with acute myeloid leukemia. *N Engl J Med* 1994;331:896–903.
29. Frei E III. What's in a name—neoadjuvant. *J Natl Cancer Inst* 1989;80:1088.
30. Hortobagyi GN, Buzdar AU. Current status of adjuvant systemic therapy for primary breast cancer: progress and controversy. *CA Cancer J Clin* 1995;45:199–226.
31. McGuire WL. Adjuvant therapy of node-negative breast cancer [editorial]. *N Engl J Med* 1989;320:525–7.
32. Moertel CG, Fleming TR, Macdonald JS, et al. Fluorouracil plus levamisole as effective adjuvant therapy after resection of stage III colon carcinoma: a final report. *Ann Intern Med* 1995;122:321–26.
33. Kirkwood JM, Strawderman MH, Ernstoff MS, et al. Interferon alfa-2b adjuvant therapy of high-risk resected cutaneous melanoma: the Eastern Cooperative Oncology Group trial EST 1684. *J Clin Oncol* 1996;14:7–17.
34. Goldie JH, Coldman AJ. A mathematical model for relating the drug sensitivity of tumors to their spontaneous mutation rate. *Cancer Treat Rep* 1979;63:1727–33.
35. Fidler IJ, Poste G. The cellular heterogeneity of malignant neoplasm: implications for adjuvant chemotherapy. *Semin Oncol* 1985;12:207–21.
36. DeVita VT Jr. The relationship between tumor mass and resistance to chemotherapy: implications for surgical adjuvant treatment of cancer. *Cancer* 1983;51:1209–20.

SELF-STUDY QUESTIONS

1. A small tumor mass increases in size from 4 cells to 16 cells in one year. What is the tumor's doubling time?

    a. 3 months
    b. 4 months
    c. 6 months
    d. 12 months

2. When most of the cells in a tumor mass are actively dividing, the tumor is said to have:

a. a high growth fraction.
b. a low growth fraction.
c. plateau phase of growth.
d. metastasized.

3. Draw a Gompertzian growth curve for a typical solid tumor and describe the tumor growth patterns that account for its shape.

4. Most of a tumor's doublings in size occur before the mass is clinically detectable.

    a. true
    b. false

5. Select the true statement.

    a. Cells cannot shed from tumor surfaces to produce metastases until the tumor mass is at least 3 cm in diameter.
    b. Liver, lungs, bones, and brain are common metastatic sites for solid tumors.
    c. The doubling times for hematological malignancies are usually longer than those for solid tumors.
    d. All of the cells that shed from a tumor produce metastatic lesions.

6. If patients would cooperate fully with aggressive cancer treatment as recommended by their physicians, any patient could be cured of cancer.

    a. true
    b. false

7. HJ is a 73-year-old female with metastatic breast cancer that is causing severe shortness of breath. She cannot walk across the room without stopping to rest. Her physician has recommended a chemotherapy treatment to help her breathe more easily. The goal of this cancer treatment is to:

    a. cure the cancer.
    b. prolong her life.
    c. palliate her symptoms.
    d. determine a safe dose of a new drug.

8. A chemotherapy regimen that produces severe side effects is most likely to be acceptable if the goal of cancer treatment for that patient is to:

    a. cure.
    b. prolong life.
    c. palliate symptoms.
    d. determine the safe dose of a new drug.

9. Of the major modalities of cancer treatment, which modality produces the most cancer cures?

    a. surgery
    b. radiation therapy
    c. chemotherapy
    d. immunotherapy

10. Select the true statement:

    a. Surgery and radiation therapy are primarily used to manage patients with disseminated cancers.
    b. Administering radiation therapy in a single large dose to increase the tumor damage is called fractionating the dose.
    c. Most radiation therapy is given by external beam techniques.
    d. The preferred unit for measuring radiation therapy doses is "rads."

11. The role(s) of surgery in patients with cancer include:

    a. cancer diagnosis and staging.
    b. cure of disease.
    c. relief of symptoms.
    d. all of the above.

12. List two nononcological uses for chemotherapy drugs.

13. EG recently had a tumor removed from his colon. It had invaded his lymph nodes, but his surgeon is confident he "got it all." To EG's surprise, the medical oncologist wants to give EG chemotherapy to decrease the chance of recurrence, even though the surgeon said there was no trace of cancer left. This use of chemotherapy is called _____.

14. Some patients receive adjuvant chemotherapy needlessly, because they were cured of their cancer by surgical removal of the primary tumor. Explain why this may occur and how it can be minimized.

15. Name two cancers for which adjuvant therapy has been proved to increase the number of patients cured of cancer.

16. AR's lung cancer could be seen as a mass on his chest X-ray. After treatment with chemotherapy, the radiology report of his next chest X-ray stated that the lung mass had decreased by about two thirds. This response to treatment is called:

    a. complete response.
    b. partial response.
    c. stable disease.
    d. progression.

17. At AR's next evaluation, his lung mass on chest X-ray appeared to have increased very slightly in size, by about

5–10%, despite continued chemotherapy. Compared with the previous chest X-ray, this response to treatment is called:

   a. complete response.
   b. partial response.
   c. stable disease.
   d. progression.

18. Name two common cancers for which hormonal therapies are cornerstones of cancer treatment.

19. The least toxic form of cancer drug therapy is:

   a. chemotherapy.
   b. hormonal therapy.
   c. immunotherapy.
   d. all of the above are very toxic treatments.

20. Define the term "response rate" as used in oncology.

21. From the following list, select the cancer treatment that has had the greatest impact on cancer patient outcomes.

   a. Regimen A produces a response rate of 50% and decreases overall survival by 1 month because of severe toxicity.
   b. Regimen B produces a response rate of 50% and does not change overall survival.
   c. Regimen C produces a response rate of 35% and increases overall survival by 6 months.
   d. Regimen D produces a 90% response rate and does not change overall survival.

Chapter 3
The Pharmacology of Cytotoxic Chemotherapy I

Rebecca S. Finley, Pharm.D., M.S.
Chair and Associate Professor
Department of Pharmacy Practice and Pharmacy Administration
Philadelphia College of Pharmacy
Philadelphia, Pennsylvania

Biochemistry	34
Nucleic Acid Synthesis	34
Topoisomerase Enzymes	36
Specificity of Cancer Chemotherapy	36
Alkylating Agents	37
Classic Alkylating Agents	37
Resistance	38
Mechlorethamine	39
Cyclophosphamide and Ifosfamide	39
Melphalan	40
Chlorambucil	40
Thiotepa	40
Busulfan	40
Nitrosoureas	40
Miscellaneous Alkylator-Like Agents	41
Platinum Analogues	41
Cisplatin	41
Carboplatin	41
Procarbazine	42
Dacarbazine	42
Altretamine	42
Antitumor Antibiotics and Anthracenediones	42
Anthracyclines	43
Resistance	44
Liposomal Products	44
Mitoxantrone	45
Bleomycin	45
Dactinomycin	46
Mitomycin	46
References	46
Self-Study Questions	48

The most fundamental objective of providing pharmaceutical care is to ensure that every patient receives rational drug therapy to maximize the likelihood of achieving desired outcomes. In the oncology setting, understanding how chemotherapy works at the cellular level is the first step toward accomplishing this objective. An in-depth understanding of the pharmacology of cytotoxic drugs enables pharmacists to contribute to the drug therapy management of patients receiving chemotherapy. For example, knowing how the drug is eliminated from the body helps pharmacists identify patients at risk for serious toxicities and then make informed decisions about dosage adjustments in the face of significant organ dysfunction. Understanding the pharmacology of cytotoxic drugs also helps pharmacists understand the factors that influence chemotherapy effectiveness and toxicity and gives them insight into the rationale used in designing combination chemotherapy regimens.

Because of the volume of information pertaining to the pharmacology of cytotoxics, this material has been divided into two chapters to permit the reader to complete each chapter and its assessment in a reasonable amount of time. Chapter 3 briefly reviews the biochemistry of deoxyribonucleic acid (DNA) and ribonucleic acid (RNA) to illustrate the various mechanisms by which cytotoxic chemotherapy damages cells. A general pharmacologic overview of each of the classes of cytotoxic drugs is provided. These classes include the alkylating agents, antitumor antibiotics, antimetabolites, plant alkaloids, and miscellaneous drugs. The mechanism each class uses to produce lethal damage to the cancer cell is described, and the pharmacologic characteristics that influence the use of many individual drugs are reviewed. Factors that may alter the pharmacokinetics and necessitate dose adjustments, such as liver and kidney dysfunction, are discussed. These chapters include only the basics of pharmacology of the cytotoxics; all readers are encouraged to consult the cited references and suggested reference texts for more comprehensive information.

After completing this chapter, the reader should be able to:

1. Describe the mechanisms of action of the various cytotoxic classes and list examples from each class.
2. Discuss the importance of the topoisomerase enzymes in relation to cytotoxic activity of various chemotherapy classes.
3. Given a specific cytotoxic drug, identify aspects of its pharmacology that influence its therapeutic applications.
4. Describe the mechanisms of at least two chemoprotective or rescue strategies.
5. Given a class of cytotoxic drugs, list toxicities that are common to the class and toxicities that are unique to specific drugs within the class.

BIOCHEMISTRY

Most cytotoxic chemotherapy drugs damage cancer cells by either interfering with the synthesis of the precursors of DNA or chemically interacting with the DNA itself to interfere with the process of cellular division. Therefore, an understanding of nucleic acid synthesis and DNA structure is essential to comprehending how cytotoxic drugs interact at the cellular level to ultimately cause the death of the cell.

The nucleic acids DNA and RNA have the same functions in all cells: the storage, transmission, and translation of all genetic information. DNA is the repository of genetic information, whereas various kinds of RNAs assist in translating this information into protein structure. The proteins are responsible for all the functions necessary for life.

Nucleic Acid Synthesis

DNA and RNA are long chains of nucleotides; the sequence of these nucleotides determines genetic information in the cell (Figure 3-1). Synthesis of both DNA and RNA requires two purine and two pyrimidine nucleoside triphosphates, each of which can be derived from either a de novo (newly made) pathway or a salvage (recycling of partially degraded nucleotides) pathway. It appears that malignant cells rely more heavily on the de novo purine synthesis pathway, so this pathway is a common therapeutic target.[1] Each nucleotide is composed of (1) a nitrogenous organic base, (2) a five-carbon sugar (deoxy-D-ribose in DNA and D-ribose in RNA), and (3) a phosphoric acid that serves as a bridge between the successive nucleotides. The nitrogenous bases are derivatives of pyrimidine (cytosine, thymine, and uracil) or purine (adenine and guanine). DNA contains adenine, guanine, cytosine, and thymine; RNA contains adenine, guanine, cytosine, and uracil.

Figure 3-2 provides a simplified schematic of the steps of DNA and RNA synthesis. It also demonstrates where some of the antimetabolite drugs exert their inhibitory effects on purine and pyrimidine synthesis.

The DNA molecule consists of two strands that wind around each other in the form of a double helix. These two strands are held together by hydrogen bonding between the bases; adenine always bonds to thymine, and guanine always bonds to cytosine. The two strands of the double helix are therefore not identical but complementary. As mentioned above, DNA is the repository of all genetic information. Whereas the antimetabolite drugs interfere with cellular division by disrupting nucleotide assembly, other drugs (e.g., alkylating agents and antitumor antibiotics) interfere with cellular division by binding to and damaging the DNA. In some cases, this results in irreparable damage that leads to cell death; in other cases, it may prevent DNA synthesis or DNA-directed RNA and protein synthesis. RNA consists of long, single

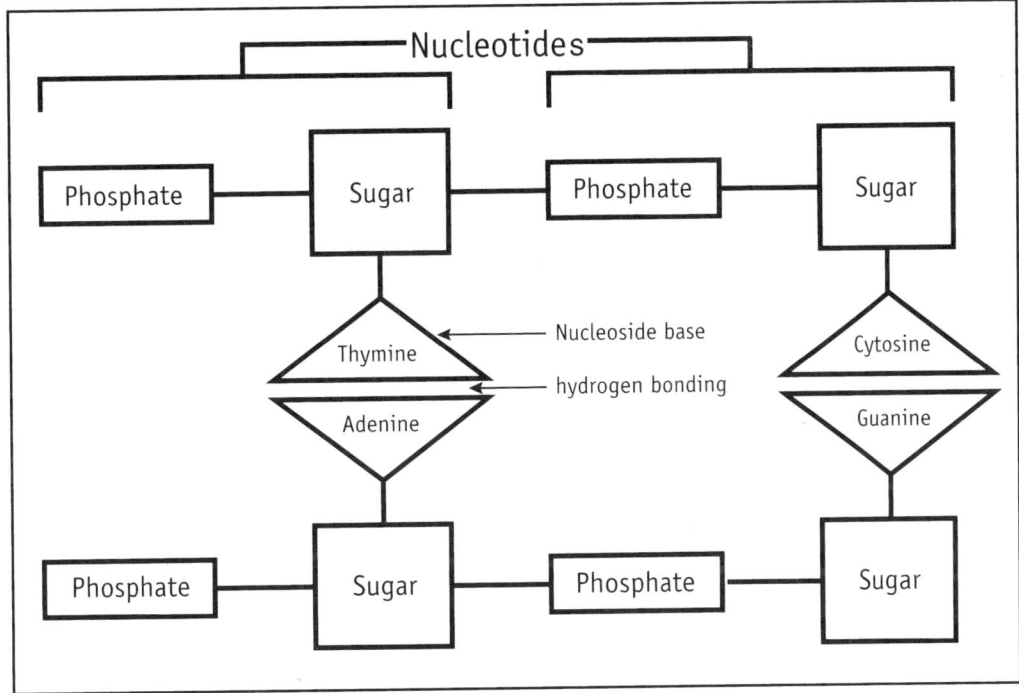

Figure 3-1. Organization of DNA. RNA is single stranded, with uracil replacing thymine.

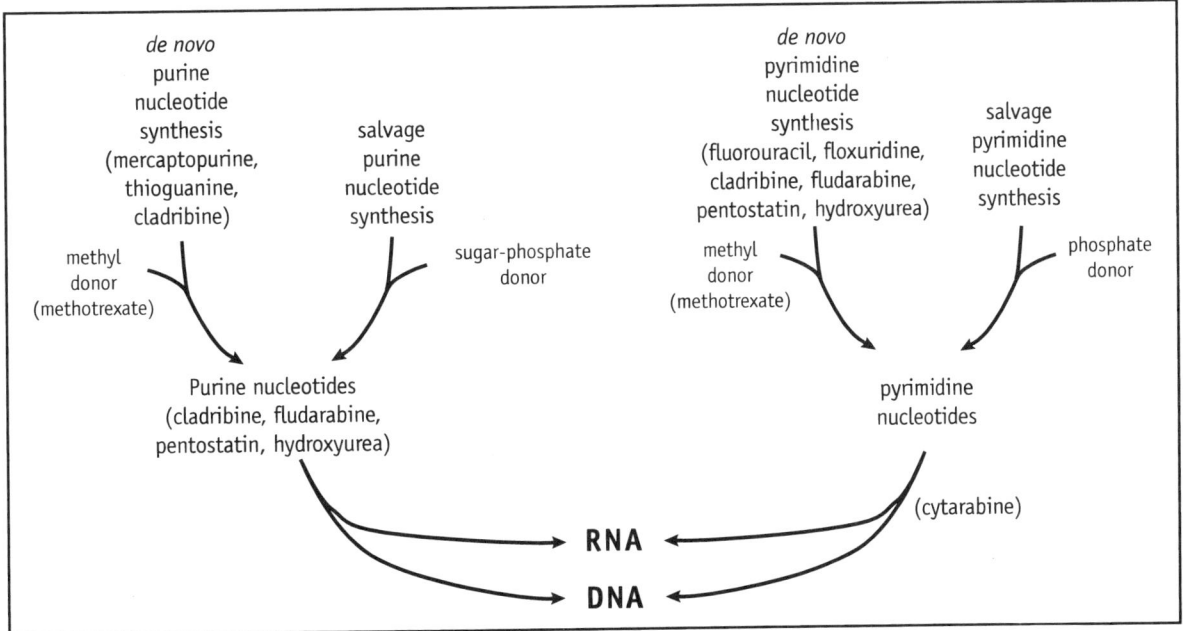

Figure 3-2. Simplified pathways of DNA and RNA synthesis
SOURCE: Adapted with permission from Pratt WB, Ruddon RW, Ensminger WD, et al., editors. *The Anticancer Drugs*. 2nd ed. New York: Oxford Univ Pr; 1994. Chapter 5, Antimetabolites. p. 70.

strands of ribonucleotides and serves as the messenger system through which DNA controls protein synthesis. Many different enzymes also are vital to the survival and function of the cell and are thus potential targets for anticancer drugs.

Topoisomerase Enzymes

Synthesis of DNA and messenger RNA requires the unwinding, separation, and orderly rejoining of complementary DNA strands. Topoisomerases are enzymes that facilitate this process, and their activity is essential for cell viability. Two classes of topoisomerases have been identified. Type I topoisomerase acts to relax the supercoiled, double-stranded DNA above and below the site that is unwinding, which allows the cleaving and resealing of a single strand of DNA during nucleic acid synthesis.[2] Although it is postulated that topoisomerase I functions primarily to allow transcription during RNA synthesis, the enzyme appears to be expressed during all phases of the cell cycle, implying that it may also serve other functions during cell replication.[3,4] The camptothecins are a new class of anticancer drugs that inhibit the type I topoisomerases.

Whereas topoisomerase I facilitates transient single-strand breaks (to allow for transcription) in DNA, topoisomerase II facilitates double-strand breaks by catalyzing the relaxation and swiveling of the supercoiled helix during DNA synthesis.[5] Relaxation and swiveling allow the creation of a double-strand break in the DNA helix, crossing over of a second DNA segment at the cleavage site, and resealing of the helix (Figure 3-3). Thus, topoisomerase II is necessary for replication of DNA, and its activity is maximal during the S phase of the cell cycle. It is postulated that topoisomerase II also contributes to the separation of the two daughter DNA molecules at the end of DNA synthesis, in preparation for mitosis, because increased levels are also found during the G_2 phase.[5] At least two classes of drugs (intercalators and epipodophyllotoxins) not only cause breaks in DNA, but also stabilize the cleavage in the DNA strands produced by type II topoisomerases and prevent resealing, thus leading to cell death.

Specificity of Cancer Chemotherapy

Unfortunately, existing cytotoxic drugs cannot distinguish between the DNA of a malignant cell and that of a normal cell; thus, these agents are capable of producing considerable toxicity to normal organs and tissues. Because cancer cells are more likely to be undergoing cellular division (i.e., the characteristic uncontrolled cellular growth), they may be more sensitive to the damaging effects of cytotoxic drugs. Not surprisingly, normal cells that are commonly undergoing cellular division—such as those of the bone marrow, the epithelial lining of the gastrointestinal tract, and the hair follicles—are also more likely to be damaged.

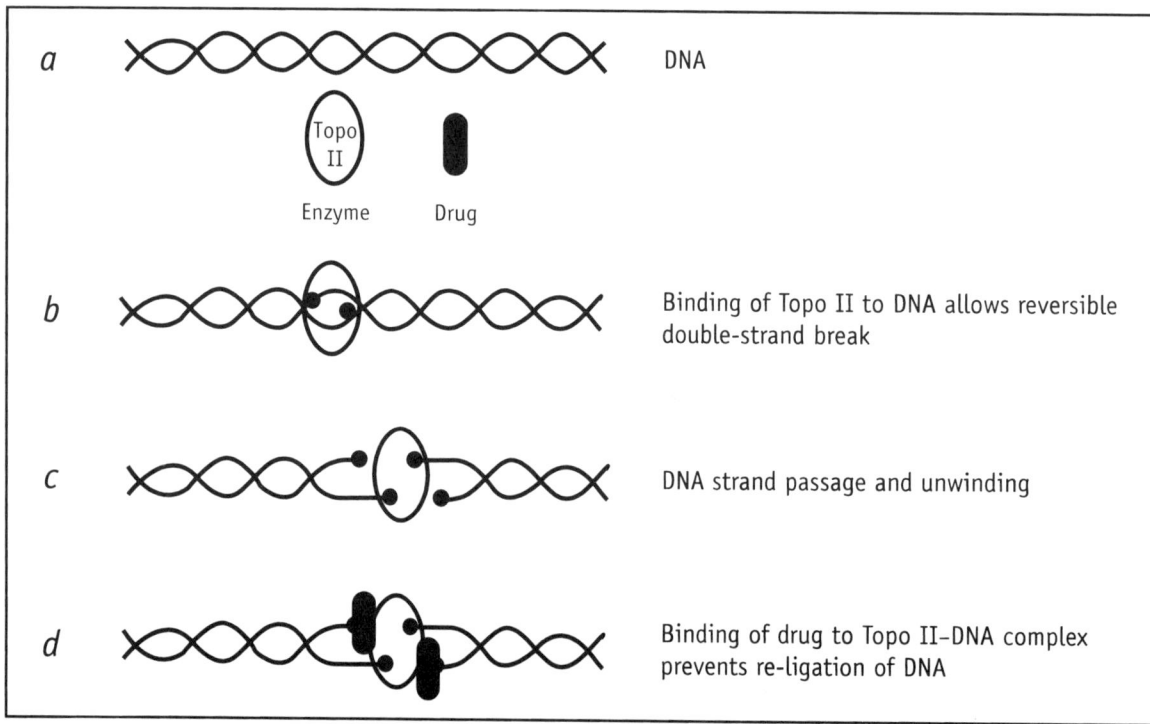

Figure 3-3. Interaction of topoisomerase II (Topo II) with DNA and the mechanism by which some drugs interact with the enzyme–DNA complex to cause double-strand breaks in DNA

SOURCE: reprinted with permission from Tannock IF, Hill RP, editors. *The Basic Science of Oncology.* 2nd ed. New York: Pergamon; 1992. p. 346.

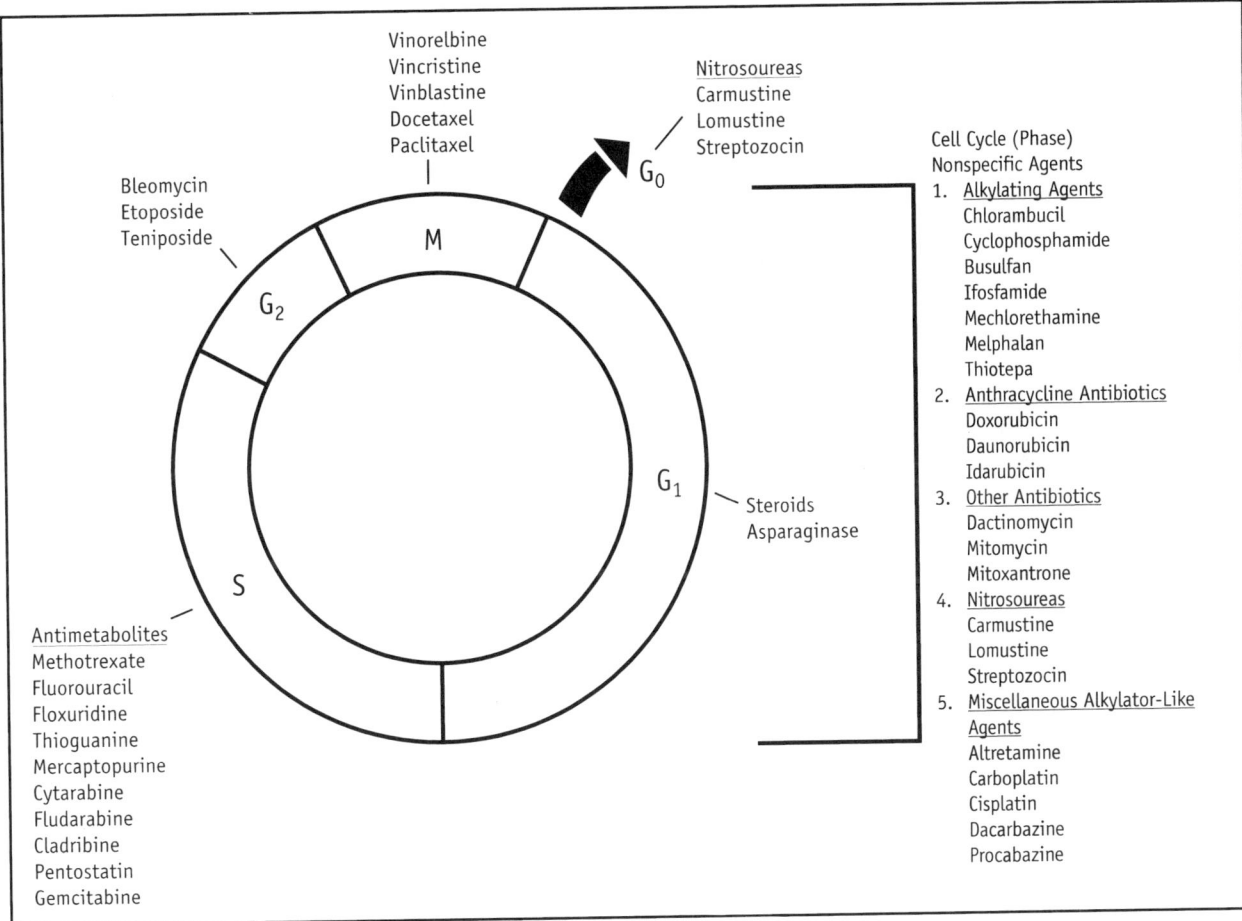

Figure 3-4. Cell cycle specificity of anticancer drugs
SOURCE: references 6 and 37.

In recent years, advances in molecular biology have further elucidated how these drugs work and, in some cases, how they do not work. This has led to greater emphasis on targeting chemotherapy to the unique biochemical or molecular characteristics of cancer cells. It is hoped that cytotoxic drugs in the very near future may be much more selective in their lethal actions and avoid much of the toxic impact on normal cells.

Cytotoxic drugs are commonly divided into groups based on their mode of action and on the phase of the cell cycle in which they are active. These classifications should not be considered absolute, because the precise mechanism or mechanisms of some agents are not known. As you read about the mechanisms of the various cytotoxic agents, you may wish to refer to Appendix I, The Mammalian Cell Cycle, and Figure 3-4, which indicates where each drug exerts its action during the cell cycle.

ALKYLATING AGENTS

The alkylating agents currently in clinical use in the United States (Table 3-1) are used to treat a wide spectrum of malignancies, including both solid tumors and hematological malignancies. Table 3-2 summarizes the toxicities common to this class of drugs, as well as toxicities unique to specific agents. Chapters 7, 8, and 9 provide more in-depth explanation of many of the major toxicities that complicate treatment with these drugs.

Classic Alkylating Agents

Alkylating agents undergo transformation to produce highly reactive, positively charged (i.e., electron-deficient) ions. These ions can then form covalent bonds with electron-rich sites on biological molecules, such as nucleic acids, proteins, and amino acids. The process of substitution of an alkyl group for a hydrogen atom in an organic compound is referred to as alkylation (Figure 3-5). Although there are sites suitable for alkylation on almost all biological molecules, the binding of drugs to DNA appears to be the predominant cause of cell death.[6]

There are three possible outcomes of alkylating reactions. First, the template (the DNA strand being replicated) may be misread or mispaired during DNA synthesis. Second, cross-linking may prevent the DNA strands from unwinding, which would hinder the replication process. Third, the alkylating agents may produce either single- or double-strand

Table 3-1. Alkylating Agents in Clinical Use in the United States

Generic Name	Trade Name	Other Synonyms
Classic Alkylators		
Busulfan	Myleran	
Chlorambucil	Leukeran	
Cyclophosphamide	Cytoxan	CTX
Ifosfamide	Ifex	Isophosphamide, IFX
Mechlorethamine	Mustargen	Nitrogen mustard, HN_2 Mustine
Melphalan	Alkeran	L-phenylalamine mustard, L-PAM
Thiotepa	Thioplex	Triethylene-thiophosphoramide
Nitrosoureas		
Carmustine	BiCNU	BCNU
Lomustine	CeeNu	CCNU
Streptozocin	Zanosar	Streptozotocin
Miscellaneous Alkylator-Like Agents		
Altretamine	Hexalen	Hexamethylmelamine
Carboplatin	Paraplatin	CBDCA, JM8
Cisplatin	Platinol	DDP, *cis*-diamminedichloroplatinum
Dacarbazine	DTIC-Dome	Dimethyl triazeno imidazole carboxamide
Procarbazine	Matulane	

breaks in the DNA. Any of these actions inhibits synthesis of DNA, RNA, or protein. Because of their propensity to alter DNA, all of these agents should be considered mutagenic. Several of the alkylating agents have also been shown to be carcinogenic in animal studies and in humans receiving therapeutic doses.

It is known that certain sites on DNA bases are more vulnerable to this reaction: the N7 position on guanine; the N1, N3, and N7 positions on adenine; and the N3 position on cytosine. It is not precisely known which sites are most important to produce misreading of the DNA template or breaking of a DNA strand. Alkylating agents have one (monofunctional) or two (bifunctional) reactive groups on each molecule, which may alkylate different nucleotide bases. Bifunctional alkylating agents (Figure 3-6) can bind with adjacent nucleotide bases, forming interstrand cross-links between the two strands of DNA. Cross-linking is believed to be responsible for much of the cellular toxicity of the alkylating agents.[6] In fact, the degree of interstrand cross-linking in tumor cells has been shown to have direct correlation to the cytotoxic response, both in vitro and in vivo.[7-9] Many of the alkylating agents in clinical use—such as mechlorethamine, cyclophosphamide, ifosfamide, melphalan, and chlorambucil—are bifunctional.

Table 3-2. Toxicities Associated with Alkylating Agents

Toxicities common to most alkylating agents:	
Nausea and vomiting	
Myelosuppression	
Alopecia	
Sterility/infertility	
Second malignancies (rare)	
Toxicities unique to specific alkylating agents:	
Hemorrhagic cystitis	cyclophosphamide, ifosfamide
Neurotoxicity	ifosfamide, cisplatin
SIADH	cyclophosphamide, ifosfamide
Nephrotoxicity	cisplatin

SIADH, syndrome of inappropriate secretion of antidiuretic hormone.

Resistance

Alkylating agents may bind to DNA during any phase of the cell cycle, but they exert their cytotoxic effects when the cell attempts to proceed through the cell cycle. Their greatest cytotoxic effect is on rapidly dividing cells, presumably because those cells have less time to repair damage before entering the vulnerable DNA synthesis phase. Cellular repair is a capacity common to all mammalian cells and is a mechanism that enables cells to resist the lethal effects of chemotherapy agents.[10] Conversely, it has been observed that cells deficient in enzymes required for DNA repair exhibit increased susceptibility to alkylating agents. Other mechanisms that result in clinically important resistance to alkylating drugs are increased drug inactivation due to reactions with cellular thiol compounds and decreased drug uptake by tumor cells. It is likely

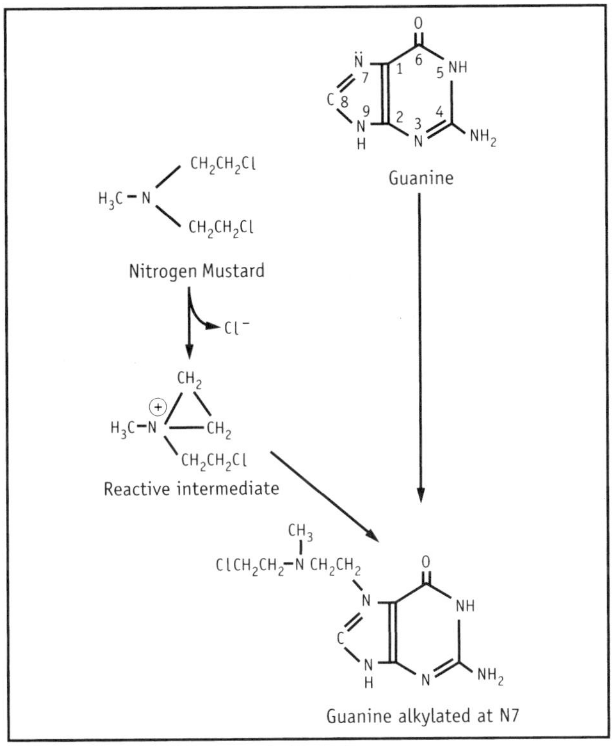

Figure 3-5. The process of alkylation

SOURCE: reprinted with permission from Erlichman C. The pharmacology of anticancer drugs. In: Tannock IF, Hill RP, editors. *The Basic Science of Oncology*. 2nd ed. New York: Pergamon; 1992. p. 322.

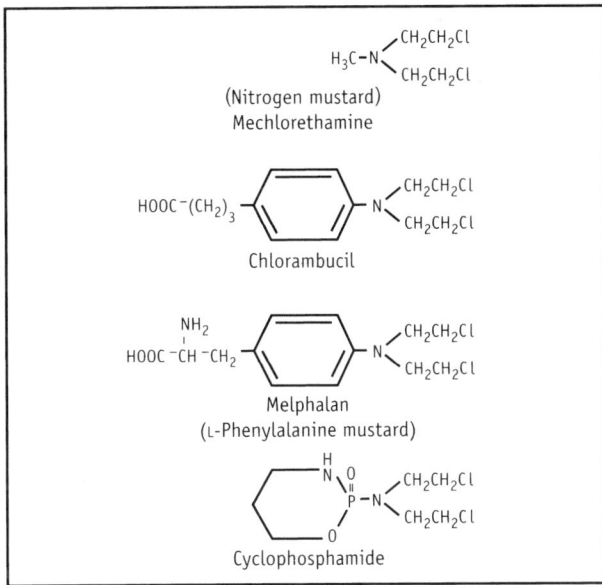

Figure 3-6. Structures of bifunctional alkylating agents

SOURCE: reprinted with permission from Erlichman C. The pharmacology of anticancer drugs. In: Tannock IF, Hill RP, editors. *The Basic Science of Oncology*. New York: Pergamon; 1987. p. 322.

that, in many cases, multiple mechanisms account for the overall resistance of a particular tumor cell line.

Mechlorethamine

Mechlorethamine (Mustargen), often called nitrogen mustard, was the first classic alkylating agent available for clinical use. Today it is used mostly for the treatment of Hodgkin's disease. Mechlorethamine's high degree of chemical instability has limited its clinical usefulness. It is recommended that mechlorethamine be used within 15 minutes of reconstitution. Furthermore, 90% of mechlorethamine is cleared from the plasma within 4 minutes of injection.[11] Mechlorethamine is also a potent vesicant if extravasated. Alterations in the drug's structure (e.g., addition of an aromatic ring) have improved its chemical stability, pharmacokinetics, and cytotoxicity and resulted in several additional clinically useful drugs, including cyclophosphamide, chlorambucil, ifosfamide, and melphalan.

Cyclophosphamide and Ifosfamide

Cyclophosphamide (Cytoxan) is now the most widely used alkylating agent. It is used to treat lymphomas and many solid tumors, including breast, ovarian, and lung cancers. Because of its immunosuppressive effects, cyclophosphamide has also been used to prevent transplantation rejection following organ, allogeneic bone marrow, or peripheral blood stem cell transplantation. Cyclophosphamide is also used in the treatment of nonmalignant, immune-mediated diseases, such as rheumatoid arthritis, Wegener's granulomatosis, idiopathic thrombocytopenic purpura, and glomerulonephritis.

The parent drug is not an active cytotoxic compound. Hepatic microsomal enzymes initially convert cyclophosphamide to 4-hydroxycyclophosphamide and aldophosphamide. After entering the cell, aldophosphamide is converted to acrolein and phosphoramide mustard. Phosphoramide mustard produces alkylation with DNA (Figure 3-5).[12] Acrolein is excreted in the urine and may cause hemorrhagic cystitis, a form of severe bladder toxicity. Hemorrhagic cystitis is a dose-related toxicity, and adequate hydration and frequent urinary voiding may prevent serious toxicity in patients receiving high doses. With very high doses (>2 g/m^2), 2-mercaptoethanesulfonate (mesna) may be given to prevent damage to the bladder. Cyclophosphamide is well absorbed after oral administration and is available in tablet and parenteral formulations.[12] The major site of clearance is the liver, but the metabolites and some of the parent compound are excreted by the kidneys. The renal clearance of the parent compound is quite low (<15%), and cyclophosphamide has been safely administered without excessive toxicity to patients with significant renal dysfunction.[13]

Ifosfamide (Ifex), a structural analogue of cyclophosphamide, has been approved for third-line therapy of germ cell testicular cancer. It is also commonly used in the treatment of lung cancer, lymphomas, and sarcomas. Like cyclophosphamide, ifosfamide is activated by hepatic microsomal enzymes and eventually converted to acrolein and ifosfamide mustard. Ifosfamide has less affinity for the activating microsomal enzymes, and an equivalent dose (in terms of alkylating activity and myelosuppression) is three to four times that of cyclophosphamide. As a result, more acrolein is produced, and the potential for severe bladder toxicity is much greater.[14]

To safely administer ifosfamide in therapeutic doses, it must be administered with a uroprotectant, such as mesna. Mesna contains a free sulfhydryl group that binds to the acrolein in urine in the bladder to form a nontoxic compound that is then excreted. Because mesna remains intravascular until it reaches the kidneys, it does not jeopardize the cytotoxic activity of ifosfamide. Mesna is very effective in preventing hemorrhagic cystitis but is not helpful in alleviating it once it has occurred. Therefore, prophylaxis is very important.

Ifosfamide also produces neurotoxicity characterized by a change in mental status, lethargy, and even coma. This neurotoxicity may be related to accumulation of chloroacetaldehyde in the bloodstream. Administration should be discontinued at the first evidence of neurological impairment, and this impairment is usually reversible.

Because cyclophosphamide and ifosfamide are both activated by the hepatic microsomal enzymes, it would be expected that they may be subject to drug interactions. In humans, cyclophosphamide can induce its own rate of metabolism, which may account for some of the variability in reported half-lives for the drug.[15-17] Although changes in half-lives have been reported when cyclophosphamide was preceded by drugs known to induce microsomal metabolism (e.g., phenobarbital or allopurinol), its toxic and therapeutic effects are not altered appreciably.[15,16,18]

Melphalan

Melphalan (Alkeran) is a bifunctional alkylating agent that has antitumor activity in lymphomas, breast and ovarian carcinomas, and multiple myeloma. Available formulations include an intravenous injection and an oral tablet that has demonstrated low and variable oral bioavailability.[19,20] Food decreases the tablet form's absorption, and melphalan's bioavailability may be further reduced by concomitant administration of cimetidine.[21] Bioavailability has also been shown to increase with successive courses of administration.[22] For this reason, oral doses should be titrated according to the degree of bone marrow suppression. Myelosuppression is enhanced in patients with renal dysfunction.[23]

Chlorambucil

Chlorambucil (Leukeran) is structurally similar to melphalan and is administered orally. It is used primarily as first-line treatment for chronic lymphocytic leukemia. Chlorambucil's pharmacokinetics are poorly understood, but it appears to undergo hepatic metabolism. Less than 1% of the administered dose is reported to be excreted in the urine as either the parent compound or the principal phenylacetic acid metabolite.[24] Oral chlorambucil appears to be absorbed more completely (80%) and rapidly than oral melphalan, and its peak plasma concentrations are reduced when taken with food.[25] Myelosuppression is the most common toxicity of chlorambucil, and pulmonary toxicity has been reported with long-term use.

Thiotepa

Thiotepa (Thioplex) is a polyfunctioning alkylating agent that, following metabolism, interacts with DNA much like the classic alkylating agents. The principal use of thiotepa is in the intravesical treatment of superficial bladder cancer. It is also used in combination chemotherapy regimens for treating breast cancer and in high-dose therapy with autologous or allogeneic bone marrow transplantation or peripheral blood stem cell rescue. After intravenous administration, about 24% of the parent compound and the major metabolite are recovered in the urine.

Busulfan

Busulfan (Myleran), an oral alkylating agent, is used primarily to lower WBC counts during the initial phase of chronic myelogenous leukemia. It has the advantage of reducing the granulocyte count while selectively sparing platelets to some degree. Following oral administration, busulfan is well absorbed and is eliminated by hepatic metabolism.[12,26] Less than 1% of the intact drug is excreted in the urine. The clearance of busulfan is greater for patients under age 18, who require higher doses per kilogram of body weight to achieve the same cytotoxic effect.[27] It is also used in very large doses (e.g., 16 mg/kg) to treat other leukemias when combined with stem cell rescue. To optimize high-dose therapy and minimize risk of severe nonmyelosuppressive toxicities, such as hepatic veno-occlusive disease and seizures, recommendations have been made for attaining specific area under the serum concentration versus time curves (AUCs).[28,29] Growchow and colleagues[28] reported that in patients receiving 4 mg/kg per day for 4 days (16 mg/kg total), the AUCs were significantly greater in patients developing hepatic veno-occlusive disease than in patients without hepatotoxicity.

Nitrosoureas

The nitrosoureas (carmustine [BiCNU], lomustine [CeeNU], and streptozocin [Zanosar]) also are believed to exert their lethal effects by alkylation with DNA. Carmustine is a bifunctional alkylating agent that forms DNA cross-links after activation. Although lomustine is monofunctional, it also can form interstrand cross-links in DNA.[6,30] Evidence suggests that the nitrosoureas may preferentially bind to different sites on the nucleoside bases than the classic alkylating agents.[31] Because carmustine and lomustine are lipid-soluble drugs that penetrate into the central nervous system, they are most often used to treat central nervous system malignancies. These drugs are also used to treat malignant lymphomas, melanomas, and some gastrointestinal tumors. High doses of carmustine are also used in preparative regimens for patients undergoing stem cell transplantation. Carmustine must be administered intravenously, but lomustine is rapidly and completely absorbed after oral administration. These agents disappear rapidly from the plasma because of hepatic microsomal activation. The active metabolites of carmustine have prolonged plasma and tissue levels, which may be due to enterohepatic recirculation or uptake and release from lipid storage sites.

Myelosuppression (primarily leukopenia) is the major dose-limiting toxicity of both carmustine and lomustine. It characteristically is delayed, occurring 3–5 weeks after administration. Both drugs also cause nausea and vomiting; premedication with antiemetics is recommended. Pulmonary toxicity has been reported with long-term carmustine use, and both renal and hepatic effects have been reported occasionally. Optic and other neurological complications have also been described.[32]

The Gliadel wafer is a biodegradable polymer wafer saturated with 7.7 mg of carmustine for use in patients undergoing surgical resection for recurrent glioblastoma multiforme. The wafers are inserted into the cavity created by the surgical resection, and the polymer erodes, releasing carmustine into the tumor bed. Approximately 70% of the carmustine is released in 3 weeks, and up to eight wafers may be placed in the cavity if size permits. The most frequent side effects are seizures, hemiplegia, and headache. However, all of the patients studied had undergone extensive surgery, and the effects could also be attributed to the surgery or underlying disease as well as the drug.

Miscellaneous Alkylator-Like Agents

In addition to the classic alkylating agents listed in Table 3-1, several cytotoxic agents are believed to exert their cytotoxic activity via alkylation.

Platinum Analogues

The platinum analogues cisplatin (Platinol) and carboplatin (Paraplatin) act by a mechanism similar to that of the alkylating agents. With cisplatin (Figure 3-7), both chloride ions undergo a slow displacement by water to generate a positively charged, aquated complex. In blood, the high chloride concentration keeps cisplatin in an unchanged form. The low-chloride environment inside cells accelerates the displacement process. The activated complex can then interact (at the two sites where the chloride ions were) with intracellular nucleophilic sites on DNA, RNA, or protein to form interstrand cross-links analogous to alkylating reactions. The reactions also may produce intrastrand links or adducts in addition to cross-links and changes in the conformation of DNA. Any of these reactions may result in inhibition of DNA synthesis. In vitro, the degree of cytotoxicity correlates well with the total platinum binding to DNA, with interstrand cross-links, and with the formation of intrastrand adducts.[33-35] Clinical responses also have been correlated with adduct formation in both tumor cells and the peripheral blood leukocytes of patients receiving cisplatin.[36] This suggests that substances found in leukocytes and tumor cells are capable of preventing DNA binding or repairing intrastrand adduct formation in resistant cells. Several other mechanisms of resistance to the platinum analogues have also been described. In addition, resistant cells may have a decreased ability to form interstrand cross-links, more rapid and efficient DNA repair, reduced intracellular concentrations of the drug, or quenching (binding) of active, unbound drug molecules by glutathione or sulfhydrl-containing proteins.[37-40]

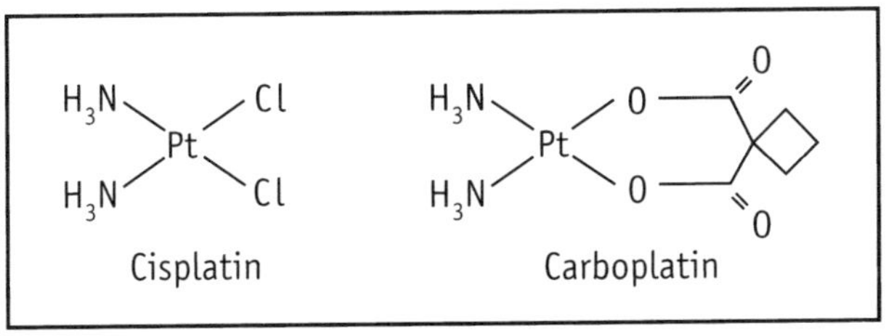

Cisplatin

Cisplatin is widely used in the treatment of testicular, ovarian, lung, and head and neck cancers. Cisplatin solutions must be admixed in a chloride-containing solution, such as saline. In solutions without chloride ions, the drug is converted to a biologically inactive form.[41] After administration, cisplatin is rapidly and tightly bound to plasma proteins. More than 90% of the free (unbound) cisplatin is lost during the first 2 hours. Platinum bound to plasma proteins disappears more slowly, having a half-life of 1–3 days. Cisplatin is excreted primarily by the kidneys, both by glomerular filtration and tubular secretion.[42] Dose-related renal toxicity has been the major dose-limiting toxicity caused by cisplatin. It manifests as reversible renal tubular damage. Administration with aggressive hydration (sometimes accompanied by osmotic diuresis) is used to maintain adequate renal blood flow and decrease the risk of nephrotoxicity. Other toxicities of cisplatin include severe nausea and vomiting, ototoxicity, peripheral neuropathy, and hypomagnesemia. Myelosuppression is pronounced only at higher dosages. Anemia is more common and more severe following cisplatin therapy than with most other chemotherapy drugs. Anemia occurs as a result of direct suppression of erythrocyte precursors in the bone marrow and secondary to damage to the kidneys, a source of erythropoietin.

Carboplatin

Carboplatin (Figure 3-7), an analogue of cisplatin, has a carboxycyclobutane moiety that replaces the chloride ions on the parent compound. The antitumor activity of carboplatin appears equivalent to cisplatin in ovarian carcinoma, and the drug is also widely used in the treatment of lung and head and neck tumors. The mechanism of action is similar to that of cisplatin, except that cross-links are formed later. Carboplatin is cleared renally. An important distinction is that cisplatin is filtered by the glomeruli and concentrated by the tubules and appears to be incompletely cleared. Carboplatin is not concentrated by the tubules and is cleared more

Figure 3-7. Structures of cisplatin and carboplatin

efficiently, with twice as much carboplatin (60–70%) recovered in the urine in the first 24 hours.[34,43,44] These differences are believed to account for carboplatin's apparent lack of renal toxicity.[45]

Carboplatin causes much more myelosuppression, predominantly thrombocytopenia, than cisplatin. Several investigators have shown that the amount of exposure to carboplatin (the AUC) correlates with renal function and can be used to predict the severity of myelosuppression. This led to the publication of several dosage adjustment guidelines.[46,47] In the Calvert formula, dose adjustment is based on the creatinine clearance or glomerular filtration rate (GFR) and a desired AUC. For carboplatin monotherapy, the suggested target AUCs are 4–6 mg/ml per minute for previously treated patients (who may be more sensitive to the myelosuppressive effects) and 6–8 mg/ml per minute for previously untreated patients. For patients receiving concomitant therapy with other myelosuppressive cytotoxics or radiation therapy, the lower end of the target AUC range may be recommended. The formula for dose calculation is:

$$\text{dose (in mg)} = \text{target AUC (in mg/ml per min)} \times [\text{GFR (in ml/min)} + 25]$$

Although Calvert and colleagues used actual ethylenediaminetetraacetic acid (EDTA) clearance to measure GFR, measured or estimated creatinine clearance may be used in the equation.

Procarbazine

Procarbazine (Matulane), a synthetic derivative of hydrazine, is used to treat Hodgkin's disease, other lymphomas, and, occasionally, brain tumors. Following oral administration, procarbazine is rapidly and completely absorbed. It does penetrate into the central nervous system.[48] Procarbazine undergoes extensive metabolism and activation by the cytochrome P-450 system in the liver. The end product is probably an alkylating agent.

Procarbazine inhibits monoamine oxidase and thus has a propensity to amplify the effects of sympathomimetic drugs, tricyclic antidepressants, and tyramine (contained in many food products). It may also produce a disulfiram-like reaction when ingested with alcohol.

Dacarbazine

Dacarbazine (DTIC-Dome) was originally synthesized as an antimetabolite. Researchers then discovered that it is metabolized (probably hepatically) to a compound with alkylating properties. Dacarbazine is used to treat melanomas, Hodgkin's disease, and some sarcomas. Following intravenous administration, up to 50% of a dose is excreted, either as the parent drug or as the (inactive) *N*-demethylated metabolite, in the urine. A prolonged half-life has been observed in patients with renal and hepatic dysfunction.[49]

Altretamine

Although the exact mechanism of action of altretamine (Hexalen) is unknown, it is generally included in this group because of its structural similarity to triethylenemelamine, an alkylating compound. Altretamine is known to undergo metabolic activation by microsomal enzymes to a compound capable of binding to DNA.[50] Its clinical use, at this time, is largely limited to the treatment of refractory ovarian cancer. Altretamine is only available in 50-mg oral capsules, and oral bioavailability appears to be variable. Approximately 60% of the oral dose is excreted as metabolites in the urine during the first 24 hours.[51,52] Gastrointestinal intolerance, including nausea, vomiting, cramping, and diarrhea, is the most common dose-limiting toxicity. Occasionally, neurotoxicity (manifested by peripheral neuropathies, confusion, and agitation) has been observed.

ANTITUMOR ANTIBIOTICS AND ANTHRACENEDIONES

The antitumor antibiotics (Table 3-3) are each fermentation products of some *Streptomyces* species. Most agents in this class appear to act by several different mechanisms, including:

- binding to DNA by either alkylation or a process called intercalation, which is the insertion of the drug molecule between the two strands of DNA;
- interaction with topoisomerase II;
- generation of free radicals, which damage cell membranes; or
- interaction with the signal transduction pathways that are responsible for communication between the cell surface and the nucleus.

The anthracenedione mitoxantrone, a synthetic product designed to structurally resemble the anthracyclines,

Table 3-3. Antitumor Antibiotics in Clinical Use in the United States

Generic Name	Trade Name	Other Synonyms
Anthracyclines		
Daunorubicin	Cerubidine	Rubidomycin, Daunomycin
Doxorubicin	Adriamycin	Hydroxydaunorubicin
Idarubicin	Idamycin	
Other		
Bleomycin	Blenoxane	
Dactinomycin	Cosmegen	Actinomycin D
Mitomycin	Mutamycin	Mitomycin C
Mitoxantrone	Novantrone	Dihydro-anthracenedione (DHAD)

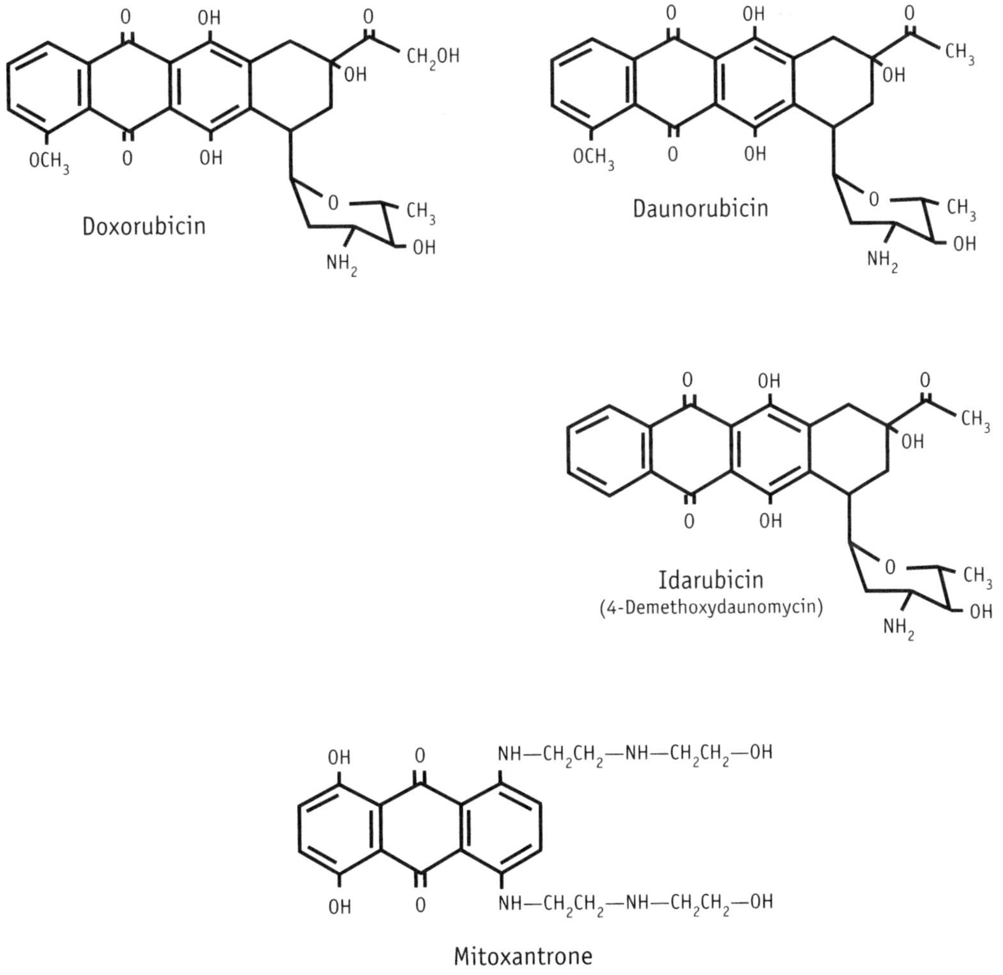

Figure 3-8. Structures of anthracycline drugs and the related anthracenedione compound mitoxantrone

SOURCE: reprinted with permission from Doroshow JH. Anthracyclines and anthracenediones. In: Chabner BA, Longo DL, editors. *Cancer Chemotherapy and Biotherapy.* 2nd ed. Philadelphia, PA: Lippincott-Raven; 1996. p. 411, 428.

is frequently grouped with the anthracyclines for purposes of discussion.

Anthracyclines

The anthracyclines doxorubicin (Adriamycin RDF, Rubex) and daunorubicin (Cerubidine) are identical except for the presence of a hydroxyl group at the C14 position on doxorubicin (Figure 3-8). In acronyms for some combination therapies, doxorubicin is sometimes referred to by an *H*, for hydroxydaunorubicin. The third anthracycline, idarubicin (Idamycin), differs from daunorubicin by lacking a methoxy group at the C4 position.

Several distinct mechanisms of action have been demonstrated for the anthracyclines, and there is much controversy regarding which is the predominant cytotoxic effect. Historically, it was first demonstrated that anthracyclines act as intercalators by sliding their planar ring structure perpendicularly between the nucleotide pairs of the DNA helix. The B and C rings appeared to be buried within the helix, with the A and D rings projecting out on either side. This process results in distortion of the shape and a partial uncoiling of the helix due to separation of the DNA bases by the drug molecule. Both single- and double-strand breaks may also occur.

Although there is no question that a portion of the anthracycline dose intercalates within cellular DNA, it now appears that concentrations of intercalated drug are not sufficient to produce the predominant cytotoxic effect.[53] Perhaps more important is the discovery that the anthracyclines also complex with nuclear enzymes called helicases that act to dissociate duplex DNA into single strands. This complex hinders the strand separation process and limits cellular replication.[54,55]

The anthracyclines also form a complex with topoisomerase II, interfering with the DNA strand breakage-reunion reaction mediated by that enzyme.[56] The result is a blockade of DNA, RNA, or protein synthesis, or all three. The anthracyclines' amino sugar appears to add stability to the DNA binding through its interaction with the sugar-phosphate backbone of the DNA.

The anthracyclines may also form a drug-iron-DNA complex that catalyzes the transfer of electrons from glutathione to oxygen, generating superoxide radicals. These radicals may produce damage to cellular constituents, predominantly DNA single-strand breaks, and alter cell membrane functions.[57] Evidence suggests that the free radical generation may contribute to, but is not predominantly accountable for, the antitumor effects.[58] There is also evidence that this process contributes to the cardiac toxicity produced by the anthracyclines. These agents may also produce lethal damage by binding to the cell membrane.[59]

It is now appreciated that the overall effects of the anthracyclines on the cell membrane may relate to DNA damage and subsequent cytotoxicity. Communication between the cell membrane and the nucleus, crucial to cellular growth and viability, is facilitated by various signal-transduction pathways. Via interaction with the cell membrane, anthracyclines appear to activate the protein kinase C pathway, one of the most crucial signal-transduction pathways. Protein kinase C can phosphorylate topoisomerase II and thus regulate anthracycline-mediated DNA damage.[53,60] It is likely therefore that a combination of the cell-damaging effects of the anthracyclines are ultimately responsible for their cytotoxicity.

Daunorubicin and idarubicin are among the most effective agents available for managing acute leukemia, and doxorubicin is used extensively in treating leukemias, lymphomas, and many solid tumors, including breast, lung, and ovarian carcinomas, as well as sarcomas. All three anthracyclines are administered intravenously, and if the drug extravasates, severe tissue damage may result (see chapter 10). After administration, the drugs are converted by the liver to several metabolites, some of which retain cytotoxic activity. All of these drugs have a long (15- to 50-hour) β elimination phase, which is probably due to the slow release from tissue depots, where they are largely intercalated in the DNA. The extensive tissue binding accounts for the large apparent volume of distribution (about 25 L/kg for doxorubicin). The parent drugs and the metabolites are excreted in the bile, thus necessitating dose reductions in patients with biliary obstruction.

Dose-related myelosuppression, nausea, and vomiting are characteristic toxicities of the anthracyclines (Table 3-4). A unique cumulative dose-dependent cardiotoxicity is also well described. As mentioned above, it is believed that the generation of oxygen free radicals is responsible for the toxic effects to the myocardium. Recently, dexrazoxane (Zinecard), a strong iron chelator, has been approved in the United States for prevention of doxorubicin-induced cardiotoxicity. Dexrazoxane, administered before doxorubicin, removes the iron from the drug complex and reduces the generation of oxygen free radicals.[61] Anthracycline cardiac toxicity is discussed in more detail in chapter 8.

Table 3-4. Toxicities Associated with Antitumor Antibiotics

Toxicities common to most antitumor antibiotics:	
Myelosuppression (except bleomycin)	
Mucositis	
Nausea and vomiting (except bleomycin)	
Alopecia	
Vesicant (except bleomycin and mitoxantrone)	

Toxicities unique to specific antitumor antibiotics:	
Pulmonary toxicity	bleomycin, mitomycin
Skin changes	bleomycin
Radiation recall	doxorubicin, daunorubicin
Fever	bleomycin
Cardiac toxicity	daunorubicin, doxorubicin, idarubicin
Hemolytic uremic syndrome	mitomycin

Resistance

Although the anthracyclines, especially doxorubicin, are among the most clinically useful antineoplastic drugs, resistance to anthracycline cytotoxic activity is well documented and clinical progression of many common tumors is often attributed to the development of resistance. The most frequent mechanism of anthracycline resistance in tumor cells in vitro is increased drug efflux due to amplification of the gene for P-glycoprotein, a multidrug cell membrane transporter. Cells developing anthracycline resistance through this mechanism are also usually resistant to other antineoplastics derived from natural products (see chapter 6). Other mechanisms of anthracycline resistance include decreased topoisomerase II activity[62-64] and increased capacity to detoxify reactive oxygen.[65]

Liposomal Products

Both doxorubicin (Doxil) and daunorubicin (DaunoXome) are also available in liposomal products for the treatment of AIDS-related Kaposi's sarcoma. These formulations prolong the plasma circulation time of the drug and result in increased tumor concentrations. Both products have demonstrated responses in patients whose cancers had previously progressed while receiving combination chemotherapy and in patients unable to tolerate other regimens. Neither liposomal anthracycline product has been studied extensively in patients with hepatic dysfunction; therefore, both manufacturers recommend that the same dosage adjustment guidelines be used as for the conventional formulations.

Doxil liposomes are formulated with surface-bound methoxypolyethylene glycol to protect the liposomes from detection by mononuclear phagocytes. This patented Stealth technology has demonstrated prolonged circulation of doxorubicin. Whereas the elimination half-life of conventional doxorubicin is 30.1 hours, the half-life for Doxil is 52–55 hours. The AUC was increased over 100-fold. In addition to the typical side effects associated with liposomal therapy (flushing, shortness of breath, facial swelling, headache, chills, back pain, chest tightness and hypotension), Doxil infusions have also been associated with severe erythema and skin sloughing of the palms of the hands and soles of the feet.

DaunoXome liposomes are composed of a single bilayer membrane of phospholipids and cholesterol. It has a longer apparent half-life than conventional daunorubicin, and DaunoXome's AUC is approximately 36-fold greater than the conventional formulation. Toxicities associated with DaunoXome include those associated with conventional daunorubicin as well as infusion reactions similar to those described for Doxil.

Mitoxantrone

Mitoxantrone (Novantrone), an anthracenedione, is a synthetic compound consisting of a three-ring structure with two side chains (Figure 3-8). Like the anthracyclines, mitoxantrone intercalates DNA and ultimately interferes with topoisomerase II function, thereby preventing strand recoiling. Mitoxantrone lacks the ability to produce free radicals and therefore has far less inherent cardiotoxicity than doxorubicin. Cardiac toxicity is rare, except in patients who have received prior anthracycline therapy. Although cumulative doses of 120–160 mg/m^2 were initially reported to be the threshold for clinically significant cardiac toxicity, most clinicians now believe that there are no obvious dose limitations.[53]

Mitoxantrone is approved for use in treating acute myelogenous leukemia and is also used to treat other leukemias, lymphomas, and breast cancer. The drug is highly bound to plasma proteins, reflected by its large volume of distribution. Mitoxantrone is metabolized by the liver, and significant amounts of the parent compound and its metabolites are excreted in the feces, indicating a biliary route of elimination. The rate of elimination may be decreased in patients with severely impaired liver function. Although specific dosage guidelines are not available, some clinicians have recommended the same percentage dose reduction recommended for doxorubicin.[66] Chlebowski et al.[67] have suggested a full dose (14 mg/m^2) for patients with a modest increase in serum bilirubin (<3.5 mg/dl) and 8 mg/m^2 for patients with severe cholestasis (bilirubin ≥3.5 mg/dl). Urinary excretion is low.[68]

Bleomycin

Bleomycin (Blenoxane), which is derived from fungal cultures, has a very complex structure (Figure 3-9). A portion of the bleomycin molecule (the S peptide) intercalates four or five base pairs of DNA, producing single- and double-strand breaks in DNA and unwinding of the helix.[69,70] The result is inhibi-

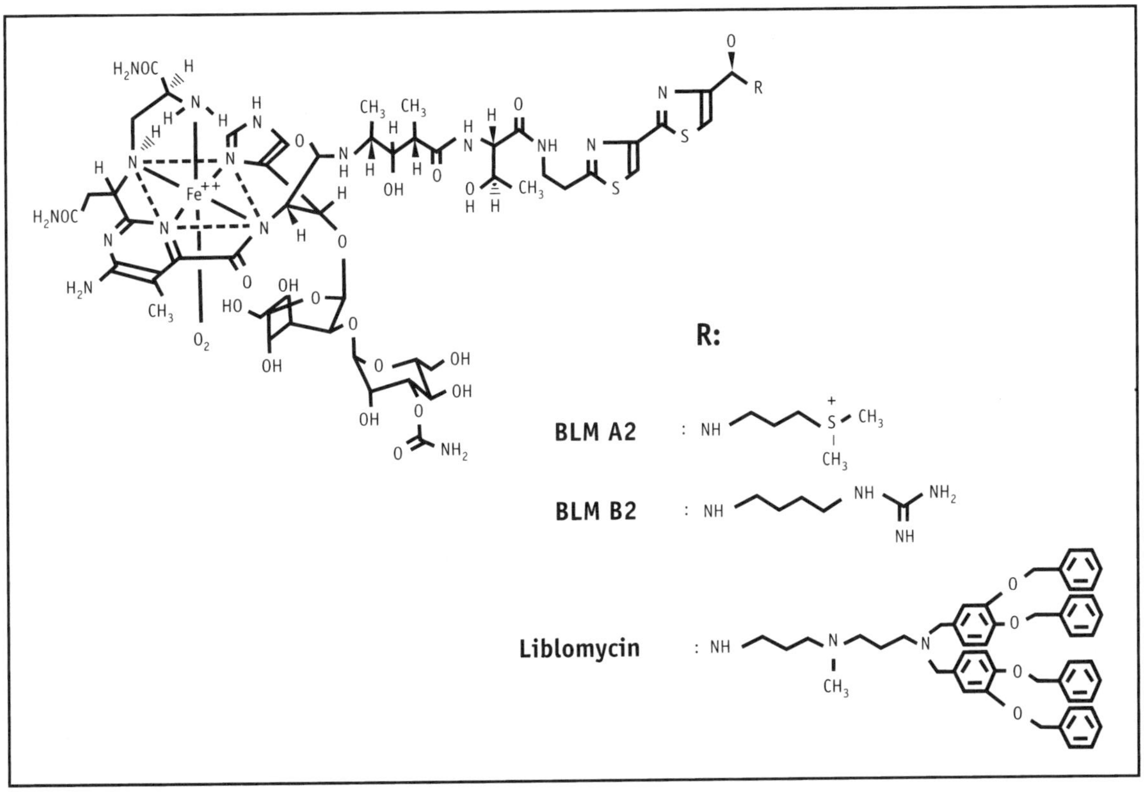

Figure 3-9. Structure of bleomycin

SOURCE: reprinted with permission from Lazo JS, Chabner BA. Bleomycin. In: Chabner BA, Longo DL, editors. *Cancer Chemotherapy and Biotherapy.* 2nd ed. Philadelphia, PA: Lippincott-Raven; 1996. p. 380.

tion of DNA synthesis. Bleomycin forms an activated complex with iron, oxygen, and DNA, which generates free radicals that may increase damage to DNA. This drug acts primarily in the G_2 phase of the cell cycle, but it also may damage cells in other phases.

Bleomycin is used to treat testicular cancer, lymphomas, and head and neck tumors. It may be given by intravenous, intramuscular, or subcutaneous injection and is also used locally to sclerose the pleural space in patients with malignant pleural effusions. Bleomycin is primarily (45–70%) excreted unchanged in the urine, and doses should be reduced in patients with severely impaired renal function.[71] Increased serum half-life due to decreased glomerular filtration (<35 ml/min) has been associated with an increased risk of pulmonary toxicity.[72,73] A bleomycin-inactivating enzyme has been found in most tissues except the lungs and the skin.[74] This enzyme dramatically reduces the formation of the activated ternary iron-oxygen-bleomycin complex, with a resulting decrease in free radical generation.[75] The deaminated bleomycin metabolite that is formed has less antitumor activity and much less pulmonary toxicity than the parent drug.[76,77]

Unlike most antineoplastics, bleomycin rarely causes myelosuppression, nausea, or vomiting. The most severe toxicity of bleomycin is a cumulative dose-dependent pulmonary toxicity that may be fatal (see chapter 8). Besides renal dysfunction, prior chest irradiation and exposure to prolonged high concentrations of oxygen appear to increase the risk of pulmonary toxicity. Dose-related mucositis is also common. This drug also frequently causes a fever within a few hours of injection and a spectrum of cutaneous effects.

Dactinomycin

Dactinomycin (Cosmegen), also called actinomycin D, is believed to intercalate base pairs of DNA. When dactinomycin binds to DNA, it permits initiation of the messenger RNA chain but blocks chain elongation by inhibiting DNA-directed RNA synthesis. Dactinomycin is used to treat several pediatric tumors (Wilms' tumor, Ewing's sarcoma, and embryonal rhabdomyosarcoma). It is given intravenously and is excreted mainly as the parent drug in urine.[78] Extravasation during administration can result in severe tissue damage. Other common toxicities include dose-related myelosuppression, mucositis, nausea, and vomiting.

Mitomycin

The mitomycin (Mutamycin) molecule can form DNA crosslinks and contains several groups that exert cytotoxic activity. A quinone group participates in free radical reactions similar to those of the anthracyclines, and the azididine ring and carbamate groups function as alkylators, following metabolism in all tissues.[79,80] Because of the ubiquitous metabolism, clearance of mitomycin is rapid. Mitomycin is given by intravenous injection and, like the anthracyclines, may cause severe tissue damage if extravasated. It also may be administered by direct instillation in the bladder for treating superficial bladder tumors. Mitomycin causes dose-related myelosuppression, stomatitis, diarrhea, nausea, and vomiting. In addition, pneumonitis, cardiotoxicity, or nephrotoxicity occur rarely in some patients.

REFERENCES

1. Pratt WB, Ruddon RW, Ensminger WD, et al., editors. *The Anticancer Drugs.* 2nd ed. New York: Oxford Univ Pr; 1994. Chapter 5, Antimetabolites. p. 69–107.
2. Wang JC. DNA topoisomerases: why so many? *J Biol Chem* 1991;266:6659–92.
3. Zhang H, Wang J, Liu L. Involvement of DNA topoisomerase in transcription of human ribosomal RNA genes. *Proc Natl Acad Sci USA* 1988;85:1060–4.
4. Takimoto CH, Arbuck SG. The camptothecins. In: Chabner BA, Longo DL. *Cancer Chemotherapy and Biotherapy.* 2nd ed. Philadelphia, PA: Lippincott-Raven; 1996. p. 463–84.
5. Pommier Y, Fesen MR, Goldwasser F. Topoisomerase II inhibitors: the epipodophyllotoxins, m-AMSA, and the ellipticine derivatives. In: Chabner BA, Longo DL. *Cancer Chemotherapy and Biotherapy.* 2nd ed. Philadelphia, PA: Lippincott-Raven; 1996. p. 435–62.
6. Erlichman C. The pharmacology of anticancer drugs. In: Tannock IF, Hill RP, editors. *The Basic Science of Oncology.* New York: Pergamon; 1987. p. 292–307.
7. Erickson LC, Bradley MO, Ducore JM. DNA crosslinking and cytotoxicity in normal and transformed human cells treated with antitumor nitrosoureas [abstract]. *Proc Natl Acad Sci USA* 1980;77:467.
8. Garcia ST, McQuillan A, Panasci L. Correlation between the cytotoxicity of melphalan and DNA crosslinks as detected by the ethidium bromide fluorescence assay in the F_1 variant of B_{16} melanoma cells. *Biochem Pharmacol* 1988;37:3189–92.
9. Thomas CB, Osieka R, Kohn KW. DNA cross-linking by *in vivo* treatment with 1-(2-chloroethyl)-3-(4-methylcyclohexyl)-1-nitrosourea of sensitive and resistant human colon carcinoma xenografts in nude mice. *Cancer Res* 1978;38:2448–54.
10. Ewig RAG, Kohn KW. DNA damage and repair in mouse leukemia L1210 cells: treatment with nitrogen mustard, 1,3-bis(2-chloroethyl)-nitrosourea, and other nitrosoureas. *Cancer Res* 1977;37:2114–22.
11. Oliverio VT, Zubrod CG. Clinical pharmacology of the effective antitumor drugs. *Ann Rev Pharmacol* 1965;5:335–52.
12. Tew KD, Colvin M, Chabner BA. Alkylating agents. In: Chabner BA, Longo DL, editors. *Cancer Chemotherapy and Biotherapy.* 2nd ed. Philadelphia, PA: Lippincott-Raven; 1996. p. 297–332.
13. Grochow LB, Colvin M. Clinical pharmacokinetics of cyclophosphamide. *Clin Pharmacokinet* 1983;4:380–94.
14. Sarosy G. Ifosfamide—pharmacologic overview. *Semin Oncol* 1989;16(*Suppl* 3):2–8.
15. Bagley CM Jr, Bostick FW, DeVita VT. Clinical pharmacology of cyclophosphamide. *Cancer Res* 1973;33:226–33.
16. Sladek NE, Doeden D, Powers JF, et al. Plasma concentrations of 4-hydroxycyclophosphamide and phosphoramide mustard in patients repeatedly given high doses of cyclophosphamide in preparation for bone marrow transplantation. *Cancer Treat Rep* 1984;68:1247–54.

17. Moore MJ, Hardy RW, Thiessen JJ, et al. Rapid development of enhanced clearance after high-dose cyclophosphamide. *Clin Pharmacol Ther* 1988;44:622–8.
18. Sladek NE. Therapeutic efficacy of cyclophosphamide as a function of its metabolism. *Cancer Res* 1972;32:535–42.
19. Tattersall MN, Jarman M, Newlands ES, et al. Pharmacokinetics of melphalan following oral or intravenous administration in patients with malignant disease. *Eur J Cancer* 1978;14:507–14.
20. Alberts DS, Chang SY, Chen H-SG, et al. Comparative pharmacokinetics of chlorambucil and melphalan in man. *Recent Results Cancer Res* 1980;74:124.
21. Sviland L, Robinson A, Proctor SJ, et al. Interaction of cimetidine with oral melphalan: a pharmacokinetics study. *Cancer Chemother Pharmacol* 1987;20:173–5.
22. Loos U, Musch E, Engel M, et al. The pharmacokinetics of melphalan during intermittent therapy of multiple myeloma. *Eur J Clin Pharmacol* 1985;35:187–93.
23. Cornwell GG III, Pajak TF, McIntyre OR, et al. Influence of renal failure on myelosuppressive effects of melphalan: Cancer and Leukemia Group B experience. *Cancer Treat Rep* 1982;66:475–81.
24. McClean A. Pharmacokinetics and metabolism of chlorambucil in patients with malignant diseases. *Cancer Treat Rev* 1978;6(Suppl):33–42.
25. Adair CG, Bridges JM, Desai ZR. Can food affect the bioavailability of chlorambucil in patients with haematological malignancies? *Cancer Chemother Pharmacol* 1986;17:99–102.
26. Ehrsson H, Hassan M, Ehrnebo M. Busulfan kinetics. *Clin Pharmacol Ther* 1983;34:86–9.
27. Vassal G, Fischer A, Chaline D, et al. Busulfan disposition below the age of three: alterations in children with lysosomal storage disease. *Blood* 1993;82:1030–6.
28. Grochow LB, Jones RJ, Brundrett RB, et al. Pharmacokinetics of busulfan: correlation with veno-occlusive disease in cancer patients undergoing bone marrow transplantation. *Cancer Chemother Pharmacol* 1989;25:55–61.
29. Vassal G, Deroussent A, Hartman O, et al. Dose-dependent neurotoxicity of high-dose busulfan in children: a clinical and pharmacological study. *Cancer Res* 1990;50:6203–7.
30. Kohn KW. Interstrand cross-linking of DNA by 1,3-bis(2-chloroethyl)-1-nitrosourea and other 1-(ω-haloethyl)-1-nitrosoureas. *Cancer Res* 1977;37:1450–3.
31. Briscoe WT, Anderson SP, May HE. Base sequence specificity of three 2-chloroethylnitrosoureas. *Biochem Pharmacol* 1990;40:1201–6.
32. Dorr RT, Von Hoff DD, editors. *Cancer Chemotherapy Handbook*. 2nd ed. Norwalk, CT: Appleton & Lange; 1994. p. 267–75, 644–9.
33. Roberts JJ, Knox RJ, Pera MF, et al. The role of platinum-DNA interactions in the cellular toxicity and anti-tumor effects of platinum coordination compounds. In: Nicolini M, editor. *Platinum and Other Metal Coordination Compounds in Cancer Chemotherapy*. Boston, MA: Marinus Nijhoff; 1988. p. 16.
34. Zwelling LA, Michaels S, Schwartz H, et al. DNA cross-linking as an indicator of sensitivity and resistance of mouse L1210 leukemia cells to *cis*-diamminedichloroplatinum(II) and L-phenylalanine mustard. *Cancer Res* 1981;41:640–7.
35. Reed E, Behrens BS, Yuspa SH, et al. Differences in cisplatin-DNA adduct formation in sensitive and resistant cell lines of human ovarian cancer cells [abstract]. *Proc Am Assoc Cancer Res* 1986;27:285.
36. Reed E, Parker RJ, Gill IK, et al. Platinum-DNA adduct in leukocyte DNA of a cohort of 49 patients with 24 different types of malignancies. *Cancer Res* 1993;53:3694–9.
37. Fox M. Drug resistance and DNA repair. In: Fox BW, Fox M, editors. *Antitumor Drug Resistance*. Berlin: Springer-Verlag; 1984. p. 335–69.
38. Tashiro T, Sato Y. Characterization of acquired resistance to *cis*-diamminedichloroplatinum(II) in mouse leukemia cell lines. *Jpn J Cancer Res* 1992;83:219–25.
39. Godwin AK, Meister A, O'Dwyer PJ, et al. High resistance to cisplatin in human ovarian cancer cell lines is associated with marked increased of glutathione synthesis. *Proc Natl Acad Sci USA* 1992;89:3070.
40. Hrubisko M, McGown AT, Fox BW. The role of metallothionein, glutathione, glutathione S-transferases and DNA repair in resistance to platinum drugs in a series of L1210 cell lines made resistant to anticancer platinum agents. *Biochem Pharmacol* 1993;45:253–61.
41. Earhart RH. Instability of *cis*-dichlorodiammine platinum in dextrose solution. *Cancer Treat Rep* 1978;62:1105–6.
42. Litterst CL, LeRoy AF, Guarino AM. The disposition and distribution of platinum following parenteral administration to animals of *cis*-dichlorodiammineplatinum (II). *Cancer Treat Rep* 1979;63:1485–92.
43. Reece PA, Bishop JF, Olver IN, et al. Pharmacokinetics of unchanged carboplatin (CBDCA) in patients with small cell lung carcinoma. *Cancer Chemother Pharmacol* 1987;19:326–30.
44. Oguri S, Sakaibara T, Mase H, et al. Clinical pharmacokinetics of carboplatin. *J Clin Pharmacol* 1988;28:208–15.
45. Ewen C, Perera A, Hendry JH, et al. An autoradiographic study of the intrarenal localization and retention of cisplatin, iproplatin, and paraplatin. *Cancer Chemother Pharmacol* 1988;22:241–5.
46. Egorin MJ, Van Echo DA, Tipping SJ, et al. Pharmacokinetics and dosage reduction of carboplatin in patients with impaired renal function. *Cancer Res* 1984;44:5432–8.
47. Calvert AH, Newell DR, Gumbrell LA, et al. Carboplatin dosage: prospective evaluation of a simple formula based on renal function. *J Clin Oncol* 1989;7:1748–56.
48. Schwartz DE, Bollag W, Obrecht P. Distribution and excretion studies of procarbazine in animals and man. *Arzneim Forsch* 1967;17:1389–93.
49. Loo TL, Householder CE, Gerulath AH, et al. Mechanism of action and pharmacology studies with DTIC (NSC-45399). *Cancer Treat Rep* 1976;60:149–52.
50. Ames MM, Sanders ME, Tiede WS. Role of *N*-methylopentamethylmelamine in the metabolic activation of hexamethylmelamine. *Cancer Res* 1983;43:500–4.
51. Bryan GT, Worzalla JF, Gorski AL, et al. Plasma levels and urinary excretion of hexamethylmelamine following oral administration to human subjects with cancer. *Clin Pharmacol Ther* 1968;9:777–82.
52. D'Incalci MD, Bolis G, Mangioni C, et al. Variable oral absorption of hexamethylmelamine in man. *Cancer Treat Rep* 1978;62:2117–9.
53. Doroshow JH. Anthracyclines and anthracenediones. In:

Chabner BA, Longo DL. *Cancer Chemotherapy and Biotherapy.* 2nd ed. Philadelphia, PA: Lippincott-Raven; 1996. p. 411, 428.

54. Bachur NR, Yu F, Johnson R, et al. Helicase inhibition by anthracycline anticancer drugs. *Mol Pharmacol* 1992;41:993–8.
55. Bachur NR, Johnson R, Yu F, et al. Anthracycline antihelicase action: new mechanism with implication for guanosine-cytidine intercalation specificity. In: Priebe W, editor. *Anthracycline Antibiotics: New Analogues, Methods of Delivery, and Mechanisms of Action.* Washington, DC: American Chemical Society; 1995. p. 204
56. Tewey KM, Chen GL, Nelson EM, et al. Intercalative antitumor drugs interfere with the breakage-reunion reaction of mammalian DNA topoisomerase II. *J Biol Chem* 1984;259: 9182–7.
57. Bachur NR, Gordon SL, Gee MV. Anthracycline antibiotic augmentation of microsomal electron transport and free radical formation. *Mol Pharmacol* 1977;13:901–10.
58. Doroshow JH. Role of hydrogen peroxide and hydroxyl radical formation in the killing of Ehrlich tumor cells by anticancer quinones. *Proc Natl Acad Sci USA* 1986;83:4514–8.
59. Tritton TR, Yee GC. The anticancer agent adriamycin can be actively cytotoxic without entering cells. *Science* 1982;217:248–50.
60. Sahyoun N, Wolf M, Besterman J, et al. Protein kinase C phosphorylates topoisomerase II: topoisomerase activation and its possible role in phorbol ester-induced differentiation of HL60 cells [abstract]. *Proc Natl Acad Sci USA* 1986;83:1806.
61. Hasinoff BB. The interaction of the cardioprotective agent ICRF-187 ((+)-1,2-bis(3,5-dioxopiperazinyl-1-yl)propane); its hydrolysis product (ICRF-198); and other chelating agents with the Fe(III) and Cu(II) complexes of adriamycin. *Agents Actions* 1989;26:378–85.
62. Glisson B, Gupta R, Hodges P, et al. Cross-resistance to intercalating agents in an epipodophyllotoxin-resistant Chinese hamster ovary cell line: evidence for a common intracellular target. *Cancer Res* 1986;46:1939–42.
63. Pommier Y, Kerrigan D, Schwartz RE, et al. Altered DNA topoisomerase II activity in Chinese hamster cells resistant to topoisomerase II inhibitors. *Cancer Res* 1986;46:3075–81.
64. Deffie AM, Batra JK, Goldenberg GJ. Direct correlation between DNA topoisomerase II activity and cytotoxicity in adriamycin-sensitive and -resistant P388 leukemia cell lines. *Cancer Res* 1989;49:58–62.
65. Batist G, Tulpule A, Sinha BK, et al. Overexpression of a novel anionic glutathione transferase in multidrug-resistant human breast cancer cells. *J Biol Chem* 1986;261:15544–9.
66. Dorr RT, Von Hoff DD, editors. Mitoxantrone. *Cancer Chemotherapy Handbook.* 2nd ed. Norwalk, CT: Appleton & Lange; 1994. p. 730–5.
67. Chlebowski RT, Bulcavage L, Henderson IC, et al. Mitoxantrone use in breast cancer patients with elevated bilirubicin. *Breast Cancer Res Treat* 1989;14:267–4.
68. Koeller J, Eble M. Mitoxantrone: a novel anthracycline derivative. *Clin Pharm* 1988;7:574–81.
69. Muller WEG, Zahn RK. Bleomycin, an antibiotic that removes thymine from double-stranded DNA. In: Cohn, WE, editor. *Progress in Nucleic Acid Research and Molecular Biology.* New York: Academic Pr; 1977. p. 21–57.
70. Takeshita M, Horwitz, SB, Grollman AP. Bleomycin, an inhibitor of vaccinia virus replication. *Virology* 1974;60:455.
71. Lazo JS, Chabner BA. Bleomycin. In: Chabner BA, Longo DL, editors. *Cancer Chemotherapy and Biotherapy: Principles and Practice.* Philadelphia, PA: Lippincott-Raven; 1996. p. 379–93.
72. Crooke ST, Comis RL, Einhorn LH, et al. Effects of variations in renal function on the clinical pharmacology of bleomycin administered as an iv bolus. *Cancer Treat Rep* 1977;61:1631–6.
73. Dalgleish AG, Woods RL, Levi JA. Bleomycin pulmonary toxicity: its relationship to renal dysfunction. *Med Pediatr Oncol* 1984;12:313–7.
74. Umezawa H, Takeuchi T, Hori S, et al. Studies on the mechanism of antitumor effect of bleomycin on squamous cell carcinoma. *J Antibiot (Tokyo)* 1972;25:409–20.
75. Lazo JS, Mignano JE, Sebti SM. Pulmonary metabolic inactivation of bleomycin and protection from drug-induced lung injury. In: Hacker MP, Lazo JS, Tritton TR, editors. *Organ Directed Toxicities of Anticancer Drugs.* Boston: Martinus Nijhoff; 1987. p. 128–39.
76. Sebti SM, DeLeon JC, Ma LT, et al. Substrate specificity of bleomycin hydrolase. *Biochem Pharmacol* 1989;38:141–7.
77. Lazo JS, Humphreys CJ. Lack of metabolism as the biochemical basis of bleomycin-induced pulmonary toxicity [abstract]. *Proc Natl Acad Sci USA* 1983;80:3064.
78. Tattersall MHN, Sodegren JE, Sergupta SK, et al. Pharmacokinetics of actinomycin D in patients with malignant melanoma. *Clin Pharmacol Ther* 1975;17:701–8.
79. Teicher BA. Antitumor alkylating agents. In: DeVita VT, Hellman S, Rosenberg SA, editors. *Cancer: Principles and Practice of Oncology.* 5th ed. Philadelphia, PA: Lippincott-Raven; 1997. p. 405–18.
80. Bachur NR, Gordon SL, Gee RV. A general mechanism for microsomal activation of quinone agents to free radicals. *Cancer Res* 1978;38:1745–50.

SELF-STUDY QUESTIONS

1. List at least four alkylating agents and describe the three possible cytotoxic outcomes that are caused by alkylating agents.

2. Alkylating agents are an example of a class of cytotoxics that are:

    a. cell cycle (phase) specific.
    b. cell cycle (phase) nonspecific.
    c. nonmyelosuppressive.
    d. both b and c are correct.

3. Which of the following statements are true regarding ifosfamide and cyclophosphamide hemorrhagic cystitis?

    i. It is dose related.
    ii. It is caused by an alteration in pH of the urine produced by the drug and its diluent and can be

prevented by administering sodium bicarbonate prior to treatment.

iii. On a milligram-to-milligram basis, it is more common with ifosfamide.

iv. It can be effectively prevented by administering mesna prior to and following ifosfamide/cyclophosphamide administration.

v. If it occurs, it can be treated by administering mesna.

a. All of the above are true.
b. Only i, ii, and iv are true.
c. Only i, iii, and iv are true.
d. Only i, iv, and v are true.
e. Only i and iv are true.

4. It is believed that doxorubicin exerts is cytotoxic effects by:

a. intercalation.
b. alkylation.
c. complexation with nuclear helicases.
d. complexation with topoisomerase II.
e. all of the above.

5. Which of the following statements is true regarding dexrazoxane?

a. It prevents anthracycline-related myelosuppression.
b. It prevents anthracycline-related cardiac damage.
c. It can be used to treat doxorubicin extravasations.
d. It is a liposomal product.
e. All of the above statements are true.

6. In patients with severe renal impairment, the dose of bleomycin should be _____.

7. Bleomycin pulmonary toxicity may be severe and is considered an idiosyncratic reaction.

a. true
b. false

8. Which of the following can cause severe tissue damage if extravasated?

a. doxorubicin
b. mitomycin
c. dactinomycin
d. only a and c
e. all of the above

9. Describe the functions of topoisomerases I and II.

10. The risk of hepatic veno-occlusive disease associated with busulfan therapy has been correlated with:

a. concomitant therapy with steroids.
b. higher areas under the serum concentration versus time curves (AUCs).
c. renal impairment.
d. only a and b.
e. all of the above.

11. Cisplatin and carboplatin act by forming:

a. interstrand cross-links.
b. intrastrand adducts.
c. changes in the DNA conformation.
d. only a and c.
e. all of the above.

12. Clinical responses to cisplatin have been correlated with:

a. the severity of renal toxicity.
b. the degree of thrombocytopenia.
c. adduct formation in peripheral blood leukocytes.
d. peak serum concentrations.
e. magnesium supplement requirements.

13. The most significant dose-related toxicity of carboplatin is:

a. nephrotoxicity.
b. ototoxicity.
c. thrombocytopenia.
d. stomatitis.
e. hepatic veno-occlusive disease.

14. Describe the most common mechanism of resistance to anthracyclines.

15. In which of the following situations is it recommended to reduce the dose of doxorubicin?

a. elevated serum creatinine
b. biliary obstruction
c. congestive heart failure
d. acidic urine
e. decreased pulmonary function tests

Chapter 4
The Pharmacology of Cytotoxic Chemotherapy II

Rebecca S. Finley, Pharm.D., M.S.
Chair and Associate Professor
Department of Pharmacy Practice and Pharmacy Administration
Philadelphia College of Pharmacy
Philadelphia, Pennsylvania

Antimetabolites 52
    Methotrexate 52
        Leucovorin Rescue 52
    Cytarabine 54
    Fludarabine 55
    Gemcitabine 55
    Fluoropyrimidines (Fluorouracil and Floxuridine) 56
    Purine Analogues (Mercaptopurine and Thioguanine) 57
    Cladribine 57
    Pentostatin 57
Plant Alkaloids 58
    Vinca Alkaloids 58
    Epipodophyllotoxins 58
        Etoposide 58
        Teniposide 58
    Taxanes 59
        Paclitaxel 59
        Docetaxel 60
    Camptothecins 60
        Topotecan 61
        Irinotecan 61
Miscellaneous Agents 61
    Asparaginase 61
    Hydroxyurea 62
Summary 62
References 62
    Suggested Reference Texts 64
Self-Study Questions 64

This chapter will review the general pharmacologic activity of the antimetabolites, plant alkaloids, asparaginase, and hydroxyurea. The mechanism of cytotoxicity, pharmacologic characteristics, and the general pharmacokinetics of each class of cancer chemotherapy agents will be discussed.

After completing this chapter, the reader should be able to:

1. Describe the mechanisms of action of the various cytotoxic classes and list examples from each class.
2. Given a specific cytotoxic drug, identify aspects of its pharmacology that influence its therapeutic applications.
3. Describe the rationale for administering high-dose methotrexate versus conventional-dose therapy.
4. Given a class of cytoxic drugs, list toxicities that are common to the class and toxicities that are unique to specific drugs within the class.

ANTIMETABOLITES

Typically, the antimetabolites (Table 4-1) are structural analogues of naturally occurring substances required for specific biochemical reactions. Antimetabolites interfere with the normal synthesis of nucleic acids in one of two ways. They can fraudulently substitute themselves for purines or pyrimidines, or they can inhibit critical enzymes that are involved in nucleic acid synthesis. They affect DNA, RNA, protein synthesis, and, ultimately, cellular replication. Antimetabolites tend to be cell cycle specific, exerting most of their cytotoxic effects during the S phase.

Methotrexate

Folic acid is not biologically useful in its fully oxidized state. It must be reduced by the enzyme dihydrofolate reductase (DHFR) to 5,6,7,8-tetrahydrofolate. This reduced folate functions as a carrier of one-carbon (methyl) groups that are required for synthesis of purine nucleotides and thymidylate (Figure 4-1). Methotrexate (Folex), an analogue of folic acid, binds to and inhibits DHFR, preventing the formation of reduced folate. The result is inhibition of DNA synthesis because thymidylate synthase or purines or both are unavailable (Figure 4-2), and cell death results.

Methotrexate is widely used in managing lymphocytic leukemias, lymphomas, and a variety of solid tumors. High-dose therapy with leucovorin rescue is controversial and is thought to be superior to conventional doses in some non-Hodgkin's lymphomas and osteogenic sarcomas. Methotrexate is occasionally used to treat some nonmalignant conditions, including rheumatoid arthritis, psoriasis, and asthma. Methotrexate has also been used to induce abortions.

Following conventional doses (i.e., <100 mg/m^2), methotrexate enters the cell primarily by a saturable active transport mechanism. Some methotrexate molecules may also diffuse passively through the cell membrane if the extracellular concentrations of methotrexate are very high (e.g., after high-dose therapy). Once inside the cell, methotrexate may be metabolized to a polyglutamate form, which inhibits DHFR like the parent drug. Because the polyglutamatized forms are usually large, they are unable to exit the cell by passive diffusion or via the folate efflux transport system like unchanged methotrexate.[1] Methotrexate exerts its activity on dividing cells during the S phase, and it appears that a threshold concentration of 10^{-8}–10^{-7}M is required for cytotoxicity.[2]

Leucovorin Rescue

Methotrexate cytotoxicity may be reversed by administering a reduced folate necessary for DNA synthesis—one that does not require activation by DHFR, such as leucovorin, a D,L-N^5-formyl-tetrahydrofolic acid. This antidote has allowed doses of methotrexate that exceed conventional doses by 10- to 100-fold to be used. High-dose methotrexate (100–12,000 mg/m^2) is thought to (1) produce higher intracellular concentrations because of increased passive diffusion of methotrexate through the cell membrane,

Table 4-1. Antimetabolite Cytotoxic Drugs in Clinical Use in the United States

Generic Name	Trade Name	Other Synonyms
Folate Antagonist		
Methotrexate	Folex	MTX
Pyrimidine Antagonists		
Cytarabine	Cytosar	Cytosine arabinoside, Ara-C
Floxuridine		FUDR
Fludarabine	Fludara	
Fluorouracil	Adrucil	5-FU
Gemcitabine	Gemzar	
Purine Antagonists		
Cladribine	Leustatin	2-CdA; 2´-chloro-2´-deoxyadenosine
Mercaptopurine	Purinethol	6-MP
Thioguanine	Tabloid	6-TG
Adenosine Deaminase Inhibitor		
Pentostatin	Nipent	2´-deoxycoformycin

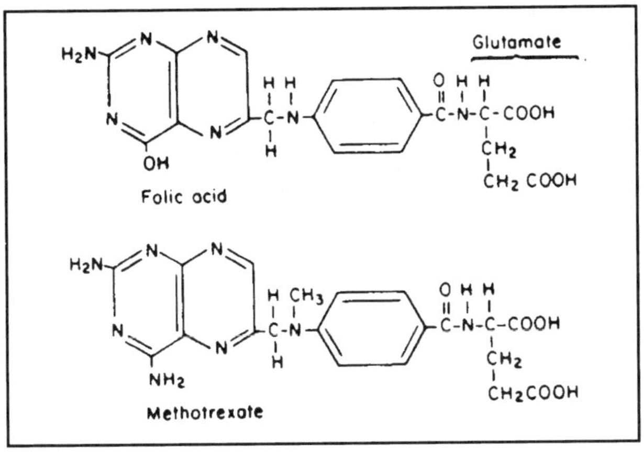

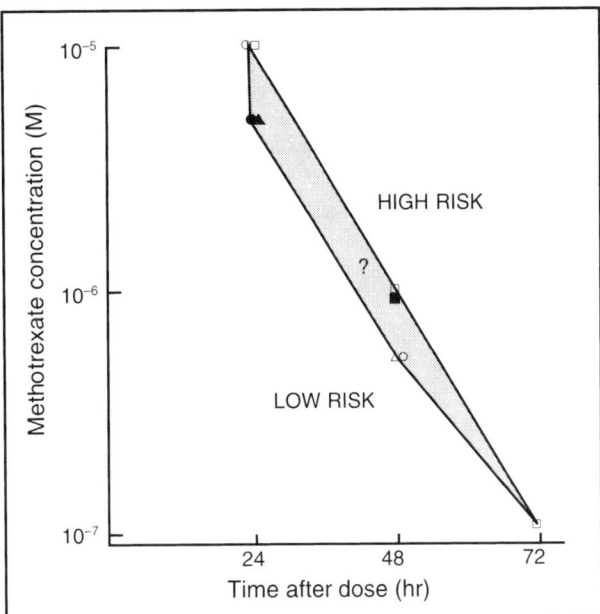

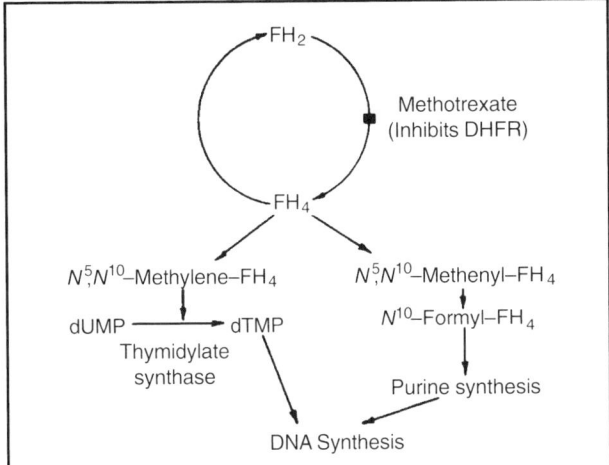

Figure 4-1. Structures of folic acid and its analogue, methotrexate

and (2) increase the amount of methotrexate that penetrates the blood-brain barrier.

It is believed that high-dose methotrexate followed by leucovorin (leucovorin rescue) preferentially kills cancer cells over normal cells for the following reasons. In normal cells, there is less accumulation of the polyglutamates, so administration of leucovorin can produce sufficient intracellular concentrations to regenerate DHFR activity and "rescue" these normal cells. Tumor cells, however, accumulate high concentrations of methotrexate polyglutamates and displacement by leucovorin is minimized, so the cells are more likely to be mortally damaged.[3]

Figure 4-2. Utilization of reduced folates in the synthesis of DNA and the inhibitory effect of methotrexate. FH_2, dihydrofolate; FH_4, tetrahydrofolate; DHFR, dihydrofolate reductase; dUMP, deoxyuridine monophosphate; dTMP, thymidylate.

SOURCE: reprinted with permission from Erlichman C. Pharmacology of anticancer drugs. In: Tannock IF, Hill RP, editors. *The Basic Science of Oncology.* 2nd ed. New York: McGraw-Hill; 1992. p. 300

Figure 4-3. Serum methotrexate concentrations that identify patients at high risk for severe toxicity

SOURCE: reprinted with permission from Crom WR, Evans WE. Methothrexate. In: Evans WE, Schentag JJ, Jusko WR, editors. *Applied Pharmacokinetics.* 3rd ed. Vancouver, WA: Applied Therapeutics; 1992. p. 531.

Clearance of methotrexate and serum concentrations following high-dose therapy reliably predict which patients will experience severe or even fatal myelosuppression and mucosal damage if appropriate leucovorin rescue is not administered (Figure 4-3). The dose of leucovorin required to reverse methotrexate cellular toxicity has been correlated with the concentration of methotrexate at the time of leucovorin administration.[1] Appropriate leucovorin rescue will prevent any significant toxicity. Most of a methotrexate dose is excreted by the kidneys, so creatinine clearance should be ≥60 ml/min before methotrexate is initiated. For patients with renal function below this level, methotrexate should only be considered when no alternative therapy is feasible or when the methotrexate therapy is likely to result in significant improvement in renal function (e.g., when a tumor mass is causing obstruction of a renal artery). It is always necessary to monitor methotrexate serum concentrations after high-dose methotrexate as well as in patients receiving conventional doses who have significant renal dysfunction; these patients are at high risk for toxicity. Both enzymatic assay and immunoassay techniques are used. Guidelines are available for interpreting methotrexate serum concentrations and administering leucovorin rescue (Table 4-2).[5] Early detection of high methotrexate serum concentrations allows for initiation of appropriate rescue measures. If the urine is too acidic following high-dose therapy, methotrexate can precipitate in the renal tubules and cause severe and irreversible renal failure. Both the drug and its metabolites are more soluble in alkaline pH. The risk of

Table 4-2. General Guidelines for Modification of Leucovorin Dosage Following High-Dose Methotrexate in High-Risk Patients

Methotrexate Serum Concentration (μM)[a]		Desired TRF Concentration (μM)[b]	Approximate Leucovorin Dose Required[c]
20–50	=	200–500	500 mg/m² IV q6hr
10–20	=	100–200	200 mg/m² IV q6hr
5–10	=	50–100	100 mg/m² IV q6hr
1–5	=	5–10	30 mg/m² IV or PO q6hr
0.6–1	=	0.6–1	15 mg/m² PO q6hr
0.1–0.5	=	0.1–0.5	15 mg/m² PO q12hr
0.05–0.1	=	0.05–0.1	5–10 mg/m² PO q12hr

[a] Concentrations ≥42 hr after beginning of methotrexate infusion.
[b] Total reduced folates (active) are 1-formyl tetrahydrofolate and 5-methyl-tetrahydrofolate.
[c] Methotrexate concentrations should be monitored and leucovorin administration should be continued in high-risk patients until methotrexate serum concentrations are <0.05 μM. Leucovorin dosages may be reduced, as indicated, as methotrexate serum concentrations decrease.

SOURCE: reprinted with permission from Crom WR, Evans WE. Methotrexate. In: Evans WE, Schentag JJ, Jusko WR, editors. *Applied Pharmacokinetics*. 3rd ed. Vancouver, WA: Applied Therapeutics; 1992. p. 532.

nephrotoxicity can be minimized by alkalinizing the urine and maintaining good urine output (≥100 ml/hr) immediately prior to, during, and for up to 24–48 hours after high-dose therapy.

Although methotrexate is excreted predominantly as the unchanged drug via the kidney by both glomerular filtration and active tubular transport, some methotrexate is metabolized by the liver. Both metabolites and the parent drug are excreted by the active process in the renal tubules. This active transport mechanism may be inhibited by penicillin, aspirin, and other nonsteroidal anti-inflammatory drugs, including ibuprofen and ketoprofen, which can result in increased methotrexate toxicity. Aspirin may also displace methotrexate from plasma protein binding sites.

Methotrexate may accumulate in fluid-filled spaces, such as pleural effusions and ascites. Slow efflux from these sites may produce prolonged toxicities, especially after high-dose therapy. Such fluid accumulations should be drained before methotrexate therapy. Methotrexate also penetrates the cerebrospinal fluid to some extent, but cytotoxic concentrations are achieved only after high-dose administration.[6]

Systemic methotrexate may be given orally or by intramuscular or intravenous injection. Oral absorption occurs via an active transport mechanism that becomes saturated when doses of ≥25 mg are given. Erratic absorption can result, limiting the usefulness of oral administration in the treatment of most cancers.[6] Methotrexate may also be administered intrathecally or intraventricularly.

The other major toxicities associated with methotrexate are dose-related myelosuppression and stomatitis. It can also cause reversible pulmonary toxicity and elevation of hepatic transaminases. Table 4-3 lists toxicities common to antimetabolites and toxicities unique to specific drugs of this class.

Cytarabine

Cytarabine (Cytosar-U), an analogue of deoxycytidine, penetrates cells and is rapidly phosphorylated to cytosine arabinoside triphosphate (Ara-CTP). Ara-CTP is a competitive inhibitor of DNA polymerases, the enzymes responsible for matching complementary nucleotide base pairs during DNA synthesis. When this reaction occurs, replicating cells may die. Most important, cytosine arabinoside is incorporated into DNA, leading to the inhibition of DNA synthesis.[7] Resistance to

Table 4-3. Toxicities Associated with Antimetabolite Cytotoxics

Toxicities common to most antimetabolites:
  Myelosuppression
  Mucositis
  Mild nausea and vomiting (high-dose cytarabine and high-dose methotrexate may cause moderate to severe emetic complications)

Toxicities unique to specific antimetabolites:

Neurotoxicity	high-dose cytarabine
Nephrotoxicity	high-dose methotrexate
Hepatic toxicity	chronic methotrexate administration
Rash or skin changes	cladribine, cytarabine
Cardiac toxicity	fluorouracil

cytosine arabinoside has been associated with decreased transport into cells and increased inactivation of the drug.

Cytarabine is used to treat several types of leukemia and is considered part of the standard induction therapy for newly diagnosed acute myelogenous leukemia. It may also be given intrathecally or intraventricularly to treat meningeal leukemia. Cytarabine may be used subcutaneously in low doses for palliative regimens and in high intravenous doses (2–3 g/m^2) for refractory leukemias and for postremission intensification. Current information suggests that administration of high-dose cytarabine significantly decreases the relapse rate and prolongs disease-free survival.

Cytarabine is destroyed rapidly in the plasma and has a half-life of 7–20 minutes. Conventional regimens administer 100–200 mg/m^2 daily via continuous infusion for 5–10 days. Because of the possibility of clinical resistance due to decreased influx of drug into cells, high-dose regimens were developed in which 2–3 g/m^2 is given in short infusions every 12 hours for up to 6 days.[8] These schedules maintain plasma concentrations at a level at which active transport does not limit uptake. Metabolic deamination accounts for 70–90% of cytosine arabinoside elimination, with most of the drug being excreted as an inactive metabolite, uracil arabinoside.[9] Elimination kinetics appear to be similar following conventional and high-dose therapy.[8,10] Cytarabine is not absorbed orally. Simultaneous cerebrospinal fluid levels reach 50% of plasma levels within 2 hours after intravenous administration.[11]

Myelosuppression is the most predominant dose-related toxicity of cytarabine. Because cytarabine is most commonly used in the treatment of acute leukemia, in which the therapeutic goal is ablation of the bone marrow, the myelosuppression is not usually considered to be dose limiting. Other dose-related toxicities include nausea, vomiting (which can be severe with high-dose therapy), stomatitis, and diarrhea. Following high-dose therapy, cerebellar dysfunction (slurring of speech, nystagmus, and inability to articulate thoughts) is the most significant dose-limiting toxicity. Renal dysfunction and age >50 years appear to predispose patients to this toxicity.[12–14] Conjunctivitis can also be a problem following high-dose therapy; it can be prevented by the use of corticosteroid eye drops throughout treatment.

Fludarabine

Fludarabine (Fludara), a nucleotide analogue of the antiviral agent vidarabine, also closely resembles cytarabine (Figure 4-4). Like cytarabine, fludarabine is rapidly phosphorylated intracellularly and inhibits DNA synthesis (and repair) by inhibition of DNA polymerases. It also exerts cytotoxicity by incorporation into the DNA strand, leading to chain termination.[15,16]

Fludarabine is most widely used for the treatment of chronic lymphocytic leukemia (CLL). It is usually administered as a 30-minute infusion on 5 consecutive days each month. Although it is not appreciably excreted by the kidneys, patients with poor renal function have a low tolerance for the drug.[17,18] This low tolerance may be due to renal elimination of a toxic metabolite. Fludarabine is reasonably well-tolerated, which is important because CLL occurs predominantly in patients >60 years old. Myelosuppression is the dose-limiting toxicity, although neurotoxicity and pulmonary toxicity have been observed. Neurotoxicity has been seen primarily in clinical trials for other types of leukemia in which doses far exceeded the standard CLL dose. However, the drug should be used cautiously in treating any patient with prior neurological problems. An interstitial pneumonitis in which patients initially present with cough, dyspnea, hypoxia, and fever is also well described. This effect does not appear to be dose related and is seen in patients receiving conventional dosages. The pneumonitis is usually reversible and spontaneously resolves over several weeks with or without the use of corticosteroids.[19] Many patients experiencing pulmonary toxicity have had prior treatment with chlorambucil, which is also toxic to the lungs.

Gemcitabine

Gemcitabine (Gemzar) is a synthetically prepared pyrimidine nucleoside with a structure very similar to that of deoxycytidine and cytarabine (Figure 4-4). The primary difference in the

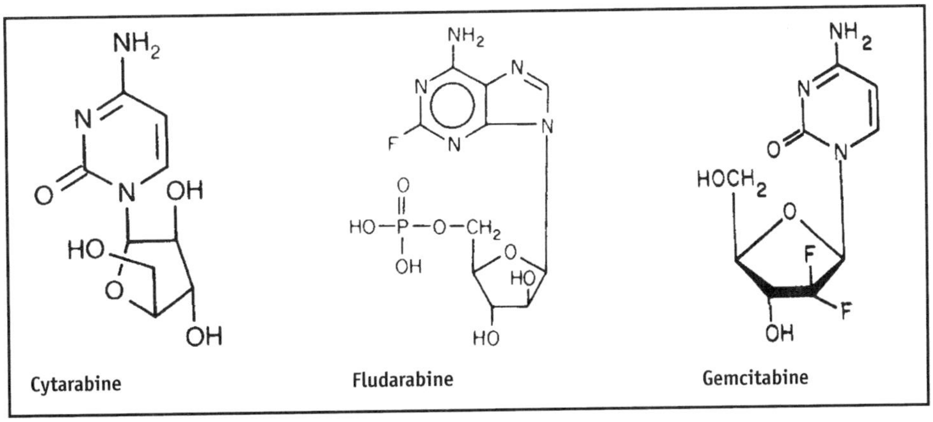

Figure 4-4. Structures of cytarabine, fludarabine, and gemcitabine

structure is that two fluorine atoms are appended at the 2′ position of the oxyribose sugar ring.

Gemcitabine is used to treat locally advanced or metastatic pancreatic cancer. In the clinical trials, benefit following gemcitabine administration was assessed on the basis of patient's perception of pain, intake of analgesics, weight gain, and Karnofsky performance scores. The recommended dose is 1 g/m² over 30 minutes every week for up to 7 weeks, followed by a week of rest. Subsequent cycles should be given every 3 or 4 weeks. Studies to determine whether dosage adjustment is necessary for renal or hepatic dysfunction are under way.

Like cytarabine, phosphorylation is essential for the cytotoxic activity of gemcitabine. Gemcitabine is first phosphorylated intracellularly to the monophosphate by deoxycytidine kinase and subsequently to the di- and triphosphate forms by other kinases.[20] It is the triphosphate of gemcitabine that inhibits DNA polymerases and is incorporated into DNA strands, leading to termination of DNA chain elongation. In addition, gemcitabine diphosphate inhibits ribonucleotide reductase, an enzyme that converts ribonucleotides to deoxynucleotides. This inhibition depletes key deoxynucleotide pools that are also necessary for DNA synthesis.[21] In vitro activity of gemcitabine is significantly greater than that of cytarabine in many systems. Explanations for the enhanced cytotoxicity include greater intracellular accumulation of the gemcitabine triphosphate, greater effectiveness of gemcitabine phosphorylation, and significantly longer intracellular retention.

Gemcitabine pharmacokinetics are linear and best described by a two-compartment model. It is believed that soon after injection gemcitabine is rapidly deaminated in the liver and kidney by deoxycytidine deaminases to 2′,2′-difluorodeoxyuridine (dFdU), which has only minimal cytotoxic activity. Gemcitabine is eliminated almost completely, either as the parent compound (5%) or as the primary metabolite (77%) in the urine.[22] The pharmacokinetics of gemcitabine are influenced by age, gender, and infusion duration. Clearance is lower in women and elderly patients. The half-life for short infusions ranges from 32 to 94 minutes, and the half-life for long infusions is 245–638 minutes.[23]

Gemcitabine is generally well tolerated by most patients. Myelosuppression is the most significant dose-limiting toxicity, with 25% of patients experiencing World Health Organization grade 3 or 4 neutropenia following the recommended dose. The nadir generally occurs between days 8 and 15. Anemia and thrombocytopenia are rare. Other adverse effects include mild to moderate nausea, vomiting, fever, edema, rash, and flu-like symptoms. Mild proteinuria and hematuria have also been reported. Up to one third of patients have transient elevations in serum transaminases. The rise in transaminases typically occurs early in therapy, peaks by cycle 2, and returns to baseline by the end of therapy. In the single-agent trials, gemcitabine was rarely discontinued because of toxicity, and there was no evidence of cumulative adverse effects.

Fluoropyrimidines (Fluorouracil and Floxuridine)

Fluorouracil (Adrucil) resembles the pyrimidine bases uracil (a component of RNA) and thymine (a component of DNA).[6] After administration, fluorouracil penetrates cells, where it is metabolized to nucleoside forms and phosphorylated to 5-fluorouridine triphosphate (5-FUTP) and 5-fluorodeoxyuridine monophosphate (5-FdUMP). 5-FUTP may be erroneously incorporated into RNA in the place of uridine triphosphate, which may cause errors during RNA transcription. An enzyme called thymidylate synthase (TS) ordinarily catalyzes the methylation of deoxyuridine monophosphate (dUMP) during DNA synthesis. When TS attempts to use FdUMP instead, the process is inhibited and the enzyme, FdUMP, and the folate cofactor (the source of the methyl group) are trapped in a ternary complex that dissociates very slowly. DNA synthesis is inhibited as a consequence (Figure 4-5). Incorporation of 5-FUTP into RNA occurs throughout the cell cycle, but inhibition of TS occurs only during the S phase. Both mechanisms probably account for the cytotoxicity of fluorouracil, although one of the mechanisms may predominate in different types of cells. Evidence suggests that TS inhibition is the predominant mechanism, however; in vitro and in vivo data demonstrate that an improved therapeutic effect is observed when leucovorin is combined with fluorouracil. Administration of exogenous leucovorin increases the formation of the ternary complex, enhancing the cytotoxicity of fluorouracil.[24]

Breast, colon, and head and neck tumors are among

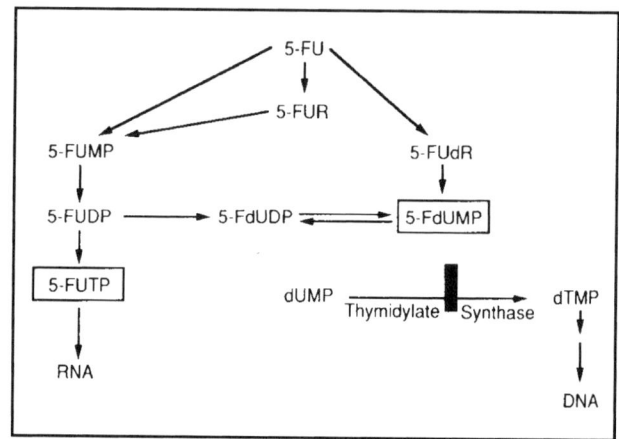

Figure 4-5. Metabolic activation of fluorouracil (5-FU). 5-FUR, 5-fluorouridine; 5-FUMP, 5-fluorouridine-5′-monophosphate; 5-FUdR, 5-fluorodeoxyuridine; 5-FUDP, 5-fluorouridine-5′-diphosphate; 5-FdUDP, 5-fluoro-2-deoxyuridine-5-diphosphate; 5-FdUMP, 5-fluorodeoxyuridine monophosphate; 5-FUTP, 5-fluorouridine triphosphate; dUMP, deoxyuridine-5′-monophosphate; dTMP, thymidylate.

SOURCE: reprinted with permission from Erlichman C. Pharmacology of anticancer drugs. In: Tannock IF, Hill RP, editors. *The Basic Science of Oncology.* 2nd ed. New York: McGraw-Hill; 1992. p. 326

the solid tumors that fluorouracil is commonly used to treat. Intravenous administration is customary for fluorouracil because oral bioavailability is quite variable. Fluorouracil is eliminated rapidly from the plasma by breakdown in the liver and other tissues; its half-life is about 10–20 minutes. Because it is active predominantly in the S phase of the cell cycle, many regimens have been designed to optimize exposure to fluorouracil by providing a prolonged concentration as cells cycle through the S phase. It is often given by prolonged infusions. Fluorouracil has also been given by intra-arterial and intra-peritoneal infusions. Because it is metabolized by the liver, it can be infused into the hepatic artery or portal vein to treat hepatic metastases, and only small amounts of fluorouracil reach the systemic circulation.[6] This method of administration is discussed further in chapter 10.

Fluorouracil and leucovorin have been studied in many combinations, varying doses and schedules of administration, as a treatment for colon cancer. Data from randomized trials report that weekly high-dose intravenous leucovorin (e.g., 500 mg/m^2) with fluorouracil (600 mg/m^2) as well as those using 5 consecutive days of low-dose leucovorin (e.g., 20 mg/m^2 per day) with fluorouracil (370–475 mg/m^2) have shown the highest response rates.[25-27]

Floxuridine (FUDR), which is structurally similar to its prodrug, fluoruracil, is phosphorylated to 5-FdUMP and also inhibits TS. It may also be administered by intravenous bolus or infusion, but it is most commonly administered directly into the hepatic artery for managing primary and metastatic liver tumors.

The toxicities of fluorouracil and floxuridine are influenced by the dose, schedule, and route of administration. When given as a monthly bolus injection, the most common dose-limiting toxicity is myelosuppression. When the dose is given as a continuous infusion over several days, the dose-limiting toxicity is usually mucositis or diarrhea. Nausea and vomiting are generally mild. Although both drugs can cause hepatic damage when given intra-arterially, this route may result in fewer systemic toxicities.

Purine Analogues (Mercaptopurine and Thioguanine)

Mercaptopurine (Purinethol) and thioguanine (Thioguanine Tabloid) are purine analogues that are used primarily in treating leukemias. Thioguanine structurally resembles guanine, and mercaptopurine resembles hypoxanthine. After administration they are metabolized and incorporated erroneously into DNA and RNA. Both agents are given orally. Mercaptopurine undergoes substantial first-pass metabolism, which is highly variable among patients.[28] Mercaptopurine is metabolized by xanthine oxidase, an enzyme that is inhibited by allopurinol. Therefore, a 75% dose reduction is recommended for patients who are receiving both mercaptopurine and allopurinol. The toxicities associated with mercaptopurine are usually mild, including myelosuppression (e.g., leukopenia). Cholestatic liver dysfunction, characterized by increased bilirubin and/or transaminases, is frequently the dose-limiting toxicity. Mild to moderate nausea, vomiting, stomatitis, and diarrhea may also occur.

Cladribine

Cladribine (Leustatin) causes extensive DNA damage. Several distinct mechanisms of cytotoxicity have been proposed. Following administration, the drug is phosphorylated intracellularly to its triphosphate form, cladribine triphosphate (CdATP), which (like gemcitabine) inhibits ribonucleotide reductase. CdATP, also inhibits DNA strand elongation by causing strand breaks and inhibiting enzymes (e.g., DNA polymerases and ligases) necessary for DNA repair. Cladribine can also cause death in resting cells (those not undergoing division). It has also been proposed that it produces nucleotide imbalances that may trigger programmed cell death (apoptosis).[29-31]

Cladribine is indicated for the treatment of hairy cell leukemia and has also been used in the management of other hematological diseases, including non-Hodgkin's lymphomas, myelogenous leukemias, pediatric leukemias, and CLL. Cladribine is administered by intravenous infusion. Most regimens use a 7-day continuous infusion, although other schedules have been used. The drug is rapidly phosphorylated, its half-life is 35 minutes, and all drug and metabolites are cleared from the body within 1–3 days after completion of the infusion.[32]

Cladribine at recommended doses has a rather mild toxicity profile when compared with many of the other antineoplastic drugs, and it can be safely administered as an ambulatory infusion. Neutropenia is generally mild, although most patients experience a suppression of circulating lymphocytes that may increase the risk of opportunistic infections. Fever, a common occurrence among patients receiving cladribine, is usually due to cell lysis and the release of endogenous pyrogens.[33] Unfortunately, these fevers are difficult to differentiate from infectious complications, and many patients receive antibiotic therapy until infection can be ruled out. Skin rashes also occur in about 50% of patients.[34]

Pentostatin

Adenosine deaminase (ADA) is an enzyme that regulates intracellular adenosine levels. ADA levels are highest in lymphatic cells and tissues. Pentostatin (Nipent), an irreversible inhibitor of ADA, causes intracellular accumulation of adenine deoxynucleotides (e.g., dATP) that, in turn, inhibits ribonucleotide reductase and subsequent DNA synthesis. Other mechanisms of action have been proposed that include depletion of ATP, inhibition of DNA repair, induction of strand breaks, and inhibition of RNA transcription.[35-37]

Pentostatin is administered intravenously. It is usually given as a single dose weekly for up to 3 consecutive weeks, followed by 1–2 weeks off therapy. Most of a pentostatin dose is excreted unchanged in the urine, and significant dose reductions are necessary for patients with renal insufficiency. Guidelines for dosage reduction have been published, but they have not been prospectively validated.[38] In addition, the dose-limiting toxicity of pentostatin is renal tubular damage that can progress to acute renal failure. Adequate hydration and avoidance of other nephrotoxic drugs are recommended to minimize the risk of pentostatin-induced renal tubular damage. Dose-related neurological toxicity and bone marrow suppression are also well described. The neurological effects present with lethargy and fatigue that can occasionally progress to coma. Myelosuppression is evidenced by granulocytopenia, thrombocytopenia, and lymphopenia (which is part of the desired therapeutic activity). Fever and infection commonly complicate pentostatin therapy. Mild to moderate nausea, vomiting, dry skin, and conjunctivitis are also reported.

PLANT ALKALOIDS

Vinca Alkaloids

The vinca alkaloids (vincristine [Oncovin], vinblastine [Velban], and vinorelbine [Navelbine]) are derived from the periwinkle plant and exert their cytotoxic activity by binding to tubulin (Table 4-4). Tubulin is found in the cytoplasm of all cells; the polymerized form makes up the microtubular apparatus that forms the spindle along which chromosomes migrate during mitosis. The microtubules are also responsible for maintaining cellular structure and transport functions in nerve axons. Vinca alkaloids act by preventing the polymerization of tubulin; this inhibits the assembly of the microtubules and results in dissolution of the mitotic spindle.[39] Consequently, cells are arrested during the metaphase of mitosis.

The vinca alkaloids are used primarily to treat hematological malignancies and lung cancer. Vinblastine is also used to treat testicular cancer. Vinorelbine, the most recently marketed vinca alkaloid in the United States, is approved for use in non-small cell lung cancer. The vinca alkaloids are given intravenously and are excreted mainly through the biliary tract or via hepatic metabolism.[6]

All three vinca alkaloids are rapidly cleared from the plasma but slowly eliminated from the body; the slow elimination may be related to extensive tissue binding. Vincristine and vinblastine are extensively excreted through biliary mechanisms, so dose adjustments may be warranted for patients with severe obstructive liver disease.

Neurotoxicity and myelosuppression are the most common toxicities associated with the vinca alkaloids. The relative incidence and severity of these toxicities appears to differ among the three drugs and may be related to the dose, schedule of administration, and concomitant chemotherapy drugs. Myelosuppression is usually the most prominent toxicity associated with vinblastine and vinorelbine, whereas neurotoxicity is more common with vincristine. All of the available vinca alkaloids are vesicants if extravasated.

Epipodophyllotoxins

Etoposide (VePesid) and teniposide (Vumon) are semisynthetic derivatives of podophyllotoxin that are derived from the mandrake plant. Although podophyllotoxin binds to tubulin like the vinca alkaloids, etoposide does not appear to alter microtubule assembly. The epipodophyllotoxins are potent inhibitors of type II DNA topoisomerase, acting in the late portion of the S or early G_2 phase and preventing cells from entering mitosis.[40] These agents also produce protein-associated DNA double strand breaks. Dose-related myelosuppression is the most common toxicity associated with these drugs. Secondary leukemias have also been reported.

Etoposide

Etoposide is most widely used in the treatment of lymphomas and lung and testicular cancers. Etoposide may be administered intravenously or orally. About 45% of the drug is excreted in the urine (some as metabolites) and 15% in the feces. Dosage attenuation is recommended for patients with severe hepatic dysfunction.[6] Because oral bioavailability is about 50%, the usual oral dose is twice the intravenous dose. Intravenous doses should be administered over 60 minutes because rapid injection may produce hypotension.

Teniposide

Teniposide is used primarily in the treatment of pediatric leukemias. It is only available as an intravenous formulation and is eliminated much more slowly than etoposide. Over 80% of the dose is metabolized, and <15% has been reported to ultimately be eliminated in the urine.[41-43] As with etoposide, hypotension has

Table 4-4. Plant Alkaloids Used as Anticancer Drugs

Generic Name	Trade Name	Other Synonyms
Vinca alkaloids		
Vinblastine	Velban	VBL
Vincristine	Oncovin	VCR
Vinorelbine	Navelbine	
Epipodophyllotoxins		
Etoposide	VePesid	VP-16, VP-16-2123
Teniposide	Vumon	VM-26
Taxanes		
Docetaxel	Taxotere	
Paclitaxel	Taxol	

been associated with rapid infusions. Hypersensitivity reactions appear to be more common with teniposide than with etoposide and have been attributed to the high concentration of polyethoxylated castor oil (Cremophor EL) in the formulation.[44]

Taxanes

Paclitaxel

Paclitaxel (Taxol) is derived from the bark of the Western (Pacific) yew (*Taxus brevifolia*) or produced semisynthetically from a compound found in the needles and twigs of a more prevalent yew (*Taxus baccata*). It was the first of the taxanes to be approved for use in the United States. Paclitaxel has a unique structure; studies have shown that both the taxane ring and the ester side chain are necessary for the cytotoxic effect (Figure 4-6).

In contrast to the vinca alkaloids, paclitaxel promotes microtubule assembly and binds to stabilized microtubules once they have been formed, even under conditions that generally promote disassembly.[45] The net effect is arrest of the normal mitotic cellular division and subsequent cell death. Paclitaxel can also inhibit cells in the G_2 phase.[46]

Paclitaxel is used to treat lung, ovarian, and breast cancers and is being widely evaluated for use against many other types of cancer. Following intravenous administration, clearance is rapid, but this clearance is not due to urinary excretion. Hepatic extraction and biliary secretion probably account for most of paclitaxel's elimination. The major metabolite appears to be relatively inactive. Paclitaxel exhibits nonlinear pharmacokinetics.[47] Because of this characteristic, standard (percentage-based) incremental increases in dose may result in unacceptable toxicity. Conversely, dosage attenuation based on percentage may dramatically diminish exposure to paclitaxel.

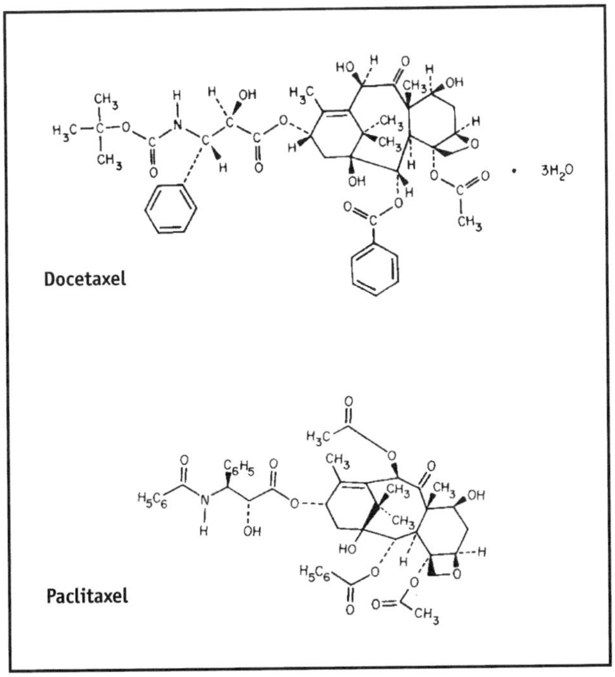

Paclitaxel's major dose-limiting toxicity is neutropenia. The duration of paclitaxel exposure above a critical plasma concentration may be more important in determining the severity of neutropenia than absolute dose or peak serum concentration.[47–50] This may have important implications for administration, suggesting that toxicity may be greater for 24-hour infusions than for 3-hour infusions.

Cardiac disturbances, especially bradycardia, and neurotoxicity have also been well described. Cardiac toxicity has ranged from asymptomatic bradycardia to myocardial infarction and sudden death. In most cases, bradycardia is benign and rarely requires interruption of the infusion, but special caution should be used when treating patients receiving medications that slow conduction (e.g., beta-adrenergic blockers, calcium channel blockers, or digoxin).

The neurotoxicity of paclitaxel appears to be cumulative and is characterized by paresthesia, usually beginning symmetrically in both the upper and lower extremities. This effect is reversible, with complete resolution within 3–6 months for most patients. Myalgias and arthralgias sometimes occur 48–72 hours after infusion and resolve within 5–7 days; nonsteroidal anti-inflammatory drugs may alleviate this discomfort. Nausea and vomiting are usually mild to moderate, and mucositis has been reported at higher dose levels. Several cases of severe local tissue damage have been reported following extravasation (see chapter 10).[51–53] Cellulitis is common following extravasation.

Hypersensitivity reactions were common during early paclitaxel clinical trials. These reactions ranged from flushing and mild dyspnea (with or without bronchospasm) to anaphylaxis and death in a few cases. It is not certain whether these reactions were caused by the drug or the polyethoxylated castor oil diluent. These reactions usually occur during the first 10 minutes of infusions and have been observed with the first or second dose, although occasionally they are reported with subsequent infusions. Pretreatment with dexamethasone, diphenhydramine, and an H_2 antagonist (such as cimetidine or ranitidine) has dramatically reduced the incidence of hypersensitivity reactions.

Because of the low solubility of paclitaxel in aqueous solutions, the commercial formulation is solubilized in polyethoxylated castor oil and dehydrated alcohol, USP. Polyethoxylated castor oil can cause leaching of plasticizers in polyvinyl chloride (PVC) bags and IV tubing, so paclitaxel must be admixed in glass, polypropylene, or polyolefin containers and infused through non-PVC tubing, such as that used for nitroglycerin infusions. Small fibers have also been observed in paclitaxel admixtures; it is recommended that this drug be administered through a hydrophilic 0.22-micron filter. Admixtures should always be visually inspected for particulate matter and discoloration before administration.

Figure 4-6. Structures of docetaxel and paclitaxel

Docetaxel

In 1996, Docetaxel (Taxotere) was approved for marketing in the United States for the treatment of patients with locally advanced or metastatic breast cancer who have progressed during anthracycline-based therapy or who have relapsed during anthracycline-based adjuvant therapy. Unlike paclitaxel, which is derived from the needles and bark of the *Taxus baccata* and the *Taxus brevifolia* respectively, docetaxel is semisynthetically produced from inactive precursors extracted only from the renewable needles of the European yew, *Taxus baccata*.[54] Docetaxel also has a complex structure that includes the unsaturated taxane ring linked to a four-membered oxetane ring at positions C4 and C5 and to a bulky ester side chain at C13 (Figure 4-6). The oxetane ring and the ester side chain at C13 are associated with the cytotoxic action of docetaxel,[55,56] and the ester side chain at C13 structurally differentiates docetaxel from paclitaxel.

Like paclitaxel, tubulin is the intracellular target for docetaxel. Both taxanes promote the formation of stable microtubules that resist disassembly by physiological stimuli, but docetaxel possesses a higher binding affinity for the tubulin subunit and produces microtubules of a slightly different size than paclitaxel does. In addition, docetaxel has a longer intracellular retention time.[54] Whereas paclitaxel appears to act primarily in the G_2 and M phases of the cell cycle, docetaxel's activity also is evident in the S phase. Paclitaxel acts primarily via damage to the mitotic spindle; docetaxel acts by inhibiting centrosome organization, which aborts mitosis, inducing cell death.[57]

Paclitaxel exhibits complex, nonlinear pharmacokinetics. Docetaxel appears to have linear pharmacokinetics, and its clearance is not dependent on infusion duration or dose.[58] Docetaxel is extensively metabolized and is excreted mainly in the feces via biliary elimination. The clearance of docetaxel by the liver is reduced by 25–30% in patients who have liver transaminase levels >1.5 times the upper limit of normal associated with alkaline phosphatase levels >2.5 times the upper limit of normal.[58,59] Dosage reductions are recommended for patients with serum bilirubin levels above the normal range and for those with liver transaminases >1.5 times normal plus alkaline phosphatase >2.5 times the upper limit of normal range. Myelosuppression and mucositis are more severe in patients with hepatic dysfunction.

Like paclitaxel, the major dose-limiting toxicity of docetaxel is neutropenia.[60,61] When paclitaxel is used at the recommended dose of 100 mg/m^2, the majority of patients experience neutropenia that persists for 7–8 days. Thrombocytopenia is usually not clinically significant. Fluid retention is a rather unique toxicity associated with the cumulative dose of docetaxel. Early studies reported onset of peripheral edema and weight gain (which is sometimes associated with pleural effusion) at cumulative doses of 400–500 mg/m^2. Corticosteroids, which were initially administered to prevent hypersensitivity reactions, appeared to delay the onset of fluid retention. Current recommendations include administering dexamethasone 8 mg BID PO for 3–5 days beginning the day before docetaxel administration. This corticosteroid regimen delays the onset of symptoms to a median cumulative dose of about 750 mg/m^2.[59] The etiology of this syndrome is unclear, although it does not appear to be related to renal, cardiac, pulmonary, endocrine, or hepatic dysfunction. Diuretics are often useful in alleviating symptoms. After discontinuation of docetaxel, peripheral edema and diuretic requirements resolve gradually over several months.

Skin and nail effects are also prominent with docetaxel and have included nonpruritic erythema (usually of the neck, upper torso, arms, and hands), maculopapular eruptions (which may be associated with desquamation), nail changes, and total alopecia (all body hair, not just scalp hair). Noninfectious conjunctivitis may also occur. Other toxicities associated with docetaxel include neurosensory (e.g., paresthesias) and neuromuscular (e.g., decreased deep tendon reflexes) manifestations, asthenia, myalgias, and occasional hypersensitivity reactions. Pre-existing neurological conditions secondary to disease (e.g., diabetes) or drugs (e.g., cisplatin) may increase the risk of docetaxel-induced neurotoxicity. Although docetaxel is formulated in polysorbate 80 (Tween 80) rather than polyethoxylated castor oil, hypersensitivity reactions were reported during phase I trials. The use of corticosteroids has decreased the incidence of hypersensitivity reactions. Nausea and vomiting are generally mild, and prophylactic antiemetics are not recommended unless the patient has had emetic complications with prior chemotherapy.

Like paclitaxel, docetaxel is practically insoluble in water, and polysorbate 80 is added to the formulation as a surfactant. Addition of the provided diluent may cause foaming of the solution. Gentle manual rotation of the solution for at least 15 seconds will assure full mixture with minimal foaming, although not all foam must dissipate before the preparation process is continued. Docetaxel may be admixed in either 0.9% saline or 5% dextrose in water, and the final concentration should not exceed 0.9 mg/ml. It is not necessary to filter docetaxel during administration, but the solution should be clear and without precipitate.

Camptothecins

The camptothecins are a class of cytotoxic drugs derived from plants such as the *Camptotheca acuminata*. They exert their activity by inhibiting type I DNA topoisomerase. Type I topoisomerase relieves torsion strain in DNA by inducing reversible single strand breaks. The camptothecins bind to the type I DNA topoisomerase–DNA complex and prevent resealing of the single strand breaks. This activity is believed to occur predominantly in the S phase of the cell cycle.[62] Topotecan (Hycamtin) and irinotecan (Camptosar) are the two camptothecins currently available in the United States.

Topotecan

Topotecan is currently indicated for the treatment of small cell lung cancer and metastatic ovarian cancer in patients who have failed first-line or subsequent cisplatin-based chemotherapy. Following administration, topotecan undergoes hydrolysis of its pharmacologically active lactone moiety to a ring-opened hydroxy acid form. This hydrolysis is pH dependent, and at physiological pH the ring-opened form predominates.[63] About 30% of the dose is excreted in the urine. The terminal half-life is 2–3 hours.[64] The manufacturer recommends that the dose be decreased by 50% for patients with moderate renal dysfunction (20–39 ml/min). There is insufficient information to recommend a specific dose adjustment for patients with severe renal dysfunction. Although plasma clearance is decreased in patients with hepatic impairment, patients with serum bilirubin levels between 1.7 and 15 mg/dl appeared to tolerate the drug normally.[65]

The primary dose-limiting toxicity associated with topotecan is myelosuppression manifested as neutropenia, thrombocytopenia, and anemia. This effect does not appear to be cumulative. Emetic complications are generally mild, and prophylactic antiemetics are not generally necessary unless the patient has a history of nausea and vomiting with prior chemotherapy.

Irinotecan

Irinotecan is used to treat patients with metastatic carcinoma of the colon or rectum whose disease has recurred or progressed following a fluorouracil-based chemotherapy regimen. Following administration, irinotecan is converted to an active metabolite, SN-38, in the liver. The SN-38 metabolite subsequently undergoes conjugation to form an inactive glucuronide.[66] Like topotecan, both the parent drug and the SN-38 metabolite exist in an active lactone form and an inactive hydroxy acid anion form; an acidic pH promotes formation of the lactone. The half-life of the parent drug is about 6 hours, and the half-life of the SN-38 metabolite is about 10 hours. (The half-lives of the lactone and hydroxy acid forms do not differ.) Urinary excretion accounts for only a small percentage of irinotecan elimination. Biliary elimination appears to be more important, although specific recommendations for dosage adjustment in patients with this type of hepatic impairment have not been made.[67]

Irinotecan produces significant dose-related myelosuppression, but severe diarrhea is considered the major dose-limiting toxicity. Both early (during the first 24 hours) and late diarrhea may occur. It is usually preceded by abdominal cramping and diaphoresis. The early diarrhea is believed to be a cholinergic effect and typically responds to atropine. Although early diarrhea is generally transient, the late form can be prolonged and result in life-threatening dehydration and electrolyte imbalances. Elderly patients and patients who have previously undergone pelvic irradiation may be at increased risk for this toxicity. Patients with late diarrhea should be carefully monitored and treated with loperamide.[66-68] Patients should be well educated about this toxicity and instructed to keep loperamide on hand and begin treatment at the first episode of diarrhea (see chapter 9). Other medications that may exacerbate diarrhea should be avoided if possible. Fluid and electrolyte replacement therapy should be given whenever necessary. Toxic deaths have resulted from severe irinotecan-induced diarrhea. For patients who experience severe diarrhea, the dose of irinotecan for subsequent courses should be reduced.

Irinotecan is more emetogenic than topotecan, and prophylactic antiemetics (a serotonin antagonist plus dexamethasone) should be given before each course (see chapter 9).

MISCELLANEOUS AGENTS

Asparaginase

The nonessential amino acid asparagine is synthesized in vivo from aspartic acid and glutamine through the enzyme asparagine synthetase. Many lymphocytic leukemia cells lack this enzyme, so their viability depends on the availability of asparagine from the circulating amino acid pool. Asparaginase is an enzyme that causes degradation of asparagine in the circulation, inhibiting the growth of these leukemic cells.

Because asparaginase is a protein purified from bacterial sources, the major toxicity is a hypersensitivity reaction; appropriate precautions should be taken before administering it. It appears to produce fewer severe reactions when given by intramuscular or subcutaneous injection than when given intravenously.[69] Asparaginase is commercially available in the United States in two forms: asparaginase (Elspar), which is derived from *Escherichia coli*, and pegaspargase (Oncaspar). Another type, derived from *Erwinia carotovora*, is available under treatment protocol from Ogden Biosciences of Rockville, Maryland for patients who are hypersensitive to the *E. coli* preparation. Pegaspargase conjugates the asparaginase enzyme with polyethylene glycol (PEG), which extends its biological half-life to 6 days (versus about 1 day for the *E.coli* formulation) and dramatically reduces the immunogenicity of the drug. The PEG product appears to be safe and effective in patients who have had prior allergy to either the *E. coli* or the *Erwinia carotovora* asparaginase.[70]

Asparaginase is relatively nonmyelosuppressive and is used primarily to treat lymphatic malignancies, especially acute lymphocytic leukemia. Besides hypersensitivity, asparaginase may cause other problematic toxicities, including hepatic toxicity, gastrointestinal intolerance, and pancreatitis. The hepatic effects may be severe and include suppression of hepatic protein synthesis. In addition to elevated hepatic transaminases and bilirubin, patients may experience hypoalbuminemia, hypercholesterolemia (due to depressed production of proteins that carry cholesterol), and coagulation defects caused by depressed levels of hepatically produced clotting factors (including prothrombin, fibrinogen, and factors V, VII, VIII, and IX).[71] Acute pancreatitis may range from mild to life threatening. Hyperglycemia may result from depressed insulin production and necessitate exogenous insulin therapy until toxicity has resolved. A central nervous system toxicity characterized by somnolence, lethargy, or confusion may be observed in up to 25% of patients. The effects may be worse in elderly patients and may result from alterations of amino acid metabolism in the brain.

Hydroxyurea

Hydroxyurea (Hydrea) acts by inhibiting the enzyme ribonucleoside diphosphate reductase, which converts ribonucleotides to deoxyribonucleotides, and thus impairs DNA synthesis. It is available only in an oral formulation and is rapidly absorbed. Hydroxyurea is capable of rapidly killing circulating leukemic cells and is therefore used primarily for cytoreduction when leukemic cell counts are dangerously high. It is also used occasionally to treat head and neck tumors. Myelosuppression is the most common toxicity of hydroxyurea; in the treatment of hematological malignancies, however, this is usually the desired therapeutic effect. Because this is a dose-related effect, the dose must be carefully titrated to the desired level of myelosuppression. Patients may also experience mild to moderate nausea, vomiting, diarrhea, and skin rashes.

SUMMARY

Most cytotoxic chemotherapy drugs damage cancer cells by either interfering with the synthesis of the precursors of DNA or chemically interacting with the DNA itself. The alkylating agents, the intercalating agents, and the plant alkaloids cause damage directly to the DNA, whereas the antimetabolites interfere with the synthesis of DNA. Damage to DNA produced by chemotherapy drugs may include cross-links between the two strands, single or double strand breaks, or changes in the conformation. Each type of injury may result in the inability of the DNA to replicate itself, ultimately leading to cell death.

Most chemotherapy drugs are cleared from the body via either renal or hepatic mechanisms, and organ dysfunction may lead to increased concentrations and subsequent toxicities. Knowledge of drug disposition is necessary to make informed decisions about dosages in the face of significant organ dysfunction.

REFERENCES

1. Schilsky RL, Bailey BD, Chabner BA. Methotrexate polyglutamate synthesis by cultured human breast cancer cells. *Proc Natl Acad Sci USA* 1980;77:2919–22.
2. Pinedo HM, Zaharko DS, Bull JM, et al. The relative contribution of drug concentration and duration of exposure to mouse bone marrow toxicity during continuous methotrexate infusion. *Cancer Res* 1977;37:445–50.
3. Matherly LH, Barlowe CK, Goldman ID. Antifolate polyglutamylation and competitive drug displacement at dihydrofolate reductase as important elements in leucovorin rescue in L1210 cells. *Cancer Res* 1986;46:588–93.
4. Golden A, Mantel I, Greenhouse SW, et al. Effect of delayed administration of citrovorum factor on antileukemic effectiveness of aminopterin in mice. *Cancer Res* 1954;14:43–8.
5. Allegra C. Antifolates. In: Chabner BA, Collins JM, editors. *Cancer Chemotherapy: Principles and Practice.* New York: JB Lippincott; 1990. p. 110–53.
6. Erlichman C. Pharmacology of anticancer drugs. In: Tannock IF, Hill RP, editors. *The Basic Science of Oncology.* 2nd ed. New York: McGraw-Hill; 1992. p. 317–37.
7. Chabner BA. Cytidine analogues. In: Chabner BA, Longo DA, editors. *Cancer Chemotherapy and Biotherapy: Principles and Practice.* 2nd ed. Philadelphia, PA: JB Lippincott; 1996. p. 213–34.
8. Bolwell BJ, Cassileth PA, Gale RP. High dose cytarabine: a review. *Leukemia* 1988;2:253–60.
9. Harris AL, Potter C, Bunch C, et al. Pharmacokinetics of cytosine arabinoside in patients with acute myeloid leukaemia. *Br J Clin Pharmacol* 1979;8:219–26.
10. Wan SH, Huffman DH, Azarnoff DL, et al. Pharmacokinetics of 1-β-D-arabinofuanosylcytosine in humans. *Cancer Res* 1974;34:392–7.
11. Ho DHW, Frei E III. Clinical pharmacology of 1-β-D-arabinofuranosylcytosine. *Clin Pharmacol Ther* 1971;12:944–54.
12. Graves T, Hooks MA. Drug-induced toxicities associated with high-dose cytosine arabinoside infusions. *Pharmacotherapy* 1989;9:23–8.
13. Jolson HM, Bosco L, Bufton MG, et al. Clustering of adverse events: analysis of risk factors for cerebellar toxicity with high-dose cytarabine. *J Natl Cancer Inst* 1992;84:500–5.
14. Lazarus HM, Herzig RH, Herzig GP, et al. Central nervous system toxicity of high-dose systemic cytosine arabinoside. *Cancer* 1981;48:2577–82.
15. Plunkett W, Huang P, Gandhi V. Metabolism and action of fludarabine phosphate. *Semin Oncol* 1990;17(*Suppl* 5):3–17.
16. Huang P, Chubb S, Plunkett W. Termination of DNA synthesis by 9-beta-D-arabinofuranosyl-2-fluoroadenine. A mechanism for cytotoxicity. *J Biol Chem* 1990;265:16617–25.
17. Malspeis L, Grever MR, Staubus AE, et al. Pharmacokinetics of 2-F-ara-A (9-beta-D-arabinofuranosyl-2-fluoroadenine) in cancer patients during the phase I clinical investigation of fludarabine phosphate. *Semin Oncol* 1990;17:18–32.
18. Grever M, Leiby J, Kraut E, et al. A comprehensive phase I and II clinical investigation of fludarabine phosphate. *Semin Oncol* 1990;17:39–42.
19. Hood MA, Finley RS. Fludarabine: a review. *DICP* 1991;25:518–24.
20. Plunkett W, Huang P, Searcy C, et al. Gemcitabine: preclinical pharmacology and mechanisms of action. *Semin Oncol* 1996;23(*Suppl* 10):3–15.
21. Gandhi V, Plunkett W. Modulatory activity of 2′,2′-difluorodeoxycytidine on the phosphorylation and cytotoxicity of arabinosylnucleosides. *Cancer Res* 1990;50:3675–80.
22. Lund B, Kristjansen PEG, Hansen HH. Clinical and preclinical activity of 2′,2′-difluorodeoxycytidine (gemcitabine). *Can-*

cer Treat Rev 1993;19:45–55.
23. Guchelaar HJ, Richel DJ, van Knapen A. Clinical, toxicological and pharmacological aspects of gemcitabine. *Cancer Treat Rev* 1996;22:15–31.
24. Grem JL, Hoth DF, Hamilton MJ, et al. Overview of current status and future direction of clinical trials with 5-fluorouracil in combination with folinic acid. *Cancer Treat Rep* 1987;71: 1249–64.
25. Moertel CG. Chemotherapy for colorectal cancer. *N Engl J Med* 1994;330:1136–42.
26. Poon MA, O'Connell MJ, Wieand HS, et al. Biochemical modulation of fluorouracil with leucovorin; confirmatory evidence of improved therapeutic efficacy in advanced colorectal cancer. *J Clin Oncol* 1991;9:1967–72.
27. Gerstner JB. A prospective randomized clinical trial comparing 5-FU combined with either high or low dose leucovorin for the treatment of colorectal carcinoma [abstract]. *Proc Am Soc Clin Oncol* 1991;10:134.
28. Zimm S, Collins JM, Riccardi R, et al. Variable bioavailability of oral 6-mercaptopurine: is maintenance chemotherapy in acute lymphoblastic leukemia being optimally delivered? *N Engl J Med* 1983;308:1005–9.
29. Petersen AJ, Brown RD, Gibson J, et al. Nucleoside transporters, bcl-2 and apoptosis in CLL cells exposed to nucleoside analogues in vitro. *Eur J Haematol* 1996;56:213–20.
30. Arner ES. On the phosphorylation of 2-chlorodeoxyadenosine (CdA) and its correlation with clinical responses in leukemia treatment. *Leuk Lymphoma* 1996;21:225–31.
31. Szondy Z. The 2-chlorodeoxyadenosine-induced cell death signalling pathway in human thymocytes is different from that induced by 2-chloroadenosine. *Biochem J* 1995;311:585–8.
32. Carson DA, Wasson DB, Beutler E. Antileukemic and immunosuppressive activity of 2-chloro-2′-deoxyadenosine. *Proc Natl Acad Sci USA* 1984;81:2232–6.
33. Dorr RT, Von Hoff D. Cladribine. In: Dorr RT, Von Hoff D, editors. *Cancer Chemotherapy Handbook*. 2nd ed. Norwalk, CT: Appleton & Lange; 1994. p. 298–301.
34. Estey EH, Kurzock R, Kantarjian HM, et al. Treatment of hairy cell leukemia with 2-chlorodeoxyadenosine (2-Cda). *Blood* 1992;79:882–7.
35. O'Dwyer PJ, Wagner B, Leyland-Jones B, et al. 2′-deoxycoformycin (pentostatin) for lymphoid malignancies. *Ann Intern Med* 1988;108:733–43.
36. Seto S, Carrera CJ, Kubota M, et al. Mechanism of deoxyadenosine and 2-chlorodeoxyadenosine toxicity to nondividing human lymphocytes. *J Clin Invest* 1985;75:377–83.
37. Koller CA, Mitchell BS, Grever MR, et al. Treatment of acute lymphoblastic leukemia with 2′-deoxycoformycin: clinical and biochemical consequences of adenosine deaminase inhibition. *Cancer Treat Rep* 1979;63:1949–52.
38. Dorr RT, Von Hoff DD. Pentostatin. In: Dorr RT, Von Hoff DD, editors. *Cancer Chemotherapy Handbook*. 2nd ed. Norwalk, CT: Appleton & Lange; 1994. p. 774–9.
39. Owellen RJ, Hartke CA, Dickerson RM, et al. Inhibition of tubulin-microtubule polymerization by drugs of the vinca alkaloid class. *Cancer Res* 1976;36:1499–502.
40. Drewinko B, Barlogie B. Survival and cycle-progression delay of human lymphoma cells in vitro exposed to Vp-16-213. *Cancer Treat Rep* 1976;60:1295–306.
41. Allen LM, Creaven PJ. Comparison of the human pharmacokinetics of VM-26 and VP-16, two antineoplastic epipodophyllotoxin glucopyranoside derivatives. *Eur J Cancer* 1975;11:697–707.
42. Dorr RT, Von Hoff DD. Teniposide. In: Dorr RT, Von Hoff DD, editors. *Cancer Chemotherapy Handbook*. 2nd ed. Norwalk, CT: Appleton & Lange; 1994. p. 882–9.
43. Holthuis JJ. Etoposide and teniposide. Bioanalysis, metabolism and clinical pharmacokinetics. *Pharm Weekbl Sci* 1988; 10:101–16.
44. Siddal DJ, Martin J, Nunn AJ. Anaphylactic reactions to teniposide. *Lancet* 1989;1:394.
45. Gregory RE, DeLisa AF. Paclitaxel: a new antineoplastic agent for refractory ovarian cancer. *Clin Pharm* 1993;12:401–15.
46. Schiff PB, Fant J, Horwitz SB. Promotion of microtubule assembly in vitro by Taxol. *Nature* 1979;277:665–7.
47. Gianni L, Kearns CM, Giani A, et al. Nonlinear pharmacokinetics and metabolism of paclitaxel and its pharmacodynamic relationships in humans. *J Clin Oncol* 1995;13:180–90.
48. Kearns C, Gianni L, Vigano L, et al. Non-linear pharmacokinetics of Taxol in humans [abstract]. *Proc Am Soc Clin Oncol* 1993;12:135.
49. Huizing MT, Keung ACF, Rosing H, et al. Pharmacokinetics of paclitaxel and metabolites in a randomized comparative study in platinum-pretreated ovarian cancer patients. *J Clin Oncol* 1993;11:2127–35.
50. Tamura T, Sasaki Y, Nishiwaki Y, et al. Phase I and pharmacokinetic study of paclitaxel administered by 3-hour infusion [abstract]. *Proc Am Soc Clin Oncol* 1994;13:132.
51. Dorr RT, Snead K, Liddil JD. Skin ulceration potential of paclitaxel in a mouse skin model in vivo. *Cancer* 1996;78:152–6.
52. DuBois A, Fehr MK, Bochtler H, et al. Clinical course and management of paclitaxel extravasation. *Oncol Rep* 1996;3: 973–4.
53. Herrington JD, Figueroa JA. Severe necrosis due to paclitaxel extravasation. *Pharmacotherapy* 1997;17:163–5.
54. Lavelle F, Bissery MC, Combeau C, et al. Preclinical evaluation of docetaxel (Taxotere). *Semin Oncol* 1995;22(Suppl 4):3–16.
55. Gueritte-Voegelein F, Guenard D, Lavelle F, et al. Relationships between the structure of taxol analogues and their antimitotic activity. *J Med Chem* 1991;34:992–8.
56. Kingston DGI. Taxol: the chemistry and structure-activity relationships of a novel anticancer agent. *Trends Biotechnol* 1994;12:222–7.
57. Hennequin C, Giocanti N, Favaudon V. S-phase specificity of cell killing by docetaxel (Taxotere) in synchronized HeLa cells. *Br J Cancer* 1995;71;1194–8.
58. Bruno R, Hille D, Thomas L, et al. Population pharmacokinetics/pharmacodynamics (PK/PD) of docetaxel (Taxotere) in phase II studies [abstract]. *Proc Am Soc Clin Oncol* 1995;14:457.
59. Burris HA. Optimal use of docetaxel (Taxotere): maximizing its potential. *Anticancer Drugs* 1996;7(Suppl 2):25–28.
60. Ravdin PM, Burris HA, Cook G, et al. Phase II trial of docetaxel in advanced anthracycline-resistant or anthracenedione-resistant breast cancer. *J Clin Oncol* 1995;13:2879–85.
61. Valero V, Holmes FA, Walters RS. Phase II trial of docetaxel: a new, highly effective antineoplastic agent in the management of patients with anthracycline-resistant metastatic breast cancer. *J Clin Oncol* 1995;13:2886–94.
62. Dennis MJ, Beijnen JH, Grochow LB, et al. An overview of

the clinical pharmacology of topotecan. *Semin Oncol* 1997;24(*Suppl* 5):12–8.
63. Grochow LB, Rowinsky EK, Johnson R, et al. Pharmacokinetics and pharmacodynamics of topotecan in patients with advanced cancer. *Drug Metab Dispos* 1992;20:706–13.
64. Takimoto CH, Arbuck SG. The camptothecins. In: Chabner BA, Longo DL, editors. *Cancer Chemotherapy and Biotherapy: Principles and Practice*. 2nd ed. Philadelphia, PA: JB Lippincott; 1996. p. 463–84.
65. O'Reilly S, Rowinsky E, Slichenmyer W, et al. Phase I and pharmacologic study of topotecan in patients with impaired hepatic function. *J Natl Cancer Inst* 1996;88:817–24.
66. O'Reilly S, Rowinsky EK. The clinical status of irinotecan (CPT-11), a novel water soluble camptothecin analogue: 1996. *Crit Rev Hematol Oncol* 1996;24:47–70.
67. Gupta E, Lestingi TM, Mick R, et al. Metabolic fate of irinotecan in humans: correlation of glucuronidation with diarrhea. *Cancer Res* 1994;54:3723–7.
68. Rowinsky ED, Grochow LB, Ettinger DS, et al. Phase I and pharmacokinetic study of the novel topoisomerase I inhibitor 7-ethyl 1-1 0-[4-(1-piperidino)-1-piperidino] carbonyloxycampothecin (CPT-11) administered as a ninety minute infusion every 3 weeks. *Cancer Res* 1994;54:427–33.
69. Nesbit M, Karon M, Chard R, et al. Evaluation of intramuscular versus intravenous administration of L-asparaginase in childhood leukemia. *Am J Pediatr Hematol Oncol* 1979;1:9–13.
70. Capizzi RL. Asparaginase revisited. *Leuk Lymphoma* 1993;10(*Suppl*):147–50.
71. Ramsay NKC, Coccia PF, Krivit W, et al. The effect of L-asparaginase on plasma coagulation factors in acute lymphoblastic leukemia. *Cancer* 1977;40:1398–401.

Suggested Reference Texts

The following are useful reference texts that provide more in-depth information regarding cytotoxic drugs:

Dorr RT, Von Hoff DD, editors. *Cancer Chemotherapy Handbook*. 2nd ed. Norwalk, CT: Appleton & Lange; 1994.

Chabner BA, Collins JM, editors. *Cancer Chemotherapy: Principles and Practice*. Philadelphia, PA: JB Lippincott; 1990.

Perry MC, editor. *The Chemotherapy Source Book*. Baltimore, MD: Williams & Wilkins; 1992.

Pratt WB, Ruddon RW, Ensminger WD, et al., editors. *The Anticancer Drugs*. 2nd ed. New York: Oxford Pr; 1994.

SELF-STUDY QUESTIONS

1. Describe how high-dose methotrexate followed by leucovorin preferentially kills tumor cells over normal cells.

2. List at least three mechanisms by which methotrexate elimination can be slowed, resulting in prolonged drug exposure.

3. Cytarabine is retained within cells significantly longer than gemcitabine.
   a. true
   b. false

4. Which of the following should be administered with high-dose cytarabine?
   a. sodium bicarbonate
   b. corticosteroid eye drops
   c. antiemetics
   d. only b and c
   e. all of the above

5. The pulmonary toxicity associated with fludarabine is:
   a. related to the cumulative dose.
   b. seen only after high-dose therapy and is irreversible.
   c. not dose related and resolves spontaneously.
   d. a hypersensitivity reaction.

6. If a patient receiving gemcitabine therapy experiences a mild rise in serum transaminases, which of the following responses is most appropriate?
   a. Therapy should be discontinued immediately.
   b. Therapy should be continued because the effect is usually transient.
   c. The dose should be reduced by 50%.
   d. The dose should be reduced by 25%.

7. Explain the rationale for administering leucovorin with fluorouracil.

8. When fluorouracil is given by continuous infusion, the most signficant toxicity is/are:
   a. myelosuppression, predominantly leukopenia.
   b. anemia.
   c. stomatitis and diarrhea.
   d. nausea and vomiting.

9. The severity of neutropenia, the major dose-limiting toxicity of paclitaxel, is influenced by:

   a. renal function.
   b. the length of the infusion.
   c. premedication with corticosteroids.
   d. only b and c.
   e. all of the above

10. Fluid retention that may include pleural effusion following docetaxel administration is related to:

    a. renal dysfunction.
    b. congestive heart failure.
    c. hepatic dysfunction (bilirubin above normal range).
    d. cumulative dose.
    e. c and d.

11. Topotecan and irinotecan exert their cytotoxic activity by:

    a. intercalation, similar to doxorubicin.
    b. inhibition of type II DNA topoisomerase, similar to doxorubicin.
    c. inhibition of type I DNA topoisomerase, a novel mechanism.
    d. stimulation of mitotic spindle formation.

12. If patients experience diarrhea within 24 hours of irinotecan therapy, they should receive _____. If diarrhea occurs >24 hours after treatment, therapy should be immediately initiated with _____.

    a. atropine, loperamide
    b. loperamide, atropine
    c. loperamide, loperamide
    d. loperamide, Kaopectate
    e. oral vancomycin

13. Fewer severe hypersensitivity reactions are reported when asparaginase is given by intramuscular injection than when it is given by intravenous injection.

    a. true
    b. false

14. Hypotension can occur when _____ is/are infused rapidly.

    a. vincristine
    b. etoposide
    c. cytarabine
    d. fluorouracil
    e. all of the above

15. _____ and _____ are common side effects of cladribine.

    a. Severe neutropenia, hypersensitivity reactions
    b. Fever, lymphopenia
    c. Conjunctivitis, fever
    d. Neuropathy, hypersensitivity reactions
    e. Diarrhea, lymphopenia

16. Compare the mechanisms of action of the vinca alkaloids and the taxanes.

Chapter 5
Pharmacology of Immunotherapies

Carol Balmer, Pharm.D.
Associate Professor
University of Colorado School of Pharmacy
Denver, Colorado

Review of Immune Function	68
Classification of Immunotherapies	70
Interferons	71
Antitumor Mechanisms	72
Pharmacokinetics	72
Clinical Applications	72
Toxicity	73
Interleukins	73
Antitumor Mechanisms	73
Pharmacokinetics	73
Clinical Applications	74
Toxicity	74
Monoclonal Antibodies	75
Antitumor Mechanisms	75
Clinical Applications	75
Toxicity	76
Tumor Vaccines	76
Gene Therapy of Cancer	76
Alternative Cancer Therapies	77
Summary	77
References	78
Self-Study Questions	79

The immune system has long been known to be a defense against disease-causing bacteria and viruses, but it is now recognized to be an effective antitumor defense as well. The original rationale for studying the immune system as an anticancer tool was based on circumstantial evidence. Malignant cells sporadically arise in healthy bodies as a result of mutations, but not all of these malignant cells give rise to clinically evident cancers. Historically, there are rare but well-documented reports of spontaneous tumor regression in patients with metastatic cancers, particularly renal cell cancer and malignant melanoma. Distant tumor metastases have been known to regress following surgical removal of a primary tumor mass, even though the metastatic sites were not touched by the surgical procedure. The incidence of some tumors is increased in patients who are immunosuppressed, such as patients who receive chronic immunosuppressive drug therapy to prevent rejection of transplanted organs. It is also well established that cancer is more common among the elderly, who have less active immune systems than the young. It is evident from all of these facts that an intact immune system can identify malignant cells and destroy them. And, in contrast to the relatively indiscriminate effects of cytotoxic agents, the immune system can distinguish between foreign substances (such as tumor cells) and normal body tissues. Normal cells are recognized as self and are not destroyed.[1,2]

The possibility that the cancer-controlling potential of the human immune system might be harnessed and directed to destroy cancer cells has been under intense investigation for >20 years. These efforts are called by many names: biological cancer therapy, biotherapy, immunotherapy, and biological response modification. They include all cancer treatment approaches that attempt to influence the patient's immune response to a tumor. In its broadest definition, biological therapy is any therapeutic alteration in the relationship between the patient and the tumor, except direct killing of the tumor, that improves the ability of the patient to reject the tumor.[1] By this interpretation, biological therapy can include treatments to help the bone marrow recover from chemotherapy, or even chemopreventive strategies. For the purposes of this chapter, however, *biological therapy* refers to the use of immune system therapies to treat cancer.

There are many categories of biological response modifiers used for cancer immunotherapy. Agents used in biological therapy include cytokines (the protein products of immune cells), more complex proteins (monoclonal antibodies), and all or part of tumor cells (tumor vaccines or infusions of cytotoxic cells). The cytokines most commonly used in the treatment of cancer are interferon alfa (IFN-α) and interleukin 2 (aldesleukin or IL-2).

This chapter will include a brief review of the immune system, and then it will focus on IFN-α and IL-2, the most commonly used biological anticancer therapies. It will then address emerging biological therapies: monoclonal antibodies, tumor vaccines, and gene therapy. The chapter will conclude with a brief discussion of alternative cancer treatments that are claimed to work by unproven effects on the immune system.

After completing this chapter, the reader should be able to:

1. Outline the categories of biological agents used for cancer treatment, and classify each as an active or passive intervention and as a specific or nonspecific biological therapy.
2. Describe the proposed mechanisms of action and clinical uses of IFN-α and IL-2 as anticancer agents.
3. Describe general strategies to prevent or manage the side effects of IFN-α and IL-2 therapy.
4. Briefly describe the rationale, advantages, and limitations of monoclonal antibodies and immunoconjugates in the management of cancer.
5. Describe the rationale, potential roles, and limitations of tumor vaccines and gene therapy in the prevention and treatment of cancer.

REVIEW OF IMMUNE FUNCTION

The function of the immune system depends on the integrated action of many cells and their products, usually proteins, which may interact in multiple ways (Figure 5-1). Because of the complex interactions among these cells and proteins, any intervention may create more than one action within the immune system. Some of these effects may be stimulatory, but at the same time they might suppress other components of the immune system or stimulate components that were not targeted or anticipated. A brief overview of the immune system's role in cancer treatment is provided below. The reader is referred to the texts in the reference list at the end of this chapter for more detailed descriptions of immune system function.[1–4]

Tumor cells arise from normal cells that have been altered by mutagenic changes, as described in chapter 1. They are distinguished as foreign to the cells of the immune system by the presence of antigens on their surfaces. Although a variety of antigens are present on tumor cells, the tumor antigens are globally referred to as tumor-associated antigens (TAAs). Not all TAAs are truly immunogenic, because they might not be strong enough to evoke an immune response, but all are antigenic—that is, foreign when compared with normal cells of the same tissue.[1]

The immune response to tumors, like the immune response to such foreign substances as bacteria or allergens, includes a humoral (or antibody-mediated) component and a cell-mediated response. Cell-mediated immunity is more important to destruction of cancer cells than antibody-mediated responses. The most important cells in cancer surveillance and destruction are lymphocytes and macrophages.

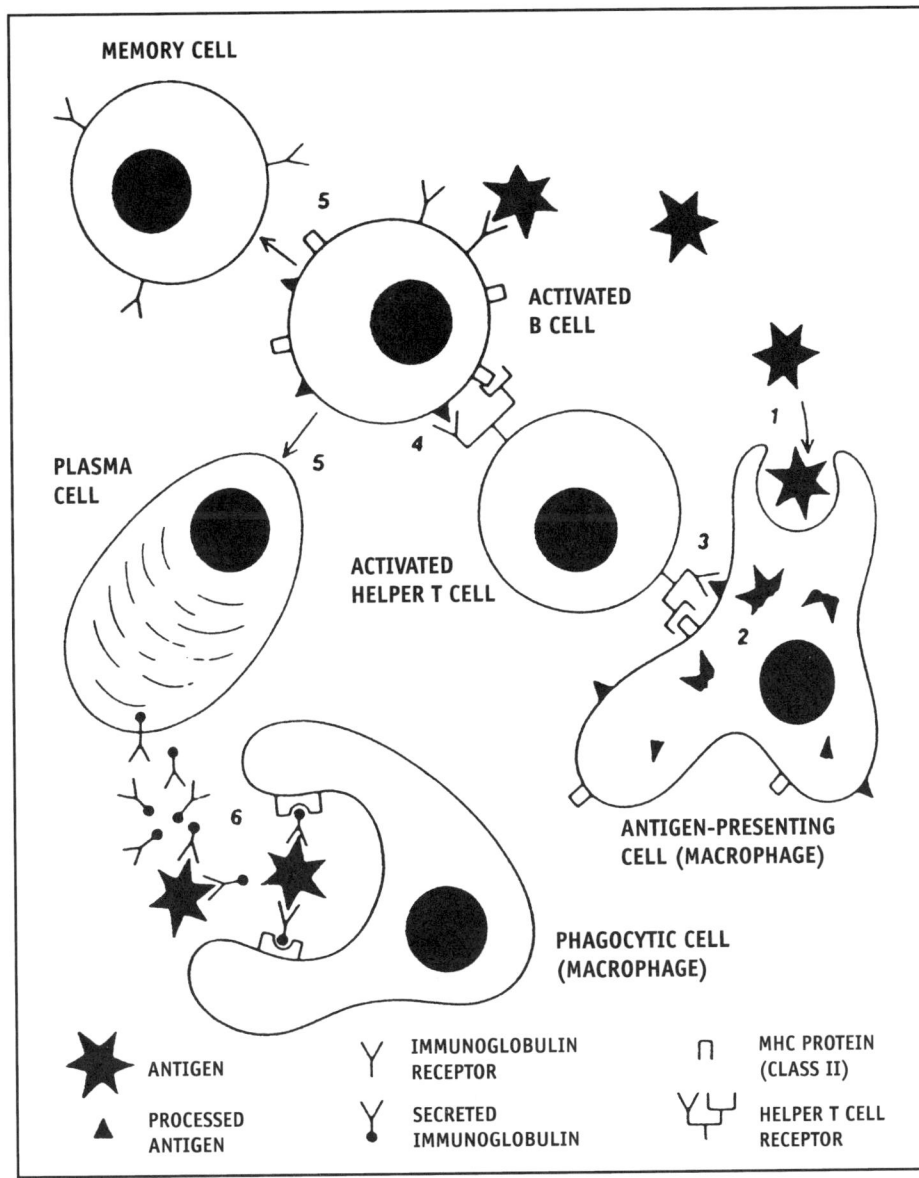

Figure 5-1. Immune system response to an antigen. First, the antigen is taken up by an antigen-presenting cell (1), such as a macrophage, which processes (2) the antigen and displays it on its surface. There it is recognized by a helper T cell, which is then activated (3) and in turn activates B cells that recognize the same antigen (4). The B lymphocytes then differentiate (5), some into memory cells and some into antibody-secreting plasma cells. The antibodies produced by those plasma cells bind to cells expressing that antigen, thereby marking the cells for destruction by other components of the immune system, such as macrophages (6). Marked cells may also be destroyed by a variety of killer cells, such as cytotoxic T lymphocytes.

SOURCE: reprinted with permission from Tonegawa S. The molecules of the immune system. *Sci Am* 1995;253:122.

Lymphocytes are classified as B, T, or null cells. T cells, or thymus-derived lymphocytes, are the most important in cancer defense. They are subdivided into helper T cells, cytotoxic T lymphocytes (CTLs or killer T cells), memory T cells, and suppressor T cells. Helper T cells have a specific receptor that is programmed to recognize a single antigen. After recognizing the antigen and receiving appropriate immune signals, helper T cells produce small peptide lymphokines (cytokines produced by lymphocytes). Lymphokines are soluble proteins that circulate within the blood and lymphatic tissue to signal other helper T cells, CTLs, and macrophages to multiply, differentiate, and mobilize against the cells displaying that specific TAA. In this way, the helper T cells act as the master controllers of the immune response, without directly attacking tumor cells. Attacking is the role of CTLs and a variety of other killer cells, such as natural killer (NK) cells. Some of the cytokines produced by T cells include interferon gamma, tumor necrosis factors (TNFs), and a variety of interleukins. CTLs are believed to kill tumor cells by releasing cytotoxic substances into the microenvironment around the tumor cells. Some of these substances destroy the tumor cell by perforating the cell membrane, resulting in cell lysis.[1-4]

The main role of suppressor T cells appears to be slowing the immune response. They stop the immune response that has been activated against a specific antigen to prevent the immune response from escalating and damaging normal cells. There is evidence that some tumors can activate suppressor T cells and suppress the immune system responses directed against the tumor.

Other important cells that are part of cell-mediated

immunity are macrophages and NK cells. Macrophages function as antigen-presenting cells. They process TAAs and present them to helper T cells to initiate an immune response against the tumor cells. Macrophages can also act as tumor cell killers, either by phagocytizing their target cells or by releasing toxic substances in close proximity to the cells. Unlike CTLs, which only destroy cells that carry a specific stimulating antigen, macrophages are nonspecific killers and, once activated by lymphokines, can kill a variety of tumor cell types.[1–4]

NK cells are large lymphocytes that are also nonspecific tumor cell killers. They can lyse tumor cells without prior exposure to TAAs. When NK cells are exposed to the lymphokine IL-2, they proliferate and become hyperactivated, which permits them to kill a wider range of tumor cells. These hyperactivated NK cells are called lymphokine-activated killer (LAK) cells. LAK cells are more efficient killers than NK cells, requiring fewer cells to destroy each tumor cell, and they can kill tumor cells that are resistant to NK cells. Tumor-infiltrating lymphocytes (TILs) are even more efficient tumor cell killers. TILs are the subpopulation of LAK cells found within a patient's tumor mass, and they are believed to be the most efficient killer cells of that tumor.[1]

B cells differentiate into plasma cells, which in turn produce antibodies. All of the plasma cells that arise from a single B cell produce identical antibody molecules (monoclonal antibodies). Each antibody reacts with a single antigen, in a unique relationship often described as a lock matched to a key. When the antibody interlocks with the antigen on a cell, it marks the cell for destruction. The actual destruction of the cell may occur in several ways. Antibodies can bind to both tumor cells and to complement proteins on the cell surface. Activation of the appropriate complement proteins in the complement cascade results ultimately in the formation of a membrane attack complex. Once the complex is inserted in the wall of the target tumor cell, it makes a channel that permits fluids and molecules to flow in and out of the cell, resulting in cell lysis. Antibodies can also function to bind cells of the cellular arm of the immune system (such as macrophages, NK cells, and LAK cells) more tightly to tumor cells. When the tumor cells are destroyed by these cytotoxic cells, with the assistance of antibodies, the process is called antibody-dependent cell-mediated cytotoxicity (ADCC).[1,3]

CLASSIFICATION OF IMMUNOTHERAPIES

As with other pharmaceutical agents, such as immunizations and vaccinations, that affect the immune system, biological response modifiers used in cancer treatment may be classified by their interaction with the immune system (active or passive) and by their degree of specificity. Active interventions attempt to stimulate the host's natural immune responses to the tumor. Passive methods transfer preformed defenses into the cancer patient. Examples of passive immunity include administration of antitumor antibodies or immune cells from other individuals to a patient. Either of these approaches can be specific or nonspecific; that is, they can focus on one or many facets of immune function. Early attempts at immunotherapy of cancer focused on nonspecific modification of the immune response with microbial agents, such as the Bacillus Calmette-Guérin (BCG) vaccine.[1,2] The rationale was that the defenses of the immune system would be mobilized to respond to the apparent tuberculosis infection caused by the vaccine and that this generalized increase in activity might

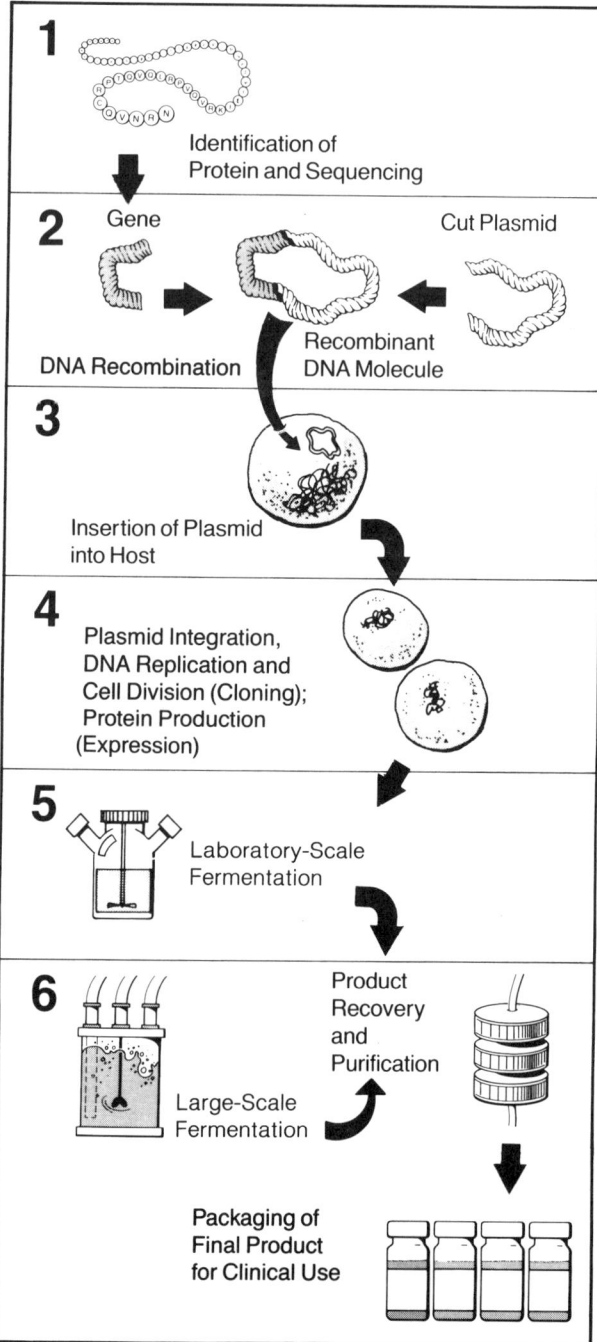

Figure 5-2. How recombinant DNA is made
SOURCE: reprinted with permission from Genentech, Inc.

result in destruction of cancer cells as well. Because of the indiscriminate action of agents such as BCG vaccine, both immune-stimulating and immunosuppressive components of the immune system are augmented. The ultimate effect on the host reflects the net effects on the immunoregulatory system and is not predictable.[1,2] BCG vaccine is still used as a bladder instillation for the treatment of localized bladder tumors, but the clinical results in treating systemic cancers with nonspecific approaches, such as BCG vaccine, have been disappointing.[5]

Scientific advances in the last two decades have permitted the development of more specific agents. One of the most important advances was recombinant DNA technology (Figure 5-2). With this technology, the gene that codes for production of a desired protein is removed from a human cell. The DNA of a simple organism, usually a bacterium or a yeast, is opened, the human gene is inserted, and the organism's DNA is recombined. The organism and all of its offspring then begin to produce the desired human protein, in addition to their normal complement of proteins. The human protein can be isolated, purified, and then packaged to be administered as a drug product.[6] Interferons, interleukins, and hematopoietic growth factors are examples of cytokine proteins used in oncology that are prepared using this technology. Recombinant DNA products are generally used to supplement the body's normal production of these cytokines, to magnify the normal effects of that cytokine within the immune system.

Recombinant DNA technology is useful for producing relatively simple proteins but cannot be used to produce more complex proteins, such as monoclonal antibodies. A second technological development, hybridoma technology, made production of pure antibodies possible. Plasma cells that produce antibodies do not normally live long in culture, but they can be made immortal by fusion with myeloma cells. Myeloma cells are long-lived, altered plasma cells. The resulting hybrid cell, a hybridoma, can be grown in the ascitic fluid of mice or in cell culture, and its antibody products can be harvested. Hybridoma technology using mouse ascitic fluid as a culture medium is illustrated in Figure 5-3.

INTERFERONS

Interferons are the most thoroughly studied and most widely used biological response modifiers. Interferons are proteins with antiviral, immunomodulatory, and antitumor actions that are produced by nucleated cells in response to viral infection or other IFN-inducers. Interferons were discovered almost accidentally in the late 1950s when two scientists studying viruses noticed that the growth of one virus in tissue could

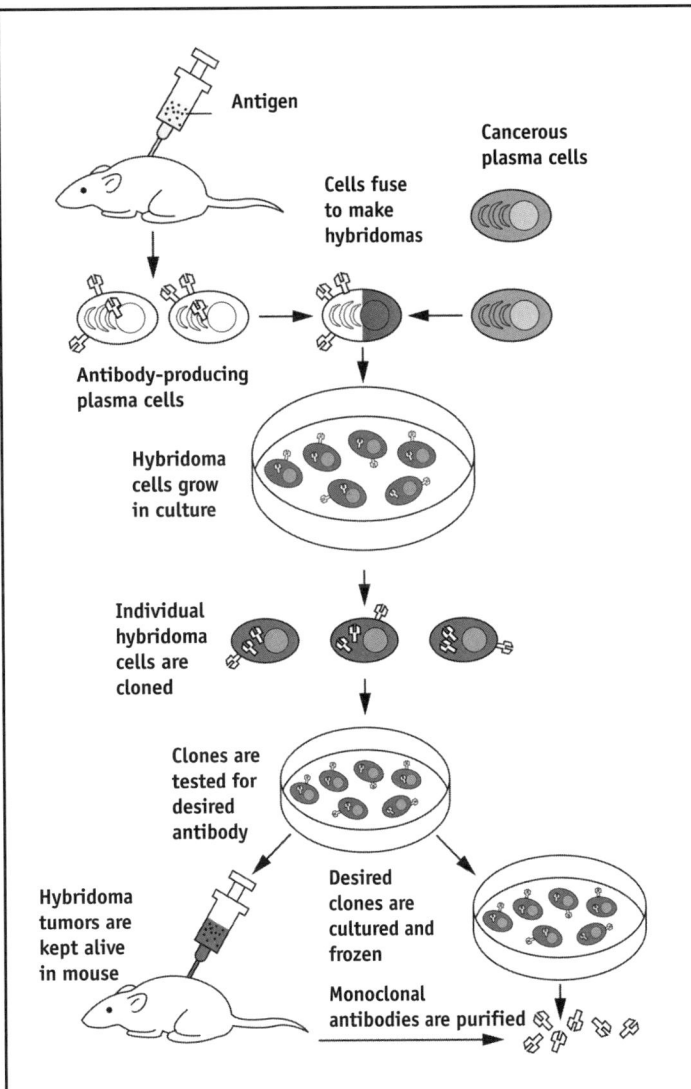

Figure 5-3. Using hybridoma technology to make monoclonal antibodies
SOURCE: Schlinder LW. Understanding the immune system [monograph]. Bethesda, MD: National Cancer Institute; 1993. NIH Publication No. 93-529.

interfere with the growth of another virus in the same tissue. They called the substance that caused this viral growth inhibition *interferon*. It was not until 20 years later that the antitumor activity of interferons was discovered, making them the first human proteins proven effective in cancer treatment.[7-9]

The three major classes of interferons vary in their antigenic makeup, biological actions, and pharmacologic properties. The largest and best-studied class is interferon alpha (IFN-α), also called *leukocyte interferon* because it is produced by human leukocytes. There are more than fifteen subtypes of IFN-α. Interferon alpha-2 (or interferon alfa-2b, USAN) and interferon alpha-A (interferon alfa-2a, USAN) are pure preparations of single alpha subtypes and have been commercially available in recombinant forms for >10 years. These two products differ in the sequence of two amino acids. Other IFN-α products are polyclonal mixtures of alpha subtypes. Interferon doses are usually measured in megaunits (million units or 10^6 units) of antiviral activity.

Interferons beta and gamma are also commercially available. Two forms of IFN-β are approved for use in treating multiple sclerosis. IFN-γ is indicated for management of chronic granulomatous disease. Neither of these interferons is approved by the FDA for anticancer use or widely used for investigational anticancer treatments. IFN-β and IFN-γ will not be addressed in this chapter.

Antitumor Mechanisms

Precisely how interferons function as antitumor agents is unknown, although their antiviral mechanism of action is well characterized. Their effects on tumor cells are believed to be a combination of several mechanisms (Figure 5-4). Interferons were first believed to function as antitumor agents by stimulating or activating effector cells in the immune system. This mechanism is still recognized as a component of their antitumor action: IFN-α is known to enhance the killing activity of NK cells, and CTLs, and to increase macrophage activity and ADCC. However, several other actions are now recognized to be of equal or greater importance. IFN-α enhances the expression of a variety of antigens on the tumor cell surface, including TAAs and major histocompatibility (MHC) class I antigens, that are important in recognition of self. The net result of these effects on surface antigens is to make the tumor cells appear more immunogenic, or more foreign, so that they are more easily recognized by effector cells of the immune system. Other pharmacologic actions of the interferons include antiproliferative effects, caused by a lengthening of all phases of the cell cycle, and modulation of the expression of oncogenes. Interferons also induce several enzymes, such as 2,5A synthetase, protein kinase, and phosphodiesterase enzymes, that together inhibit RNA, DNA, and protein synthesis. Although enzyme induction is critical to the antiviral mechanism of action of interferons, it is important in antitumor actions as well. Interferons can also interfere with angiogenesis, the growth of new blood vessels needed to support tumor growth, and can induce tumor cell differentiation.[3,7-9]

Pharmacokinetics

Interferons, like most immunotherapies, are proteins, which are destroyed by digestive enzymes and must therefore be administered parenterally. They are well absorbed after intramuscular or subcutaneous administration, although peak plasma concentrations are delayed for about 4–7 hours. The interferons penetrate the central nervous system very poorly. They have short terminal half-lives of about 4–5 hours. Renal secretion and catabolism are believed to be responsible for interferon elimination. Hepatic metabolism is considered minor.[7,8]

Clinical Applications

The commercially available IFN-α preparations have their best

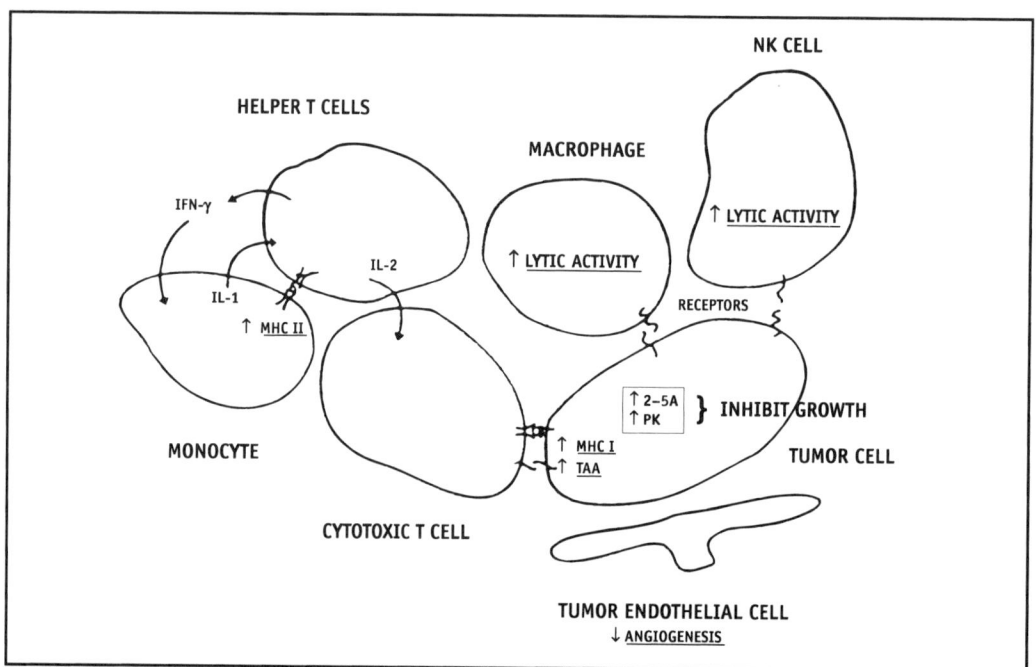

Figure 5-4. Interferon antitumor mechanisms. Boxed items are direct mechanisms; underlined items are indirect mechanisms. IFN-γ, interferon gamma; IL-1, interleukin 1; IL-2, interleukin 2; MHC-I, major histocompatibility complex I; MHC-II, major histocompatibility complex II; NK, natural killer cell; PK, protein kinase; TAA, tumor-associated antigen; 2–5A, 2,5A synthetase.

SOURCE: adapted with permission from reference 7, p. 597.

established antitumor activity in the management of hematological malignancies. They were first approved for management of hairy cell leukemia, a rare leukemia that responds poorly to the effects of conventional antileukemic drugs. IFN-α was the first drug found to be effective in the management of hairy cell leukemia and formed the cornerstone for treatment of this disorder for nearly a decade. Its use has recently been displaced by new purine analogues, such as cladribine.

At present, the most important clinical uses of IFN-α are in the management of patients with chronic myelogenous leukemia and in the adjuvant treatment of patients with surgically resected malignant melanoma at high risk of recurrence. IFN-α is also of clinical value in the management of patients with multiple myeloma, low-grade lymphomas, Kaposi's sarcoma, or renal cell cancer.[7–10]

Toxicity

The most common toxicity of the interferons is an acute flu-like syndrome of fever, muscle aches, chills, and headaches that persist for several hours after drug administration. These symptoms may be prevented or relieved with acetaminophen. They are also subjectively less troublesome when IFN-α is administered in the evening hours, which allows the patient to sleep through the period of discomfort. Rapid tolerance to the flu-like symptoms develops with daily or every-other-day administration. The other characteristic syndrome is a neurological complex of weakness, lethargy, and fatigue that can be dose limiting. When disabling, this syndrome can be managed by withholding doses until symptoms have decreased, then reinstituting therapy at a reduced dose. Leukopenia, thrombocytopenia, nausea, vomiting, and alopecia may also occur. In contrast to conventional cytotoxics, these are rarely severe, except at high doses. Liver transaminase increases are common but rarely severe.[7–9] However, careful monitoring of liver function tests is essential, especially with patients receiving high-dose regimens. Two patients died of liver failure in a recent study of high-dose IFN-α administered for adjuvant treatment of melanoma.[10]

INTERLEUKINS

Interleukins are lymphokines with biological effects on themselves or on other cells. More than a dozen interleukins have been identified, but the most widely studied, and the only interleukin approved for treatment of cancer, is interleukin 2 (aldesleukin, IL-2). IL-2 was originally called T-cell growth factor because it aids the growth and differentiation of T cells.

Antitumor Mechanisms

The most direct action of IL-2 as an antitumor agent is stimulating the growth of killer lymphocytes, including LAK cells and TILs, that recognize and destroy tumor cells. IL-2 binds to the IL-2 receptors of lymphocytes, especially T cells

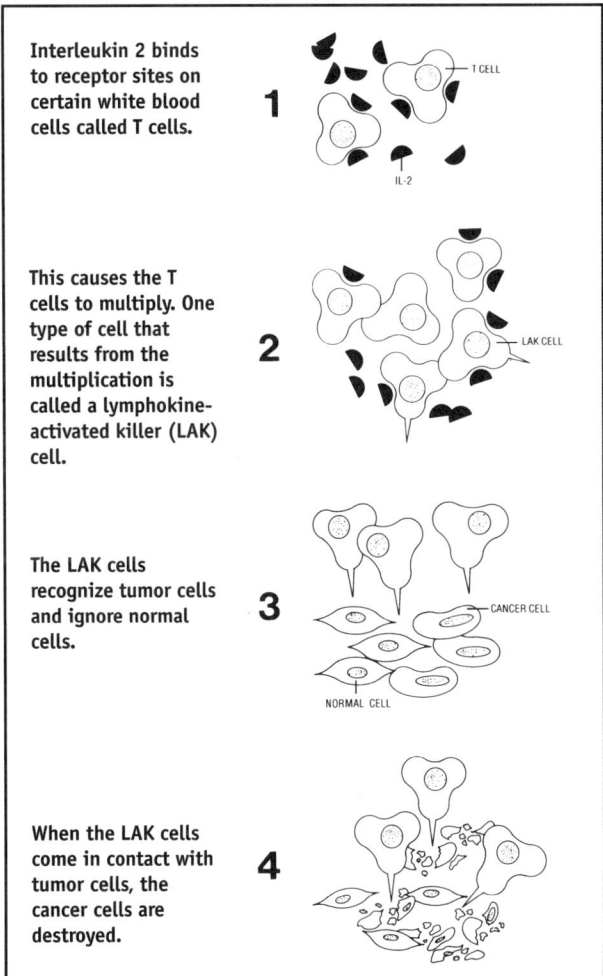

Figure 5-5. Antitumor mechanism of interleukin 2

SOURCE: reprinted with permission from Cetus Corporation, Emeryville, CA.

and NK cells. Binding promotes proliferation of antigen-specific activated T cells and potentiates their cytotoxic activity. IL-2 also enhances the cytotoxic activity of NK cells, which then become LAK cells or TILs. The process of cell destruction is illustrated in Figure 5-5. IL-2 also stimulates the formation of proteins involved in the cell-killing process, such as proteins that perforate the tumor cell membranes to cause their lysis.[11–13]

Killer cell growth may be stimulated in vivo or in vitro. When lymphocytes are taken from the patient, incubated with IL-2, and then reinfused into the patient, the process becomes a form of adoptive immunotherapy, because the patient "adopts" the immune cells that were grown in culture.

Pharmacokinetics

Pharmacokinetics of IL-2 follow a two-compartment model, with rapid distribution to extravascular compartments and a beta half-life of 30–120 minutes. IL-2 is metabolized in cells lining the proximal tubules of the kidneys and is eliminated primarily by renal tubular filtration. Bioavailability following intramuscular administration is about 37%.[13]

Clinical Applications

IL-2 therapy can produce antitumor responses in patients with some tumor types that are highly resistant to treatment with conventional cytotoxic drugs, particularly malignant melanoma and renal cell carcinoma. Although the number of patients with these cancers who respond to IL-2 treatment is small (approximately 15–20%), some responses are complete and may persist for several years. Encouraging results have also been produced when IL-2 is combined with other biological therapies, such as interferon therapy. The combination of IL-2 with interferon is theoretically appealing. One proposed action of IFN-α is enhanced expression of TAAs, which makes the tumor cells more antigenic. The enhanced expression of TAAs increases the likelihood that killer cells, whose growth and proliferation is stimulated by IL-2 administration, will recognize the tumor cells and destroy them.[14,15]

Toxicity

IL-2 therapy is frequently complicated by severe toxicity. In addition to fever, chills, rash, fatigue, hepatotoxicity, and eosinophilia in most patients, IL-2 produces a characteristic capillary or vascular leak syndrome that leads to loss of intravascular fluid into soft tissues. Together with a decrease in systemic vascular resistance and resulting renal damage, this

Table 5-1. Guidelines for Withholding IL-2 Therapy

Organ System	Hold Dose For	Restart If
Cardiovascular	Atrial fibrillation, ventricular tachycardia, bradycardia that requires treatment or is recurrent or persistent	Patient asymptomatic with full recovery to normal sinus rhythm
	Systolic pressure <90 mmHg with increasing requirement for pressors	Systolic pressure ≥90 mmHg and stable or improving pressor requirement
	Any ECG change consistent with MI or ischemia with or without chest pain; suspicion of cardiac ischemia	Patient asymptomatic, MI ruled out, clinical suspicion of angina low
Pulmonary	O_2 saturation <94% on room air or <90% with 2 L O_2 by nasal prongs	O_2 saturation ≥94% on room air or ≥90% with 2 L O_2 by nasal prongs
CNS	Mental status changes, including moderate confusion or agitation	Mental status changes resolved
Systemic	Sepsis syndrome, patient clinically unstable	Sepsis syndrome resolved, patient clinically stable, infection under treatment
Renal	Serum creatinine ≥4.5 mg/dl, or ≥4 mg/dl in presence of severe volume overload, acidosis, or hyperkalemia	Serum creatinine <4 mg/dl and fluid and electrolyte status stable
	Persistent oliguria, urine output ≤10 ml/hr for 16–24 hr with rising serum creatinine	Urine output >10 ml/hr with decrease of serum creatinine ≤1.5 mg/dl or normalization
Hepatic	Signs of hepatic failure, including encephalopathy, increasing ascites, liver pain, hypoglycemia	All signs of hepatic failure resolved[a]
Gastrointestinal	Stool guaiac repeatedly ≥3+	Stool guaiac negative
Skin	Bullous dermatitis or marked worsening of pre-existing skin condition (avoid topical steroid therapy)	Resolution of all signs of bullous dermatitis

SOURCE: reprinted with permission from Bruton JK, Koeller JM. Recombinant interleukin-2. *Pharmacotherapy* 1994;14:635–56. IL-2, interleukin 2; ECG, electrocardiogram; MI, myocardial infarction; CNS, central nervous system.
[a]Discontinue all further treatment for that course. Consider starting a new course of treatment at least 7 weeks after cessation of adverse event and hospital discharge.

syndrome produces hypotension and potentially dramatic fluid weight gain and can lead to respiratory distress, congestive heart failure, arrhythmia, or myocardial infarction. The effects are similar to the early stages of septic shock and may be caused by direct damage to endothelial cells lining capillaries, or by the release of other cytokines that indirectly damage these cells.[12–14]

The hypotension resulting from IL-2–induced capillary leak syndrome should be managed with careful fluid administration and early institution of low-dose dopamine infusions. Low-dose dopamine helps maintain blood pressure, minimizes the risks of fluid overload, and supports renal perfusion to decrease the incidence of renal failure.[12–14] Serious toxicities of IL-2 that cannot be managed symptomatically require withholding until the toxicity resolves, then restarting doses (Table 5-1).

Toxicity from IL-2 is dose related, and serious toxicities leading to life-threatening consequences are unlikely with low-dose IL-2 regimens (i.e., 1–3 MIU/m^2 per day). They are common with high-dose regimens (i.e., 9 MIU/m^2 q8hr for 4–5 days).

The death rate due to toxicity during treatment with full FDA-approved doses of IL-2 is about 4%.[14] In lower-dose regimens, mortality is typically 1–1.5%. Careful patient selection to screen for cardiovascular and pulmonary risk factors can minimize the morbidity and mortality associated with therapy. Although IL-2 toxicity is rapidly reversible when treatment is stopped, it requires close patient monitoring and vigorous supportive care.

MONOCLONAL ANTIBODIES

Nearly 100 years ago, Paul Erlich, a German scientist, proposed the use of "bodies which possess a particular affinity for a certain organ" to deliver therapeutic agents to tumors without damaging normal host cells. His vision is closer to reality today, with the use of monoclonal antibodies (MoAbs).

Antitumor Mechanisms

The term *monoclonal* means that all of the antibodies produced by one plasma cell react against a single antigen. The MoAbs used in cancer treatment are directed against TAAs. Because of this specific interaction, MoAbs offer the advantage of relative selectivity—they interact primarily with cells that express their matching antigen. They may be used alone (as naked antibodies) to activate the cell destruction components of the immune system described previously. They may also be conjugated with other therapeutic agents to function as carriers to more directly target tumor cells. These complexes are called immunoconjugates. Some therapeutic agents that can be conjugated to MoAbs include cytotoxic drugs, toxins (creating immunotoxins), or radioisotopes (Figure 5-6).[16–18] Because MoAbs are transferred to patients as preformed antibodies (as opposed to stimulating the body's production of antibodies), they are considered a form of passive immunotherapy.

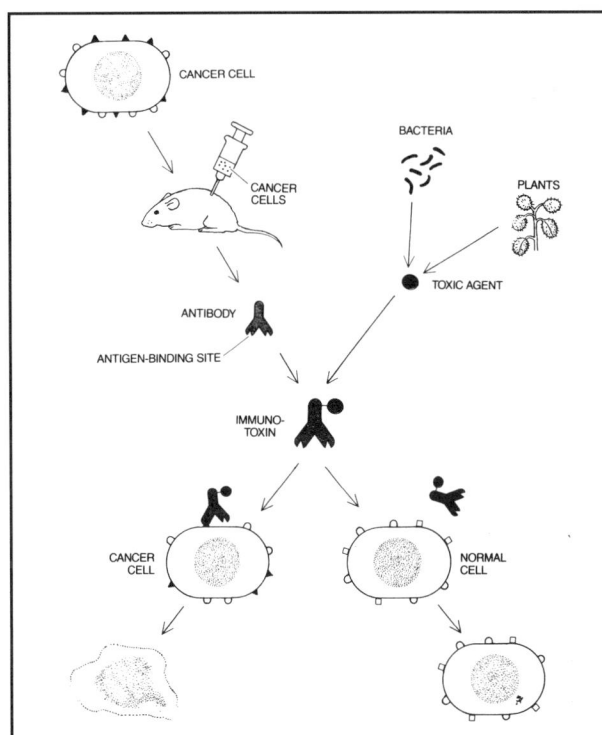

Figure 5-6. Concept of immunoconjugates, illustrated using an immunotoxin example

SOURCE: reprinted with permission from Collier RJ, Kaplan DA. Immunotoxins. *Sci Am* 1984;251:56.

Clinical Applications

MoAbs are currently used primarily for detection of cancer and for screening high-risk populations. The use of radioisotope conjugates for diagnosis is called RAID (radioimmunodetection). RAID may be clinically useful for pre- and post-surgical evaluation of patients, for detection of recurrence, for confirmation of diagnoses made by other methods, and to differentiate tumor tissue from scar tissue. Some of the FDA-approved agents for RAID are listed in Table 5-2. Radioconjugates for treatment of cancer are not as well developed. Their use is referred to as RAIT (radioimmunotherapy).[16]

The first MoAb for the treatment of cancer, rituximab (IDEC C2B8), was approved by the FDA in late 1997 for

Table 5-2. Examples of FDA-Approved Cancer Detection Agents

Trademarked Name	Cancer
OncoScint CR/OV	Colorectal and ovarian cancers
CEA-Scan	Colorectal cancer
Verluma	Small cell lung cancer
Prostascint	Prostate cancer

treatment of patients with relapsed low-grade or follicular lymphomas. It reacts with CD20 (cluster of differentiation 20), a B lymphocyte surface antigen. Administration of rituximab depletes normal and malignant B cells; it also binds complement and increases ADCC. Rituximab can produce clinical responses in up to 50% of patients with low-grade B-cell non-Hodgkin's lymphomas who have relapsed after treatment with chemotherapy. Infusions may be given as outpatient therapy and can produce prolonged remissions.[19]

Antibody directed against *HER/2* (also called *erb-2, neu,* or *HER/2-neu*) receptors on some breast cancer cells is a very promising immunotherapy for breast cancer patients who have failed hormonal therapy and chemotherapy. *HER/2* is a member of the epidermal growth factor receptor family. Its overexpression suggests a poor prognosis for breast cancer patients, with a more aggressive disease course and resistance to many chemotherapy agents. MoAbs directed against these growth factor receptors can interfere with the growth of breast cancer cells and produce clinical responses in patients with this disease.[20,21]

Toxicity

MoAbs are relatively nontoxic when used in their unconjugated form. Most patients experience no severe side effects. Because many of the MoAbs in clinical trials are derived from mice, allergic reactions may occur. The most common side effects are fever, chills, and flushing. Bronchospasm and hypotension have followed rapid infusion. These immune reactions to mouse antigens are called human anti-mouse antibody (HAMA) reactions. Partly humanized (chimeric) antibodies and fully humanized formulations greatly decrease the risk of allergic reactions. Toxicity of conjugated antibodies is determined by the substance that is attached. Administration of antibodies conjugated with plant toxins, for example, may produce a capillary leak syndrome characterized by edema and hypotension similar to the one produced by IL-2.[16-20]

Despite the low toxicity, there are still many problems with the use of MoAbs in cancer treatment. These MoAbs are specific for a single antigen, but sometimes antigens very similar to TAAs are expressed on the surfaces of normal cells as well. Because of tumor heterogeneity, all tumor cells in the same patient may not express the same TAAs. Developing more specific MoAbs and multiple-MoAb combinations ("MoAb cocktails") may solve these problems. In a process called antigenic modulation, antigens are sometimes lost from the tumor cell surfaces. Antigenic modulation prevents the MoAb from recognizing and attaching to the tumor cell. Because the reticuloendothelial system is responsible for removing antibodies from the body, these MoAbs and any drugs or radioisotopes they are carrying may collect in the liver and the spleen and damage those organs. If these limitations can be resolved, the unique specificity of MoAbs holds exciting potential for both diagnosis and treatment of cancer.[16-18]

TUMOR VACCINES

Tumor vaccines are an attempt to stimulate the immune system to mount a specific immune response against the tumor. The most common use of tumor vaccines involves administration of cancer cells, or parts of cancer cells, that have been irradiated to render the cells incapable of further proliferation or growth. The patient's own cells or cells from other patients with the same type of cancer may be used. The cancer cells may be made more antigenic than the patient's own cancer cells by a variety of techniques. Tumor vaccines may be used alone or with other agents that bolster the immune response. Although vaccines are traditionally used in infectious disease management to prevent rather than treat infection, the use of tumor vaccines has generally been limited to the treatment of patients with established cancers. In these patients the tumor burden is often high. It is likely that tumor vaccines will ultimately have their most effective use in the prevention of cancers or in the management of micrometastatic disease. They have been most widely studied in the management of malignant melanoma and have shown some clinical efficacy, especially as adjuvant therapy.[3,22]

GENE THERAPY OF CANCER

One new area of intense research and clinical interest that overlaps with the realm of biological therapy is the rapidly emerging area of gene therapy for cancer. Gene therapy is a technique by which a functioning gene is inserted into a human cell to correct a genetic error or introduce a new function to the cell. Gene therapy can be seen as a form of drug delivery that uses the patient's cells to produce a therapeutic agent. Target cells are removed from the host and maintained in cell culture. Additional genes are introduced into the cells by a variety of biological vectors or carriers. Harmless viruses are often used as vectors because viruses easily invade mammalian cells. Once the desired genes have been introduced, the altered cells are readministered to the patient. When the altered cells are readministered to the patient, they target the site of the cancer.

Several therapeutic strategies can be applied to gene therapy. Normal genes can be introduced to replace abnormal or absent genes, such as tumor suppressor genes, that suppress cancer growth. More commonly, genes that program the cell to produce cytotoxic substances, such as IL-2, are introduced into the cell's DNA. They produce the effects that are programmed by the inserted genes (e.g., if a gene for a cytokine were introduced, it would produce a cytotoxic substance to kill or inhibit the growth of the cancer cells). All the cells of a tumor mass do not need to be genetically altered. A bystander effect is recognized, in which tumor regression occurs, even when only a fraction of the tumor mass is genetically modified.[23-25]

Table 5-3. Alternative Cancer Therapies

Therapy	Proposed Immunologic Role
Antineoplastons	Polypeptides discovered in human urine that serve as biochemical switches to turn off cancer genes by interrupting signals for cells to multiply.
Cancell	Based on the theory that cancer is a disease of altered cellular energy states. Cancell is a mixture of chemicals, combined on the basis of electrical properties, that deprives cancer cells of their ability to obtain energy.
Fresh cell therapy	Fresh embryonic animal cells that correspond to the cancerous organ or tissue in the patient are injected into the patient, where they are transported to the diseased tissue and repair the diseased cells.
Greek cancer cure	Administration of "serums" that stimulate the immune system, following a diagnostic blood test that indicates the location and extent of the cancer.
Hyperoxygenation therapy	Based on the theory that cancerous tissues grow best under hypoxic conditions. Hydrogen peroxide, germanium salts, or ozone are administered to kill cancer cells by supplying more oxygen than the cells can tolerate.
Immunoaugmentative therapy	Immunity-modulating agent restores an imbalance of serum factors involved in immune system surveillance. Based on the theory that an imbalance permits cancer growth.
Livingston-Wheeler vaccines	Based on the theory that cancer is caused by mycobacterium. Vaccines derived from this mycobacterium are administered to stimulate antibody formation against it.
Shark cartilage	Inhibits angiogenesis, the formation of new blood vessels needed to supply nutrients to tumors.

SOURCE: references 26 and 27. The effects of these therapies on the immune system have not been proved.

ALTERNATIVE CANCER THERAPIES

Alternative cancer therapies, also called *unproven* or *unorthodox therapies*, is a broad term that refers to treatment methods that are not approved by the FDA and are not recognized as part of conventional medical therapy for the treatment of cancer. The terms *complementary therapy* and *integrative therapy* are used to describe therapies that are used in conjunction with conventional medical treatments but do not replace those therapies.[26,27] Although a thorough discussion of alternative cancer therapies is beyond the scope of this chapter, most alternative or complementary cancer treatments claim to affect the immune system's interaction with tumor cells, so they will, for the purposes of this chapter, be considered a form of biological cancer therapy. Efficacy claims for these alternative cancer therapies are not currently supported by objective, controlled clinical trials.[26,27] Representative alternative cancer treatments and their claimed effects on the immune system are outlined in Table 5-3. Further clinical studies will be needed to document the efficacy of any of these agents.

SUMMARY

The immune system can recognize and destroy cancer cells. Biological cancer therapy, biotherapy, immunotherapy, and biological response modification are all terms that are used to describe efforts to prevent or treat cancer by harnessing the resources of the immune system. The agents most commonly used in biological therapy are cytokines, antibodies, and whole or parts of tumor cells.

Interferons are proteins with antiviral, immunomodulatory, and antitumor actions. They are believed to function as antitumor agents by stimulating the actions of several immune cell types, by increasing the expression of tumor-associated antigens, by lengthening all phases of the cell cycle, by modulating the expression of oncogenes, and by interfering with angiogenesis. They are clinically useful for the treatment of patients with hairy cell leukemia, chronic myelogenous leukemia, low-grade lymphomas, renal cell carcinoma, melanoma, and several other tumor types. Their most common toxicity is a flu-like syndrome, to which tolerance develops with continued administration. Tolerance does not develop to fatigue, which is often dose limiting.

Interleukin 2 stimulates the growth of killer lymphocytes that can recognize and destroy tumor cells. It has been most efficacious in treating renal cell carcinoma and malignant melanoma. Its clinical use is complicated by fluid retention and hypotension, which result from a capillary leak syndrome and the loss of intravascular fluid into soft tissues. Hypotension should be managed with careful fluid replacement and low-dose dopamine.

Monoclonal antibodies may be used alone or conjugated with cytotoxic drugs, toxins, or radioisotopes for the diagnosis and treatment of cancer. Rituximab, an unconjugated antibody that depletes B cells, was the first monoclonal antibody approved for cancer treatment. Several antibody radioimmunoconjugates are approved for primary diagnosis of cancer or for detection of cancer recurrence.

Other promising biological therapies include the use of tumor vaccines to actively stimulate a host's antitumor response to tumor cells, and gene therapies of cancer, in which host cells are genetically altered to correct a genetic error or to introduce new cellular functions. Most commonly, genes that program cells to produce cytotoxic substances are introduced into the cancer cell's genome.

Many alternative cancer therapies are claimed to exert their antitumor effects by biological effects on the immune system. Their use is not currently supported by objective, controlled clinical trials and cannot be recommended.

REFERENCES

1. Quan WD Jr, Mitchell MS. Principles of biologic therapy. In: Haskell CM, editor. *Cancer Treatment*. 4th ed. Philadelphia, PA: WB Saunders; 1995. p. 57–69.
2. Rosenberg SA. Principles of cancer management: biologic therapy. In: DeVita VT Jr, Hellman S, Rosenberg SA, editors. *Cancer: Principles and Practice of Oncology*. 5th ed. Philadelphia, PA: Lippincott-Raven; 1997. p. 349–73.
3. Bruton JK. Immunotherapy of cancer. In: *Concepts in Immunology and Immunotherapeutics*. 3rd ed. Bethesda, MD: ASHP; 1997. p. 229–68.
4. Schlinder LW. Understanding the immune system [monograph]. Bethesda, MD: National Cancer Institute; 1993. NIH Publication No. 93-529.
5. Moss JT, Kadmon D. BCG and the treatment of superficial bladder cancer. *DICP* 1991;25:1355–67.
6. Black WJ. Drug products of recombinant DNA technology. *Am J Hosp Pharm* 1989;46:1834–44.
7. Witt PL, Lindner DJ, D'Cunha J, et al. Pharmacology of interferons: induced proteins, cell activation, and antitumor activity. In: Chabner BA, Longo DL, editors. *Cancer Chemotherapy and Biotherapy*. 2nd ed. Philadelphia, PA: Lippincott-Raven; 1996. p. 585–607.
8. Dorr RT. Interferon-alfa in malignant and viral diseases: a review. *Drugs* 1993;45:177–211.
9. Rosenberg SA. Principles of cancer management: biologic therapy. In: DeVita VT Jr, Hellman S, Rosenberg SA. *Cancer: Principles and Practice of Oncology*. 5th ed. Philadelphia, PA: Lippincott-Raven; 1997. p. 349–73.
10. Kirkwood JM, Strawderman MH, Ernstoff MS, et al. Interferon alfa-2b adjuvant therapy of high-risk resected cutaneous melanoma: the eastern cooperative oncology group trial EST 1684. *J Clin Oncol* 1996;14:7–17.
11. Bukowski RM, McLain D, Finke J. Clinical pharmacokinetics of interleukin 1, interleukin 2, interleukin 4, tumor necrosis factor, and macrophage colony-stimualting factor. In: Chabner BA, Longo DL, editors. *Cancer Chemotherapy and Biotherapy*. 2nd ed. Philadelphia, PA: Lippincott-Raven; 1996. p. 609–38.
12. Whittington R, Faulds D. Interleukin-2: a review of its pharmacologic properties and therapeutic use in patients with cancer. *Drugs* 1993;46:446–514.
13. Bruton JK, Koeller JM. Recombinant interleukin-2. *Pharmacotherapy* 1994;14:635–56.
14. Fyfe G, Fisher RI, Rosenberg SA, et al. Results of treatment of 255 patients with metastatic renal cell carcinoma who received high-dose recombinant interleukin-2 therapy. *J Clin Oncol* 1995;13:688–96.
15. Marincola FM, White DE, Wise AP, et al. Combination therapy with interferon alfa-2a and interleukin-2 for the treatment of metastatic cancer. *J Clin Oncol* 1995;13:1110–22.
16. Goldenberg DM. New developments in monoconal antibodies for cancer detection and therapy. *CA Cancer J Clin* 1994;44:43–64.
17. Dillman RO. Antibodies as cytotoxic therapy. *J Clin Oncol* 1994;12:1497–515.
18. Junghans RP, Scouros G, Scheinberg DA. Antibody-based immunotherapies for cancer. In: Chabner BA, Longo DL, editors. *Cancer Chemotherapy and Biotherapy*. 2nd ed. Philadelphia, PA: Lippincott-Raven; 1996. p. 655–89.
19. McLaughlin P, Cabanillas F, Grill-Lopez AJ, et al. IDEC-C2B8 anti-CD20 antibody: final report on a phase III pivotal trial in patients with relapsed low-grade or follicular lymphoma [abstract]. *Blood* 1996;88:90A.
20. Basselga J, Tripathy D, Mendelsohn J, et al. Phase II study of weekly intravenous recombinant humanized anti-p185HE 2 monoclonal antibody in patients with HER2/neu overexpressing metastatic breast cancer. *J Clin Oncol* 1996;14:737–44.
21. Slamon D, Leyland-Jones B, Shak S, et al. Addition of Herceptin® (humanized anti-Her2 antibody) to first line chemotherapy for Her2 overexpressing metastatic breast cancer (Her2 +/MBC) markedly increases anticancer activity [abstract]. *Proc Am Soc Clin Oncol Ann Mtg* 1998;17:A377.
22. Morton DL, Barth A. Vaccine therapy for malignant melanoma. *CA Cancer J Clin* 1997;46:225–44.
23. Blau HM. Gene therapy—a novel form of drug delivery. *N Engl J Med* 1995;333:1204–7.
24. Goldspiel BR, Green L, Calis KA. Human gene therapy. *Clin Pharm* 1993;12:488–505.
25. Freeman SM, Whartenby KA, Freeman JL, et al. In situ use of suicide genes for cancer therapy. *Semin Oncol* 1996;23:31–45.
26. Nelson WK. Alternative methods of cancer treatment available beyond the United States borders. *Highlights Oncol Pract* 1997;15(4):85–93.
27. Cassileth BR, Chapman CC. Alternative and complementary cancer therapies. *Cancer* 1996;77:1026–34.

SELF-STUDY QUESTIONS

1. The interaction of monoclonal antibodies (MoAbs) with the immune system is classified as:

    a. active and specific.
    b. active and nonspecific.
    c. passive and specific.
    d. passive and nonspecific.

2. The interaction of Bacillus Calmette-Guérin (BCG) vaccine with the immune system is classified as:

    a. active and specific.
    b. active and nonspecific.
    c. passive and specific.
    d. passive and nonspecific.

3. Which of the following immunotherapies are considered cytokines?

    a. interferon and interleukin 2 (IL-2)
    b. interferon and MoAbs
    c. MoAbs and IL-2
    d. tumor vaccines and interferon

4. Active immune interventions stimulate the host's natural immune response to the tumor.

    a. true
    b. false

5. Which of the following hematological malignancies represents an important clinical use of interferon alfa (IFN-α)?

    a. acute myelogenous leukemia
    b. Hodgkin's disease
    c. chronic myelogenous leukemia
    d. acute lymphocytic leukemia

6. Which of the following solid tumors represents an important clinical use of IFN-α?

    a. breast cancer
    b. prostate cancer
    c. lung cancer
    d. malignant melanoma

7. The most important clinical applications of IL-2 are:

    a. breast and prostate cancers.
    b. renal cell cancer and malignant melanoma.
    c. lung and colon cancers.
    d. acute myelogenous leukemia and Hodgkin's disease.

8. Which of the following is/are believed to be important in the antitumor action of IFN-α?

    a. stimulation of effector cells in the immune system
    b. increasing expression of antigens on tumor cell surfaces
    c. lengthening all phases of the tumor cell cycle
    d. all of the above

9. Which of the following immunotherapies has/have antiviral action in addition to its antitumor effects?

    a. IL-2
    b. BCG vaccine
    c. IFN-α
    d. all of the above

10. Which of the following cytokines stimulates the activity of lymphokine-activated killer (LAK) cells, tumor-infiltrating lymphocytes (TILs), and cytotoxic T lymphocytes (CTLs)?

    a. IL-2
    b. IFN-α
    c. IL-2 and IFN-α
    d. none of the above

11. The most common and characteristic side effect of IFN-α therapy is:

    a. capillary leak syndrome.
    b. fatigue.
    c. flu-like syndrome.
    d. human antimouse antibody (HAMA) reaction.

12. The most common and characteristic dose-limiting toxicity of IFN-α therapy is:

    a. capillary leak syndrome.
    b. fatigue.
    c. flu-like syndrome.
    d. HAMA reaction.

13. The most common and characteristic toxicity of IL-2 therapy is:

    a. capillary leak syndrome.
    b. fatigue.
    c. flu-like syndrome.
    d. HAMA reaction.

14. Hypotension secondary to treatment with IL-2 is best managed by aggressive fluid replacement.

    a. true
    b. false

15. Mrs. K. had her first prescription for IFN-α injections filled in your pharmacy yesterday. Today she calls, complaining of fever and chills, and says she will not be able to continue treatment because of this side effect. What is the most appropriate counseling that you can provide to her at this time?

    a. Discontinue therapy; the fever and chills represent an allergic reaction to this therapy.
    b. Discontinue therapy until the side effect disappears, then reinstitute therapy at half the initial dose.
    c. Take acetaminophen before each dose and administer doses at bedtime; although the side effects are unpleasant, it is important to learn to live with them.
    d. Take acetaminophen before each dose and administer doses at bedtime; tolerance will develop to this side effect with 1–2 weeks of continued use.

16. The most important potential advantage of MoAbs in the treatment of cancer is:

    a. specificity.
    b. passivity.
    c. multiplicity.
    d. longevity.

17. Which of the following compounds can be conjugated to MoAbs?

    a. plant toxins
    b. conventional cytotoxic drugs
    c. radioisotopes
    d. all of the above

18. Rituximab is a MoAb approved for the management of:

    a. breast cancer.
    b. non-Hodgkin's lymphoma.
    c. acute myelogenous leukemia.
    d. colorectal cancer.

19. HAMA reactions to MoAbs can be minimized by:

    a. development of chimeric antibodies.
    b. use of recombinant DNA technology.
    c. conjugation of proteins with plant toxins.
    d. radioimmunodetection.

20. Limitations to the use of MoAbs in cancer therapy include:

    a. antigenic modulation.
    b. tumor heterogeneity.
    c. damage to the liver and spleen.
    d. all of the above.

21. Administration of disabled cancer cells or parts of cells to cancer patients to stimulate the immune system to mount an immune response against the tumor describes the use of:

    a. MoAbs.
    b. cytokines.
    c. tumor vaccines.
    d. BCG vaccine.

22. Tumor vaccines are expected to have their greatest clinical application in adjuvant treatment of cancer or in cancer prevention.

    a. true
    b. false

23. A therapeutic approach that consists of insertion of a functioning gene into a human cell to correct a genetic error or to introduce a new function to the cell is called:

    a. recombinant DNA.
    b. hybridoma.
    c. gene therapy.
    d. MoAb therapy.

24. All the cells in a tumor mass need not be genetically altered to produce a desirable effect in gene therapy. This phenomenon is called the _____.

25. Unproven cancer therapies that are used in conjunction with, rather than instead of conventional therapies, are called:

    a. unorthodox therapies.
    b. complementary therapies.
    c. gene therapies.
    d. investigational therapies.

Chapter 6

Optimizing Chemotherapy Outcomes

Rebecca S. Finley, Pharm.D., M.S.
Chair and Associate Professor
Department of Pharmacy Practice and
  Pharmacy Administration
Philadelphia College of Pharmacy
Philadelphia, Pennsylvania

Carol Balmer, Pharm.D.
Associate Professor
University of Colorado School of Pharmacy
Denver, Colorado

Tumor-Related Factors 82
    Tumor Growth Kinetics 82
    Tumor Size or Tumor Burden 83
    Site of Tumor and Tumor Vascularization 83
    Antineoplastic Drug Resistance 84
Drug-Related Factors 86
    Pharmacokinetics and Cytotoxic Effect 86
    Combination Chemotherapy 86
        Multipronged Attacks on Biochemical Pathways 87
        Manipulation of Drug Transport Mechanisms 88
        Rescue Techniques 88
        Metabolic Modulation or Biomodulation 88
        Advantages and Disadvantages of Drug Combinations 89
        Guidelines for Developing Drug Combinations 89
            Effective Drug Use 89
            Overlapping Toxicity 90
            Optimal Dose and Schedule of Administration 90
Patient-Related Factors 94
    Immunocompetence 94
    Renal and Hepatic Function 94
    Prior Exposure to Chemotherapy and Radiation Therapy 94
    Nutritional Status 94
    Age 94
Selection of Chemotherapy Regimens 95
Summary 96
References 96
Self-Study Questions 97

As you learned in the preceding chapters, cancer chemotherapy attacks tumors at the cellular level by interrupting processes or inhibiting substances necessary for cellular replication and life. Although some types of cancer can be cured with the judicious use of chemotherapy (e.g., childhood leukemia, testicular cancer, and Hodgkin's disease), it is obvious that chemotherapy is often not successful in curing many types of advanced cancer (e.g., cancers of the colon, lung, prostate, or breast). However, even for the many cancers that cannot be cured, the use of chemotherapy may produce some positive outcomes, including the relief of symptoms such as pain or dyspnea caused by the tumor. Chemotherapy may also prolong survival and slow the progression of some advanced cancers, enabling patients to experience an improved quality of life. But why is chemotherapy effective for some types of cancer and not others? Why do some patients initially respond (i.e., their tumors clearly regress) only to have the cancer begin to grow again despite continued chemotherapy?

We now appreciate that there are many tumor-, drug-, and patient-related factors or variables that may influence the outcomes of chemotherapy. A comprehensive understanding of these variables and how they relate to each other is the foundation for optimization of therapeutic outcomes and minimization of the toxic effects of chemotherapy.

This chapter will help the reader integrate information learned about cancer and cancer drugs in the previous chapters and assist in identifying factors that will influence the outcomes for specific patients. In the treatment of cancer, understanding and applying this information in a rational manner is just as important as the discovery of new antineoplastic drugs. Some of the most important therapeutic advances over the past two decades were the result of improving the clinical use of existing anticancer drugs through changes in the dose or schedule based on pharmacokinetic and pharmacodynamic observations or by modulating the activity through the design of more rational combination regimens. This knowledge leads us to effective treatment and also helps explain why chemotherapy may fail.

After completing this chapter, the reader should be able to:

1. Describe how tumor growth kinetics influence chemotherapy effectiveness.
2. Discuss the influence of drug resistance on the selection of specific chemotherapy regimens.
3. Discuss how the pharmacokinetics of a specific drug may limit or enhance its effectiveness.
4. Describe the importance of combination chemotherapy and discuss the influence of dose and schedule of administration on chemotherapy effectiveness.
5. Describe patient-related factors that influence chemotherapy effectiveness.

In addition to comprehension of the information provided in the preceding chapters, an understanding of the mammalian cell cycle (Appendix I) is essential to appreciating the complexities and interrelationships of the many variables that affect a patient's response to chemotherapy. Variables that influence the effectiveness of chemotherapy are discussed separately as tumor-related, drug-related, or patient-related factors. Most of these factors have an impact on the treatment plans of every patient, so it is not surprising that it is difficult to predict what a patient's response will be.

The ultimate goal of chemotherapy is to deliver a sufficient concentration of an agent to the target site, usually the tumor cells, to produce a lethal effect without producing excessive or undesired toxicity to the normal surrounding tissues. Several considerations determine which therapy is the most effective for a given tumor:

- How much of the drugs should be administered?
- How frequently should the drugs be administered?
- What are the safest and most effective methods of administering them?

Most antineoplastic drugs have a steep dose-response curve, so even small increases in the dose can result in significant enhancement of both the therapeutic and toxic effects. Although it is tempting to decrease the dose if toxicity occurs, decreasing the dose may also compromise the effectiveness of the therapy. Therefore, optimal therapy is frequently considered to be the highest possible dose that does not produce life-threatening toxicity (the maximum tolerated dose).

TUMOR-RELATED FACTORS
Tumor Growth Kinetics
As stated in chapter 1, neoplastic cells have several properties that distinguish them from normal cells. One of these properties is uncontrolled growth, which makes the malignant cells more susceptible to the cytotoxic effects of many anticancer drugs than normal cells. The rate at which tumor cells replicate and expand the tumor mass is referred to as *growth kinetics*.

Most chemotherapy drugs are capable of killing only dividing cells, so they are most effective when the tumor mass is small and the growth fraction is high. Therefore, small but rapidly growing tumors are most susceptible to chemotherapy. Unfortunately, a tumor mass usually cannot be detected by physical examination or radiological studies until it is about 1 cm in diameter. By this time, approximately a billion cells are present and the growth curve may have progressed to the plateau phase, meaning that fewer cancer cells are actively dividing and are likely to be affected by chemotherapy.

The growth fraction of most human tumors ranges from 20 to 70%. To eradicate all the cells, the nondividing cells

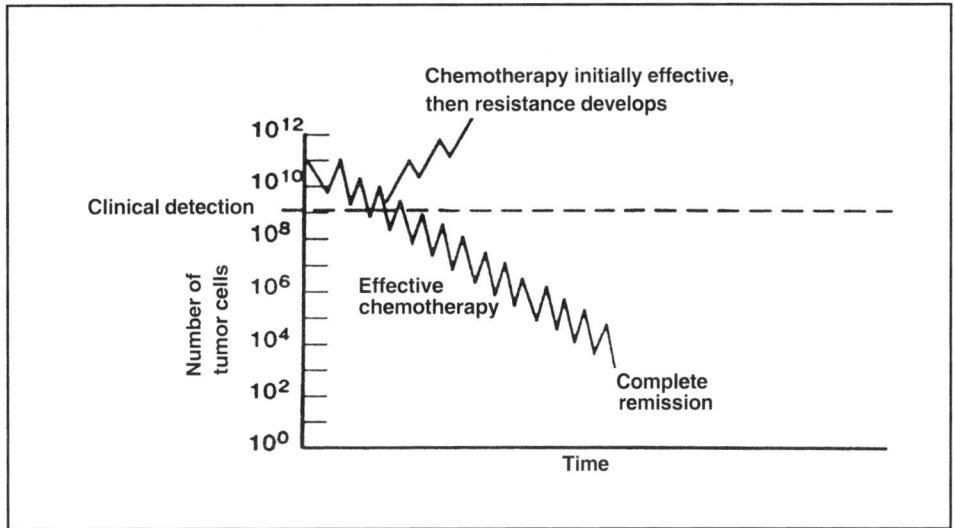

Figure 6-1. Effects of chemotherapy on tumor growth and regression
SOURCE: adapted from Dorr RT, Fritz WL. *Cancer Chemotherapy Handbook.* New York: Elsevier Science; 1980. p. 3–20.

must either be removed or be stimulated to begin dividing again. Effective treatment for this situation may be to decrease the size of the tumor with surgery or to reduce the tumor burden with chemotherapy or radiation. Either strategy may shift the growth curve toward a higher growth fraction by stimulating cells that were resting to re-enter the cell cycle and start proliferating again. This strategy is sometimes referred to as *recruitment*.

In theory, the effects of cancer chemotherapy on a mass of tumor cells follow first-order kinetic principles; that is, the absolute number of cells killed by a chemotherapy regimen is proportional to the dose administered (Figure 6-1). A constant fraction of cells is killed rather than a constant number. The predictable logarithmic reduction of tumor mass shown in Figure 6-1 would only occur under ideal circumstances: if all the cells were equally susceptible to the cytotoxic effects (i.e., if the cells were homogenous); if all the cells were actively dividing; if all cells were equally accessible to the drug molecules; and if all the cells had equal access to oxygen, nutrients, and growth factors. Under normal circumstances, however, the cells of a tumor mass are heterogeneous, and as the tumor grows, more cells enter a resting phase that makes them impervious to chemotherapy. As the tumor mass grows, the distribution of blood becomes less uniform as well. The net effect is that reduction of tumor mass may be unpredictable, and the tumor frequently appears stable between cycles of chemotherapy.

Tumor Size or Tumor Burden

As mentioned above, the size of a tumor mass can be a limiting factor to successful chemotherapy. In large, bulky tumors, a high fraction of the cells are typically in the resting phase and are less susceptible to the cytotoxic effects. Because of the lack of uniform blood supply, chemotherapy drugs may not be able to penetrate the mass and produce sufficient intracellular concentrations. In addition, the larger the tumor mass, the more likely it is that it has already metastasized to other sites. For example, Table 6-1 shows that for breast cancer the larger the diameter of the tumor, the more likely it is that axillary lymph nodes will show evidence of tumor spread.

Site of Tumor and Tumor Vascularization

The site where a tumor develops, or the sites to which it metastasizes, may also influence its response to chemotherapy. Getting a drug to the tumor site may be impossible if the tumor is located in a drug sanctuary (an anatomical location where

Table 6-1. Breast Cancer: 10-Year Survival (%) Related to Size of Primary Tumor and Lymph Node Involvement

Axillary Node Status	<2 cm	2–5 cm	>5 cm	Total
Negative	82	65	44	72
Positive, proximal only	73	74	39	65
Positive, middle or distal	a	28	37	31
Positive, all	68	51	37	

SOURCE: Schottenfeld D, Nash AG, Robbins GF, et al. Ten-year results of the treatment of primary operable breast carcinoma. *Cancer* 1978;38:1001–7.
aInsufficient data

drug penetration is usually poor, such as the central nervous system). Techniques for administering chemotherapy that deliver the agent directly to the site of the tumor are described in chapter 10.

The amount of blood that reaches or penetrates the tumor also influences the response to chemotherapy. Even if tumor cells are very sensitive to the drug, they cannot be destroyed by drugs unless they have a good blood supply. As mentioned above, large, bulky tumors often do not have constant blood supply throughout because of poor vascularization and/or variations in hydrostatic pressure between various areas of the tumor. Consequently, the cytotoxic drugs, which are carried in the blood, are unable to reach the tumor. Differences in microcirculation between tumors makes it even more difficult to predict how different tumors will respond. Microcirculation also affects how effectively cells and mediators of the immune system penetrate the tumor. One area of cancer research is the development of drugs to inhibit angiogenesis of newly forming tumors.

Antineoplastic Drug Resistance

Drug resistance of tumors is the most frequent reason that chemotherapy treatment fails. Resistance to chemotherapy can be influenced by the tumor's cellular kinetics, site, or vascularization. Pharmacokinetic and other drug-related properties (which are discussed later) can also have an impact. Many types of cancer (e.g., colon cancer, non-small cell lung cancer, renal cancer, and melanoma) are usually resistant to available chemotherapy agents at first exposure (a property termed *intrinsic resistance*). Other tumors, however, are sensitive to chemotherapy at first but acquire resistance after being exposed to chemotherapy.

Intrinsic resistance is largely due to the heterogeneity of cells in the tumor mass. Normal cells are genetically stable and reproduce consistently, with daughter cells identical to parent cells. Tumor cells, in contrast, are genetically unstable and have a higher mutation rate than normal cells. The result is an ever-changing tumor mass composed of many different but related tumor cell lines or clones. These clones may differ in one or many characteristics, such as chromosome number, histology, metastatic potential, and, most important, drug resistance and response. The theory that mutational changes result in varying patterns of drug resistance within a patient's tumor mass (somatic or growth mutation theory) was proposed by Goldie and Coldman in 1979.[2]

This genetically controlled variability in drug response makes the tumor a moving target for drug therapy, and it is the tumor's best defense against cancer treatment. Mutations might produce clones that (1) are missing a drug-activating enzyme, (2) overproduce enzymes responsible for drug destruction, (3) have faulty transport mechanisms for a drug, (4) actively transport a drug out of the cell, or (5) are resistant in other ways to at least one of the antineoplastic agents available.[3-6] Tumor heterogeneity and the drug-resistant offspring that result (clonal expansion) are illustrated in Figure 6-2. Because of genetic in-

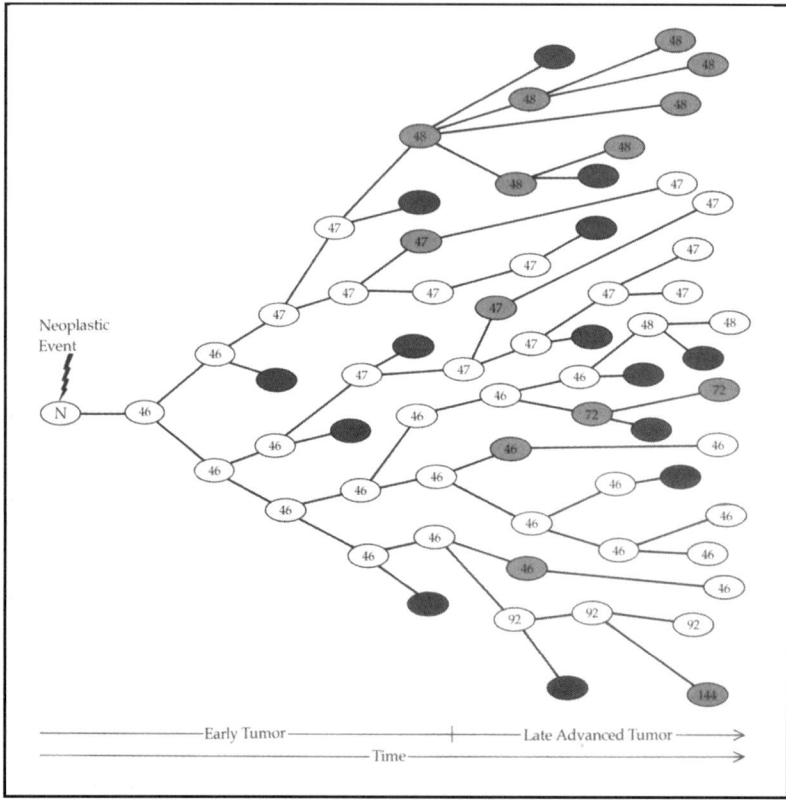

Figure 6-2. A single cell transformed by a neoplastic event undergoes clonal expansion. For the purposes of illustration, a mutation rate of 1 in 4 is depicted; actual mutation rates are much lower.

SOURCE: reprinted with permission from reference 5, Sec. 12, Subsection III. © 1986, Scientific American, Inc. All rights reserved.

Table 6-2. Mechanisms of Tumor Cell Resistance to Antineoplastic Drugs

Mechanism	Examples of Drugs
Decrease in cellular uptake or increase in efflux of drug	Daunorubicin, doxorubicin, melphalan, methotrexate, vincristine, vinblastine, taxanes
Decrease in drug activation	Cytarabine, doxorubicin, fluorouracil, mercaptopurine, thioguanine
Increase in drug degradation	Bleomycin, cytarabine, mercaptopurine
Increased ability to repair DNA	Cisplatin, cyclophosphamide, melphalan, mitomycin, mechlorethamine, nitrosoureas
Use of alternate biochemical pathways	Cytarabine

SOURCE: DeVita VT, Schein PS. The use of drugs in combination for the treatment of cancer. N Engl J Med 1973;288:998–1006.

stability, drug-resistant clones evolve. Note that although not all mutations cause drug resistance, most cells in the mature tumor are different from the original parent cell. Although the mutation rate of 1 in 4 used in Figure 6-2 is artificially high for the sake of illustration, an accurate mutation rate probably still results in at least 100 different clones among the billion cells that make up a tiny 1-g tumor mass. The number of clones may be ≥100,000 in larger masses.[3] Given this great diversity within a tumor, it is no surprise that treatment with a single cancer drug cannot eliminate all the tumor cells. The tumor may appear to respond at first and even shrink below clinically detectable levels, but millions of cells may survive to multiply and ultimately overwhelm the host.

Mechanisms of tumor cell resistance to antineoplastic drugs are summarized in Table 6-2. These mechanisms of resistance may occur as a result of somatic mutations due to genetic instability, or mutations may be induced through exposure to chemotherapy or radiation. Many anticancer drugs are known to be mutagenic and may produce changes in the genetic material of tumor cells that result in drug resistance. In the case of acquired resistance, there is usually an initial decrease in the tumor mass when treatment begins, but eventually tumor growth resumes despite continued treatment.

Besides induced mutations, tumor cells may also undergo gene amplification as a result of chemotherapy. In this situation, the gene for a normal protein becomes multiplied, and these cells then produce more of the protein. If this protein is normally a target enzyme for the chemotherapy drug, then the increased concentrations of the protein may enable the cell to survive despite continued chemotherapy. For example, if exposure to chemotherapy caused amplification of the gene that encodes for dihydrofolate reductase (DHFR, see chapter 4), then these cells could easily become resistant to methotrexate.

Perhaps the most clinically significant form of antineoplastic resistance is referred to as *multidrug resistance* (MDR) or *pleiotropic drug resistance*. This resistance is a result of amplification of a gene that encodes for a protein (P170 or P-glycoprotein) found in the cell membrane that pumps drugs out of the cell.[7] The result is a lower intracellular concentration of drug and a shorter duration of exposure to the drug's lethal effects within the cell. This MDR mechanism confers cross-resistance to many antineoplastics derived from plants and to the antitumor antibiotics, even though these drugs have distinct chemical structures and exert their activity through very different mechanisms (Table 6-3). The only common features are that all these drugs have a hydrophobic aromatic ring, tend to be positively charged at neutral pH, and, most important, enter cells via passive diffusion and exit via an energy-dependent process.[8,9] The amount of P-glycoprotein production correlates directly with the degree of resistance.[10,11] It is now known that other substances may compete with these antineoplastics for efflux from cells. Verapamil, quinidine, and trifluoperazine are agents that have been shown to increase the intracellular concentrations of these antineoplastics by competing for P-glycoprotein binding. Unfortunately, the concentrations of these competitors that are necessary to block antineoplastic efflux produce significantly harmful side effects. The inert isomer of verapamil, dexverapamil, is being studied as a modulator of MDR.[12]

Other recognized mechanisms of resistance to antineoplastics are described in Table 6-2. For example, the tumor cell may begin to produce enzymes that can degrade the drug rapidly. In other cases, the drug may require some enzymatic activation in the cell that the cell is unable to produce, leaving the drug in its inactive form. Perhaps one of the most common mechanisms of drug resistance is the ability of the tumor cell to repair damage inflicted by a chemotherapy agent. Tumor cells may also be able to circumvent the biochemical damage and use alternate mechanisms to continue their cellular division.

Table 6-3. Examples of Antineoplastic Drugs Cross-Resistant via the P-Glycoprotein–Mediated Multidrug Resistance Mechanism

Vinca alkaloids (vincristine, vinblastine, vinorelbine)

Anthracyclines (doxorubicin, daunorubicin, idarubicin)

Taxanes (paclitaxel, docetaxel)

Epipodophyllotoxins (etoposide, teniposide)

Recognition of some of these mechanisms has led to the development of strategies to overcome the problem of resistance. These strategies include developing new (non-cross-resistant) agents, modulating agents to overcome the resistance mechanism, and using different dosages and schedules of administration.

DRUG-RELATED FACTORS

Pharmacokinetics and Cytotoxic Effect

The effectiveness of some drugs is influenced by the stage in the cell cycle at which they exert their effect. Drugs can be cell cycle specific or cell cycle nonspecific, and that specificity and the drug's pharmacokinetic properties can influence how the drug should be administered. If a drug exerts activity in a specific phase of the cell cycle and has a very short half-life, it will not be in contact with the tumor for very long and most tumor cells are unlikely to be in the target phase of the cell cycle during drug exposure (see Appendix I, The Mammalian Cell Cycle).

The importance of the interaction between pharmacokinetics and phase specificity has been demonstrated in the clinical use of cytarabine in the treatment of acute myelogenous leukemia. During its early clinical development, cytarabine, which has a short half-life (about 10 minutes), was administered as a bolus injection in doses of up to 4.2 g/m^2 but did not produce significant bone marrow suppression. However, when the drug was administered by continuous infusion over 48 hours, only 1 g/m^2 could be tolerated.[1] Low doses administered to mice three times daily proved to be more effective than a larger, once-a-day bolus injection.[13] The schedule dependency of cytarabine's antileukemic activity was demonstrated in an early study that compared the effects of the same dose given over either 48 or 120 hours. An increase in the complete responses from 20 to 38% was found with the prolonged infusion.[14] Currently, cytarabine is given as a continuous infusion for 5–10 days. Substantial antileukemic effects are seen with doses of 100–200 mg/m^2 per day. When it is combined with other agents, such as daunorubicin, mitoxantrone, or idarubicin, 60–80% of patients have a complete response to therapy.

As the cytarabine example demonstrates, you must consider the pharmacokinetic properties of an antineoplastic agent when striving for optimal drug effectiveness. In addition to drug half-life, drug distribution characteristics are important in determining whether the drug can reach the tumor site in sufficient concentration. For example, cytarabine is very active in the treatment of acute myelogenous leukemia, but at regular doses, cytarabine does not distribute well into the central nervous system and may not be effective in treating leukemic meningitis. Therefore, intrathecal injections of cytarabine may be needed.

The rate at which the cytotoxic agent is cleared via metabolism or renal and hepatic mechanisms influences the serum concentration and may influence the exposure of the tumor to the agent. Renal or hepatic impairment may result in higher concentrations both in the blood and at the site of the tumor. However, the exposure of normal cells would also be increased, leading to enhanced toxicity. Inversely, enhanced clearance may result in decreased exposure. Similarly, some cytotoxics (e.g., cyclophosphamide and ifosfamide) may require activation (metabolism) by the liver or other tissue. The rate of activation may also influence tumor exposure to the drug.

Several antineoplastics are administered orally. Factors that may impair or limit the rate of absorption influence systemic availability of the drug and, hence, its effectiveness (see chapter 10).

Combination Chemotherapy

The activity of a particular antineoplastic agent against different tumor types is assessed through a series of carefully designed clinical trials. The information gathered from these trials is probably the most valuable tool in predicting a response to a particular therapy. Early in the clinical use of chemotherapy it was realized that few patients are cured with the use of just one antineoplastic drug (single-agent therapy). Single-agent therapy is limited by the heterogeneity of the cells in the tumor mass, with their differing intrinsic sensitivities, as well as by the development of acquired resistance. To increase the likelihood of affecting more clones and killing more tumor cells, it has become customary to combine several agents that have activity against a particular tumor type when developing a regimen.

Several clones of a single tumor are pictured in Figure 6-3, each demonstrating a continuum of sensitivity to three chemotherapy agents. For each drug, some clones fall beyond the normal tissue tolerance barrier and are considered resistant to that drug. The resistant clones cannot be eradicated with that drug alone without jeopardizing the patient's life. However, every clone shown is sensitive to at least one of the drugs in tolerable doses. All the clones can therefore be destroyed by this combination regimen, and the patient can potentially be cured.

Figure 6-3 illustrates a few other useful points about drug resistance and combination regimens. Note that sensitivity to one agent does not depend on sensitivity to another agent. The response patterns depend on the individual drug and are unpredictable, although MDR affects many unrelated drugs.[6] Second, some clones are resistant to more than one drug (MDR). Third, collateral drug sensitivity occurs; that is, more than one drug may be attacking certain sensitive subpopulations simultaneously.[3]

The clinical situation of a patient with cancer is more complex than shown in Figure 6-3. There are many, perhaps hundreds or thousands, of tumor subpopulations, each of which falls somewhere on the continuum of sensitivity for each of the approximately 50 anticancer drugs commercially available. If the right selection is made among the drugs avail-

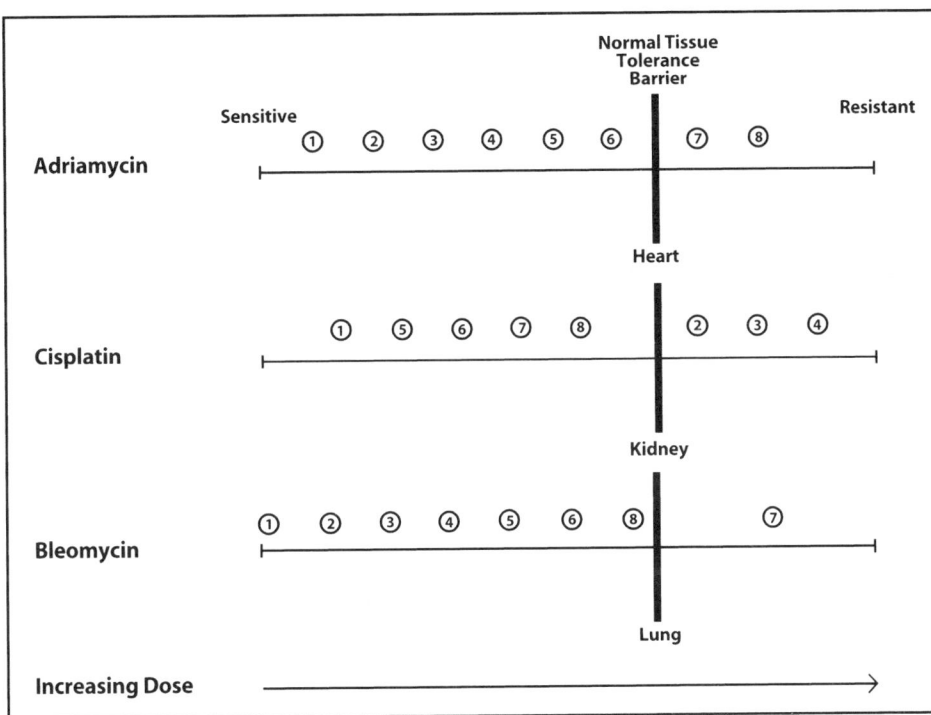

Figure 6-3. Response continuum of tumors to combination chemotherapy regimens. Numbers in circles represent different clones.

SOURCE: reprinted with permission from Dexter DL, Leith JT. Tumor heterogeneity and drug resistance. *J Clin Oncol* 1986;4:244–57.

able, it is possible that the patient's tumor can be eliminated. But time is limited for that patient, and so many drugs are available that the number of permutations of drug combinations is very high. With random selection, the odds are heavy against choosing the right combination for that patient's unique and ever-changing tumor mass before the patient dies of the disease.[3,4]

Yet combination therapy regimens do cure some patients. Components of combination regimens are selected because they have demonstrated activity against a certain tumor type when given as single agents. As biochemical and pharmacokinetic characteristics of the drugs have become better understood, combinations have been developed for more sophisticated rationales. Several of these are described elsewhere in this chapter.

Multipronged Attacks on Biochemical Pathways

The strategy of multiple insults is to combine drugs with different mechanisms of action to attack the tumor from several biochemical directions.[15,16] Several categories of approaches use this strategy (Figure 6-4). In sequential blockade, two or more drugs that block a single critical metabolic pathway at different sites are used together, eliminating the essential pathway from the cancer cell's metabolism. This is a familiar strategy in antibiotic therapy; the combination of trimethoprim and sulfamethoxazole interferes at two different steps in folate synthesis in bacterial cells. An example of sequential blockade used in cancer treatment is the combination of fluorouracil and methotrexate. Both of these antineoplastic agents inter-

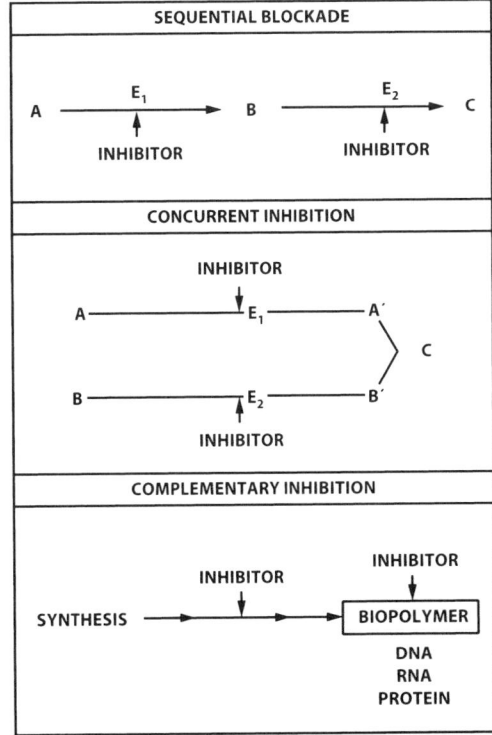

Figure 6-4. Theoretical points of blockade of metabolic pathways by drugs. A, B, and C, proteins; A' and B', activated proteins; E_1 and E_2, enzymes.

SOURCES: reprinted with permission from reference 16 and DeVita VT, Schein PS. The use of drugs in combination for the treatment of cancer. *N Engl J Med* 1973;288:998–1006.

fere with the biosynthesis of thymidine, which is required for DNA synthesis.

Concurrent inhibition, in which two or more parallel pathways leading to synthesis of DNA are interfered with at the same time, is common in oncology practice. Regimens that include two antimetabolites, such as a purine and a pyrimidine antagonist, are exploiting this method. Another approach is complementary inhibition. In this strategy, an agent that inhibits a pathway contributing to DNA synthesis (an antimetabolite) is combined with one that reacts directly with the product of that pathway, the DNA itself. Alkylators, which react directly with DNA, are combined with antimetabolites in some of the most common chemotherapy regimens. In the CMF chemotherapy regimen for breast cancer, for example, the alkylator cyclophosphamide is combined with two antimetabolites, methotrexate and fluorouracil.

Manipulation of Drug Transport Mechanisms

Most cytotoxic drugs act on the nuclear material of cancer cells, particularly DNA and its components. For these cytotoxic effects to take place, the cytotoxic agent must be transported from the extracellular fluid to the interior of the cancer cells, through the cell membrane. It also must remain in the cell long enough to damage or destroy the cell. As mentioned above, some cancer cells are resistant to particular cancer drugs because they possess transport mechanisms that actively pump drugs out of the cell. The use of other, noncytotoxic drugs to block the efflux is an example of this type of modulation.

Rescue Techniques

In general, chemotherapy regimens aim for the maximum tolerated dose, as discussed previously. One exception to that practice is the use of rescue techniques. The strategy of rescue is that one agent, which may or may not be an antineoplastic agent, is supplied to rescue normal cells (but not tumor cells) from the toxic effects of the cytotoxic agent. The most important example is leucovorin rescue after administration of high-dose methotrexate. Methotrexate poisons the enzyme system responsible for producing the reduced form of folic acid (leucovorin) that is required as a cofactor in numerous metabolic pathways in the cell. Large doses of methotrexate or decreased elimination of methotrexate from the body can cause lethal toxicity from methotrexate's poisonous effects on normal cells. These normal cells are rescued from death by leucovorin, the end product of the poisoned pathway, bypassing the need for folinic acid production in the cell. Tumor cells may lack the mechanisms required for transporting leucovorin into the cell or produce higher concentrations of active methotrexate forms; if they do, they are less easily rescued.

Metabolic Modulation or Biomodulation

In this combination drug strategy, an agent, which need not be cytotoxic itself, is administered to increase either the antitumor effects or the selectivity for tumor cells of an active

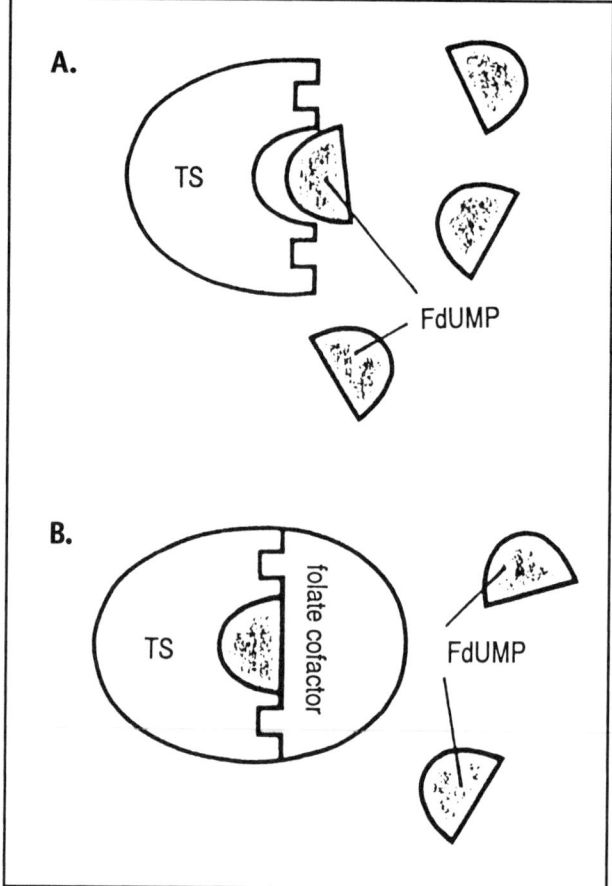

Figure 6-5. Biomodulation of fluorouracil action by leucovorin. *A*, binding of 5-fluorodeoxyuridine monophosphate (FdUMP) to thymidylate synthase (TS) in the absence of folate cofactor. *B*, binding of FdUMP to TS in the presence of folate cofactor.

SOURCE: reprinted with permission from Bertino JR, Knobf T, Remington JS. Leucovorin: interaction of leucovorin with 5-fluorouracil. Monograph 2. Research Triangle Park, NC: Burroughs Wellcome; 1985.

antineoplastic agent.[17,18] This strategy is the basis for the combination of leucovorin and fluorouracil. An active metabolite of fluorouracil, 5-fluorodeoxyuridine monophosphate (FdUMP), is responsible for much of fluorouracil's antitumor activity. In the presence of a folate cofactor, FdUMP binds to the enzyme thymidylate synthase (TS) and inhibits its action. TS is essential for production of thymidine, a key building block of DNA. When the folate cofactor is present in normal body concentrations, FdUMP binds very poorly to TS, inhibiting DNA synthesis only slightly (Figure 6-5). When high concentrations of folate cofactor are provided by administering leucovorin before fluorouracil (Figure 6-5), a very stable complex of TS and FdUMP is formed, making TS unavailable for DNA synthesis and potentially killing more cancer cells than fluorouracil alone.[18] Although leucovorin itself has no anticancer activity in this example, sometimes both drugs used for biomodulation are cytotoxic.

Advantages and Disadvantages of Drug Combinations

The advantages of cytotoxic drug combinations are compelling (Table 6-4).[4] Several agents can be administered concurrently at full therapeutic doses, provided that the potential life-threatening toxicities of the selected chemotherapy agents do not overlap. The result is the maximum possible destruction of tumor cells within the range of toxicity tolerated by the host for each individual drug. A broader range of coverage is provided against the cell lines in the heterogeneous tumor mass when agents are chosen with different mechanisms of action. When several agents are given, the odds favor more cell lines responding to at least one of the cytotoxic agents.

Combination therapy may also prevent or slow the emergence of new resistant cell lines during therapy, prolonging the usefulness of those particular drugs against the tumor. Although new mutations continue throughout the life of the tumor, a single new mutation is unlikely to create a cell line resistant to all components of any multidrug regimen. The new clones are then likely to be destroyed before reproducing significantly. Regimens that cause dramatic cell destruction early in therapy also discourage new mutations by reducing the number of cell-doubling opportunities, because dead cells cannot mutate into drug-resistant cells.

Despite these important advantages, combination chemotherapy regimens have serious disadvantages (Table 6-4). Most important, although the drugs chosen do not have additive life-threatening toxicities, no cytotoxic drug is without some significant adverse effects. Multiplying the number of drugs multiplies the toxicities as well. (Many of these toxicities are described in chapters 7–9.) For the benefit of greater cell destruction with relative safety, the patient is subjected to the unpleasant trade-off of potential drug-induced damage to many organ systems. This point is illustrated by the CAP regimen (Table 6-5), a combination of cyclophosphamide, Adriamycin (doxorubicin), and Platinol (cisplatin) used to treat gynecological cancers. The net result is a high degree of discomfort, but the risk of major toxicities that could lead to death is reduced.

Safe combination chemotherapy depends on the ability to combine drugs with noncumulative serious toxicity. In reality, doing so is difficult. Bone marrow suppression in particular, with its risks of serious infection and bleeding, is the rule rather than the exception among antineoplastic agents. The few drugs that do not cause myelosuppression are not active against all cancer types. Despite improvements in supportive care, doses of drugs given in combinations may need to be reduced below single-agent dose amounts to decrease the risk of life-threatening bone marrow suppression. Some sacrifice in efficacy because of these dose reductions is inescapable and may compromise the cure rates of the chemotherapy regimen. This phenomenon is called the *dose effect*.[6,19,20]

Combination regimens are complicated therapies for both patients and physicians because of the broad range of toxicities, the potential for drug interactions among the agents, and the need for optimal scheduling of drug doses. Patients require close monitoring, which means a major commitment of time and health resources, resulting in high costs. Combination therapy typically requires more clinic visits, more extensive patient monitoring, and greater drug expense and is generally more debilitating for the patient than single-agent therapy. The expense and risks are justified if combination therapy achieves its goals of increased response rate and survival without compromising patient safety.

Table 6-5. Potential Toxicities of the CAP Regimen

Toxicity	Responsible Drug
Alopecia	C,A
Ototoxicity	P
Stomatitis	A
Cardiotoxicity	A
Skin ulceration	A
Nausea and vomiting	C,A,P
Myelosuppression	C,A
Nephrotoxicity	P
Bladder toxicity	C
Neuropathy	P

SOURCE: DeVita VT, Schein PS. The use of drugs in combination for the treatment of cancer. *N Engl J Med* 1973;288:998–1006. C, cyclophosphamide; A, Adriamycin (doxorubicin); P, Platinol (cisplatin).

Table 6-4. Advantages and Disadvantages of Combination Chemotherapy

Advantages
1. Maximum cell kill within acceptable toxicity
2. Broad coverage against multiple cell lines
3. Slow emergence of resistant strains

Disadvantages
1. Multiple toxicities with greater patient discomfort
2. Impact of dose effect
3. Complicated to administer
4. Expensive

Guidelines for Developing Drug Combinations

The optimal combination of drugs for the treatment of any cancer is not and may never be known because the tumor heterogeneity of the same cancer may vary substantially among patients. However, much has been learned in the past 30 years about effective design and administration of cytotoxic combinations, and some general guidelines can be suggested.

Effective Drug Use

Only drugs that are effective when used alone against a particular tumor type should be used in combinations. Ideally, each of these drugs should be able to produce at least a small percentage of complete responses when used alone. With rare exceptions, agents that produce only low incidences (10–20%) of partial responses rather than complete responses generally contribute little to a regimen except toxicity. Combinations of inactive drugs cannot convert a refractory tumor into a curable one. Unfortunately, the lack of effective cytotoxic agents is still the basic cause of failure in cancer chemotherapy.

The drugs chosen should work by different mechanisms of action to deliver multiple insults to the tumor and permit independent cell destruction by each agent. This strategy also decreases the likelihood that new somatic mutations in the tumor masses will produce resistance to more than one agent simultaneously (cross-resistance). For the same reasons, drugs known to show cross-resistance (e.g., drugs that require the same enzyme for activation) should not be used together, because a single mutation could make both agents useless.

Truly synergistic combinations, if they exist for a given tumor, provide an added advantage. In oncology practice, therapeutic synergy exists if a drug combination produces a greater response rate or survival time than is possible with each drug used alone at its optimum dose.[6] Therapeutic synergy was demonstrated in early combination therapy trials of childhood acute leukemia when the combination of mercaptopurine and prednisone, which should have added up to a 40–50% complete response rate, induced complete responses in 82% of treated children. Unfortunately, true synergism is only rarely documented.

Combinations should include the greatest number of effective drugs possible. Because the major reason for the success of combination therapy is coverage of multiple resistant cell lines within the tumor, Goldie and Coldman's[2] mathematical model predicts the maximal chance of cure if all available effective drugs are given simultaneously. This is rarely possible, because of additive toxicities, but several approaches increase the number of drugs that can be given in a short period of time. One option is to administer alternating cycles of equally effective non-cross-resistant drug combinations. This method has been best studied in the treatment of Hodgkin's disease with alternating cycles of MOPP (*m*echlorethamine, vincristine [*O*ncovin], *p*rocarbazine, and *p*rednisone) and ABVD (doxorubicin [*A*driamycin], *b*leomycin, *v*inblastine, and *d*acarbazine) (Table 6-6). In the course of 2 months, eight effective drugs are targeted at the cancer. Another technique being tested is the use of hybrid combinations (Table 6-6). Half the scheduled number of doses of two different effective combinations are given over the time usually occupied by a single cycle. This approach results in tumor exposure to twice as many effective drugs at full doses in half the time.[4]

Table 6-6. An Alternating Regimen Compared with a Hybrid Combination

Agent	Dose	Schedule
MOPP-ABVD[a]		
Cycle 1		
Mechlorethamine (M)	6 mg/m²	Days 1 and 8
Vincristine (Oncovin) (O)	1.4 mg/m²	Days 1 and 8
Procarbazine (P)	100 mg/m²	Days 1–14
Prednisone (P)	40 mg/m²	Days 1–14
Cycle 2		
Doxorubicin (Adriamycin) (A)	25 mg/m²	Days 1 and 15
Bleomycin (B)	10 units/m²	Days 1 and 15
Vinblastine (V)	6 mg/m²	Days 1 and 15
Dacarbazine (D)	375 mg/m²	Days 1 and 15
MOPP-ABV Hybrid[b]		
Mechlorethamine	6 mg/m²	Day 1
Vincristine	1.4 mg/m²	Day 1
Procarbazine	100 mg/m²	Days 1–7
Prednisone	40 mg/m²	Days 1–14
Doxorubicin	35 mg/m²	Day 8
Bleomycin	10 units/m²	Day 8
Vinblastine	6 mg/m²	Day 8

SOURCE: reference 19.
[a]Give MOPP and ABVD on alternate months.
[b]Repeat all drugs each month.

Overlapping Toxicity

The problem of selecting drugs that do not produce an additive risk of life-threatening toxicity has been addressed (see Tables 6-4 and 6-5), but its importance in patient protection cannot be overemphasized. Such selection leads to a greater range of side effects and more patient discomfort, but it permits higher doses of individual agents and, accordingly, a greater chance of cure. Toxicity that is directly attributable to a drug is not a sufficient reason to eliminate the drug from the therapy. The pattern of toxicity of chemotherapy drugs must be very well known before they can be safely incorporated into a combination regimen. Dehydration from nausea and vomiting, for example, may increase the potential for bladder toxicity from cyclophosphamide, because prevention of bladder damage depends on high urine output. Attention must also be given to the potential for pharmacokinetic drug interactions when drugs are combined. For example, drugs that cause nephrotoxicity may increase the toxic and therapeutic effects of drugs excreted renally, such as methotrexate.

Optimal Dose and Schedule of Administration

The dosage of most chemotherapy agents is calculated on the basis of the patient's body surface area (BSA). The dosage is usually reported as milligrams, grams, or units of drug per square meter of BSA (e.g., 100 mg/m²). BSA has been chosen rather than body weight as the standard unit of comparison for two reasons. First, BSA has been demonstrated to provide a more accurate cross-species comparison of activity and toxicity for many drugs. These comparisons have held true in preclinical animal studies and early clinical trials. Second, BSA can be more closely correlated with cardiac output, which determines the blood flow to the liver and kidneys and subsequently influences drug elimination. The BSA may be calculated with a nomogram (Figures 6-6 and 6-7) or the following formula (the average adult male BSA is 1.7 m²):

$$BSA\ (m^2) = weight\ (kg)^{0.425} \times height\ (cm)^{0.725} \times 0.007184$$

The most common reason for treatment failure (apart from inherent inactivity of available drugs) probably is failure to maintain frequent doses at maximum tolerated levels. It is a very human tendency on the part of both patients and clinicians to delay or decrease doses. Patients may want to get their strength back or feel really well for a while before being knocked down from receiving toxic chemotherapy again, or they may want to delay treatment until after a special social event. Physicians tend to decrease doses arbitrarily for elderly patients, although it is not well established that this population's tolerance of chemotherapy is any worse than that of younger

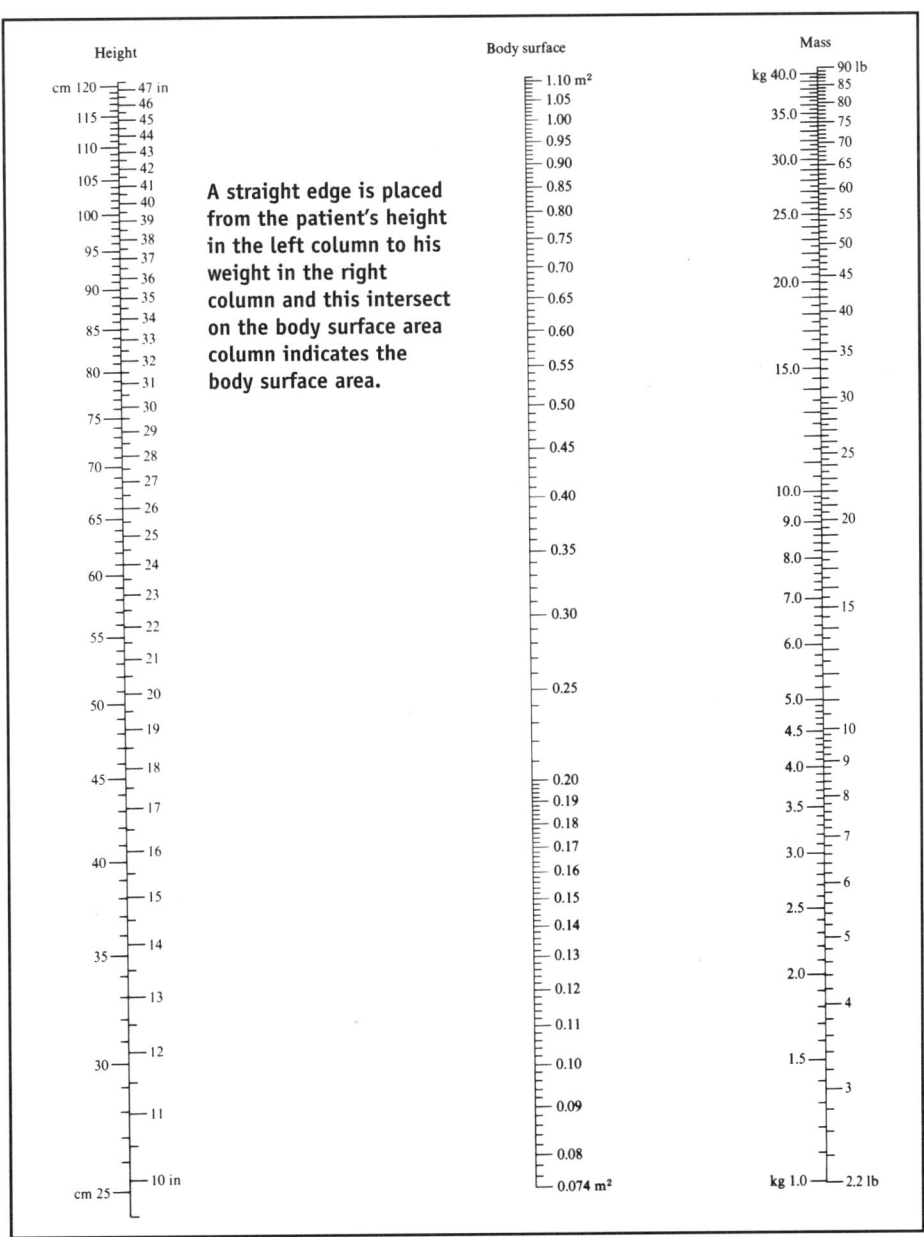

Figure 6-6. Body surface area of children
SOURCE: reprinted with permission from Lentner C, editor. *Geigy Scientific Tables*. Vol. 1. 8th ed. Basel, Switzerland: Ciba-Geigy; 1981. p. 226.

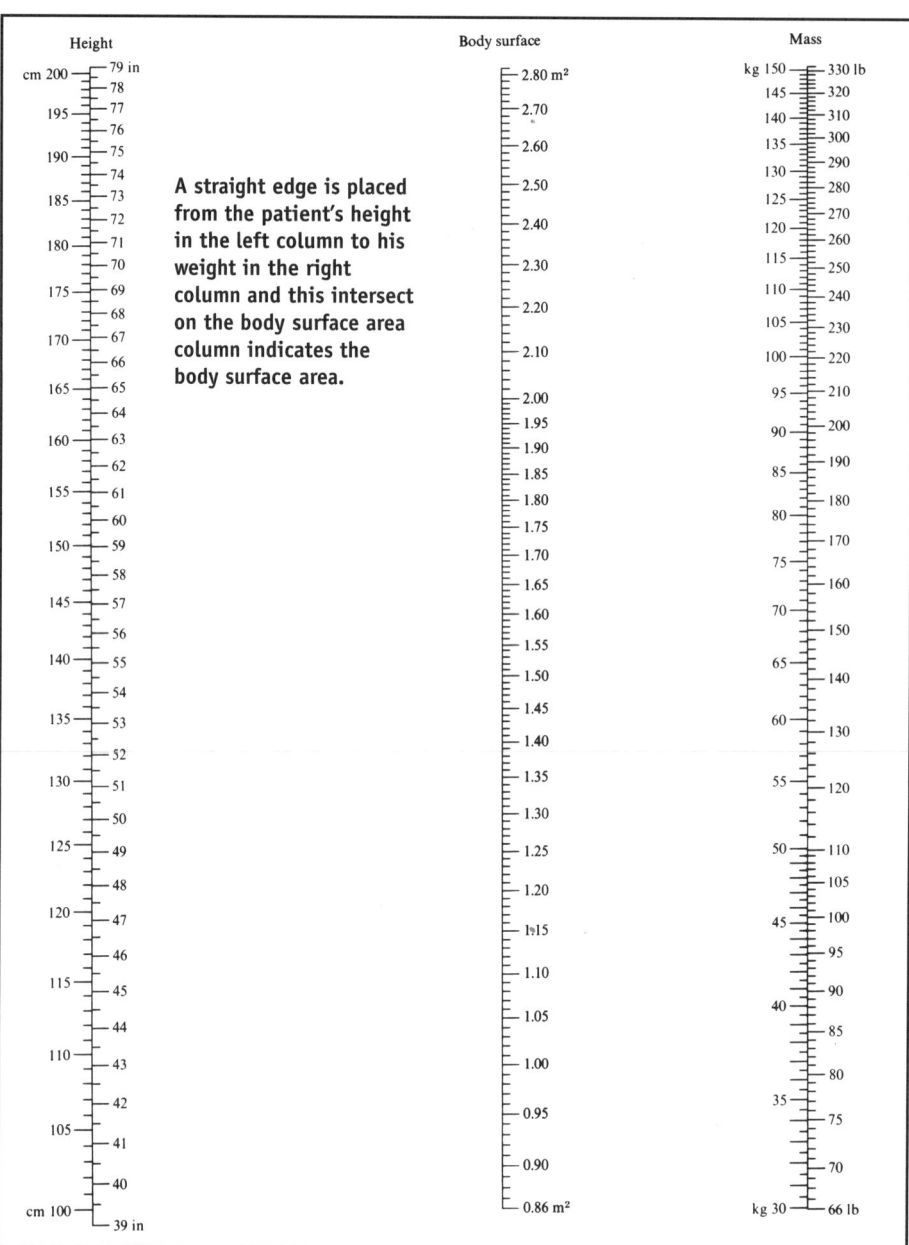

Figure 6-7. Body surface area of adults
SOURCE: reprinted with permission from Lenter C, editor. *Geigy Scientific Tables*. Vol. 1. 8th ed. Basel, Switzerland: Ciba-Geigy; 1981. p. 227.

adults.[4,19,20] Doctors may seek to minimize risk of infection when patients live long distances from medical care facilities or are unreliable. Despite the apparently compassionate reasons for reducing doses, a high price may be paid in compromised efficacy of the chemotherapy regimen.

The amount of drug given per unit of time, called the *dose rate* or *dose intensity*,[19,20] has a profound influence on outcome. This point was dramatically illustrated when a multigroup study of acute myelogenous leukemia chemotherapy regimens by the Southwest Oncology Group found that discrepancies in the dose rate caused a major variation in the response rate among institutions.[4,19] Experienced institutions with better supportive care facilities repeated treatment courses at the prescribed 2-week intervals, despite low white blood cell counts and high risks of complications. Less experienced centers tended to extend the interval to 3 weeks, a 50% decrease in dose rate, although all doses were eventually given. The impact of this change was a halving of the response rate; the complete response rate dropped from 53 to 25%.

Some dose adjustments and delays are required to ensure patient safety because interpatient variability in drug pharmacokinetics and dynamics demonstrates that all patients

Table 6-7. MOPP Chemotherapy Regimen Dose Adjustment Guideline

Leukocyte Count	Platelet Count	Dose Adjustment
>4000/mm^3	100,000/mm^3	100% all drugs
3000–4000/mm^3	100,000/mm^3	100% vincristine, 50% mechlorethamine and procarbazine
2000–3000/mm^3	50,000–100,000/mm^3	100% vincristine, 25% mechlorethamine and procarbazine
1000–2000/mm^3	50,000/mm^3	50% vincristine, 25% mechlorethamine and procarbazine
<1000/mm^3	50,000/mm^3	No therapy

SOURCE: Hellman S, Jaffe ES, DeVita VT. Hodgkin's disease. In: DeVita VT, Hellman S, Rosenberg SA, editors. *Cancer: Principles and Practice of Oncology*. 3rd ed. Philadelphia, PA: JB Lippincott; 1989. p. 1718.

cannot be optimally dosed by any single arbitrary regimen. It is important, however, that dose adjustment guidelines for particular regimens be followed so that doses are adjusted no more than absolutely necessary.[4,20] An example of such a guideline, for MOPP, is given in Table 6-7.[4] Subsequent doses may be increased if toxicity is minimal, so that underdosing is avoided and maximum dose intensity is achieved. When dose adjustment is required, every attempt should be made to give at least partial doses of all the drugs in the combination to avoid negating the strategy that directed their selection. This point is particularly true if the components of the combination interact mechanistically on the tumor cells. It is imperative that strong supportive care systems be available to treat both the predictable effects of myelosuppression and the unforeseen life-threatening toxicities that are always a risk with these dangerous agents.

Appropriate scheduling is another way to achieve optimal therapeutic benefit from the drugs in a combination regimen with minimal toxicity. The most common concern is hematological toxicity—the most difficult toxicity to avoid, because nearly all of the antineoplastic agents available cause myelosuppression. To minimize this risk, bone marrow-sparing drugs are given between courses of myelotoxic chemotherapy in some regimens. This method gives added insults to the tumor without prolonging the period of myelosuppression, but its utility is limited by the sensitivity of the tumor to bone marrow-sparing agents. Fortunately, the pattern of recovery of normal bone marrow tissue is fairly consistent. Neutropenia and thrombocytopenia typically do not appear until 7–10 days after myelotoxic chemotherapy, because the bone marrow has a storage reserve of cells. The lowest trough of blood cell counts (the nadir) is reached at about 16 days in many commonly used combination regimens. Hematological recovery usually begins within 3 weeks and is complete within 4 weeks.[4] This consistent pattern of bone marrow suppression and recovery makes another common approach feasible. A second full dose of myelotoxic drugs can be given on day eight of a chemotherapy cycle, just as the white blood cell count is beginning to drop from the first dose. By the time the full effects of the second dose are felt, the bone marrow is beginning to recover from the first insult. Although the nadir period may be prolonged, it is usually well tolerated as long as the degree of white blood cell count depression is not extreme.[4] The use of hematopoietic growth factors may also attenuate the myelosuppressive effects. Growth factors that modulate the granulocyte (filgrastim and sargramostim), macrophage (sargramostim), and megakaryocyte (oprelvekin) cell lineages are available. The use of hematopoietic growth factors must be scheduled carefully to avoid additive myelosuppressive effects. If blood cell precursors are being stimulated by the use of CSFs and myelotoxic chemotherapy is administered concomitantly, enhanced myelosuppression may occur.

Another important consideration in drug scheduling is drug interactions involving cell cycle kinetics, which were referred to in the discussion of strategies for combination therapy. Treatment is frequently begun with cell-cycle-nonspecific agents, such as alkylators, which can kill even resting cells. These indiscriminate killers decrease tumor bulk and recruit more cells into active division to make them more susceptible to cell-cycle-specific drugs that are given later. Sequential fluorouracil and methotrexate dosing is a good example of the importance of cell cycle kinetic scheduling. Other strategies that require careful attention to scheduling are tumor priming and rescue of normal cells with an antidote. When the mechanisms of drug action and interaction are better understood, more scheduling guidelines of this nature will likely be developed.

It is important to note that the toxicity pattern may also change considerably if the schedule of administration is altered. For example, if fluorouracil is administered as a single bolus injection each week, the most significant toxicity is usually myelosuppression. However, the most significant toxicity of fluorouracil when it is given as a continuous infusion over 4–5 days is ulceration of the mucosal lining of the mouth (stomatitis) or lower gastrointestinal tract. The latter results in severe diarrhea.

Attention has been given to the administration of some agents at particular times during the 24-hour day according to biological rhythms (circadian timing). This scheduling method is based on the premise that normal tissues in the body vary in their metabolism and proliferation in response to the daily rhythm of hormone and growth factor release, whereas malignant tissues are less dependent on these daily cycles. Chronobiotic trials in animals first demonstrated that the time of day of administration of some antineoplastics affected their therapeutic activity and toxicity. For example, doxorubicin toxicity is greatest in rodents when the drug is given late in the daily activity cycle, and cisplatin toxicity is greatest when given early in the daily cycle. Clinical trials continue to investigate these principles in the hope of augmenting the activity of some therapies or diminishing serious toxicities. One limited clinical study demonstrated that toxicity of doxorubicin and cisplatin was decreased when the doxorubicin was administered in the morning and the cisplatin in the evening rather than the reverse.[21] In some cases, altering the schedule to alleviate some toxicity may be tempting. However, such changes should not be made indiscriminately, because the activity of the drug may be lessened. Randomized clinical trials must be completed to ascertain whether the overall effectiveness is superior for either schedule.

PATIENT-RELATED FACTORS

A number of host-related factors influence the patient's response to chemotherapy. The most important is the patient's general health status and ability to withstand the toxicities associated with cancer chemotherapy. One method to subjectively evaluate the patient's overall status is the use of performance status criteria. Appendix III describes the Karnofsky Performance Status Criteria. Application of these criteria prior to and periodically throughout the treatment helps clinicians determine whether the patient's general condition is worsening. This information, used in conjunction with objective evaluation of tumor response (i.e., complete response, partial response, stable disease, or progression), can guide treatment decisions.

As mentioned previously, it is extremely important to recognize general health status factors as well as the more specific factors detailed below that influence a patient's ability to withstand treatment and to attenuate dosages only when necessary to avoid life-threatening toxicities. Any reduction in dosage may also compromise antitumor activity, so such reductions must be weighed carefully.

Immunocompetence

Although it is difficult to quantitate the importance of the immune system response to malignant cells, it is well appreciated that both cellular and humoral factors play an important role in fighting cancer. Several studies have shown that patients with different types of cancer are less likely to respond to chemotherapy if their cell-mediated immunity is impaired. In addition, as the cancer progresses it may cause further deterioration of the immune system, and both chemotherapy and radiation therapy may also impair the immune system. Therefore, it is difficult to judge whether the patient's lack of response is a result of a deteriorating immune system or the cause of the immune system's deterioration. Either way, it is important to avoid unnecessary insults to the immune system, such as the use of immunosuppressants (e.g., corticosteroids for minor disorders).

Renal and Hepatic Function

Like almost all other drugs, most antineoplastic agents are eliminated by either renal or hepatic mechanisms. Prolonged systemic exposure to the drug may occur if the patient has significant impairment of the organ that is primarily responsible for eliminating that drug. This prolonged exposure often results in increased toxicity. It is important to evaluate a patient's renal and hepatic function before starting chemotherapy and periodically between courses of chemotherapy. A sudden impairment in hepatic or renal function means the patient should be monitored for signs of toxicity. Unfortunately, clearly defined guidelines for dosage reduction in renal and hepatic dysfunction are available for only a few of the cytotoxic drugs. Therefore, in many instances empiric adjustments must be made. Table 6-8 lists some of the recommended dosage guidelines. A patient's ability to tolerate further chemotherapy may also be limited by major organ toxicity caused by previous administration of cytotoxic drugs. Many of these toxicities are described in chapters 7–9.

Prior Exposure to Chemotherapy and Radiation Therapy

Myelosuppression is the most significant dose-limiting toxicity of many of the antineoplastic agents. The bone marrow stem cells, from which new blood cells are formed, are damaged by radiation and chemotherapy. Because there is only a limited number of bone marrow stem cells, repeated insults from radiation and chemotherapy may result in progressively lower blood cell counts and longer periods until recovery. For adults, much of the blood-cell-producing bone marrow is located in the sternum and pelvic bones, and radiation to these areas can have profound effects on the circulating blood counts. For patients who have had extensive prior chemotherapy or radiation treatment, it may be necessary to lower dosages or lengthen the interval between courses or both to avoid life-threatening aplasia.

Nutritional Status

It has been recognized for some time that patients who are in a good nutritional state have less severe myelosuppression than those who are nutritionally depleted. The severity of mucositis and other toxicities may also depend on the nutritional status of the patient. High nutritional standards for patients receiving chemotherapy aid in safely administering optimal chemotherapy dosages (see chapter 18).

Age

Much controversy has been generated about the ability of elderly patients to withstand the debilitating effects of chemotherapy. In some elderly patients, bone marrow recovery may be prolonged because of the toxic effects of chemo-

Table 6-8. Recommended Dose Adjustments of Cytotoxics for Organ Dysfunction

Agents	Organ Dysfunction	Suggested Dose Modification
Methotrexate	Renal	Decrease dose in proportion to decrease in Cl_{creat} (normal 60 ml/m² per min).[a] Monitor serum levels after treatment and administer appropriate leucovorin rescue.
Cyclosphosphamide/ ifosfamide	Renal (Cl_{creat} <25 ml/min)	Dose reduction of 50%.[a]
Cisplatin	Renal (Cl_{creat} <60 ml/min)	Decrease dose in proportion to Cl_{creat}.[a]
Carboplatin	Renal (Cl_{creat} <60 ml/min)	Cl_{creat} of 41–49 ml/min: give 250 mg/m²; 16–40 ml/min: give 200 mg/m²; <15 ml/min: treatment not recommended or target AUC of 5–7 mg/ml per min.[b]
Bleomycin	Renal (Cl_{creat} ≤25 ml/min)	Dose reduction of 50–70%.[a]
Streptozocin	Renal (Cl_{creat} <25 ml/min)	Same as bleomycin.
Vincristine, vinblastine, vinorelbine	Hepatic	Bilirubin >1.5 mg/100 ml: reduce initial dose by 50%; >3.0 mg/100 ml: reduce initial dose by 75% (approximate guidelines).[a]
Etopisde	Renal	In proportion to Cl_{creat}/100 when Cl_{creat} is <60 ml/min.
Fludarabine	Renal	Same as etoposide.
Pentostatin	Renal	Same as etoposide.
Cladribine	Renal	Same as etoposide.
Docetaxel	Hepatic	Per package insert.
Paclitaxel	Hepatic	Dose reduction of 25–50% for patients with hepatic metastases >2 cm.

Cl_{creat}, creatinine clearance; AUC, area under concentration-versus-time curve [AUC = Dose/(Cl_{creat} + 25)].
[a]SOURCE: Chabner BA, Myers CE. Clinical pharmacology of cancer chemotherapy. In: DeVita VT, Hellman S, Rosenberg SA, editors. *Cancer: Principles and Practice of Oncology.* 3rd ed. Philadelphia, PA: JB Lippincott; 1989. p. 349–95.
[b]SOURCE: Paraplatin package insert. Evansville, IN: Bristol-Myers; February 1989.

therapy. However, if kidney, liver, heart, and lung functions are intact and the patient's nutritional status is good, administering full doses of chemotherapy is usually safe. A patient with concomitant diseases may be at higher risk of experiencing serious complications, however.

SELECTION OF CHEMOTHERAPY REGIMENS

Many factors influence whether an individual patient will respond to chemotherapy. The selection of a particular regimen for a patient must be based on a careful and comprehensive assessment of each of these factors. The histological documentation of tumor type and stage of the disease are the most important determinants of therapeutic options (Table 6-9). When these variables have been confirmed, determination of other prognostic variables should further delineate treatment options.

For example, as shown in Figure 6-8, in the case of a woman with breast cancer recently diagnosed from a biopsy sample, the next step should be to assess whether she has metastases. If none are apparent, then axillary lymph nodes must be exam-

Table 6-9. Steps in Selection of a Chemotherapy Regimen

1. Determination of histological diagnosis, tumor stage, and prognostic variables
2. Identification of treatment options and determination of benefits
3. Assessment of comorbid conditions and psychosocial environment
4. Determination of treatment-related risks
5. Assessment of risk versus benefit
6. Selection of therapeutic regimen

```
Biopsy breast lump: malignant
            ↓
History and physical: to assess for tumor spread
            ↓
Assess other prognostic variables: lymph node
involvement, menopausal status, estrogen
receptor status, S phase fraction,
HER/2-neu status
            ↓
Define treatment options and benefits:
radiation, adjuvant therapy, hormonal therapy,
or chemotherapy
            ↓
Assess comorbid conditions: organ function,
concomitant disease states, compliance,
psychosocial environment and stability,
cultural barriers
            ↓
Delineate treatment-related risks: short- and
long-term toxicities
            ↓
Risk-vs.-benefit assessment (e.g., risk of
endometrial cancer secondary to tamoxifen
treatment vs. decreased likelihood of breast
cancer recurrence)
            ↓
Treatment selection
```

Figure 6-8. Algorithm of treatment decisions in early-stage breast cancer

ined at the time of surgery to remove the localized tumor. Once the stage of the disease is determined, other disease-related factors that influence treatment outcomes must be considered. In the case of breast cancer, this may include such information as the woman's menopausal status, the presence of estrogen receptors, and the fraction of cells in the S phase (see chapter 12). This information will help to determine whether cytotoxic or hormonal therapy is indicated. The next step must evaluate any comorbid conditions (patient-related variables) that may affect either the patient's ability to tolerate therapy or the likelihood of response to therapy. This process should also consider any social, economic, cultural, or lifestyle barriers to the recommended treatment. For example, if the recommended therapy would necessitate frequent visits to a clinic or physician's office and the patient is unable or unwilling to comply, then an alternate treatment plan may be advisable.

To enable the patient to make an informed decision regarding treatment alternatives, the potential benefits of treatment must be presented from a balanced perspective along with the potential serious risks (e.g., life-threatening toxicities) associated with treatment. The patient must also be provided with a realistic plan for treatment that delineates what responsibilities will be placed on the patient. These responsibilities may include frequent clinic visits, invasive procedures, financial obligations, self-monitoring for toxicities, and other details that could affect the patient's physical, psychosocial, or financial well-being. When all of this information has been properly considered, the patient and the clinicians should mutually decide on a treatment plan that has the best chance of optimal outcomes in terms of cancer treatment, toxic effects, and quality of life.

SUMMARY

Many factors influence whether a patient will respond to chemotherapy. The inherent heterogeneity of tumor cells presents the greatest challenge to successful therapy. The use of combination chemotherapy with non-cross-resistant agents has clear advantages over single-agent therapy. A steep dose-response curve apparently exists for most chemotherapy agents. However, most of the serious toxicities associated with these drugs are dose related as well. Therefore, optimal therapy is usually defined as the maximum tolerated dose. Other factors—such as the schedule of administration, cellular kinetics, the site and vascularity of the tumor, the pharmacokinetic characteristics of the agent or agents, and the patient's immune function—may influence the effectiveness of the therapy. A patient's physical conditions may also limit his or her ability to tolerate aggressive chemotherapy and therefore compromise optimal therapy. The choice of therapy requires consideration of each variable that affects outcome as well as careful assessment of the potential risks and benefits of treatment. Regardless of the variables under consideration, the patient must be an active participant in all treatment decisions.

REFERENCES

1. Frei E III, Bickers JN, Hewlett JS, et al. Dose schedule and antitumor studies of arabinosyl cytosine (NSC 63878). *Cancer Res* 1969;29:1325–32.
2. Goldie JH, Coldman AJ. A mathematical model for relating the drug sensitivity of tumors to the spontaneous mutation rate. *Cancer Treat Rep* 1979;63:1727–33.
3. Dexter DL, Leith JT. Tumor heterogeneity and drug resistance. *J Clin Oncol* 1986;4:244–57.
4. Beck WT, Dalton WS. Mechanisms of drug resistance In: DeVita VT Jr, Hellman S, Rosenberg SA, editors. *Cancer: Principles and Practice of Oncology.* 5th ed. Philadelphia, PA: Lippincott-Raven; 1997. p. 498–512.
5. Frei E III. Pathobiology of cancer. In: Rubenstein E, Federman DD, editors. *Scientific American Medicine.* New York: Scientific American; 1986. p. 1–17.
6. Deuchars KL, Ling V. P-glycoprotein and multidrug resistance

7. Roninson IB, Abelson HT, Hausman DE, et al. Amplification of specific DNA sequences correlates with multidrug resistance in Chinese hamster cells. *Nature* 1984;309:626–31.
8. Borst P. DNA amplification and multidrug resistance. *Nature* 1984;309:580–7.
9. Ling V, Juranka PF, Endicott JA, et al. Multidrug resistance and P-glycoprotein expression. In: Woolley PV, Tew KD, editors. Mechanisms of drug resistance in neoplastic cells. New York: Academic Pr; 1988. p. 197–209.
10. Kartner ND, Evernden-Porelle G, Bradley G, et al. Detection of P-glycoprotein in multidrug-resistant cell lines by monoclonal antibodies. *Nature* 1985;316:820.
11. Robertson SM, Ling V, Stanners CP. Coamplification of double minute chromosomes, multiple drug resistance and cell surface P-glycoprotein in DNA-mediated transformants of mouse cells. *Mol Cell Biol* 1984;4:500–5.
12. Gruber A, Peterson C, Reizensteil P. D-verapamil and L-verapamil are equally effective in increasing vincristine accumulation in leukemic cells in vitro. *Int J Cancer* 1988; 41:224–9.
13. Skipper HE, Schabel FM, Wilcox WS. Experimental evaluation of potential anticancer agents, XXI: Scheduling of arabinosyl cytosine to take advantage of its S-phase specificity against leukemia cells. *Cancer Chemother Rep* 1967;51:125–41.
14. Southwest Oncology Group. Cytarabine for acute leukemia in adults: effect of schedule on therapeutic response. *Arch Intern Med* 1974;133:251–9.
15. Wittes RE, Goldin A. Unresolved issues in combination chemotherapy. *Cancer Treat Rep* 1986;70:105–21.
16. Pitot HC. Some principles of cancer chemotherapy. In: Pitot HC, editor. *Fundamentals of Oncology*. 2nd ed. New York: Marcel Dekker; 1981. p. 245–58.
17. Leyland-Jones B, O'Dwyer PJ. Biochemical modulation: application of laboratory models to the clinic. *Cancer Treat Rep* 1986;70:219–29.
18. Grem JL. 5-fluoropyrimidines. In: Chabner BA, Longo DL, editors. *Cancer Chemotherapy and Biotherapy*. 2nd ed. Philadelphia, PA: Lippincott-Raven; 1996. p. 149–212.
19. Frei E III, Canellos GP. Dose: a critical factor in cancer chemotherapy. *Am J Med* 1980;69:585–94.
20. Hryniuk WM. The importance of dose intensity in the outcome of chemotherapy. In: Hellman S, DeVita V, Rosenberg S, editors. *Important Advances in Oncology 1988*. Philadelphia, PA: JB Lippincott; 1988. p. 121–41.
21. Hrushesky WJM. Circadian timing of cancer chemotherapy. *Science* 1985;228:73–8.

SELF-STUDY QUESTIONS

1. Explain why chemotherapy doses should not be arbitrarily reduced for less serious toxicities.

2. Small cell lung cancer is characterized by very rapid cellular proliferation, whereas non-small cell lung cancer is characterized by much slower proliferation. Which of these types of lung cancer may be most sensitive to chemotherapy? Explain your rationale.

3. At the time of earliest clinical detection, when it is about 1 cm in diameter, a tumor typically already has about _____ cells.
   a. 100,000
   b. 1,000,000
   c. 100,000,000
   d. 1,000,000,000

4. Once the growth of a tumor mass has reached a plateau phase, _____.
   a. fewer cells are dividing and it becomes easier to manage with chemotherapy
   b. more cells are dividing and it becomes easier to manage with chemotherapy
   c. fewer cells are dividing and it becomes more difficult to manage with chemotherapy
   d. more cells are dividing and it becomes more difficult to manage with chemotherapy

5. Theoretically, the effects of chemotherapy on a mass of tumor cells follow _____ kinetics, meaning that _____.

6. In reality, the effect of chemotherapy on a mass of tumor cells may be unpredictable because _____.

7. The heterogeneity of cells in a tumor mass is a result of the _____.
   a. polyclonal origin of cells
   b. monoclonal origin of cells
   c. toxic effect of chemotherapy
   d. genetic instability of tumor cells
   e. both a and d are correct

8. Describe at least three mechanisms of antineoplastic drug resistance.

9. Exposure of tumor cells to chemotherapy may cause _____ or _____, which may result in drug resistance.

10. _____ is synonymous with multidrug resistance.
    a. Heterogeneity
    b. Pleiotropic drug resistance
    c. Intrinsic drug resistance
    d. Acquired drug resistance

11. The multidrug resistance mechanism usually confers cross-resistance to _____.

    a. all alkylating agents
    b. antitumor antibiotics
    c. many antineoplastics derived from plants
    d. all of the above
    e. only b and c

12. _____ is known to compete for P-glycoprotein binding, reversing multidrug resistance in vitro.

    a. Propranolol
    b. Verapamil
    c. Enalapril
    d. All of the above
    e. None of the above

13. Cytarabine is relatively ineffective when given as a bolus injection because _____.

14. The tumor exposure and cytotoxicity of cyclophosphamide are influenced by its rate of elimination as well as its rate of _____.

15. Explain why combinations of chemotherapy drugs are generally more successful than single agents.

16. Concomitant administration of methotrexate and fluorouracil is an example of _____.

    a. concurrent inhibition
    b. sequential blockade
    c. complementary inhibition
    d. competitive inhibition

17. Leucovorin acts as a _____ agent when given with methotrexate and a _____ agent when given with fluorouracil.

    a. biomodulating, rescue
    b. biomodulating, biomodulating
    c. rescue, biomodulating
    d. rescue, rescue

18. Describe four potential disadvantages of combination chemotherapy.

19. List the principles for developing combination chemotherapy regimens.

20. Describe three strategies that have been used with combination chemotherapy to minimize dose-related neutropenia while maintaining effectiveness.

21. Age >70 years is a relative contraindication for chemotherapy because of the risk of severe toxicity.

    a. true
    b. false

22. A 43-year-old woman receiving chemotherapy for ovarian cancer develops allergic dermatitis. Oral prednisone for 7 days is ordered to treat the reaction. Is this appropriate? Discuss your rationale.

Chapter 7: Systemic Toxicity

Carol Balmer, Pharm.D.
Associate Professor
University of Colorado School of Pharmacy
Denver, Colorado

Rebecca S. Finley, Pharm.D., M.S.
Chair and Associate Professor
Department of Pharmacy Practice
and Pharmacy Administration
Philadelphia College of Pharmacy
Philadelphia, Pennsylvania

Hematological Toxicity 100
   Neutropenia 101
   Thrombocytopenia 103
      Treatment of Thrombocytopenia 104
         Types and Risks of Platelet Transfusions 104
         Thrombopoietic Growth Factors 104
   Anemia 105
   Other Hematological Toxicities 106
Dermatological Reactions 106
   Drug Reactions 106
   Photosensitivity Reactions 109
   Radiation and Chemotherapy Reactions 109
   Recombinant Cytokine Reactions 109
   Nonchemotherapy Drug Reactions 109
   Alopecia 109
Hypersensitivity Reactions 110
Late Complications of Cancer Therapy 111
   Secondary Malignancies 111
      Radiation Therapy 111
         Factors Affecting Radiation-Induced Carcinogenicity 112
      Chemotherapy 112
   Gonadal Dysfunction and Infertility 113
      Effects of Cytotoxic Agents on Male Fertility 113
      Effects of Cytotoxic Agents on Female Fertility 115
      Prevention of Gonadal Damage 115
Summary 116
References 116
Self-Study Questions 118

The contributions made by Robert H. Hoy, Pharm.D., and Helen M. McFarland, Pharm.D., to this chapter are gratefully acknowledged.

One of the greatest challenges of cancer treatment is the prevention and management of cytotoxic drug damage to normal cells. Although some cancer cells have characteristics that make them more sensitive to the action of cytotoxic drugs, no cytotoxic drug is specific enough to selectively destroy cancer cells without causing any toxicity to the host.

Adverse effects of cytotoxic drugs are divided into the two general categories of systemic toxicity and major organ toxicity. Effects on major organs, such as the heart, liver, lungs, and nervous system, are detailed in chapter 8. Damage to the gastrointestinal tract is a component of major organ damage and is reviewed separately in chapter 9. This chapter addresses systemic toxicity, damage that occurs throughout the body, including hematological toxicity and dermatological and hypersensitivity reactions. Late complications of cancer therapy, including secondary malignancies and infertility, are also discussed in this chapter because carcinogenesis and the control of fertility may depend on the interactions of many components of the body.

After completing this chapter, the reader should be able to:

1. Outline the time course, potential sequelae, and risk factors for three common hematological toxicities: neutropenia, thrombocytopenia, and anemia.
2. Describe the role and rational use of hematopoietic growth factors in the prevention and management of neutropenia, thrombocytopenia, and anemia.
3. For each of the following subtypes of dermatological side effects of cytotoxic therapy, list commonly used cytotoxic agents that cause that effect, and recommend guidelines for management of that effect: rash, alopecia, photosensitivity reactions, hyperpigmentation, and hand-foot syndrome.
4. Compare the leukemia caused by anthracyclines with that caused by topoisomerase inhibitors.
5. Outline the effects of cytotoxic drugs on fertility and gonadal function in males and females, including the agents with most serious effects, the impact of age, reversibility, and management guidelines.

HEMATOLOGICAL TOXICITY

Myelosuppression, or bone marrow suppression, is the most pervasive toxicity of cancer chemotherapy. Myelosuppression, defined as the suppression of bone marrow activity, results in a reduced number of platelets, red cells, and white cells. It is the most common cause of chemotherapy treatment delays and dose reductions. These delays and reductions can compromise a patient's treatment plan, diminishing the patient's chance of treatment response and, in chemotherapy-sensitive malignancies, the chance of cure. The degree and severity of myelosuppression depend not only on the selection and dose of the cytotoxic drugs but also on patient-specific factors, such as age, degree of bone marrow reserve, or bone marrow compromise from previous chemotherapy or radiation therapy, and nutritional status.[1]

Cancer treatment often causes a confusing mix of desired and undesired pharmacologic effects. Chemotherapy used to treat solid tumors (e.g., breast, lung, prostate, and colon cancers that arise from solid tissues) has undesirable side effects on the bone marrow. In the treatment of hematological malignancies, such as leukemia, in which cancer cells may infiltrate the bone marrow, the toxic effects of chemotherapy on the bone marrow are the desired therapeutic actions.

All blood cells are produced in the bone marrow and

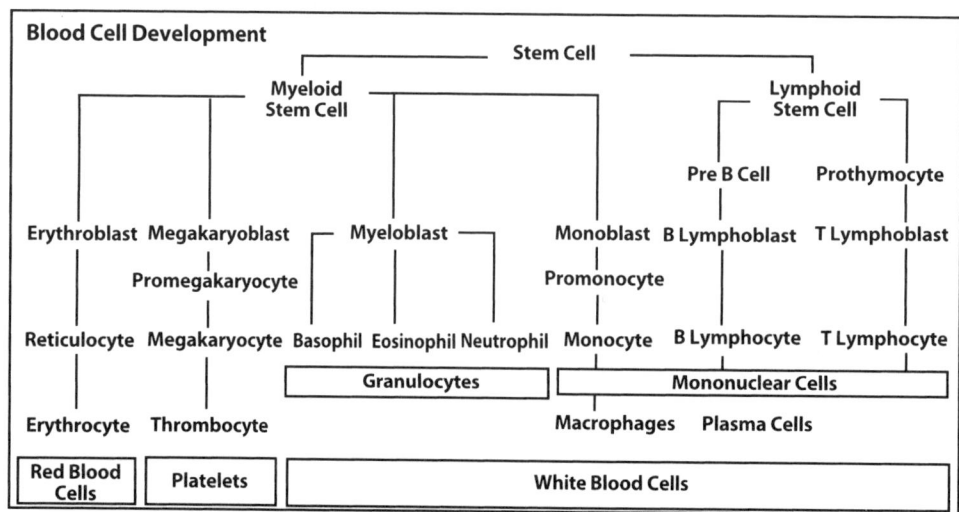

Figure 7-1. Blood cell development

arise from pluripotent stem cells (Figure 7-1). Stem cells have a lifelong ability to replicate and produce differentiated cells. The growth and differentiation of all blood cells are regulated by hematopoietic growth factors. These growth factors are cytokines that interact with specific receptors on hematopoietic cells to stimulate growth. Stem cells differentiate first into one of two types of committed stem cells, lymphoid and myeloid stem cells, that ultimately give rise to all circulating blood cells.[2] Lymphoid stem cells give rise to B and T lymphocytes. The role of lymphoid cells in the treatment of cancer with biological therapies is discussed in chapter 5. Lymphoid cell suppression is not a dose-limiting side effect of chemotherapy, but it can increase the patient's susceptibility to opportunistic infections (see chapter 15).[3]

Myeloid stem cells differentiate into all other blood cells: granulocytes (neutrophils, eosinophils, and basophils), monocytes, platelets, and red blood cells (RBCs). Suppression of neutrophils (neutropenia) and platelets (thrombocytopenia) is critical in the dosing of chemotherapy drugs because the risks of infection and bleeding that result from their suppression may be life threatening. Anemia, or too few RBCs, develops more slowly than neutropenia or thrombocytopenia, but it can seriously impact quality of life by contributing to pervasive weakness and fatigue.

Neutropenia

Neutrophils are phagocytic cells that destroy bacteria in the blood stream and in tissues. They are loosely (but not always correctly) referred to by several names: granulocytes (grans), polymorphonuclear leukocytes (PMNs or polys), or segs. Neutrophils normally make up >95% of granulocytes, the remainder being eosinophils and basophils. All neutrophils are granulocytes, but not all granulocytes are neutrophils. The terms *polymorphonuclear leukocytes* (*PMNs* or *polys*) and *segs* refer to the neutrophil's nucleus, which typically has several segments (segs) and can change shape (is polymorphic). These characteristics enable neutrophils to squeeze through small spaces between endothelial cells in blood vessel walls and enter tissues to destroy bacterial invaders.

Neutrophils are the cells most sensitive to the damaging effects of myelosuppressive chemotherapy. Two factors account for this susceptibility. The first is that neutrophils are very short-lived cells. They mature for 9–10 days in the bone marrow but live <1 day after they are released into the circulation. The average neutrophil's circulating half-life is about 6 hours. Second, neutrophils are also very plentiful, making up about 60% of the total white blood cell (WBC) count. Under normal conditions, neutrophil turnover is tremendous, with billions of new neutrophils being released into the circulating blood each day. Rapid turnover and a high growth fraction account for the sensitivity of neutrophils to the cytotoxic effects of chemotherapy.[4]

The normal absolute neutrophil count (ANC) averages 3000–7000 neutrophils/mm^3. To obtain the ANC you need the patient's complete blood count (CBC) with differential. The CBC provides the total WBC count, and the differential lists percentages for each type of WBC. Multiply the total WBC count by the percentage of neutrophils plus the percentage of bands (immature neutrophils).

Some drugs (e.g., corticosteroids, hormonal agents, bleomycin, vincristine, moderate doses of cisplatin [≤50 mg/m^2], asparaginase, and methotrexate with leucovorin rescue) produce little or no hematological toxicity, but most other cytotoxic drugs cause dose-related myelosuppression. The severity and pattern of myelosuppression produced by chemotherapy drugs are determined by pharmacologic and pharmacokinetic factors. Most chemotherapy agents have their greatest effects on rapidly growing cells, so they interfere with the growth of any neutrophils produced while sufficient concentrations of chemotherapy drugs are present. Other chemotherapy drugs kill cells in all phases of growth. Knowing the pharmacology and pharmacokinetics of the specific agents will help identify the pattern of myelosuppression that the patient is most likely to experience with therapy (see chapters 3 and 4).

The nadir of the WBC count is the lowest concentration of WBCs in the peripheral blood after cytotoxic chemotherapy. The nadir is usually reached 7–14 days after drug administration and corresponds with the decreased production of neutrophils, which normally take about 10 days to mature, that results from the cytotoxic effects of chemotherapy. The usual pattern of WBC suppression and recovery, when plotted on a graph, resembles in the shape of a valley (Figure 7-2). The magnitude of the toxic effect (depth of the valley or nadir) is proportional to the dose of the drug. The duration of neutropenia is related to pharmacokinetic factors that control drug concentration and elimination as well as to the schedule of cytotoxic drug administration. Nadirs are usually longer when cytotoxic drugs are administered each day for several days than when the full cytotoxic dose is administered on one day.

Normal ANCs provide a wide margin of safety against bacterial disease. ANCs are much higher during periods of active bacterial infection and may reach ≥90% of the total WBC count. The degree of risk of infectious complications secondary to neutropenia can be estimated from the ANC. The risk of infection is inversely proportional to the ANC, so the lower the ANC, the greater the risk of infection. In addition to how low the ANC goes, the risk of infectious complications is also affected by the duration of neutropenia.

A patient is said to be neutropenic when the ANC is <500 cells/mm^3 (or <1000 cells/mm^3, depending on institutional guidelines). Neutropenic patients should be watched closely for symptoms of infections, such as fever, chills, or sore throat. Fever is the most reliable sign of infection in neutropenic patients because it does not depend on the presence of neutrophils. Because the neutrophils are a critical component of the body's defenses against life-threatening bacterial and fungal infections, fever in a neutropenic patient must be

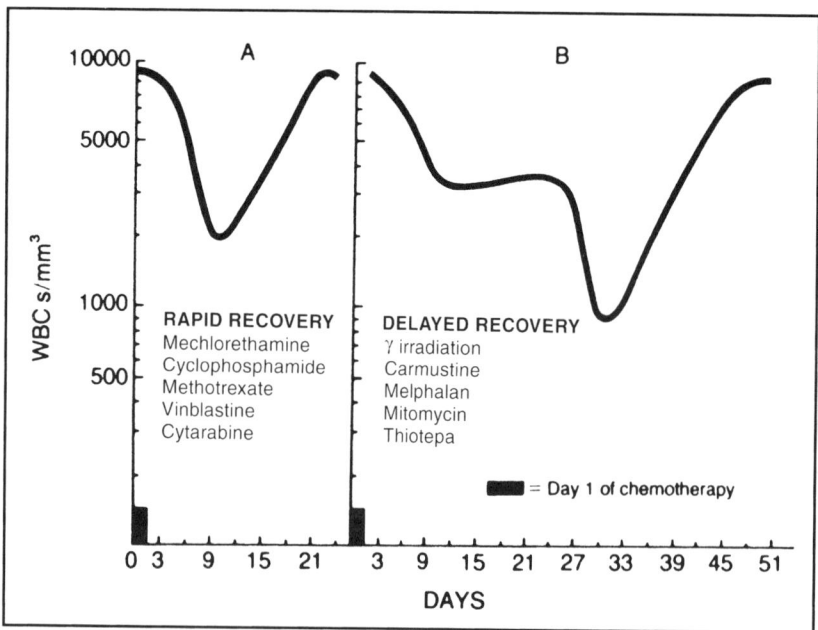

Figure 7-2. Patterns of chemotherapy myelosuppression
SOURCE: reprinted with permission from Young LY, Koda-Kimble MA, editors. *Applied Therapeutics*. Vancouver, WA: Applied Therapeutics; 1988. p. 1095.

treated as a medical emergency.[4] Management of infections in neutropenic patients is discussed in chapter 15.

The occurrence of neutropenic fever during one chemotherapy cycle requires that an intervention be made on subsequent cycles to decrease the risk of additional life-threatening neutropenic febrile events. A major exception to this general rule occurs in the treatment of acute leukemic patients for whom current cancer chemotherapy requires bone marrow ablation, despite risk of infection. Until recently, the only intervention that decreased the risk of neutropenic febrile events on subsequent chemotherapy cycles was reduction of the dose of the myelosuppresive agents. This compromise in dose can also compromise the patient's chances of tumor response and, in some situations, cure. Transfusion of neutrophils from donors to neutropenic patients is rarely a treatment option, because of the short life span of circulating neutrophils; transfused cells live only a few hours in the recipient.

Two neutrophil growth factors that decrease the clinical risks of neutropenia are commercially available: granulocyte colony-stimulating factor (G-CSF or filgrastim) and granulocyte-macrophage colony-stimulating factor (GM-CSF or sargramostim). G-CSF is a specific stimulant of neutrophil growth and differentiation. GM-CSF has broader effects and is considered a multilineage hematopoietic growth factor; it stimulates the growth and differentiation of neutrophils, eosinophils, and macrophages (monocytes). Because deficiencies of eosinophils and macrophages are not known to be clinically important as side effects of cancer chemotherapy, GM-CSF is administered for the same single purpose as G-CSF: to shorten the severity and duration of neutropenia that results from myelosuppressive chemotherapy administration. Food and Drug Administration (FDA)–approved indications for G-CSF and GM-CSF are listed in Table 7-1.[2,4,5]

CSFs may be administered to patients at high risk of febrile neutropenia on the first cycle of chemotherapy (primary administration), but they are more widely used to reduce the risk of febrile neutropenia following a cycle that is complicated by febrile neutropenia or neutropenia-induced treatment delays (secondary administration). Several randomized trials have shown a reduction in the duration of neutropenia, days on antibiotics, and days of hospitalization with use of these agents.[6]

Use of CSFs has had a major impact on the management of neutropenia as a dose-limiting systemic side effect of cytotoxic cancer treatment, but CSF use is quite costly. The average wholesale drug cost for a 10-day treatment course of CSFs for an adult of average size is more than $1500 for

Table 7-1. FDA-Approved Indications for Clinical Use of G-CSF and GM-CSF

Indication	G-CSF	GM-CSF
Acceleration of myeloid recovery in patients with NHL, Hodgkin's disease, and ALL undergoing ABMT		X
Congenital, cyclic, or idiopathic neutropenia	X	
Myelosuppressive chemotherapy	X	
BMT failure of engraftment		X
Induction chemotherapy in AML (GM-CSF approved for patients >55 years of age)	X	X
Peripheral blood progenitor cell mobilization	X	X

SOURCE: product package inserts (indication as of 8/98). FDA, U.S. Food and Drug Administration; G-CSF, granulocyte colony-stimulating factor (filgrastim); GM-CSF, granulocyte-macrophage colony-stimulating factor (sargramostim); NHL, non-Hodgkin's lymphoma; ALL, acute lymphocytic leukemia; ABMT, autologous bone marrow transplantation; BMT, bone marrow transplantation; AML, acute myelogenous leukemia.

Table 7-2. Summary of ASCO Recommendations for Use of Hematopoietic CSFs

Primary administration:	Administration of CSFs on the first cycle of chemotherapy should be reserved for patients with an expected incidence of febrile neutropenia comparable to or >40%. Exceptions to this may include patients at higher risk for chemotherapy-induced complications, such as patients with pre-existing neutropenia, a history of recurrent febrile neutropenia when receiving regimens of similar or less neutropenic potential, or conditions that increase the risks of serious infection (e.g., open wounds, decreased immune function, active tissue infections, poor performance status, and more advanced cancer).
Secondary administration:	Administration of CSFs on subsequent chemotherapy cycles is appropriate for patients with documented occurrence of febrile neutropenia in an earlier chemotherapy cycle, or if prolonged neutropenia causes excessive dose reduction or treatment delays.
Afebrile patients:	Use of CSFs is not recommended in afebrile neutropenic patients.
Febrile patients:	Administration of CSFs in addition to antibiotic therapy is not recommended, except in patients with pneumonia, hypotension, multiorgan dysfunction, or fungal infection.
Myeloid malignancies:	CSFs can reduce the morbidity of chemotherapy in patients >55 years of age after completion of induction chemotherapy. Their use in younger patients should be confined to clinical trials.
Radiation therapy:	CSFs should not be administered to patients receiving chemotherapy and radiation concomitantly.
Dosing and route:	Dose escalation above 5 µg/kg per day for G-CSF or 250 µg/m² per day for GM-CSF is not recommended. Doses may be rounded to the nearest vial size to reduce costs.
Initiation and duration:	Begin CSF treatment between 24 and 72 hours after chemotherapy is completed. Continue until ANC reaches 10,000 cells/µl or a lower limit specified in institutional guidelines.

SOURCE: references 6–8. ASCO, American Society of Clinical Oncology; CSFs, colony-stimulating factors.

each chemotherapy cycle. As with other costly drug resources, institutions commonly develop or adopt guidelines to limit inappropriate use and contain drug costs. The American Society of Clinical Oncology (ASCO) has published recommendations for the cost-effective use of these agents (Table 7-2).[6–8]

Thrombocytopenia

Thrombocytopenia has many potential causes in cancer patients, but the most common cause is chemotherapy (Table 7-3). Platelets, also called thrombocytes, are the second-most-sensitive cells to the effects of myelosuppressive chemotherapy. The aggregation or clumping of platelets is the body's first line of defense against bleeding. In the process of coagulation following vascular injury, platelets adhere to collagen fibers and aggregate to form the first stage of the clot. The release of platelet mediators then results in irreversible platelet aggregation. Platelets provide a receptor site for clotting factors and provide the phospholipid surface that is needed to convert prothrombin to thrombin in the formation of a stable fibrin cross-linked clot. Thrombocytopenia therefore increases the risk of severe bleeding and is a common cause of delays and/or dose reductions in the administration of subsequent chemotherapy treatments.[9]

Circulating platelets are non-nucleated cells that are fragments of mature megakaryocytes, large cells that develop from myeloid precursors. Normal peripheral platelet counts range from about 150,000 to 450,000 platelets/µl. As with ANCs, normal platelet counts provide a large margin of safety. Although bleeding times become progressively longer as platelet counts fall below 100,000 platelets/µl, increased bleeding with trauma or surgery does not usually occur until the platelet count is <50,000 platelets/µl. Spontaneous bleeding does not usually occur until the platelet count drops to 10,000–15,000 platelets/µl.[10,11] However, there is no well-established, safe threshold at which severe bleeding cannot occur.

The pattern of thrombocytopenia following chemotherapy administration is similar to that of neutropenia. The average platelet life span is approximately 1 week. Following cytotoxic chemotherapy, platelet counts decrease gradually to a nadir, which occurs at about the same time as the neutrophil nadir. Recovery to normal counts usually takes 3–4 weeks. A few chemotherapy agents, most notably carboplatin,

Table 7-3. Common Causes of Thrombocytopenia in Cancer Patients

> Bone marrow infiltration with malignant cells
> Disseminated intravascular coagulation
> Marrow aplasia or fibrosis
> Medications (e.g., amphotericin B, cimetidine, heparin, and thiazide diuretics)
> Myelosuppressive chemotherapy
> Radiation therapy
> Splenomegaly

nitrosoureas, and mitomycin, produce prolonged thrombocytopenia. Chemotherapy guidelines usually require patients to have platelet counts of >100,000 platelets/µl before receiving full doses of chemotherapy.

Treatment of Thrombocytopenia

Persistent or severe thrombocytopenia may require the use of platelet transfusions. Transfusing patients with donor platelets has been the only intervention for management of severe thrombocytopenia since it was first attempted in the early 1900s. Historically, the most commonly used threshold to trigger prophylactic platelet transfusions for patients with thrombocytopenia, in the absence of bleeding, is 20,000 platelets/µl.[10] There is recent evidence that the use of platelet transfusions can be decreased without a corresponding increase in the incidence of life-threatening bleeding episodes if platelet transfusions are reserved for patients whose platelet count is <10,000 platelets/µl.[12,13]

Types and Risks of Platelet Transfusions

Most patients receive random-donor platelets, platelet concentrates that are separated by centrifugation from several units of donated whole blood. These are the least expensive platelet transfusions, but because they come from many donors, they carry the greatest risk of infection from contamination. The risk of bacterial overgrowth is a concern because platelets must be stored at room temperature to preserve their ability to aggregate. Random-donor platelets also have the greatest risk of transfusion reactions, such as fevers, chills, and rigors. These are attributed to cytokines released by donor WBCs that remain in the platelet transfusions. Many patients eventually become refractory to the beneficial effects of random-donor platelet transfusions, meaning their platelet counts do not improve with subsequent transfusions. The main reason for this reaction is alloimmunization—the formation of antibodies against human leukocyte antigens (HLAs) found on donor blood cells. Exposure to simultaneously infused WBCs is probably the cause of the alloimmunization, because platelets themselves do not carry the HLAs that are required to cause primary immunization reactions. Alloimmunized patients may achieve a better clinical response from single-donor platelets, especially if the donor is HLA-matched to the patient. Unfortunately, single-donor platelets and HLA-matched platelets are much more expensive than random-donor platelet transfusions. Other common reasons for platelet refractoriness are sepsis and severe, continuous bleeding.[9,10]

Thrombopoietic Growth Factors

The first thrombopoietic growth factor, oprelvekin (interleukin 11 [IL-11]), was approved by the FDA in 1997, providing an alternative to platelet transfusions. It is indicated for prophylactic administration to reduce the need for platelet transfusions in patients at high risk for severe thrombocytopenia secondary to myelosuppressive chemotherapy. Use of oprelvekin is not indicated for use in patients with myeloid malignancies, such as acute myelogenous leukemia or chronic myelogenous leukemia, because it has the theoretical but unproven potential to stimulate myeloid precursors. It is feared that its use could stimulate the growth of myeloid leukemic cells. It is also not indicated for treatment of established thrombocytopenia.

Oprelvekin's approval was supported by two randomized, placebo-controlled trials. In the first trial, patients who had required platelet transfusions for severe thrombocytopenia during prior chemotherapy cycles were randomized to receive one of two oprelvekin doses or placebo. Their chemotherapy doses were not reduced. Thirty percent of patients who received the higher dose (50 µg/kg per day) were able to avoid platelet transfusion on this cycle of chemotherapy, compared with only 4% of patients who received placebo. Some efficacy was also documented with the lower dose (25 µg/kg per day).[14]

The second trial compared oprelvekin at doses of 50 µg/kg per day with a placebo in preventing the need for platelet transfusions in women with breast cancer who were receiving their first two cycles of a high-dose cyclophosphamide (3200 mg/m^2) and doxorubicin (75 mg/m^2) regimen, which was expected to produce a high degree of thrombocytopenia. Sixty-eight percent of patients who received oprelvekin did not require platelet transfusions, compared with 41% of patients who received the placebo. The total number of platelet transfusions required in the assessable subgroup and the time to platelet recovery were also significantly decreased.[15]

The FDA-approved dose of oprelvekin is 50 µg/kg per day. Dosing should begin 6–24 hours after completion of chemotherapy and continue past the platelet nadir until the platelet count has recovered to >50,000 platelets/µl. This will usually require 10–21 days of oprelvekin administration. The initial average wholesale price for 10 days of oprelvekin administration is about $1800.[16] The estimated cost of treating an episode of thrombocytopenia with platelet transfusions is $2600 per episode.[17] In addition to the financial costs of thrombopoietic growth factors, there is also a cost in toxicity. Oprelvekin causes fluid retention in >50% of patients, which typically manifests as edema and dyspnea on exertion, but the incidence of pleural effusions, atrial arrhythmias, syncope, fatigue, and reddened conjunctiva are also increased in patients receiving oprelvekin when compared with placebo.[14,15] Administration of diuretics to manage edema may help modify the toxicity of oprelvekin. Evidence-based practice guidelines for optimal utilization of this useful but expensive resource have not yet been published.

Other thrombopoietic growth factors that are under investigation include thrombopoietin, megakaryocyte growth and development factor (MGDF), and interleukin 6 (IL-6). These thrombopoietic growth factors are being evaluated in studies of patients with severe thrombocytopenia secondary to chemotherapy administration.[9,18] The chemoprotectant amifostine may provide another alternative therapy for thrombocytopenia management. In a recent randomized trial, amifostine attenuated the thrombocytopenia caused by carboplatin administration.[19] Together, these new developments in the management of thrombocytopenia give confidence that this dose-limiting side effect of cancer chemotherapy will soon be manageable with less dependence on platelet transfusions and, as a result, fewer complications.

Anemia

Like thrombocytopenia, anemia usually has many potential causes in patients with cancer. RBC levels may be affected by low production of hormonal signals for RBC production, tumor infiltration of the bone marrow, damage from prior chemotherapy or radiation therapy, hemolysis, blood loss, poor nutrition, or by the anemia of chronic disease, in addition to the direct chemotherapy-induced myelosuppression.[20] Cisplatin is the cytotoxic agent that produces the highest risk of anemia.

RBCs are much longer lived than neutrophils or platelets, with an average circulating life span of about 3 months. Consequently, anemia as a manifestation of myelosuppression is less common than neutropenia or thrombocytopenia, takes a greater number of chemotherapy cycles to develop, and is less likely to cause chemotherapy dose reductions or dose delays. Despite this, anemia is a significant contributing factor to symptoms of fatigue and weakness among patients receiving chemotherapy.

Clinically significant anemia is managed in most cancer patients by transfusion of packed RBCs. Retrospective studies indicate that about 18% of patients with solid tumors, 25% of patients with lymphoma, and >75% of patients with leukemia require RBC transfusions because of the toxicity of chemotherapy agents used to treat these diseases.[21] RBC transfusions share many of the risks of platelet transfusions, such as the risks of transfusion-related reactions and infections. Fluid overload is also a common problem because of the volume of the RBCs transfused and the necessity of administering fluids concomitantly.

Normal RBC production is regulated by endogenous erythropoietin production. Erythropoietin, a hematopoietic growth factor, is produced by the kidneys in response to low blood oxygen concentrations. Increased erythropoietin secretion results in an increased concentration of RBCs, with a correspondingly greater amount of hemoglobin that can carry oxygen to the tissues. It is an indirect but effective feedback system. Epoetin alfa (Epogen, Procrit) is a recombinant hematopoietic growth factor for RBC production. Chronic administration of epoetin alfa diminishes the need for RBC transfusions in patients with renal failure–induced anemia. Because the kidneys of patients receiving chemotherapy are usually functional, endogenous erythropoietin levels are usually not greatly diminished, compared with the very low levels in patients with chronic renal failure. The erythropoietin levels of cancer patients are generally slightly lower than those of normal controls, and cancer patients often demonstrate a decreased erythropoietin response. Epoetin alfa administration is clinically useful in treating cancer patients, but the responses in chemotherapy patients are less dramatic than those seen in patients with anemia of renal failure.[20] High doses of epoetin alfa (150–300 units/kg three times weekly) are required to increase RBC production in chemotherapy patients, and they

Table 7-4. Nonmyelosuppressive Hematological Toxicity of Chemotherapy Agents

Agent	Toxicity
Asparaginase	Clotting or bleeding abnormalities caused by decreased synthesis of clotting factors or natural anticoagulants
Cisplatin	Hemolytic anemia
Estrogens (males)	Increased incidence of thromboembolic effects
Fludarabine	Lymphocytopenia with opportunistic infections
Interleukin 2	Anemia; thrombocytopenia; coagulopathy; severe lymphocytopenia within first 24 hours, followed by rebound after stopping therapy
Mitomycin	Hemolytic uremic syndrome
Paclitaxel	Severe lymphocytopenia and opportunistic infections when combined with radiation therapy
Tamoxifen	Increased incidence of thromboembolic effects, especially in combination with chemotherapy

SOURCE: references 25–27.

have been proven to significantly reduce transfusion requirements.[2,5,21-23] What is perhaps more important is that epoetin alfa therapy significantly improves patients' self-rated scores for energy level, activity level, and overall quality of life. This improvement in functional status corresponds to increases in hemoglobin and is independent of tumor response.[24] The toxic effects of epoetin alfa in cancer patients are generally minimal and are limited to mild symptoms, such as low-grade fevers. Hypertension and seizures that have been associated with rapid increases in hematocrit in patients with chronic renal failure treated with epoetin alfa are rarely seen in cancer patients. Although epoetin alfa is nontoxic in cancer patients, it is costly therapy. Treatment should not be continued beyond 2–3 months in patients who fail to respond—those who lack objective increases in hematocrit or decreases in transfusion requirements or subjective decreases in anemia-related symptoms within 2 months. Optimal doses, schedules, and durations of therapy required to maximize therapeutic benefits in cancer patients remain to be defined.

Other Hematological Toxicities

Neutropenia, thrombocytopenia, and anemia are the most common hematological side effects of chemotherapy administration, but there are also many other effects on blood components and function. Some of the more established nonmyelosuppressive hematological toxicities of chemotherapy are outlined in Table 7-4.[25-27]

DERMATOLOGICAL REACTIONS

This section will provide a broad overview of the dermatological reactions that occur among patients with cancer, emphasizing reactions that commonly occur following chemotherapy. An exhaustive review of the dermatological complications of cancer is beyond the scope of this chapter, but comprehensive reviews are listed in the references.[28,29]

Dermatological complications of cancer range from mild erythema to rashes to widespread sloughing of dermal tissue; the severity of these complications ranges from mildly annoying to life threatening. In the broadest sense, dermatological reactions include nail and hair changes as well as skin and mucosal reactions. The potential causes of dermatological reactions in patients with cancer include drugs (both chemotherapy and nonchemotherapy drugs), the cancer itself, radiation therapy, and the manifestations of unrelated diseases. Many potential causes of problematic skin reactions are listed in Table 7-5.[29-52] Severe skin reactions can lead to secondary infections, bleeding complications (especially among thrombocytopenic patients), and delays in treatment. Skin reactions should be evaluated and managed appropriately to minimize the risk of severe complications.

When a potentially drug-related skin reaction occurs, the same steps recommended for distinguishing any adverse drug event should be taken. First, a temporal relationship with the drug or drugs in question and the appearance of the reaction should be established, and other potential causes should be ruled out. Skin biopsies and skin tests may be helpful in establishing a diagnosis, but testing patients with cancer may be problematic. Biopsies may be difficult or contraindicated in thrombocytopenic patients, and patients with depressed cellular immunity may not have reliable skin test results. If the cause of the skin reaction is not apparent, the first step should include discontinuation of any nonessential drugs that might be responsible. If those measures provide no relief, other therapies that are less likely to react with the potential culprit (i.e., a different class of drug) should be considered. In either case, comfort measures to relieve distressing symptoms and treatment of any secondary complications should be initiated immediately.

Management of dermatological reactions requires that pharmacists assist in identifying skin reactions and differentiating those related to drugs from those attributable to other causes. Pharmacists must collaborate with physicians and other health care providers in the assessment of these reactions and in the development of a care plan.

Drug Reactions

Cutaneous drug reactions are most often morbilliform or exanthematous (resembling symptoms of a viral disease). They may also have atypical presentations in patients who are immunosuppressed or thrombocytopenic. For example, in neutropenic patients, erythema associated with a skin infection (cellulitis) may be blunted or nonexistent. Similarly, profoundly suppressed cellular immunity may alter the appearance of local hypersensitivity reactions. Patients with severe thrombocytopenia may bleed into rashes or other skin eruptions, either spontaneously or as the result of scratching, and the severe hematomas that result may have an alarming appearance.

Hypersensitivity reactions are responsible for most morbilliform eruptions associated with drug therapy.[29] In addition to morbilliform eruptions, chemotherapy may also induce other types of skin changes, including hyperpigmentation, acral erythema (inflammatory redness of extremities), hidradenitis (inflammation of the sweat glands), and sclerotic plaques.

Hyperpigmentation is a result of stimulation of or toxicity to melanocytes.[28,34] This discoloration of the skin can present diffusely (e.g., after treatment with busulfan, dactinomycin, or hydroxyurea) or in localized areas (e.g., after treatment with fluorouracil or thiotepa). Patients who have received intravenous therapy with fluorouracil may notice hyperpigmented streaks overlying the veins in which the drug was administered. This condition is sometimes referred to as *roadmap veins*.[47] Other than the cosmetic concerns, hyperpigmentation is not usually a significant problem. Hyperpigmentation typically resolves gradually after the drug is stopped, but it occasionally is permanent.

Table 7-5. Potential Causes of Skin Reactions in Patients with Cancer

Cause	Reaction	Comments
Chemotherapy Drugs		
Bleomycin	Hyperpigmented linear streaks Raynaud's phenomenon Sclerotic plaques Neutrophilic apocrine hidradenitis Radiation enhancement and recall	Resemble striae
Busulfan	Hyperpigmentation	May mimic Addison's disease
Cyclophosphamide	Acral erythema Hyperpigmentation	
Cytarabine	Acral erythema (palmar-plantar erythrodyesthesia) Neutrophilic apocrine hidradenitis	
Dacarbazine	Photosensitivity reactions	
Dactinomycin	Hyperpigmentation Radiation enhancement and recall	May be accentuated by ultraviolet light
Docetaxel	Acral erythema (palmar-plantar erythrodyesthesia) Nail changes (Beau's lines) Scleroderma-like changes	Preceded by diffuse subcutaneous edema
Doxorubicin	Acral erythema (palmar-plantar erythrodyesthesia) Radiation enhancement and recall Neutrophilic apocrine hidradenitis	More common and severe with liposomal doxorubicin
Etoposide	Radiation recall	
Fluorouracil	Hyperpigmentation Radiation enhancement Photosensitivity reactions Acral erythema (palmar-plantar erythrodyesthesia)	Often causes streaks overlying veins May be accentuated by ultraviolet light
Hydroxyurea	Hyperpigmentation	Especially in traumatized areas
Ifosfamide	Hyperpigmenation	
Methotrexate	Hyperpigmentation Radiation enhancement and recall Photosensitivity reactions Acral erythema (palmar-plantar erythrodyesthesia)	May be accentuated by ultraviolet light Hyperpigmentation banding of light-colored hair
Mitoxantrone	Neutrophilic apocrine hidradenitis	
Paclitaxel	Erythematous macular lesions	In some cases they may progress to painful, vesicular exfoliative dermatitis
Thiotepa	Hyperpigmentation	
Vinblastine	Radiation recall Photosensitivity reactions	
Vincristine	Neutrophilic apocrine hidradenitis	
Recombinant Cytokines		
Filgrastim	Sweet's syndrome Vasculitis	Neutrophilic infiltration of the skin

Continued next page

Table 7-5. Potential Causes of Skin Reactions in Patients with Cancer (continued)

Cause	Reaction	Comments
Filgrastim (continued)	Folliculitis Exacerbation of pre-existing vasculitis and psoriasis	
Erythropoietin	Eczema Skin rash	Uncommon
Interferon alfa	Pruritus Rash Cutaneous vascular lesions Exacerbation of psoriasis	Uncommon
Interleukin 2	Pruritus Erythroderma Exacerbation of psoriasis Life-threatening dermatoses	
Sargramostim	Injection site reactions Folliculitis Disseminated erythematous papular eruptions Exacerbation of vasculitis	
Nonchemotherapy Drugs		
Allopurinol	Stevens-Johnson syndrome Toxic epidermal necrolysis Vasculitis	See description in text
Hydantoins	Stevens-Johnson syndrome Toxic epidermal necrolysis Vasculitis	
Carbamazepine	Stevens-Johnson syndrome Toxic epidermal necrolysis	
NSAIDs	Stevens-Johnson syndrome Toxic epidermal necrolysis	
Cephalosporins	Stevens-Johnson syndrome Toxic epidermal necrolysis	
Fluoroquinolones	Stevens-Johnson syndrome Toxic epidermal necrolysis	
Vancomycin	Stevens-Johnson syndrome Toxic epidermal necrolysis	

SOURCE: references 29–52. NSAIDs, nonsteroidal anti-inflammatory drugs.

Acral erythema is characterized by sharply demarcated, tender erythematous plaques, especially on the palms of the hand and the soles of the feet. When acral erythema occurs only on the palms and soles, it is referred to as palmar-plantar erythrodyesthesia or hand-foot syndrome. Patients may describe it as the sensation of walking on hot coals. Improvement of this condition by the addition of pyridoxine to subsequent courses of therapy has been anecdotally reported.[39,45] Acral erythema may develop following treatment with a number of chemotherapy drugs, including cytarabine, docetaxel, doxorubicin, fluorouracil, and methotrexate. It is most commonly seen following high-dose therapy or prolonged infusions.[28,42] Palmar-plantar erythrodyesthesia is common among patients receiving therapy with liposomal doxorubicin, and it has been postulated that the longer circulation time of this dosage form may increase the risk of this reaction.[41]

Hidradenitis presents as multiple red indurated papules or plaques that may be purpuric and accompanied by fever.[28] It is also called neutrophilic apocrine hidradenitis. Pathologically, it is characterized by neutrophil infiltrates around the apocrine sweat glands and ducts. This reaction has been reported following treatment with cytarabine, bleomycin, doxorubicin, and vincristine.

Photosensitivity Reactions

Several chemotherapy drugs, including fluorouracil, dacarbazine, methotrexate, and vinblastine, may cause photosensitivity reactions. Patients receiving these agents should be counseled to use sunblock and to wear protective clothing when exposed to sunlight. It is particularly important that patients be cautioned to protect the scalp area that may be exposed by chemotherapy-induced hair loss. Patients treated with porfimer (Photofrin II) as a part of photodynamic therapy regimens may be especially sensitive to sunlight. They must be counseled to avoid exposure to direct sunlight and strong indoor lighting for several weeks after drug administration.

Radiation and Chemotherapy Reactions

The combined effects of chemotherapy and radiation on skin may produce very distinct reactions. Chemotherapy is sometimes administered within a few days of radiation therapy to enhance the therapeutic effects of radiation. This procedure is referred to as chemosensitization or radiosensitization, and it is a form of combined modality therapy. The result may be not only enhancement of the desired therapeutic effect but also enhanced toxicity to other tissues, including the skin. These dermatological reactions are typically characterized by erythema, edema, and occasionally large, fluid-filled blisters or bullae, sometimes with subsequent ulcerations.[26]

Chemotherapy may also produce an inflammatory reaction in tissues that were treated with radiation therapy weeks to months before. These reactions are most commonly seen in skin, but they may also occur in lung, gastrointestinal, or cardiac tissue. These recall reactions have been most frequently reported with bleomycin, dactinomycin, and doxorubicin.

Radiation reactions of the skin should be treated symptomatically with cool compresses, gentle debridement of destroyed tissue, and monitoring for secondary infections.[28]

Recombinant Cytokine Reactions

Recombinant cytokines used in either the treatment or supportive care of cancer patients can produce skin reactions that range from minor injection site reactions, pruritus, and flushing to life-threatening autoimmune disorders, severe erythroderma, or bullous skin reactions (Table 7-5). In addition, several of these agents may cause exacerbation of pre-existing unrelated cutaneous disorders, such as vasculitis and psoriasis.

Nonchemotherapy Drug Reactions

Many nonchemotherapy drugs that are commonly administered to patients with cancer can also produce a variety of skin reactions. As with chemotherapy-induced cutaneous reactions, most skin reactions caused by nonchemotherapy drugs are also manifestations of hypersensitivity reactions. Other reactions include idiosyncratic reactions, vasculitis, Stevens-Johnson syndrome (SJS), and toxic epidermal necrolysis (TEN). Drugs that are commonly implicated in causing dermatological complications in patients with cancer include allopurinol, antibiotics (especially β-lactam antibiotics), analgesics (especially nonsteroidal anti-inflammatory drugs), and anticonvulsants.

SJS and TEN are related mucocutaneous disorders characterized by small blisters on purpuric maculae or atypical targets, areas of confluent erythema, and detachment of the skin. They differ in that TEN has >30% skin detachment, whereas SJS has ≤10%. There is considerable overlap between the two disorders. Both disorders cause mucosal lesions that can occur on any mucosal surface. Almost all cases of TENS are believed to be drug related, whereas only about 50% of SJS cases are clearly related to drug use. Drugs commonly used to treat patients with cancer that have been implicated in these reactions include the hydantoins, carbamazepine, allopurinol, cephalosporins, nonsteroidal anti-inflammatory drugs, rifampin, and fluoroquinolones. These disorders typically begin 1–3 weeks after the start of drug therapy.[50] TEN may also occur after bone marrow transplantation and may be related to either drug use or to severe graft-versus-host disease.[53]

Both SJS and TEN have high morbidity and mortality rates. Complications include massive fluid loss from denuded skin, prerenal azotemia, bacterial infection, a hypercatabolic state, and diffuse interstitial pneumonitis that may progress to adult respiratory distress syndrome. Treatment includes pain control, fluid replacement, aseptic handling, avoidance of adhesive material, and aggressive treatment of secondary infections.

Hypersensitivity syndrome refers to idiosyncratic disorders that include skin rash and fever, sometimes complicated with hepatitis, arthralgias, lymphadenopathy, or hematological abnormalities. Hypersensitivity reactions typically develop 2–6 weeks after initiation of a drug. Allopurinol, the hydantoins, and carbamazepine have all been associated with hypersensitivity reactions.

Alopecia

Alopecia, a common side effect of cancer chemotherapy, has significant psychological impact. Many patients identify hair loss as one of their major concerns when facing chemotherapy.[54,55] Scalp hair is particularly susceptible to cytotoxic effects because the hair bulb cells replicate every 12–24 hours.[28] Other body hair (such as eyebrows, eyelashes, and sexually distributed hair) is less susceptible, and patients usually only experience thinning of hair in these distributions. A few drugs, particularly the taxanes, characteristically cause total body alopecia. Hair loss secondary to cytotoxic drugs usually begins 7–10 days after chemotherapy and is prominent within 1 month.

Table 7-6 lists cytotoxic drugs that may cause alopecia. The extent of alopecia is influenced by the drug, dose, and schedule of administration.[26] Drug-induced alopecia is reversible, and regeneration begins within 1–2 months of comple-

Table 7-6. Cytotoxic Drugs That May Cause Alopecia

Bleomycin	Fluorouracil
Cyclophosphamide	Idarubicin
Cytarabine	Ifosfamide
Dactinomycin	Methotrexate
Daunorubicin	Paclitaxel
Docetaxel	Vinblastine
Doxorubicin	Vincristine
Etoposide	

tion of therapy. Hair that regrows after chemotherapy sometimes differs in color or texture from the hair that was lost.

No safe and effective measures for preventing hair loss are known. Scalp hair loss from some chemotherapy regimens may be decreased by application of ice packs (often called ice caps or cold packs) to the scalp before, during, and after chemotherapy administration. Vasoconstriction induced by the cold temperatures is believed to decrease cytotoxic drug circulation to the scalp. Sometimes scalp tourniquets are used in combination with ice caps to further decrease drug delivery to the scalp. Use of ice caps is uncomfortable and cumbersome, and it also poses the theoretical risk of creating a tumor sanctuary; during the cooling, tumor cells in the scalp would receive relatively less cytotoxic drug exposure.

The effectiveness of scalp cooling depends on the duration of drug administration and the pharmacokinetic parameters of the drug. This method can be expected to be least effective and least practical during long-term drug infusions or with the use of drugs with long circulating half-lives.

Pharmacologic measures to prevent hair loss or to speed the regrowth of hair have been disappointing. Topical application of minoxidil, which stimulates hair growth in androgenic alopecia, has not been effective in counteracting chemotherapy-induced alopecia.[56]

HYPERSENSITIVITY REACTIONS

Although there are sporadic reports of hypersensitivity reactions associated with most cytotoxic drugs, only asparaginase and the taxanes (docetaxel and paclitaxel) have caused allergic reactions in a significant proportion of patients.[57,58] These drugs most commonly stimulate type I hypersensitivity reactions, which are characterized by acute onset of wheezing, dyspnea, pruritic rash, angioedema, extremity pain, bradycardia, and hypotension.

Standard premedication regimens for docetaxel and paclitaxel have significantly reduced the incidence and severity of allergic reactions (Table 7-7).[57-65] Both docetaxel and paclitaxel, as well as the solubilizers used in their commercial formulations (Tween 80 for docetaxel and Cremophor EL for paclitaxel), have been implicated in causing these hypersensitivity reactions. In unpremedicated patients, these reactions most commonly occur after the second dose and seldom oc-

cur later than after the third course of therapy. Premedication regimens for docetaxel also reduce the incidence and severity of edema that commonly occurs as a side effect.

Patients who experience hypersensitivity reactions to taxanes but for whose cancer the taxanes are important therapeutic agents may be rechallenged with these agents under carefully controlled circumstances. Recommended methods include slow initiation of a dilute solution administered only after high repeated doses of corticosteroids.

Ten to twenty percent of patients who receive the *Escherichia coli* form of asparaginase (Elspar) experience immediate and life-threatening anaphylaxis. The incidence is lower when asparaginase is administered intramuscularly than when given intravenously. Patients who experience allergic reactions to *E. coli* asparaginase can usually be switched to either asparaginase of *Erwinia* origin or to the polyethylene glycol–protected form of the drug, pegaspargase (see chapter 4). Because of the high incidence of acute hypersensitivity reactions to asparaginase, it is recommended that emergency medications, equipment, and personnel required for the management of anaphylactic reactions be nearby during administration. Some institutions require that a physician be present during administration. It is prudent to administer a test dose of asparaginase before the patient's first dose and before any dose administered >1 week after the previous doses of asparaginase.

Although most hypersensitivity reactions to cytotoxics are type I reactions, other types have also been reported (Table 7-8).[57-63] Hypersensitivity reactions have also occurred following the administration of cytokines. At least one report has also suggested that pretreatment with interleukin 2 may sensitize patients to cisplatin or dacarbazine.[55] Cross-sensitivity between cytotoxic structural analogues has also been reported

Table 7-7. Recommended Premedication Regimens for Paclitaxel and Docetaxel

Paclitaxel
Dexamethasone 20 mg PO at 12 and 6 hr before chemotherapy
OR
Dexamethasone 20 mg IV 30 min before chemotherapy
PLUS
Diphenhydramine 50 mg IV 30 min before chemotherapy
H_2 antagonist[a] IV 30 min before chemotherapy

Docetaxel
Dexamethasone 8 mg PO BID for 1 day before day of chemotherapy treatment, on the day of treatment, and for 3 days following chemotherapy treatment (5 days total).

SOURCE: references 57–65. PO, orally; IV, intravenously; BID, twice per day.
[a]H_2 antagonist may include cimetidine 300 mg IV, famotidine 20 mg IV, or ranitidine 50 mg IV.

Table 7-8. Anticancer Drugs That Cause Hypersensitivity Reactions

Type I Hypersensitivity Reactions[a]
- Asparaginase
- Carboplatin
- Chlorambucil
- Cisplatin
- Cyclophosphamide
- Cytarabine
- Daunorubicin
- Docetaxel
- Doxorubicin
- Fluorouracil
- Ifosfamide
- Melphalan
- Mesna
- Methotrexate
- Paclitaxel
- Pentostatin
- Procarbazine
- Teniposide

Type II Hypersensitivity Reactions[b]
- Chlorambucil
- Cisplatin
- Etoposide
- Interferon alfa

Type III Hypersensitivity Reactions[c]
- Methotrexate
- Procarbazine

Type IV Hypersensitivity Reactions[d]
- Mitomycin
- Methotrexate[e]

SOURCE: references 57–63.
[a]Characterized by acute onset of wheezing, dyspnea, pruritic rash, angioedema, extremity pain, and hypotension.
[b]Characterized by hemolytic anemia.
[c]Characterized by interstitial pneumonitis and vasculitis.
[d]Characterized by erythematous, vesicular rash that is pruritic.
[e]Anaphylactoid reactions during initial exposure to drug.

(e.g., between cisplatin and carboplatin or between etoposide and teniposide).[60–61]

Hypersensitivity reactions caused by anticancer drugs should be managed like any acute hypersensitivity reaction. If a hypersensitivity reaction occurs during administration, the drug should be stopped immediately. In some cases, the patient may be receiving several medications (e.g., combination chemotherapy and antiemetics), and it may be difficult to determine which drug is producing the reaction. In such a case, all medications should be stopped until the patient is stabilized and the cause can be more clearly identified. Intravenous access should be established immediately (if it is not present), blood pressure should be carefully monitored, and epinephrine and diphenhydramine should be administered as needed. The difficult decision is whether to attempt subsequent administration of the drug with corticosteroid premedication. In some situations the potential benefit of the anticancer drug may justify the risk.

LATE COMPLICATIONS OF CANCER THERAPY

Although hematological toxicity and dermatological toxicity are important acute and subacute toxicities of cancer chemotherapy, a variety of long-term complications can affect quality of life and even survival for patients who have survived cancer. Two long-term complications are of particular importance: secondary malignancies and impaired fertility.

Secondary Malignancies

The treatment of cancer has the potential to cause the very disease that it is intended to treat; secondary malignancies may arise after treatment, and even the cure, of the primary cancer. Secondary malignancies are the most serious late complications of cancer treatment because they cause significant morbidity and mortality. Although secondary malignancies are closely linked with cytotoxic chemotherapy, radiation therapy is also an important cause of secondary cancers, especially solid tumors.

Secondary cancer risks are usually assessed by cohort studies that follow a large number of patients with a specified cancer for many years to determine the incidence of secondary cancers. The number of cancers in the cohort is then compared with the expected incidence of the same cancers among members of the general population who are matched to the cohort in age and gender. This comparison gives a relative risk figure, in which the risk in the general population equals 1. A risk in the cohort of >1 indicates an increased relative risk. The risk can also be indicated by the absolute excess risk, which estimates the number of excess cancers per 10,000 patients per year. Absolute excess risk may be a more accurate indicator of risk when the secondary cancer is rare in the general population. Leukemia, for example, is a relatively rare cancer. Multiplying a low number even many times may still result in a low actual number of leukemia cases among the cohort. In comparison, lung cancer is a common tumor, so even just doubling the number of expected lung cancer cases in a population could result in many deaths.[64]

Radiation Therapy

Ionizing radiation has been known to be carcinogenic for >50 years, as a result of follow-up studies of atomic bomb survivors in Japan following World War II. Occupational exposure, diagnostic radiation, and therapeutic radiation for malignant or nonmalignant disorders have contributed to the knowledge of radiation as a carcinogen. Radiation can cause almost any type of solid tumor or hematological malignancy, but leukemias, thyroid cancers, and breast cancers are the most thoroughly studied secondary cancers attributable to radiation. The risk of leukemias increases within a few years of exposure. It peaks at 5–9 years and then gradually declines. Solid tumors emerge more slowly. The relative risks of solid tumors do not increase for 10–15 years after exposure, but once increased, they remain elevated for many years, perhaps for life.[64]

Factors Affecting Radiation-Induced Carcinogenicity

The risk of solid tumors is closely related to the dose of radiation administered, but the dose relationship is much less consistent for leukemias. The risk of leukemias depends on exposure of active bone marrow to radiation, the percentage of bone marrow exposed, and the radiation dose rate. The patient's age at exposure to radiation does not affect the degree of risk. In contrast, age at exposure is a very strong determinant of risk of some solid tumors. Breast and thyroid cancer risks are much greater for children and adolescents exposed to radiation than for those exposed in adulthood.[64,66]

Chemotherapy

The carcinogenic potential of cytotoxic chemotherapy was not identified until the 1970s. Late recognition of this serious toxicity was a result of the long latency period of most cancers caused by cytotoxic drugs, making the toxic event (the secondary cancer) distant in time from the insult (the cytotoxic chemotherapy) by many years. The long latency period contributed in another way to the delayed recognition of malignancies as adverse effects of cancer chemotherapy; in the early years of chemotherapy, many patients did not survive the several years that were necessary for the secondary cancer to become clinically evident. In one way, secondary malignancies can be viewed as part of the success of current cancer treatments, because long-term survival from one cancer is usually required for the patient to survive long enough to demonstrate the secondary cancer effect.

Exactly how cytotoxic chemotherapy causes secondary cancers is not known. Most chemical carcinogens are electrophilic (positively charged) and react with negatively charged sites in DNA. This binding appears to initiate the development of cancer—that is, to trigger the genetic changes in a normal cell that ultimately result in what we recognize as cancer.

Acute myelogenous leukemia (AML) is the predominant malignancy associated with cytotoxic chemotherapy, which is much more potent than radiation therapy in causing leukemia. Chemotherapy-related AML accounts for 10–20% of all new AML cases.[67] Two forms of chemotherapy-induced leukemia are currently recognized. The first, or classic, type is induced by alkylating agents. The second type, more recently described, is a form of AML induced by type II topoisomerase inhibitors.[64,68] These two AML syndromes are compared in Table 7-9.[64]

Almost all alkylating agents have demonstrated an increased risk of secondary AML, although cyclophosphamide is distinctly less carcinogenic than the classic alkylators, such as melphalan, chlorambucil, mechlorethamine, or thiotepa, or the nitrosourea lomustine. The cumulative dose of the alkylator is the strongest determinant of subsequent AML risk. Age and gender do not appear to affect risk. The prognosis of AML secondary to treatment with alkylating agents is very poor; it is notoriously resistant to conventional treatments for AML.[64]

Although alkylating agents have been recognized as a cause of AML since the 1970s, the first report linking AML with type II topoisomerase inhibitors appeared in 1987.[69] In the early 1990s, AML was linked with teniposide,[68] and more recently AML has been associated with the anthracyclines (e.g., doxorubicin). It is not known whether anthracyclines alone can produce AML, because the studies to date have included combinations of anthracyclines and either radiation therapy or alkylating agents. Type II topoisomerase inhibitors induce permanent double-strand breaks in DNA as their therapeutic mechanism of action. It is theorized that this same mechanism induces chromosomal rearrangements that ultimately result in leukemic transformations. It is not yet known whether cumulative dose or schedule of the type II topoisomerase inhibitors is a more important determinant of the risk of secondary AML.[64,67] The prognosis is poor for patients who develop AML secondary to treatment with type II topoisomerase

Table 7-9. Comparison of Secondary AML Induced by Alkylating Agents and by Type II Topoisomerase Inhibitors

Characteristic	Alkylator-Induced	Topoisomerase Inhibitor-Induced
Peak incidence	5–10 years	2–3 years
Preceding MDS	Common, up to 50% of cases	Uncommon
Chromosomal abnormalities	Unbalanced, deletions of all or parts of chromosomes 5 or 7	Balanced translocations, especially 11q23 translocation
FAB subtype	M1 and M2	M4 and M5
Prognosis	Very poor	Poor

SOURCE: reference 64. MDS, myelodysplastic syndrome; FAB, French-American-British.

Table 7-10. Relative Risk of Secondary Malignancies After Hodgkin's Disease Treatment

Cancer Site or Type	Relative Risk	Absolute Excess Risk per 10,000 Patients per Year
Acute myelogenous leukemia	70.8	15.5
Non-Hodgkin's lymphoma	18.6	10.7
Lung cancer	4.2	13.5
Colon	2.9	3.0
Bone	12.2	0.8
Connective tissue	7.0	1.0
Melanoma	4.2	1.6
Breast	2.5	11.3

SOURCE: reference 64.

inhibitors. Although patients can achieve a remission, it is usually brief; allogeneic bone marrow transplantation may offer some chance of prolonged remission.[70]

Secondary malignancies have been most thoroughly studied in survivors of Hodgkin's disease, who have a high rate of cure from their primary malignancy and are often young at presentation. Hodgkin's disease patients who are treated with chemotherapy have a dramatic increase in the incidence of AML; it is approximately 70 times that of the general age-matched population. The degree of risk closely correlates with chemotherapy regimen and is much higher with the MOPP regimen (*m*echlorethamine, vincristine [*O*ncovin], *p*rocarbazine, and *p*rednisone) than with ABVD (doxorubicin [*A*driamycin], *b*leomycin, *v*inblastine, and *d*acarbazine). ABVD is as efficacious as MOPP and has therefore replaced it to a large extent in the management of Hodgkin's disease.[64] Risks of solid tumors are increased for Hodgkin's disease patients who are treated with radiation therapy. An increased risk of breast cancer has been established, with a 55- to 75-fold increase in risk of breast cancer by 40 years of age in women who received radiation therapy to the chest during adolescence.[68,71] The relative risks and absolute excess of risk for hematological and solid tumors among survivors of Hodgkin's disease are outlined in Table 7-10.[64]

Survivors of non-Hodgkin's lymphoma (NHL) demonstrate significantly increased risk of AML, melanoma, and cancers of the bladder, lung, kidneys, and brain. Testicular cancer patients have an increased risk of testicular cancer in the remaining testicle (which may not be related to the effects of cancer treatment) as well as increased risks of leukemia, sarcomas, and bladder, gastrointestinal, and lung cancers. Testicular cancer patients treated with cisplatin-based chemotherapy without radiation therapy do not appear to have an increased risk of secondary malignancies. Specific patterns of secondary malignancies are also established for survivors of breast cancer and pediatric malignancies. The occurrence of treatment-related secondary malignancies in long-term cancer survivors requires lifelong medical surveillance, with a focus on screening tests to detect the most common malignancies in each patient population.[64]

Gonadal Dysfunction and Infertility

Damage to gonadal and reproductive functions that impair the ability to conceive or father children can have a devastating impact on the quality of life for young cancer survivors. The impact of cytotoxic therapies varies based on the gender and age of the patient at the time cancer treatment is administered, as well as on the type and dose of therapy administered. In addition, some cancers directly affect reproductive function, particularly those that affect the reproductive organs or the normal control of the hypothalamic-pituitary-gonadal axis, which control hormone production.

Several methodological issues complicate the assessment of fertility and reproductive function following cancer treatment. Most patients lack a pretreatment fertility assessment, so there is no way to know whether an individual would have been fertile had cancer therapy never been administered. Studies suffer from lack of long-term follow-up, and concurrent radiation therapy often complicates evaluation of the effects of drug therapy. In addition, most data on drug effects comes from single-agent animal studies, although single agents are rarely administered in current cancer treatment regimens and animal studies are difficult to extrapolate to humans. Human data is largely limited to case reports and case series, which can provide only limited information. There is also more information available about effects on male fertility than effects on female fertility, because male fertility is more easily assessed by such noninvasive tests as assessments of sperm count and motility.[72]

Effects of Cytotoxic Agents on Male Fertility

The effects of cytotoxic therapies on males depends on the proliferation rates of the various reproductive tissues. The differentiating spermatogonia are the most actively proliferating sperm cells and are therefore the most sensitive to the effects of cytotoxic agents. Neither the interstitial cells, which produce androgens, nor the Sertoli's cells, which provide support and regulatory factors to the germ cells, are proliferative in adults, so they are relatively unaffected by most cytotoxic therapies.[73]

Table 7-11. Fertility Effects of Individual Chemotherapy Agents

Drug	Effects in Men	Effects in Women
Bleomycin	Inhibition of intermediate spermatogenesis (animal data)	Low risk of reversible amenorrhea
Busulfan	Moderate risk of azoospermia; inhibition of early spermatogenesis	High risk of amenorrhea; may be reversible in younger women
Chlorambucil	High risk of azoospermia; may be reversible up to months after therapy, particularly with cumulative doses <400 mg	Moderate risk of amenorrhea
Cisplatin	Moderate risk of dose-related azoospermia; inhibition of all stages of spermatogenesis (animal data)	Moderate risk of reversible amenorrhea
Cyclophosphamide	High risk of azoopsermia; dose and duration of therapy dependent; may be reversible	High risk of amenorrhea; highly age and dose dependent
Cytarabine	Low to moderate risk of azoospermia; inhibition of early spermatogenesis	Unknown effects
Dactinomycin	Toxic to gonadal stem cells (animal data)	Unknown effects
Doxorubicin	Moderate, sometimes reversible risk of azoospermia; effects are age related	Unknown effects
Etoposide	Unknown effects	Moderate risk of amenorrhea; reversible in younger women but irreversible if >40 years of age
Fluorouracil	Low risk of azoospermia	Low risk of amenorrhea
Interferon alfa	Low risk of azoospermia	Unknown effects
Mechlorethamine	High risk of azoospermia; inhibition of intermediate and late spermatogenesis (animal data)	High risk of amenorrhea
Melphalan	High risk of azoospermia	Age-related risk of amenorrhea; moderate risk in women <40 years of age and high risk in women ≥40 years of age
Mercaptopurine	Low risk of azoospermia	Low risk of amenorrhea
Methotrexate	Low risk with low doses and moderate risk with high doses; rapidly reversible	Low risk of amenorrhea
Mitomycin	Unknown effects	Low risk of amenorrhea
Mitoxantrone	Unknown effects	Single case report of irreversible amenorrhea
Nitrosoureas	Moderate to high risk of azoospermia; inhibition of gonadal stem cells and early spermatogenesis (animal data)	Moderate risk of amenorrhea

Continued next page

Table 7-11. Fertility Effects of Individual Chemotherapy Agents (continued)

Drug	Effects in Men	Effects in Women
Procarbazine	High risk of azoospermia, especially when used as part of MOPP	High risk of amenorrhea, especially when used as part of MOPP
Vinblastine	Low to moderate risk of azoospermia	Unknown effects
Vincristine	Low risk of azoospermia	Unknown effects

SOURCE: reprinted with permission from Lenz KL, Valley AW. Infertility after chemotherapy: a review of the risks and strategies for prevention. *J Oncol Pharm Practice* 1996;2:79. MOPP, mechlorethamine + vincristine (Oncovin) + procarbazine + prednisone.

Males usually produce >2 million spermatozoa per day. Although production decreases when cytotoxic drugs are administered, the sperm count may not be affected for the first 2 months of therapy, because the more mature sperm cells are relatively resistant. Counts usually drop by 2–3 months after chemotherapy begins, although not all forms of chemotherapy affect the sperm count. Whether the decrease in sperm production is temporary or permanent depends on whether the sperm stem cells survive and maintain their ability to proliferate and differentiate. Normal counts recover within a few months if the sperm stem cells are not damaged. Recovery usually occurs within 1–3 years after nonlethal damage to the spermatogenic stem cells, but it may take many years, and sometimes recovery does not occur. Testosterone production is usually not affected by chemotherapy.[73]

Although the man's age at treatment has little effect on the recovery of sperm production, the cytotoxic agents administered are quite important. In general, the drugs with greatest adverse effects on male fertility are the alkylating agents and cisplatin, although not all alkylating agents produce azoospermia. The effects of individual agents on male fertility are detailed in Table 7-11.[72]

Effects of Cytotoxic Agents on Female Fertility

In contrast to sperm production, which is a perpetual process after puberty in males, all of the oocytes (incompletely developed eggs or ovum) are already present in females at birth. The number of oocytes gradually decreases until menopause, which usually occurs at about 50 years of age. The oocytes are present in follicles until they are stimulated to grow and mature. An individual oocyte then develops until it either degenerates or ovulates. When maturing follicles are damaged by chemotherapy, the woman stops menstruating. Whether the amenorrhea is temporary or permanent depends on whether the number of follicles is reduced below the number needed for menstrual cycling. Because older women have fewer follicles than younger women, older women are more sensitive to follicle damage. Temporary amenorrhea may last for a few months or up to 3 years. Permanent amenorrhea may begin during chemotherapy, but sometimes several years of irregular menstrual periods occur before the onset of permanent amenorrhea.[73]

As in males, the alkylating agents produce the most severe impairment of fertility in females. The effects of individual cytotoxic agents are outlined in Table 7-11.[72]

Prevention of Gonadal Damage

Most prevention strategies have attempted to suppress spermatogenesis or oogenesis to make the gonadal cells less susceptible to damage from chemotherapy. A variety of hormonal interventions have been attempted to produce temporary hormonal castration conditions. Gonadotropin-releasing hormone (GnRH) analogues have been evaluated in both male and female patients prior to and during chemotherapy administration. Although this intervention has been effective in animal models, controlled studies in humans have failed to demonstrate protection of fertility in either male or female patients. Oral contraceptives are often prescribed for females during chemotherapy to prevent conception and help preserve fertility. Evidence that oral contraceptives preserve fertility is based on a small uncontrolled trial done in the early 1980s. No reports of larger controlled trials have been published.[72–74]

Cryopreservation of semen (sperm banking) should be offered to males undergoing chemotherapy who may wish to father children. Semen samples are collected and frozen before chemotherapy is initiated. Even semen samples with low sperm counts may be valuable when used in conjunction with assisted reproductive technologies, such as in vitro fertilization. Harvesting and freezing of oocytes is not currently practical.[67] Harvesting and freezing the ovarian tissue itself (ovary cryopreservation) is also being studied. Ovarian tissue, removed before chemotherapy is begun, is frozen and stored until the woman completes treatment and wishes to attempt pregnancy. At that time, the stored tissue is grafted to a site near the fallopian tubes, where it will begin to produce ovum.[75]

SUMMARY

Cancer chemotherapy is likely to damage normal human cells because cancer chemotherapy cannot distinguish accurately between cancer cells and normal cells. The damage produced by cytotoxic chemotherapy can be minimized by identification of known risk factors, chemotherapy pharmacology and pharmacokinetics, and preventive measures. Hematological toxicities are the most common severe toxicities, and they can compromise a cancer patient's treatment options, quality of life, and chance of cure. Cytotoxic chemotherapy can produce life-threatening neutropenia and thrombocytopenia. The management of hematological toxicities in the patient with cancer includes careful monitoring during the expected nadirs for signs and symptoms of infection and bleeding. Colony-stimulating factors are used in the prevention of neutropenia to decrease the number of days of neutropenia and to decrease the risk of infections due to neutropenia.

Certain cancer chemotherapy agents are known to produce dermatological reactions. Cancer chemotherapy agents, as well as other drugs, can also cause hypersensitivity reactions. The identification of the individual agent causing the hypersensitivity reaction can be difficult because of the number of medications a cancer patient is often taking. Hypersensitivity reactions in cancer patients are managed as they would be for any other patient, with immediate discontinuation of the suspected agent or agents and acute patient monitoring.

The late complications of cancer therapy include secondary malignancies, gonadal dysfunction, and infertility. Secondary malignancies may be seen several years after cancer chemotherapy and result in high morbidity and mortality. The identification of effective screening tests for high-risk populations will be helpful in the early diagnosis of secondary malignancies. The degree of gonadal dysfunction and infertility depends on the cytotoxic therapy used and the gender and age of the patient. Prevention has focused on preserving sperm and ovum for future reproductive uses. Patients with cancer should be counseled about the possibility of infertility, which directly affects their quality-of-life choices.

REFERENCES

1. Gastineau DA. Hematologic effects of chemotherapy. *Semin Oncol* 1992;19:543–50.
2. Bociek RG, Armitage JO. Hematopoietic growth factors. *Ca Cancer J Clin* 1996;46:165–84.
3. Sahai J, Louie SG. Overview of the immune and hematopoietic systems. *Am J Hosp Pharm* 1993;50(Suppl 3) S4–9.
4. Louie SG, Jung B. Clinical effects of biologic response modifiers. *Am J Hosp Pharm* 1993;50(Suppl 3):S10–8.
5. Rusthoven JJ. Clinical needs for hematopoietic growth factors: old and new. *Cancer Invest* 1996;14:622–34.
6. ASCO Ad Hoc Colony-Stimulating Factor Guideline Expert Panel. American Society of Clinical Oncology recommendations for the use of hematopoietic colony-stimulating factors: evidence-based, clinical practice guidelines. *J Clin Oncol* 1994;12:2471–508.
7. Ozer H, Miller LL, Schiffer CA, et al. American Society of Clinical Oncology update of recommendations for the use of hematopoietic colony-stimulating factors: evidence-based, clinical practice guidelines. *J Clin Oncol* 1996;14:1957–60.
8. American Society of Clinical Oncology. 1997 Update of recommendations for the use of hematopoietic colony-stimulating factors: evidence-based, clinical practice guidelines. *J Clin Oncol* 1997;15:3288.
9. Kaushansky K. The thrombocytopenia of cancer: prospects for effective cytokine therapy. *Hematol Oncol Clin North Am* 1996;10:431–55.
10. Kruskall MS. The perils of platelet transfusions [editorial]. *N Engl J Med* 1997;337:1914–5.
11. Rutherford CJ, Frenkel EP. Thrombocytopenia: issues in diagnosis and therapy. *Med Clin North Am* 1994;78:555–75.
12. Rebulla P, Finazzi G, Marangoni F, et al. A multicenter randomized study of the threshold for prophylactic platelet transfusions in adults with acute myeloid leukemia. *N Engl J Med* 1997;337:1870–5.
13. Heckman KD, Weiner GJ, Davis CS, et al. Randomized study of prophylactic platelet transfusion threshold during induction therapy for adult acute leukemia: 10,000/microL versus 20,000/microL. *J Clin Oncol* 1997;15:1143–9.
14. Tepler I, Elias L, Smith JW II, et al. A randomized placebo-controlled trial of recombinant human interleukin-11 in cancer patients with severe thrombocytopenia due to chemotherapy. *Blood* 1996;87:3607–14.
15. Isaacs C, Robert NJ, Bailey FA, et al. Randomized placebo-controlled study of recombinant human interleukin-11 to prevent chemotherapy-induced thrombocytopenia in patients with breast cancer receiving dose-intensive cyclophosphamide and doxorubicin. *J Clin Oncol* 1997;15:3368–77.
16. Data available from the Genetics Institute.
17. Malone D, Sullivan S, Black D, et al. The cost of treating chemotherapy-induced thrombocytopenia [abstract]. *Proc Am Soc Clin Oncol Annu Meet* 1995;14:305.
18. D'Hondt V, Humblet Y, Guillaume T, et al. Thrombopoietic effects and toxicity of interleukin-6 in patients with ovarian cancer before and after chemotherapy: a multicentric placebo-controlled, randomized phase Ib study. *Blood* 1995;85:2347–53.
19. Budd GT, Ganapathi R, Adelstein DJ, et al. Randomized trial of carboplatin plus amifostine versus carboplatin alone in patients with advanced solid tumors. *Cancer* 1997;80:1134–40.
20. Griffin JD. Hematopoietic growth factors. In: DeVita VT Jr, Hellman S, Rosenberg SA, editors. *Cancer: Principles and Practice of Oncology*. 5th ed. Philadelphia, PA: Lippincott-Raven; 1997. p. 2639–57.
21. Whitsett CF. The role of hematopoietic growth factors in transfusion medicine. *Hematol Oncol Clin North Am* 1995;9:23–68.
22. Cascinu S, Fedeli A, Del Ferro E, et al. Recombinant human erythropoietin treatment in cisplatin-associated anemia: a randomized double-blind trial with placebo. *J Clin Oncol* 1994;12:1058–62.
23. Dunphy FR, Dunleavy TL, Harrison BR, et al. Erythropoietin reduces anemia and transfusions after chemotherapy with paclitaxel and carboplatin. *Cancer* 1997;79:1623–8.
24. Glaspy J, Bukowski R, Steinberg D, et al. Impact of therapy

with epoetin alfa on clinical outcomes in patients with nonmyeloid malignancies during cancer chemotherapy in community oncology practice. *J Clin Oncol* 1997;15:1218–34.
25. Pritchard KI, Paterson AH, Paul NA, et al. Increased thromboembolic complications with concurrent tamoxifen and chemotherapy in a randomized trial of adjuvant therapy for women with breast cancer. *J Clin Oncol* 1996;14:2731–7.
26. MacFarlane MP, Yang JC, Guleria AS, et al. The hematologic toxicity of interleukin-2 in patients with metastatic melanoma and renal cell carcinoma. *Cancer* 1995;75:1030–7.
27. Reckzeh B, Merte H, Pfluger K-H, et al. Severe lymphocytopenia and interstitial pneumonia in patients treated with paclitaxel and simultaneous radiotherapy for non-small cell lung cancer. *J Clin Oncol* 1996;14:1071–6.
28. DeSpain JD. Dermatologic toxicity of chemotherapy. *Semin Oncol* 1992;19:501–7.
29. Roujeau JC, Stern RS. Severe adverse cutaneous reactions to drugs. *N Engl J Med* 1994;331:1272–85.
30. Cohen IS, Mosher MB, O'Keefe EJ, et al. Cutaneous toxicity of bleomycin therapy. *Arch Dermatol* 1973;553–5.
31. Adoue D, Arlet P. Bleomycin and Raynaud's phenomenon. *Ann Intern Med* 1984;100:770.
32. Scallan PJ, Kettler AH, Levy ML, et al. Neutrophilic eccrine hidradenitis: evidence implicating bleomycin as a causative agent. *Cancer* 1988;62:2532–36.
33. Harrold BP. Syndrome resembling Addison's disease following prolonged treatment with busulfan. *Br Med J* 1966;14:63–4.
34. Markenson AAL, Chandra M, Miller DR. Hyperpigmentation after cancer chemotherapy [letter]. *Lancet* 1975;1:128.
35. Burgdorf WH, Gilmore WA, Ganick RP. Peculiar acral erythema secondary to high dose chemotherapy for acute myelogenous leukemia. *Ann Intern Med* 1982;97:61–2.
36. Flynn TC, Harrist TJ, Murphy GF, et al. Neutrophilic eccrine hidradenitis: a distinctive rash associated with cytarabine therapy and acute leukemia. *J Am Acad Dermatol* 1984;11:584–90.
37. Beck TM, Hart NE, Smith CE. Photosensitivity reaction following DTIC administration: report of two cases. *Cancer Treat Rep* 1980;64:725–6.
38. Dorr RT, Alberts DS, Einspahr J, et al. Experimental dacarbazine antitumor activity and skin toxicity in relation to light exposure and pharmacologic antidotes. *Cancer Treat Rep* 1987;71:267–72.
39. Vukelja SJ, Baker W, Burris HA. Pyridoxine therapy for palmar-plantar erythrodysesthia associated with taxotere [letter]. *J Natl Cancer Inst* 1993;85:1432–3.
40. Battafarano DF, Zimmerman GC, Older SA, et al. Docetaxel (taxotere) associated scleroderma-like changes of the lower extremities. *Cancer* 1995;76:110–5.
41. Gordon KB, Tajuddin A, Guitart J, et al. Hand-foot syndrome associated with liposome-encapsulated doxorubicin therapy. *Cancer* 1995;75:2169–73.
42. Samuels BL, Vogelzang NJ, Ruane M, et al. Continuous venous infusion of doxorubicin in advanced sarcomas. *Cancer Treat Rep* 1987;71:971–2.
43. Greco FA, Brereton HD, Kent H, et al. Adriamycin and enhanced radiation reaction in normal esophagus and skin. *Ann Intern Med* 1976;85:294–8.
44. Fontana JA. Radiation recall associated with VP-16-213 therapy. *Cancer Treat Rep* 1979;63:224.
45. Fabian CJ, Molina R, Slavik M, et al. Pyridoxine therapy for palmar-plantar erythrodyesthesia associated with continuous 5-fluorouracil infusion. *Invest New Drugs* 1990;8:57–63.
46. Curran CF, Luce JK. Fluorouracil and palmar-plantar erythrodysesthesia [letter]. *Ann Intern Med* 1989;111:858.
47. Berstein T. Skin reactions to 5-fluorouracil. *N Engl J Med* 1977;297:337–8.
48. Teresi ME, Murry DJ, Cornelius AS. Ifosfamide-induced hyperpigmentation. *Cancer* 1993;71:2873–5.
49. Korossy KS, Hood AF. Methotrexate reactivation of sunburn reaction. *Arch Dermatol* 1981;117:310–1.
50. Wheeland RG, Burgdorf WHC, Humphrey GB. The flag sign of chemotherapy. *Cancer* 1983;51:1356–8.
51. Glantz MJ, Choy H, Kearns CM, et al. Phase I study of weekly outpatient paclitaxel and concurrent cranial irradiation in adults with astrocytomas. *J Clin Oncol* 1996;14:600–9.
52. Breza TS, Helprin KM, Taylor JR. Photosensitivity reaction to vinblastine. *Arch Dermatol* 1975;111:1168–70.
53. Villada G, Roujeau JC, Cordonnier C, et al. Toxic epidermal necrolysis after bone marrow transplantation: study of nine cases. *J Am Acad Dermatol* 1990;23:870–5.
54. Wagner WL, Bye MG. Body image and patients experiencing alopecia as a result of cancer chemotherapy. *Cancer Nurs* 1979;2:365–9.
55. Freedman TG. Social and cultural dimensions of hair loss in women treated for breast cancer. *Cancer Nurs* 1994;17:334–41.
56. Kenes AE, Seeley K. Failure of topical minoxidil to accelerate hair growth following chemotherapy [abstract]. *Proc Am Soc Clin Oncol Annu Meet* 1994;13:1539.
57. Weiss RB. Miscellaneous toxicities. In: DeVita VT Jr, Hellman S, Rosenberg SA, editors. *Cancer: Principles and Practice of Oncology*. 5th ed. Philadelphia, PA: Lippincott-Raven; 1997. p. 2796–806.
58. Weiss RB. Hypersensitivity reactions. *Semin Oncol* 1992;19:458–77.
59. Heywood GR, Rosenberg SA, Weber JS. Hypersensitivity reactions to chemotherapy agents in patients receiving chemoimmunotherapy with high-dose interleukin-2. *J Natl Cancer Inst* 1995;87:915–22.
60. Shlebak AA, Clark PI, Green JA. Hypersensitivity and cross-reactivity to cisplatin and analogues. *Cancer Chemother Pharmacol* 1995;35:349–51.
61. Kasperek C, Black CD. Two cases of suspected immunologic-based hypersensitivity reactions to etoposide therapy. *Ann Pharmacother* 1992;26:1227–30.
62. Thompson-Moya L, Martin T, Heuft HG, et al. Case report: allergic reaction with immune hemolytic anemia resulting from chlorambucil. *Am J Hematol* 1989;32:230–1.
63. Alkins SA, Byrd JC, Morgan SL, et al. Anaphylactoid reactions to methotrexate. *Cancer* 1996;77:2123–6.
64. Van Leeuwen FE. Second cancers. In: DeVita VT Jr, Hellman S, Rosenberg SA. *Cancer: Principles and Practice of Oncology*. 5th ed. Philadelphia, PA: Lippincott-Raven; 1997. p. 2773–96.
65. Markman M, Kennedy A, Webster K, et al. Simplified regimen for the prevention of paclitaxel-associated hypersensitivity reactions. *J Clin Oncol* 1997;15:3517.
66. Bhatia SM, Robison LL, Oberlin O, et al. Breast cancer and other second neoplasms after childhood Hodgkin's disease. *N*

Engl J Med 1996;334:745–51.
67. Smith MA, McCaffrey RP, Karp JE. The secondary leukemias: challenges and research directions. *J Natl Cancer Inst* 1996;88:407–18.
68. Pui C-H, Ribeiro RC, Hancock ML, et al. Acute myeloid leukemia in children treated with epipodophyllotoxins for acute lymphoblastic leukemia. *N Engl J Med* 1991;325:1682–7.
69. Ratain MJ, Kaminer LS, Bitran JD, et al. Acute non-lymphocytic leukemia following etoposide and cisplatin combination chemotherapy for advanced non-small cell carcinoma of the lung. *Blood* 1987;70:1412–7.
70. Sandler ES, Friedman DJ, Mustafa MM, et al. Treatment of children with epipodophyllotoxin-induced secondary acute myeloid leukemia. *Cancer* 1997;79:1049–54.
71. Aisenberg AC, Finkelstein DM, Dopke KP, et al. High risk of breast carcinoma after irradiation of young women with Hodgkin's disease. *Cancer* 1997;79:1203–10.
72. Lenz KL, Valley AW. Infertility after chemotherapy: a review of the risks and strategies for prevention. *J Oncol Pharm Practice* 1996;2:75–100.
73. Meistrich ML, Vassilopoulou-Sellin R, Lipshultz LI. Gonadal dysfunction. In: DeVita VT Jr, Hellman S, Rosenberg SA, editors. *Cancer: Principles and Practice of Oncology.* 5th ed. Philadelphia, PA: Lippincott-Raven; 1997. p. 2758–73.
74. Manabe F, Takeshima H, Akaza H. Protecting spermatogenesis from damage induced by doxorubicin using the luteinizing hormone-releaseing hormone agonist leuprorelin. *Cancer* 1997;79:1014–21.
75. Law C. Freezing ovary tissue may help cancer patients preserve fertility [news]. *J Natl Cancer Inst* 1996;88:1184–5.

SELF-STUDY QUESTIONS

1. Current guidelines strongly recommend premedication with corticosteroids and diphenhydramine prior to the administration of each dose of asparaginase.

    a. true
    b. false

2. Hyperpigmented streaks overlying veins may occur following administration of:

    a. methotrexate.
    b. cytarabine.
    c. fluorouracil.
    d. paclitaxel.
    e. all of the above.

3. List three drugs that have been associated with hand-foot syndrome.

4. Hematological toxicity is common to all cancer chemotherapy agents.

    a. true
    b. false

5. Which of the following blood cells are affected by cancer chemotherapy agents that produce hematological toxicities?

    a. neutrophils
    b. platelets
    c. B lymphocytes
    d. a and b only
    e. a, b, and c

6. Granulocyte-macrophage colony-stimulating factor (GM-CSF, sargramostim) is used to stimulate proliferation of which cell line?

    a. neutrophils
    b. eosinophils
    c. macrophages
    d. erythrocytes

7. Colony-stimulating factors (such as granulocyte colony-stimulating factor [G-CSF] or GM-CSF) are indicated for primary use in patients receiving cancer chemotherapy that have an expected incidence of febrile neutropenia of >25%.

    a. true
    b. false

8. Oprelvekin (IL-11) produces which of the following side effects?

    a. fluid retention
    b. bleeding
    c. seizures
    d. dry mouth

9. Which of the following cancer chemotherapy agents is associated with development of acral erythema?

    a. bleomycin
    b. daunorubicin
    c. doxorubicin
    d. cisplatin

10. Dermatological reactions from cancer chemotherapy agents only affect the appearance of cancer patients.

    a. true
    b. false

11. Asparaginase produces life-threatening anaphylaxis in 10–20% of patients.

    a. true
    b. false

12. Secondary malignancies occur most commonly after therapy for:

    a. breast cancer.
    b. Hodgkin's disease.
    c. leukemia.
    d. b and c.
    e. all of the above.

13. Compare the advantages and disadvantages of application of ice packs to the scalp to prevent alopecia.

14. Select the premedication(s) that is/are recommended prior to paclitaxel administration.

    a. dexamethasone
    b. diphenhydramine
    c. cimetidine
    d. all of the above

15. Secondary leukemias produced by alkylating agents usually appear with a lag time of:

    a. <1 year.
    b. 2–3 years.
    c. 5–10 years.
    d. >10 years.

16. Secondary leukemias can usually be easily managed by moderate doses of conventional antileukemia agents.

    a. true
    b. false

17. Patients who receive radiation and chemotherapy for treatment of Hodgkin's disease have a significantly increased risk of developing all of the following secondary malignancies *except*:

    a. endometrial cancer.
    b. breast cancer.
    c. lung cancer.
    d. leukemia.

18. If all other risk factors are identical, which of the following women has the highest risk of developing permanent infertility following chemotherapy?

    a. 35 years old; received high doses of methotrexate
    b. 35 years old; received high doses of cyclophosphamide
    c. 18 years old; received high doses of methotrexate
    d. 18 years old; received high doses of cyclophosphamide

19. The most clinically useful intervention for males who wish to father children following chemotherapy administration is:

    a. testosterone injections
    b. GnRH analogue injections
    c. sperm banking
    d. delaying chemotherapy until one child has been conceived

20. AJ is a 25-year-old male who is in the clinic today to begin his second cycle of chemotherapy for treatment of lymphoma. He is trying to deal positively with the side effects of treatment that he has experienced since he began chemotherapy 3 weeks ago. He comments that "at least my girlfriend doesn't need to use birth contol any more" because chemotherapy makes men sterile. Counsel this patient about his understanding of the effects of chemotherapy on male fertility.

Chapter 8: Major Organ Toxicity

Carol Balmer, Pharm.D.
Associate Professor
University of Colorado School of Pharmacy
Denver, Colorado

Heidi Mahay, Pharm.D.
Clinical Pharmacist, Bone Marrow Transplantation
University of Colorado Hospital
Pharmacy Department
Denver, Colorado

Cardiac Toxicity	122
Anthracyclines	122
Risk Factors	123
Mechanism of Toxicity	123
Diagnosis of Cardiotoxicity	124
Treatment	124
Prevention	124
Cyclophosphamide and Ifosfamide	125
Fluorouracil	125
Interleukin 2	126
Taxanes	126
Renal Toxicity	126
Cisplatin	126
Pathophysiology	126
Prevention of Nephrotoxicity	127
Nitrosoureas	128
Ifosfamide	128
Mitomycin	129
Interleukin 2	129
Methotrexate	129
Bladder Toxicity	129
Hepatic Toxicity	131
Cytarabine	131
Mercaptopurine	131
Asparaginase	132
Methotrexate	132
Fluorouracil and Levamisole	132
Hormonal Therapy	133
Interferon Alfa	133
Interleukin 2	133
Hepatic Veno-occlusive Disease	133
Pulmonary Toxicity	133
Busulfan	134
Bleomycin	134
Cytarabine and Gemcitabine	135
Interleukin 2	135
Tretinoin	135

Neurological Toxicity 135
    Cytarabine 136
    Ifosfamide 136
    Antimetabolites 137
    Methotrexate 137
    Interleukin 2 138
    Interferon Alfa 138
    Vinca Alkaloids 138
    Cisplatin 139
    Paclitaxel and Docetaxel 139
Special Senses 139
    Ototoxicity 139
    Ocular Toxicity 140
Summary 140
References 140
Self-Study Questions 143

All of the chemotherapy agents currently available are toxic to normal healthy cells as well as cancer cells. Cancer chemotherapy can cause cell damage, life-threatening changes, or cell death.[1] Oncologists and oncology researchers are searching for the optimum cancer chemotherapy regimen that could target cancer cells specifically without damaging normal cells.

Some chemotherapy agents produce major organ toxicity, damaging the heart, lungs, kidneys, liver, bladder, nervous system, or vital special senses. These major organ toxicities are discussed in this chapter.

After completing this chapter, the reader will be able to:

1. Compare the three patterns of cardiac toxicity produced by anthracyclines with regard to time of onset, proposed mechanism, risk factors, symptoms, preventive measures, and therapeutic management.
2. Given a patient who is about to receive cisplatin therapy, outline a treatment plan to minimize the patient's risk of renal damage and electrolyte imbalance. Include the rationale for each component of the treatment plan that you recommend.
3. Describe the mechanism, risk factors, preventive measures, and treatment for methotrexate-induced nephrotoxicity.
4. Outline a management plan for prevention of hemorrhagic cystitis in a patient about to receive conventional-dose cyclophosphamide, high-dose cyclophosphamide as part of a bone marrow transplantation regimen, or ifosfamide.
5. List five cancer chemotherapy agents that can cause hepatotoxicity and describe the characteristic pattern of hepatic damage that each of these agents produces.
6. Describe the characteristic pattern, risk factors, prevention, and treatment of pulmonary toxicity produced by bleomycin, busulfan, interleukin 2, and tretinoin.
7. Compare the neurological toxicity produced by cisplatin, vinca alkaloids, paclitaxel, cytarabine, and the purine analogues with regard to characteristic pattern of toxicity, symptoms, risk factors, and preventive measures.

Chemotherapy agents may also produce more widespread damage, such as hypersensitivity reactions, endocrine abnormalities, dermatological reactions, fatigue, secondary malignancies, and myelosuppression. These systemic toxicities were discussed in chapter 7. Gastrointestinal toxicities are addressed in chapter 9.

CARDIAC TOXICITY

A few chemotherapy agents cause dose-limiting or fatal cardiac damage. Toxicity may be seen as arrhythmias, pericarditis, ischemia, or congestive heart failure (CHF).

Anthracyclines

The antitumor agents most recognized as cardiotoxic are the anthracycline antibiotics (doxorubicin [Adriamycin], daunorubicin [Cerubidine], and idarubicin [Idamycin]). All the anthracyclines currently available are cardiotoxic. Doxorubicin is the most widely used anthracycline and so is the one most likely to be implicated in cardiac damage.[2]

Anthracyclines produce three characteristic patterns of cardiac toxicity. These patterns are distinguished by the time of onset as acute, subacute, or late effects.[3] Subacute and chronic effects are sometimes combined under the term *chronic toxicity*, but they are now recognized as distinct clinical entities.

Acute cardiotoxic effects usually occur during or within the first 24 hours following administration of anthracyclines.

These consist of transient cardiac rhythm disturbances that appear as changes on the patient's electrocardiogram (ECG). The most common dysrhythmias include nonspecific ST–T wave changes, sinus tachycardia, and increased frequency of premature ventricular beats. Dysrhythmias are common, occurring in about 40% of patients receiving doxorubicin. Dysrhythmias are independent of dosage or schedule, and they usually are not related to development of future cardiac problems.[2-4]

The pericarditis syndrome is a rare illness that also occurs soon after anthracycline administration. This acute inflammatory process is usually accompanied by fever. It occurs within several days of an anthracycline dose and may result in life-threatening CHF. No preventive measures are known.[4]

Subacute effects are the classic presentation of anthracycline cardiac toxicity. Appearance of symptoms occurs weeks to months after the last dose of anthracycline, at an average of 3 months. Patients experience increasing tachycardia and fatigue; in some, these symptoms progress to tachypnea or rapid respiratory rate, shortness of breath, and finally to CHF with low cardiac output. In early studies, patients who progressed to CHF had a very high fatality rate, but current medical management has decreased the mortality of this serious toxicity.[2-5]

Late cardiac effects appear >5 years after completion of anthracycline administration. Onset has been documented as late as 20 years following anthracycline treatment in long-term survivors of childhood cancer.[3] Unfortunately, evidence that the incidence of late-onset cardiac damage is very high, and that the damage is progressive, continues to accumulate. In one large study, decreased cardiac contractility or increased afterload (an indicator of a thin left ventricular wall) were detected in 65% of patients 4–10 years after receiving anthracyclines as treatment for acute lymphocytic leukemia. Damage was progressive in about 70% of these patients.[6]

The late form of toxicity is characterized clinically as delayed cardiac decompensation. Patients may either have recovered from subacute cardiac damage or may have never before shown any signs of cardiac toxicity.[3] In long-term survivors of childhood cancer who received anthracyclines, cardiac abnormalities may only be evident by cardiac measurements until times of increased cardiac demand, such as during weight training or pregnancy. The symptoms of late-onset toxicity are similar to those of the subacute form: tachycardia, fatigue, shortness of breath, and CHF. Serious dysrhythmias and/or syncope may also occur. Sudden death has been documented ≥15 years after anthracycline treatment in several young patients with late-onset cardiomyopathy.[3,6]

Risk Factors

The prime risk factor for the development of subacute and late forms of anthracycline-induced cardiac toxicity is the cumulative dose of anthracycline. Although subacute anthracycline-related cardiac damage can occur at any cumu-

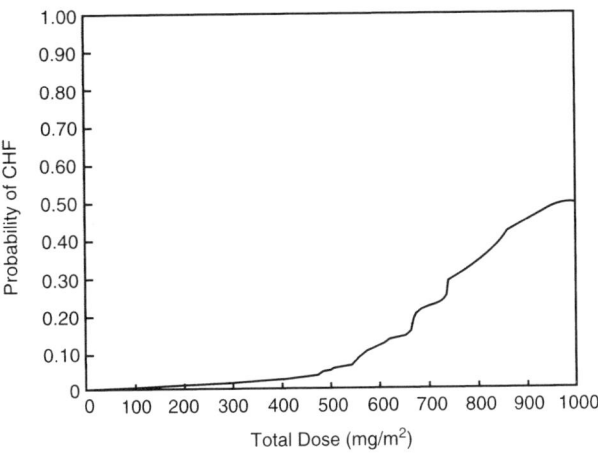

Figure 8-1. Risk of congestive heart failure (CHF) with cumulative doxorubicin doses. Doxorubicin was administered by traditional bolus dosing (approximately 60 mg/m² every 3–4 weeks).

SOURCE: reprinted with permission from Von Hoff DD, Layard MW, Basa P, et al. Risk factors for doxorubicin-induced congestive heart failure. *Ann Intern Med* 1979;91:710-7.

lative dose, the risk of CHF in adults is <5% in patients who receive a cumulative doxorubicin dose of <450–550 mg/m²; the risk of CHF rises sharply for doses above this range (Figure 8-1).[7]

The dose-response relationship is less well defined for pediatric patients than for adults. Although increasing anthracycline cumulative dose is strongly linked with late cardiac abnormalities in childhood survivors of cancer, a safe dose level has not been defined.[8] Recent evidence suggests that patients who receive cumulative doses of anthracycline of <270 mg/m² suffer less cardiotoxicity than patients who receive cumulative doses of 300–550 mg/m².[9]

Other risk factors associated with anthracycline cardiac toxicity include bolus administration schedules that result in high peak concentrations of the drug, extreme youth or advanced age, previous mediastinal radiation, malnutrition, and pre-existing cardiac disease. Females have also recently been shown to be more susceptible to anthracycline cardiac toxicity than males.[9] This gender effect is seen in children as well as adults.[8]

Mechanism of Toxicity

Dysrhythmias that occur in acute anthracycline toxicity may be caused by a sudden release of catecholamines, such as epinephrine, and histamine produced by anthracycline administration.[3] Chronic forms of anthracycline toxicity are attributed to several interrelated mechanisms. Anthracyclines are known to cause damage to mitochondrial DNA and to bind to mitochondrial membranes in heart tissue. This binding interferes with energy transfer in mitochondria and decreases contractility of cardiac muscle fibers.[3]

Anthracyclines also undergo electron reductions to free radicals. These free radicals are not important to the antitumor activity of anthracyclines, but they are closely linked to cardiac damage. Some of these highly reactive compounds are superoxide, hydrogen peroxide, and hydroxyl radicals. Free hydroxyl radicals produce additional mitochondrial membrane damage and energy disruption. Chelation of metal ions, particularly iron, by anthracyclines results in a powerfully oxidizing anthracycline–metal complex that can initiate lipid peroxidation. Lipid peroxidation of cardiac myofibrils and the contractile elements of muscle cells can directly destroy the muscle fibers. With each dose of anthracycline, there is progressive injury. The sarcoplasmic reticulum (nonfiber cytoplasm of the muscle cell) dilates, and myofibrils begin to disappear. Early in the development of the injury, these changes appear in scattered cells. As more and more myofibrils are damaged, the ability of the heart muscle to contract begins to decline. The heart's effectiveness as a pump is increasingly compromised, and clinical symptoms of CHF become evident. Late in the course of toxicity, muscle cell damage progresses to cell necrosis and loss, and widespread myocardial fibrosis occurs.[3–5,10] Heart tissue is particularly susceptible to free radical damage because it has a large number of mitochondria and low levels of the antioxidant enzymes, which normally serve as free radical scavengers.[4,10]

Diagnosis of Cardiotoxicity

Methods for early detection of anthracycline cardiotoxicity vary in their reliability, cost, and invasiveness. Serial endomyocardial biopsies in which samples of heart muscle are taken for pathological evaluation remain the standard against which other measures are compared. The morbidity and limited availability of this invasive test limit its use for routine monitoring.[1,4,11,12] The least invasive and expensive tests, such as serial chest X-rays and ECGs, are not effective predictors of doxorubicin cardiotoxicity. Echocardiograms, which produce echo images of the heart, are most useful in examining children. The echo images of children's hearts are clearer and more easily measurable than those of adults. Measurement of left ventricular ejection fraction (LVEF), although somewhat unreliable, remains the most widely used noninvasive test in adults. LVEF is the fraction of blood in the left ventricle that is pumped out with each heartbeat. It is measured by quantitating radioisotope circulation through the heart. MUGA (multiple-gated acquisition) scans are often used to measure LVEF.[2–5] Normal LVEF values are about 0.60–0.70 when measured at rest, and higher during exercise. Anthracyclines should be used cautiously if at all in patients with LVEF <0.50.[12]

Treatment

Acute rhythm disturbances associated with anthracycline administration are rarely clinically important and do not require ECG monitoring or treatment. They do not lead to chronic forms of cardiac toxicity.[3]

Clinically evident anthracycline cardiomyopathy should be managed aggressively. If anthracyclines are still being administered, they must be discontinued and no additional doses given. Useful pharmacologic interventions include inotropic support, such as administration of digoxin, to increase the contractile ability of the heart, and afterload reduction with vasodilators or angiotensin-converting enzyme (ACE) inhibitors to decrease the workload against which the heart must pump. Most patients can be stabilized and show clinical improvement with aggressive drug management. Unfortunately, pharmacologic interventions do not reverse CHF, and damage may continue to progress. Heart transplantation is an option for patients with severe cardiomyopathy who have a long expected life span.[3,4,11]

Prevention

Because doxorubicin has efficacy against a wide variety of tumor types, and because pharmacologic treatment of established cardiac damage is unsatisfactory, many methods have been studied to try to prevent cardiac toxicity.

The earliest effective strategy was to limit the cumulative dose of doxorubicin. Studies showing a very small risk of clinical CHF for patients receiving cumulative doses of <550 mg/m^2 (Figure 8-1) suggested that this was a safe dose for most adults. This strategy is the basis for recommendations to limit lifetime cumulative doses of doxorubicin to an arbitrary range of 450–550 mg/m^2. Unfortunately, variations in patient-specific tolerance mean that some patients will develop heart damage at doses below those levels. Arbitrary dose limits do not benefit patients who are more resistant to cardiotoxic effects than the average patient, because such dose limits prevent further doses of an effective antitumor drug above the arbitrary safety threshold. It must also be remembered that this dose limit reflects the risk of subacute CHF but does not address late-onset cardiac damage.[2,5,10,11] An additional reservation is that this cumulative dose level does not apply to pediatric patients. Cumulative dose limits of 250–300 mg/m^2 are recommended for children.[9]

Because subacute cardiac toxicity increases with high peak levels of anthracyclines, alteration of doxorubicin scheduling to reduce high peaks can reduce cardiac toxicity risk. High peaks can be avoided by changing traditional dose schedules, in which a large bolus of doxorubicin is given once every 3 weeks, to smaller doses given at weekly intervals, or by administering doxorubicin by prolonged continuous infusion. Antitumor effects are not compromised by these schedule changes, and patients can tolerate larger cumulative doxorubicin doses with less risk of cardiac damage.[2,5,11]

Several structural analogues of doxorubicin and daunorubicin have been developed to try to maintain their antitumor activity while reducing their cardiotoxicity. Idarubicin is the 4-demethoxy analogue of daunorubicin and is indicated for the treatment of patients with acute myelogenous leukemia. It is more potent than daunorubicin, so smaller doses may be used. At doses that produce comparable bone marrow suppression, however, the potential for cardiac damage is similar to doxorubicin and daunorubicin.[2–4,13] Mitoxantrone (Novantrone), an anthracendione structurally similar to the anthracyclines but lacking an attached sugar, has lower antitumor activity than doxorubicin in some tumors but a better safety profile. Mitoxantrone has a lower risk of cardiotoxicity than doxorubicin, probably because it has less potential to form free radicals, but it is not completely free of cardiac toxicity.[4,11,13] Epirubicin, a doxorubicin analogue that is widely used in Canada and Europe, is less cardiotoxic than doxorubicin in equivalent doses but retains some cardiac risk.[14]

Encapsulation of anthracyclines in liposomes can theoretically reduce cardiotoxicity while preserving antitumor activity. Liposomes are not taken up by the heart tissue, so anthracycline delivery to susceptible heart muscles is limited. Liposomal doxorubicin and daunorubicin are approved for use by the U.S. Food and Drug Administration (FDA). Liposomal formulations are well tolerated and appear to decrease the risk of cardiac toxicity. At present, they are much more costly than conventional anthracycline formulations and are only approved for use in patients with selected cancers.[15]

Many protective agents have been investigated for prophylaxis of doxorubicin-induced cardiotoxicity. Some of these agents include vitamin E, acetylcysteine, ascorbic acid, beta blockers, and verapamil.[11] Only one chemoprotectant, dexrazoxane (Zinecard) has been proved to be effective. Dexrazoxane was originally developed as an antitumor agent. Its active metabolite is a potent chelating agent. It is believed to protect against anthracycline-induced cardiac toxicity by binding intracellular iron that is required for free radical formation within myocardial cells.[10] Dexrazoxane has been most extensively studied in the treatment of breast cancer patients receiving doxorubicin. In prospective randomized trials in this population, the risk of cardiac events was halved in patients who received dexrazoxane. In one of these randomized trials, breast cancer patients who received dexrazoxane had a lower response rate than placebo-receiving patients, but time to progression and survival were not significantly different.[16] It is also well established that delayed administration of dexrazoxane, beginning with cumulative doxorubicin doses >300 mg/m^2, is effective as a cardioprotectant and permits higher cumulative doses of doxorubicin. Beginning dexrazoxane at this doxorubicin dose level avoids the risk of compromised efficacy of chemotherapy while offering protection before cumulative cardiac damage is likely to be clinically significant.[17] This benefit was the basis for the FDA's approval of dexrazoxane as a cardioprotectant. One small clinical trial showed similar protection against the subacute form of congestive cardiac damage in pediatric patients. The effects of dexrazoxane on development of late cardiac damage are not yet known.[18]

Cyclophosphamide and Ifosfamide

Cyclophosphamide (Cytoxan), an alkylating agent, is widely used in the management of breast cancers and lymphomas, as well as in bone marrow transplantation (BMT) procedures. Conventional doses of cyclophosphamide (500–1000 mg/m^2 IV) are not cardiotoxic. High doses, such as those used for BMT (approximately 4000 mg/m^2 for 2 days), are clearly cardiotoxic. In these doses, cyclophosphamide can cause hemorrhagic pancarditis, an acute syndrome with an onset of several days following cyclophosphamide administration. Patients develop bloody pericardial effusions, thickened heart walls with edema, and hemorrhages within the heart muscle layers. Damage typically continues to worsen for a few days and then improves over the next 3 weeks. A few patients progress rapidly to cardiac failure, shock, and death.[2,3,19] One patient died and another suffered disabling permanent cardiac damage in a widely publicized drug error in which BMT patients received quadruple overdoses of cyclophosphamide (see chapter 20).[20] Minor or asymptomatic cardiac toxicity also occurs and is seen as ECG changes, fluid retention, edema, and tachypnea.

Cardiac toxicity caused by cyclophosphamide is not related to cumulative dose. Risk is increased in patients with previous mediastinal radiation, prior anthracycline administration, and previously abnormal cardiac function. It may be increased in patients >50 years old.[2,3,19]

Treatment of cyclophosphamide-induced cardiac toxicity is supportive, with diuretics and inotropic agents (e.g., digoxin). There is currently no specific known intervention for the hemorrhagic damage, and no known prevention.[2,3,19]

Hemorrhagic pancarditis has not been recognized with ifosfamide (Ifex), a close structural analogue of cyclophosphamide, although atrial arrhythmias have been attributed to its use. Whether ifosfamide is inherently less toxic to the myocardium or whether damage has not appeared because ifosfamide is not used in high-dose regimens, such as BMT, is unknown.[3]

Fluorouracil

Fluorouracil (5-fluorouracil [5-FU] or Adrucil) was first recognized as a cardiac toxin in the mid-1970s when a low but important incidence of chest pain and ischemic damage was linked with its use. The incidence of ischemic cardiac symptoms similar to angina is about 3% in patients receiving fluorouracil by continuous intravenous infusion. It is much lower for patients who receive fluorouracil by intermittent bolus injection. Incidence is greater for patients with underlying heart disease and may be increased among patients receiving etoposide.[2,3,21,22]

Spasm of coronary blood vessels is believed to be responsible for the ischemic symptoms and damage caused by fluorouracil, but the mechanism is still unknown. Most arrhythmias caused by fluorouracil are treatable. Ischemic symptoms, such as chest pain and ECG changes, usually disappear when the fluorouracil infusion is stopped. If the symptoms respond to nitrate therapy, the infusion may be cautiously continued. Careful observation for cardiac symptoms should be maintained during fluorouracil infusions.[2,3,21,22]

Interleukin 2

Interleukin 2 (aldesleukin [IL-2]), a glycoprotein normally produced by activated lymphocytes, is commercially available through recombinant DNA technology. IL-2 administration produces widespread vascular changes, known as *capillary leak syndrome*, that result in hypotension and fluid retention. Cardiac toxicity is closely linked with IL-2's vascular toxicity. Normally, when peripheral vascular resistance decreases, cardiac output increases to maintain blood pressure and organ perfusion. In patients receiving IL-2, cardiac output does not increase appropriately to balance the decreased peripheral vascular resistance produced by the capillary leak syndrome. The poor responsiveness of the heart is referred to as *myocardial depression*. Ventricular dilation may also occur. These cardiac changes are similar to those that occur during septic shock and may be severe. The cause of the myocardial dysfunction is not known. Possible mechanisms are edema of the cardiac muscle, direct effects on the muscle fibers, indirect effects from other cytokines released by IL-2 effects, or perhaps transient cardiac ischemia.[3,23,24]

In addition to the myocardial depressant effects, arrhythmias occur in about 6% of IL-2 patients. Most of these are atrial arrhythmias and are rapidly reversible when IL-2 is discontinued. Myocardial infarctions have occurred in 2–6% of patients treated with FDA-approved doses of IL-2. Careful patient screening for cardiovascular risk factors before IL-2 treatment may decrease the incidence of severe cardiac events.[25]

Taxanes

Paclitaxel (Taxol) and docetaxel (Taxotere) are microtubule agents with excellent antitumor activity against common cancers, such as breast and lung cancers. Paclitaxel causes a variety of cardiac rhythm disturbances, most commonly sinus bradycardia. This condition occurs in up to one third of patients. Heart rates sometimes slow to 30–50 beats per minute, but the bradycardia is usually transient and asymptomatic. In the absence of hemodynamic effects, it is not an indication for discontinuing the paclitaxel. More serious bradyarrhythmias, myocardial infarction, cardiac ischemia, atrial arrhythmias, and ventricular tachycardia have also been noted, but they are rare.[3,25,26]

During early investigational studies with paclitaxel, patients were treated in cardiac units, where ECG changes could be continuously monitored. Extensive experience with paclitaxel has proved that this precaution is unnecessary for patients without a history of abnormal cardiac conduction. Routine cardiac monitoring during paclitaxel is only recommended for patients who may not be able to tolerate bradycardia.[25,26]

The closely related taxane docetaxel has a similar but less pronounced potential for cardiac rhythm disturbances than that of paclitaxel.[26]

RENAL TOXICITY

Many chemotherapy agents are excreted by the kidneys, either as unchanged drug or as metabolites, so the kidneys are vulnerable to injury from these agents. Several chemotherapy drugs can induce acute or chronic renal failure or produce lesions in the renal tubules or glomeruli that affect kidney function. No portion of the renal tubule system is free from risk (Figure 8-2).[27,28]

Cisplatin

Cisplatin (Platinol) is a heavy-metal compound that was first recognized as an effective antitumor agent in the early 1970s. Severe, dose-limiting nephrotoxicity that occurred in 25–35% of patients who received a single cisplatin dose caused suspension of clinical trials soon after they began. Several years later, the value of hydration in decreasing cisplatin nephrotoxicity was recognized, and clinical trials resumed. Nephrotoxicity is still a frequent dose-limiting toxicity, and cisplatin remains the most serious commonly used nephrotoxic agent among the antineoplastic drugs.[28–30]

Pathophysiology

Cisplatin damages the proximal and distal tubules, the loop of Henle, and the collecting ducts where secretion and absorption of water, electrolytes, and other products occur. The glomeruli are not usually affected. The greatest damage occurs in the proximal tubules, producing impaired sodium and water reabsorption that later interferes with reabsorption of potassium, magnesium, and calcium in other segments of the kidney.[27,28,31,32]

Cisplatin renal toxicity occurs in an acute form and a chronic form. Acute renal failure occurs within the first 1–2 days after drug administration. It presents as uremia (increase in blood urea nitrogen [BUN]), an increase in serum creatinine, and decreased urine output. Acute renal failure most typically occurs in the setting of inadequate hydration.[27,30,31]

Cisplatin nephrotoxicity is probably produced when intrastrand cross-links are made between cisplatin and the DNA of renal tubule cells, so it is therefore an extension of the drug's antitumor mechanism. The renal damage is characterized pathologically by altered structure of the nephron and continued impairment of its normal function. The main feature is focal acute proximal tubule necrosis.

The glomerular filtration rate (GFR) is permanently and sometimes progressively decreased in patients with cisplatin-induced renal damage, even though the serum creatinine may or may not be elevated.[29] Serum creatinine typically rises within about 1 week after drug administration, reaches a peak at about 2 weeks, and returns to pretreatment levels in cases of mild and reversible toxicity within 3–4 weeks. Although serum creatinine may return to normal over several weeks or months, it is a poor reflection of actual renal function in patients who have received cisplatin.[29] This mislead-

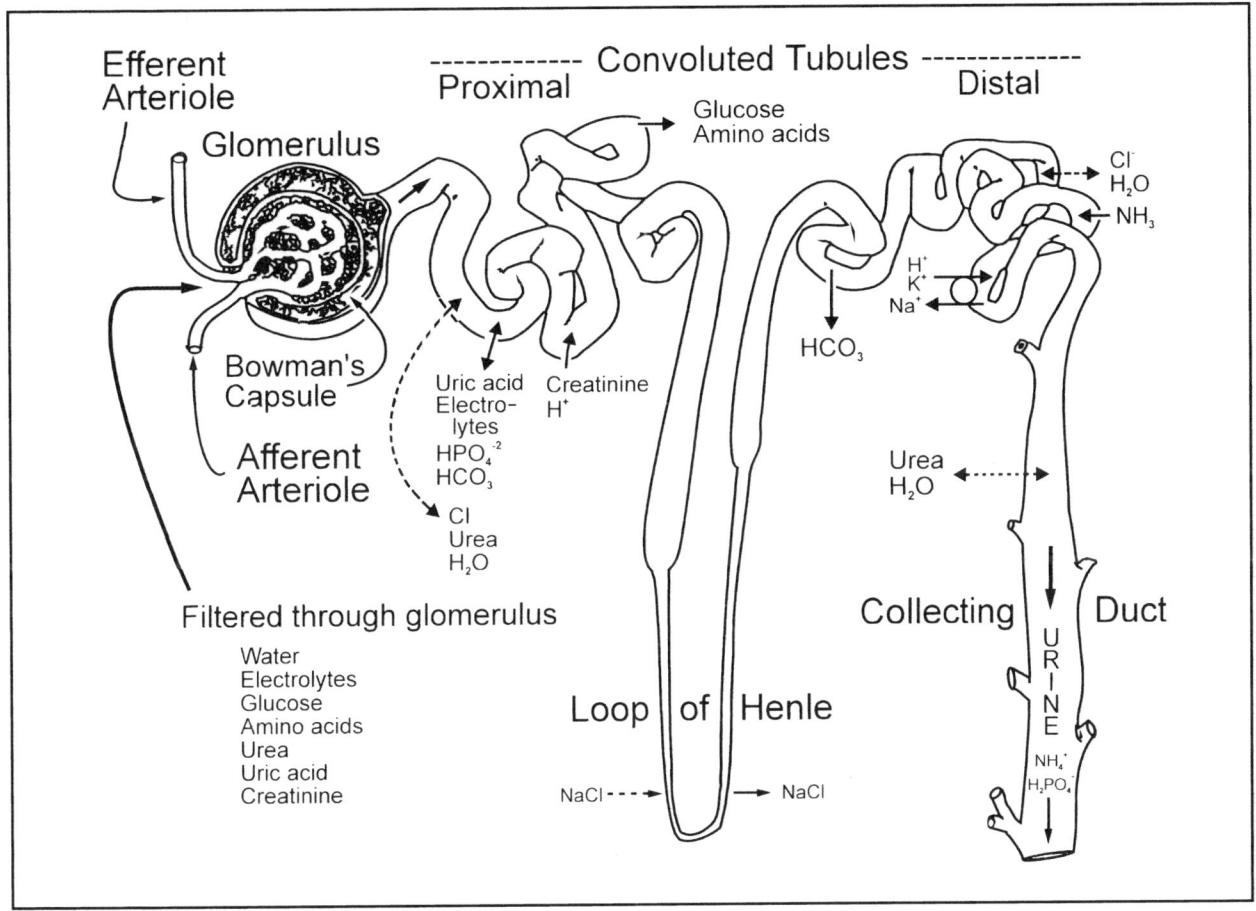

Figure 8-2. Anatomy of the renal tubules. Arrows pointing toward the nephron represent substances entering from the peritubular blood or interstitial space. Arrows heading away represent reabsorption. Solid arrows represent an active (energy-requiring) process, and dashed arrows represent a passive process.
SOURCE: reprinted with permission from Traub SL. *Basic Skills in Interpreting Laboratory Data*. 2nd ed. Bethesda, MD: American Society of Health-System Pharmacists; 1996. p. 132.

ing indicator is a particular problem for patients receiving successive cisplatin courses because cisplatin depends on the kidneys for its elimination. As renal function deteriorates, cisplatin clearance decreases concurrently, producing a greater risk of additional cisplatin toxicity with every chemotherapy cycle. This sequence is believed to occur even if no significant change in the serum creatinine (or even in measured creatinine clearance) is detectable.[33] Careful attention to dose reduction for patients with impaired renal function may help decrease the risk of additional renal damage.[28]

Electrolyte abnormalities often accompany both acute and chronic renal damage associated with cisplatin. The most well known of these abnormalities is hypomagnesemia. Magnesium loss appears to be dose related but has been reported to occur after a single cisplatin dose. Renal loss of magnesium may persist for months to years after completion of cisplatin therapy. Increased magnesium loss in the urine is evident immediately after therapy. Although decreased serum magnesium occurs in most patients, hypomagnesemia is symptomatic in only 1–10% of patients. Symptoms of hypomagnesemia include dizziness, muscle weakness, paresthesias, and tremors. Persistent orthostatic hypotension may occur.[27,34]

Cisplatin has also been associated with a defect in sodium and water handling by the kidneys, with approximately 10% of patients developing hyponatremia.[27] Potassium, sodium, and calcium loss may also be increased, and hypophosphatemia may occur.[29]

Prevention of Nephrotoxicity

The benefits of hydration, the first intervention proved to reduce cisplatin's nephrotoxicity, were recognized >20 years ago, but hydration remains the cornerstone of nephrotoxicity prevention. Hydration probably reduces renal damage by decreasing cisplatin's concentration and contact time in the renal tubules.[27,29,32] Normal saline is the preferred hydration fluid. High chloride concentrations help keep cisplatin in its nonhydrolyzed form, which is believed to be less toxic to the renal tubules than the hydrolyzed or aquated form. Aggres-

> Pre-hydration: infuse 1 L of normal saline over 2–3 hours.
>
> Confirm urine output of at least 100 ml/hr before beginning cisplatin.
>
> Mix cisplatin _____ mg/m² = _____ mg in 500 ml normal saline. Infuse over 1 hour.
>
> Post-hydration: infuse 1 L of normal saline with 20 mEq KCl and 16 mEq magnesium sulfate per liter at 500 ml/hr.

Figure 8-3. Example of cisplatin hydration regimen for outpatient administration in patients without cardiovascular compromise

sive hydration before, during, and after cisplatin administration is recommended to maintain urine output at >100 ml/hr.[28,30] An example of a hydration regimen convenient for outpatient cisplatin administration for patients with adequate cardiovascular function is outlined in Figure 8-3. Counsel patients to maintain increased oral fluid intake (2–3 L/day) for at least 24 hours after cisplatin administration.

Magnesium and potassium are usually added to either the pre- or post-hydration fluids, or both. Magnesium supplementation at the time of cisplatin administration decreases the frequency of low serum magnesium levels. There is no strong evidence that adding magnesium to the hydration fluids prevents clinical symptoms of hypomagnesemia, probably because magnesium loss is usually chronic and does not only occur during the cisplatin infusion.[34,35]

Diuretics (e.g., mannitol or furosemide) are often administered with cisplatin to increase urine output. Their use has not been shown to increase the preventive benefits of hydration alone. Mannitol acts as an osmotic diuretic and is not harmful, although its use adds to the costs and the inconvenience of cisplatin administration. Furosemide added to the risk of cisplatin nephrotoxicity in animal studies, although this risk has not been established in studies of humans. Addition of mannitol or furosemide is not recommended, except for patients who have inadequate urine output despite vigorous fluid hydration or to manage fluid overload.[28,29]

Vigorous hydration reduces but does not eliminate the risk of renal damage caused by cisplatin. Several other preventive measures have been evaluated. Intravenous thiol compounds, such as sodium thiosulfate, help counteract nephrotoxicity, especially in patients receiving intraperitoneal cisplatin. Sodium thiosulfate accumulates in the renal tubules, where it rapidly inactivates cisplatin. It does not prevent any of cisplatin's systemic toxicities, such as nausea and vomiting, and is not widely used.[31]

Amifostine (Ethyol), a thiol chemoprotectant, is approved by the FDA for prevention of cisplatin nephrotoxicity. Amifostine was originally developed as a radioprotective agent for nuclear warfare use, but it has also been proved to protect against some chemotherapy-induced major organ damage. Pretreatment with amifostine before each cycle of chemotherapy reduces cisplatin-induced nephrotoxicity without compromising antitumor activity.[36]

Amifostine is a prodrug that is rapidly metabolized to a free thiol by membrane-bound alkaline phosphatases. Free thiol binds to and detoxifies cisplatin within cells. The form of alkaline phosphatase that metabolizes amifostine is more abundant in normal cells than in tumor cells, so much higher thiol levels are attained in normal tissues. This difference may explain why amifostine protects normal tissue more than tumor cells; higher levels of thiol in normal cells make them relatively resistant to the effects of the cytotoxic agent. Amifostine may also act as a free radical scavenger, although this mechanism is not believed to be important in the prevention of cisplatin-induced nephrotoxicity. Unfortunately, amifostine is highly emetogenic, adding to the emetogenicity of cisplatin, and also causes a high incidence of hypotension.[31,32,37]

Numerous analogues of cisplatin have been developed in an attempt to preserve its therapeutic efficacy while reducing the toxicity of this valuable agent. The only analogue approved for use in the United States is carboplatin (Paraplatin). Carboplatin has a dramatically lower risk of nephrotoxicity than cisplatin, but it still has the potential to produce renal injury. Carboplatin-induced renal dysfunction is transient and rarely affects serum creatinine or creatinine clearance. It may only be detectable by means of sensitive enzyme assays or measurements of GFR.[28]

Nitrosoureas

The nitrosoureas that can cause nephrotoxicity include streptozocin (Zanosar), semustine (methyl-CCNU), and carmustine (BiCNU). Streptozocin, the most nephrotoxic nitrosourea, has very limited clinical use. It produces inflammation of the renal tubules (tubulointerstitial nephritis) and decreases tubule size (tubular atrophy), which may not produce symptoms until years after treatment. The nephrotoxicity associated with streptozocin is not clearly dose related, but it is rare at cumulative doses of <1–1.5 g/m². Renal failure associated with streptozocin can be severe and may require dialysis or cause death. No preventive measures are known, but it is recommended that renal function be monitored following administration of this agent.[27,28]

Renal dysfunction associated with the use of carmustine and semustine is similar to that of streptozocin but is much less common. It also may occur months to years following therapy. Uremia and proteinuria occur first, followed by progressive renal failure that may require dialysis. The incidence of renal failure appears to increase dramatically after a total dose of nitrosourea of 1500 mg/m².[27,28]

Ifosfamide

Ifosfamide damages both the kidneys and the bladder. Hemorrhagic cystitis, the usual form of bladder damage, is discussed below. Nephrotoxicity was apparent in early clinical studies in which ifosfamide was administered in single high doses. Fractionating the ifosfamide dose over 5 days reduces but does not eliminate the risk of renal damage. Ifosfamide-induced nephrotoxicity is more common among children and patients who have received prior cisplatin therapy or radiation to the kidneys. The risk of nephrotoxicity is not decreased by use of the bladder chemoprotectant mesna (Mesnex). Renal damage caused by ifosfamide produces tubular dysfunction and a rising serum creatinine, which is not always reversible.[28,38] Cyclophosphamide is not known to produce kidney damage, although it can cause bladder toxicity.

Mitomycin

Mitomycin (Mutamycin), an antitumor antibiotic, can produce dose-related and cumulative nephrotoxicity. Renal damage is detectable on average after 6 months of treatment and occurs in up to 20% of patients who receive total doses of 100 mg or more. Patients present with a rising BUN and serum creatinine, proteinuria, and hematuria, and they are usually hypertensive. Renal dysfunction typically occurs in conjunction with microvascular hemolysis as a component of a hemolytic uremic syndrome. The renal failure associated with mitomycin is generally reversible, but no preventive measures other than restriction of cumulative dose are known.[27,28]

Interleukin 2

Renal dysfunction is common during administration of high doses of the biological agent IL-2. The usual clinical picture is one of declining renal function, oliguria, sodium and fluid retention, and fluid-based weight gain. Together these symptoms resemble a prerenal form of acute renal failure—that is, damage to the blood supply of the kidneys rather than directly to the kidneys. The likely cause of poor renal perfusion is the hypotension that occurs as a component of IL-2's capillary leak syndrome. IL-2–induced acute renal failure is usually completely reversible within several days to weeks after IL-2 therapy is discontinued.[39] Concurrent infusion of low vasodilatory doses of dopamine (2–3 µg/kg per minute) with IL-2 infusion maintains renal blood flow and may prevent renal damage caused by poor renal perfusion.[40]

Methotrexate

Unlike cisplatin, which acts as a renal tubule poison, methotrexate damages the kidneys by a physical mechanism. Both methotrexate and its major metabolite, 7-hydroxymethotrexate, are weak bases that are eliminated renally. They must be dissolved in the urine to be excreted. When their solubility in the acidic environment of the renal tubules is exceeded, methotrexate precipitates from solution. The crystals can scrape and cut the renal tubules. Clinically, the patient demonstrates acute renal insufficiency. Serum creatinine and BUN rise rapidly, and urine output falls.[27,28,41]

Because methotrexate nephrotoxicity depends on drug solubility, it occurs only with high methotrexate doses. The risk is very low at doses of <250 mg/m^2, and nephrotoxicity is most common at doses of >1 g/m^2. Without preventive measures, the incidence of renal damage approaches 10% with high-dose methotrexate regimens. The risk of methotrexate-induced nephrotoxicity is also increased for patients with pre-existing renal impairment. This risk is best established for patients who have received prior cisplatin therapy. Concurrent administration of nonsteroidal anti-inflammatory drugs (NSAIDs) also increases the risk of nephrotoxicity, perhaps by decreasing methotrexate clearance.[27,28,41]

Prevention of methotrexate renal damage is accomplished by measures that increase the solubility of methotrexate and its metabolites in urine. Normal urine is acidic, with a pH range of 4–5. Methotrexate is in its ionized form, and is therefore much more soluble, at the pH of blood (normal physiological pH, about 7.4). For every pH unit that the urine can be increased by making the urine more alkaline, the solubility of methotrexate will increase by a factor of ten. Alkalinization can be achieved with oral or parenteral sodium bicarbonate. Urine pH should exceed 7 (some institutions specify 7.5 or 8) before methotrexate is administered, and this high pH should be maintained for several hours after methotrexate administration. Patients are also vigorously hydrated to maintain urine output at >100 ml/hr and to help flush methotrexate from the renal tubules. These preventive measures decrease the risk of renal damage to about 1%. Leucovorin rescue does not affect or prevent methotrexate nephrotoxicity.[27,28,41]

Despite careful attention to hydration and alkalinization, methotrexate renal damage may still occur. An enzyme agent, carboxypeptidase G2 (glutamate carboxypeptidase or GPDG2), has recently been evaluated for management of methotrexate-induced renal damage. Carboxypeptidase G2 cleaves methotrexate and converts it within minutes to inactive metabolites. It provides an alternate route of elimination for methotrexate for patients with impaired renal function who are accumulating toxic levels in their renal tubules. Carboxypeptidase G2 must be administered as soon as possible after nephrotoxicity is recognized to be effective. It is not available commercially but can be obtained on compassionate use basis through the National Cancer Institute.[42,43]

BLADDER TOXICITY

Damage to the urinary bladder is often confused with renal damage, but it is usually a distinct toxic process. Most bladder damage is categorized as cystitis, a general term for bladder irritation. *Hemorrhagic cystitis* refers to diffuse bleeding of the lining of the bladder. Although drug therapy is the most common cause of cystitis in cancer patients, radiation damage, antibiotics (e.g., ticarcillin and piperacillin), or viral infections may also be responsible. The chemotherapy drugs that are most commonly implicated in bladder toxicity are cyclophosphamide and ifosfamide.[44]

The incidence of chemotherapy-induced bladder damage varies by drug and regimen. Before preventive measures were known, symptoms of bladder damage occurred in up to one quarter of patients treated with cyclophosphamide and in most patients treated with ifosfamide.[19,45] Symptoms usually occur soon after parenteral drug administration, but they may occur months or years later. In a series of 100 patients with hemorrhagic cystitis, bleeding developed after a mean cumulative dose of 57 g of oral cyclophosphamide during 2 years of therapy. Prolonged administration of cyclophosphamide can result in chronic bladder fibrosis and chronic bleeding. About 5% of patients who develop hemorrhagic cystitis ultimately develop bladder cancer, with a lag time of several years.[46]

Bladder damage correlates with both high individual doses and high cumulative doses of cyclophosphamide and ifosfamide. Children develop cystitis at lower cyclophosphamide doses than adults. Other factors that increase the risk of bladder damage are dehydration, history of radiation to the bladder, and concomitant therapy with busulfan.[19,45,46]

Both cyclophosphamide and ifosfamide are metabolized to active metabolites and to the inactive metabolite acrolein, which is responsible for bladder toxicity. Acrolein binds to thiol compounds in the bladder mucosa and damages the bladder wall. Although hemorrhagic cystitis has classically been associated with cyclophosphamide, it is much more common after ifosfamide therapy, perhaps because ifosfamide is usually administered in much larger doses than cyclophosphamide, producing correspondingly greater amounts of acrolein.[19,45]

Patients with bladder toxicity experience irritative symptoms similar to those associated with urinary tract infections, such as dysuria, frequency, urgency, nocturia, and suprapubic pain. The urine may be pink-tinged with blood, or blood may only be detectable on urinalysis (microscopic hematuria). More severe damage causes visible blood in the urine, sometimes with passage of large blood clots.[19,45]

Prevention of hemorrhagic cystitis is accomplished by hydration and use of chemoprotectants. Hydration increases urine flow and decreases the contact time of acrolein with the bladder mucosa. With conventional doses of cyclophosphamide (i.e., 500–1000 mg/m^2 IV), oral hydration is usually adequate to prevent bladder damage.[19,44,45] Patients should be counseled to drink 2–3 L of fluid (eight to twelve 8-ounce glasses) on the day of cyclophosphamide administration and the day following administration. It is prudent to counsel patients to drink at least two large glasses of fluids at bedtime, so that they will need to void during the night, avoiding prolonged contact of acrolein with the bladder wall.

Oral hydration alone is not sufficient to prevent bladder damage from ifosfamide or high doses of cyclophosphamide, such as those used in BMT regimens. Very high fluid loads (hyper-hydration regimens, ≥5–6 L/day) are given to BMT patients to reduce the risk of bladder toxicity. Other BMT regimens incorporate continuous bladder irrigation to constantly wash the acrolein from the bladder.[44,45]

The chemoprotectant mesna (mercaptoethanesulfonate sodium) offers an alternative to hyper-hydration and bladder irrigation to prevent cyclophosphamide-induced bladder damage in BMT patients and patients receiving conventional doses of ifosfamide. Mesna is a sulfhydryl compound that is rapidly converted in the bloodstream to an inactive form, dimesna. Within the renal tubules, dimesna is converted again to mesna. The sulfhydryl group binds to acrolein, forming a nontoxic complex that is removed harmlessly from the bladder when the patient voids. Because mesna and dimesna are very hydrophilic, they do not pass readily into most cells of the body, so tumor cells are not protected.[19,44,45]

Mesna dosing corresponds to the dose of ifosfamide. When ifosfamide is administered as a short infusion, the total mesna dose is 60% of the ifosfamide dose. It is given in three divided doses, 20% each, before the ifosfamide infusion, and at 4 and 8 hours after the dose. The doses at 4 and 8 hours following chemotherapy are often administered orally to facilitate outpatient administration. Because the oral bioavailability of mesna is about 60%, oral doses are approximately double the intravenous dose. When ifosfamide is given by continuous infusion, the dose of mesna conventionally equals the total ifosfamide dose. Mesna may be mixed in the same infusion bag as ifosfamide. Mesna has a much shorter half-life than ifosfamide or cyclophosphamide, so it must be continued for 12–24 hours beyond the end of the chemotherapy infusion to protect the bladder mucosa throughout the entire period of exposure.[19,44,45]

Patients should be monitored with daily urinalysis or dipsticks of the urine to assess the presence of red blood cells during ifosfamide administration. If bleeding occurs, ifosfamide should be held and hydration increased, and mesna should be continued until blood is no longer detectable in the urine. Ifosfamide may then be restarted with careful attention to hydration. Increasing the mesna dose should be considered for the remainder of that chemotherapy course and for subsequent cycles.

Dosing of mesna for administration with high-dose cyclophosphamide regimens is less well established. Controlled trials have used mesna doses ranging from 100 to 200% of the cyclophosphamide dose, by either intermittent or continuous intravenous infusion. Continuous infusions maintain more consistent free thiol levels in the urine than intermittent bolus infusions.[47] Mesna protection and hyper-hydration or continuous bladder irrigation regimens are considered equivalent in efficacy for protection against hemorrhagic cystitis associated with high doses of cyclophosphamide for BMT. Mesna does not interfere with bone marrow engraftment.[48]

Hemorrhagic cystitis sometimes occurs months or years after cyclophosphamide or ifosfamide administration, despite conventional preventive measures. Mesna is not useful in the delayed-onset form of bladder damage. Mild cases of hematuria may be treated with water or saline bladder irrigation to remove clots. Astringents, such as alum or silver nitrate, may be instilled in the bladder to produce local vasoconstriction. Hemostatic agents (e.g., aminocaproic acid) inhibit fibrinolysis and help the bladder preserve clots in the bleeding areas. More severe bleeding requires transfusion of packed red blood cells to replace blood lost in the urine. Bladder instillation of prostaglandins E_2 or F_2 is often successful in stopping hematuria within 4–5 days. Prostaglandins are secreted by the kidneys and bladder and have a variety of roles in bladder function. Their effectiveness in repairing damaged bladders may come from inhibiting platelet aggregation or by causing membrane strengthening.[44,49,50]

Very severe bleeding that is unresponsive to these measures may respond to bladder instillation of formaldehyde solution (formalin) or phenol. These are toxic compounds whose painful administration requires general anesthesia. Formaldehyde and phenol hydrolyze proteins and coagulate tissues. If these measures do not stop bladder bleeding, surgical removal of the bladder may be required to prevent continued life-threatening hemorrhage.[19,44]

Although cystitis is most commonly associated with cyclophosphamide and ifosfamide, it may also occur as a result of systemic busulfan administration or from direct bladder instillation of antineoplastic agents for treatment of superficial bladder cancers. These intravesical antineoplastics include thiotepa, mitomycin, and Bacillus Calmette Guérin (BCG) vaccine. Urinary analgesics and antispasmodics are helpful in relieving the bladder discomfort caused by intravesical therapies.[45]

HEPATIC TOXICITY

The liver is closely involved in the metabolism and elimination of many antineoplastic drugs, so it is not unexpected that many of these drugs are potentially hepatotoxic. Despite this, most antineoplastic drugs are metabolized without detectable liver damage. Even agents that are well-established hepatotoxins usually produce liver damage only in a sporadic and unpredictable fashion, rather than in a uniform, dose-dependent manner.

Hepatocytes are the main cells responsible for drug metabolism and are consequently the first target site for adverse drug reactions in the liver. Typically, covalent bonds form between a reactive metabolite of the chemotherapy drug and either the cell proteins or DNA. Damage occurs to the hepatocytes, which gradually become necrotic. The direct cause of liver cell death is not clear. It may result from an increase in calcium within the hepatocyte. Calcium is a critical regulator of many hepatocellular functions, and alterations in calcium levels can compromise the integrity of the cellular membrane and skeleton.[51]

Most hepatotoxic antineoplastic drug reactions occur acutely, from a direct effect of either the parent drug or a metabolite on liver cells. Damage may occur when chemotherapy drugs produce unusual toxic byproducts (for example, in patients with rare genetic alterations in enzyme systems that permit the formation of harmful metabolites). Other reasons for hepatic toxicity include drug interactions with agents that compete for metabolizing enzymes or the depletion of enzymes that are needed to detoxify the chemotherapy drugs.[52] Chemotherapy can also cause allergic reactions through formation of toxic complexes between the drug or metabolites and hepatocellular proteins.

Levels of liver enzymes rise, sometimes to many times the upper limit of normal, as a result of direct hepatocyte damage; this rise may occur as rapidly as 1 day after drug administration. As damage progresses, fatty infiltration of the liver and obstruction of the bile ducts (cholestasis) may occur, resulting in accumulation of bile products in the blood. The serum bilirubin level increases, and the patient's sclera and skin take on the yellow-orange color of clinical jaundice. These changes in cancer patients are not specific to liver damage from chemotherapy drugs; a similar clinical picture may occur from metastases to the liver, viral hepatitis, or from other drugs (e.g., antiemetics).[28] Not all chemotherapy or nonchemotherapy drugs cause rapid changes in liver function tests. Some produce gradual progression to cirrhosis and fibrosis of liver tissue over months or years rather than acute liver damage.

Antineoplastic drugs that are commonly or consistently hepatotoxic are described in this section. Drugs that have only occasionally been implicated in hepatic damage, or that do not have frequent clinical use, are listed in Table 8-1.[52-55]

Cytarabine

Cytarabine (Cytosar-U) is the drug most commonly used for the treatment of acute myelogenous leukemia. Although liver function tests often increase in leukemic patients receiving standard-dose cytarabine chemotherapy (i.e., 100–200 mg/m^2), many competing risk factors (infection, blood transfusions, and multiple medications, for example) complicate the clinical picture. No definite evidence has been found that cytarabine contributes to liver function test abnormalities in patients receiving standard cytarabine doses. However, high-dose cytarabine (HDAC) regimens (1–3 g/m^2) are clearly hepatotoxic. Liver function tests increase in most patients who receive HDAC. Liver biopsies demonstrate drug-induced cholestasis that may be a result of injury to the hepatocyte transport system. This damage is reversible after therapy has been discontinued.[53]

Mercaptopurine

Mercaptopurine (Purinethol) is an antimetabolite that is used in the maintenance therapy of patients with acute lymphocytic leukemia. It is typically given for 2–3 years following remission induction. Liver damage presents in two patterns, either as cholestatic liver disease or as hepatocellular necrosis. Jaundice, which results from cholestatic toxicity, usually

Table 8-1. Antineoplastic Drugs That Are Only Occasionally Implicated in Hepatic Damage or That Have Infrequent Clinical Use

Drug	Reaction
Carboplatin[53]	Mild reversible increases in LFTs.
Carmustine[53]	Mild increases in LFTs are common but usually revert rapidly to normal; rare fatalities.
Cisplatin[52]	Rare increases in transaminases, sometimes with other LFTs.
Dacarbazine[53]	Several reports of hepatic vascular toxicity with clots in small veins of the liver. May cause acute hepatic failure, shock, and death.
Dactinomycin[53]	Occasional transient AST elevations in patients with previous liver radiation. May produce hepatic VOD in combination with vincristine.
Etoposide[53]	Rare reports of liver damage at standard and high doses.
Floxuridine[53]	May cause chemical hepatitis that is usually reversible or biliary sclerosis that is usually irreversible, when given intra-arterially.
Fludarabine[54]	Rare reports of increased LFTs.
Lomustine[53]	Similar to carmustine.
Paclitaxel[55]	Rare episodes of hepatic encephalopathy and hepatic necrosis leading to death, usually in patients with liver metastases.
Pentostatin[54]	Increased LFTs possible.
Plicamycin[53]	Most hepatotoxic chemotherapy drug commercially available. Rapid and sometimes enormous increases in LFTs. Currently only rare clinical use.

LFT, liver function tests; AST, aspartate aminotransferase; VOD, veno-occlusive disease.

appears 1–2 months after beginning mercaptopurine therapy, but it can occur within 1 week. It usually resolves when the drug is stopped. The hepatocellular injury causes laboratory increases in bilirubin, transaminases, and alkaline phosphatase levels. Severe hepatic necrosis can occur after high doses of mercaptopurine.[53,54]

Asparaginase

Asparaginase (Elspar), one of the most hepatotoxic antineoplastic agents, is an enzyme used in the early treatment of patients with acute lymphocytic leukemia. Asparaginase interferes with protein production in the liver, resulting in low levels of albumin, gamma globulins, transferrin, clotting and coagulation factors, and a variety of other important protein products. Laboratory studies also show increased levels of aminotransferases, bilirubin, and alkaline phosphatase. Diffuse fatty changes are evident on liver biopsy and may be due to decreased mobilization of lipids. Fatty changes have been detected at autopsy in about 40–90% of patients.[28,53]

Methotrexate

Methotrexate has a very low risk of acute liver damage, even when given in very high single or intermittent doses, as it is administered for management of most cancers. Although aminotransferases and serum lactate dehydrogenase (LDH) increases are common, liver function tests return to normal within a month of the end of therapy, and these increases do not lead to chronic liver disease.[53] However, methotrexate is clearly hepatotoxic when administered chronically in low doses. It is used in this manner for treatment of such nonmalignant conditions as psoriasis and rheumatoid arthritis. Long-term methotrexate therapy produces gradual onset of progressive cirrhosis or fibrosis, with an average of 25–33% of patients showing progressive liver changes in biopsy series.[56] Daily dosing produces more liver damage than does intermittent dosing and may be the reason for higher incidence of liver damage among patients with psoriasis than those with rheumatoid arthritis. Psoriasis patients are often treated with daily doses, whereas intermittent dosing is more commonly used for patients with rheumatoid arthritis. High cumulative doses also increase risk of hepatotoxicity; it is uncommon at cumulative doses of <2 g.[53] Patients with heavy alcohol intake have increased risk compared with patients with low intake.[56]

Methotrexate liver damage often develops over several years without symptoms and may only be detectable by liver biopsy.[51] Although liver function tests are unreliable indicators of liver damage in methotrexate patients, it is recommended that liver function tests be performed before beginning chronic methotrexate therapy, then every 4–8 weeks during therapy.[53] Hepatic fibrosis usually regresses when methotrexate is discontinued. There is no known treatment other than drug discontinuation.

Fluorouracil and Levamisole

Some antineoplastic agents are hepatotoxic in combination despite little potential for liver damage as single agents. Such is the case with the combination of fluorouracil and levamisole (Ergamisol), a drug combination that is commonly used for adjuvant treatment of colorectal cancer patients. Only rare reports of possible hepatotoxicity have been noted when fluorouracil is given alone.[53] In a large series of patients receiving fluorouracil plus levamisole, about 40% of patients showed increases in liver function tests, compared with about 15% of patients receiving levamisole alone or those receiving no adjuvant drug therapy. Alkaline phosphatase is the liver function test that is most likely to be increased. This increase may be accompanied by elevations of transaminases and bilirubin levels and occasionally by fatty changes on liver biopsy. Although increases in function tests usually are mild, are not associated with symptoms, and resolve when the drugs are stopped, caution is warranted because these changes may be misinterpreted as evidence of metastatic colon cancer rather than drug-induced toxicity.[57]

Hormonal Therapy

The hormonal anticancer agents that have been most strongly linked with hepatic toxicity are the nonsteroidal antiandrogens flutamide (Eulexin), nilutamide (Nilandron), and bicalutamide (Casodex). Liver function tests usually increase within 2 months of initiation of therapy and should be monitored at least during this time period. Rare fatalities have occurred among patients receiving continued flutamide despite increases in liver function tests. Nilutamide appears to share similar potential for hepatic damage, but there is less risk for patients receiving bicalutamide.[58]

Tamoxifen (Nolvadex) is the most widely used antiestrogen. Similar to the antiandrogens, tamoxifen can cause various hepatic abnormalities, including cholestasis, jaundice, and hepatic necrosis, that have rarely resulted in death. Tamoxifen is administered for several years as adjuvant treatment to most women with early-stage breast cancer. Despite widespread and prolonged use, very few cases of hepatic damage have been documented.[59] Monitoring of liver function tests beyond that appropriate for routine follow-up of breast cancer patients is not required.

Interferon Alfa

Mild increases in liver function tests are common in patients receiving chronic therapy with interferon alfa (IFN-α), but these increases are rarely dose limiting, except for patients receiving high doses (i.e., 20 million units/m² three to five times weekly). Hepatotoxicity is also more common in patients with abnormal liver function tests before treatment initiation. Two patients died of hepatic toxicity in a recent study of high chronic doses of IFN-α as adjuvant treatment of melanoma. Both patients had evidence of pre-existing liver disease. Careful monitoring of liver function tests is important, especially during the first several months of high-dose IFN-α treatment.[60] Interestingly, IFN-α is well established as effective therapy for patients with increased liver function tests secondary to hepatitis B and C infection, in whom liver function tests normalize with IFN-α treatment.

Interleukin 2

Cholestatic liver damage is very common in patients receiving FDA-approved doses of IL-2. Isolated increases in bilirubin occur rapidly when treatment is started, with an average increase of about five times normal levels, and they return to normal within a week when IL-2 treatment is stopped. The mechanism of hepatic damage is not known; it may be secondary to hepatic edema.[61] Recent data from animal studies suggest that IL-2 causes the release of other cytokines in the liver that cause white blood cell and platelet adhesion to the inner lining of liver blood vessels; this adhesion could physically interfere with microcirculation within the liver and result in many microscopic areas of ischemia.[62] Hepatic dysfunction is not dose limiting but requires caution in the administration of other agents that depend on the liver for elimination.

HEPATIC VENO-OCCLUSIVE DISEASE

Hepatic veno-occlusive disease (VOD) results from obstruction of blood flow in small hepatic veins. It is most commonly associated with the high doses of chemotherapy agents used in transplantation regimens and is discussed in detail in chapter 14. Hepatic VOD occasionally occurs from conventional doses of antitumor agents, including dacarbazine (DTIC-Dome), mercaptopurine, and thioguanine.[28]

Changes in liver function tests are common in cancer patients receiving systemic drug therapy. It is important that the cause of hepatic damage be evaluated and the pattern of abnormal liver function tests analyzed to assess whether any laboratory abnormalities should be attributed to drug therapy. It is also important that doses of drugs metabolized by the liver be modified for patients with compromised liver function.

PULMONARY TOXICITY

Three of the major modalities of cancer treatment are common causes of pulmonary damage. Radiation therapy is the most common cause of therapy-induced lung damage, but both chemotherapy and biological therapy can also cause pulmonary damage.

Although pulmonary toxicity can be caused by about 25 different cytotoxic drugs, most share common features (Table 8-2). Prominent exceptions are docetaxel and IL-2, whose pulmonary toxicity results primarily from the effects of fluid retention, and tretinoin (all *trans*-retinoic acid) itself, which produces the retinoic acid syndrome described later in this section.

Damage occurs in both the small blood vessels of the lungs and in the pneumocytes, the cells making up the soft tissue of the lung. Lung tissue shows an infiltration of inflammatory cells and fibrosis or stiffening from collagen deposits. A few drugs cause inflammation of the alveolar cells.[63,64] Drug-induced pulmonary toxicity almost always produces shortness of breath as the most characteristic symptom. Nonproductive cough, fatigue, and a general feeling of weakness are also common. Fever may occur, but chest pain is unusual.

Table 8-2. Antineoplastic Agents Associated with Pulmonary Toxicity

Alkylating Agents
- Busulfan
- Cyclophosphamide
- Chlorambucil
- Melphalan

Antibiotics
- Bleomycin
- Mitomycin
- Actinomycin D

Antimetabolites
- Cytarabine
- Floxuridine[65]
- Fludarabine
- Mercaptopurine
- Methotrexate

Biological Agents
- Interleukin 2
- Interferon alfa

Nitrosoureas
- Carmustine
- Lomustine

Plant Alkaloids
- Etoposide
- Teniposide
- Vinblastine

Miscellaneous Agents
- Asparaginase
- Docetaxel
- Paclitaxel
- Procarbazine
- Tamoxifen
- Tretinoin

SOURCE: references 63 and 64, except as indicated.

Symptoms generally develop over several weeks or months, although hypersensitivity reactions affecting the lungs may develop within a few hours.[63,64]

Chest X-rays usually show a reticulonodular (net-like background with scattered nodules) pattern that is seen throughout the lung fields or in the lung bases. However, chest X-rays may sometimes appear normal even in patients with well-established pulmonary toxicity. Pulmonary function tests are also nonspecific. The most common abnormalities detected are reduction in carbon monoxide diffusing capacity (DL_{CO}), a test of gas exchange across the alveolar-capillary membrane, and restrictive defects due to lung fibrosis. Because symptoms, chest X-ray, and pulmonary function tests are nonspecific, lung biopsy is required to distinguish drug-induced damage from lung infection and malignancy.[63,64]

Treatment of pulmonary toxicity is also nonspecific. The only intervention known to be effective in limiting pulmonary damage is to stop the offending agent. No clinically useful antidotes to pulmonary damage are known. High doses of corticosteroids are usually administered, but their value has not been proved in controlled human studies. Lung transplantation has been attempted in a few patients with drug-induced pulmonary damage. Unfortunately, the only truly effective way to manage pulmonary toxicity is to prevent it.[63–65]

Although pulmonary damage can be caused by many different antitumor agents, bleomycin, busulfan, and IL-2 are the antitumor agents most commonly associated with pulmonary toxicity. Recently, a distinct pulmonary toxicity syndrome has been noted in patients receiving tretinoin, and serious damage has been reported in patients receiving gemcitabine.

Busulfan

Busulfan has been recognized as a cause of pulmonary fibrosis since the early 1960s. This association is well documented and known popularly as *busulfan lung*. Busulfan lung damage occurs most typically after 3–4 years of drug administration. It is characterized by a gradual onset of fever with a nonproductive cough and shortness of breath. As toxicity progresses, the respiratory rate increases, and cyanosis appears as the lungs become more stiff and are no longer able to transport enough oxygen. Damage may progress to severe pulmonary insufficiency and death. Chest X-rays usually show either a diffuse pattern of interstitial or intra-alveolar changes, with edema and fibrosis evident in lung biopsy tissue. Pulmonary function tests may be abnormal before clinical symptoms begin. Stopping busulfan at this early stage of damage sometimes permits the lung deterioration to stabilize, but busulfan pulmonary toxicity can be rapidly fatal if not detected before the patient becomes symptomatic. The average survival time after diagnosis of busulfan lung damage is 5 months.[19,64] Busulfan, when combined with etoposide, has also been implicated in an acute form of interstitial pneumonitis in BMT patients. The contribution of each agent to this adverse effect is not established.[66]

Bleomycin

Bleomycin is the most commonly used antineoplastic agent that causes pulmonary toxicity. Lung damage has been recognized as the dose-limiting toxicity of bleomycin since early clinical trials in the 1960s. Bleomycin causes two forms of pulmonary toxicity. One form is rare and is probably a hypersensitivity reaction. The most common form is a subacute gradual progression to lung fibrosis and, in severe cases, to death. It is this form of bleomycin toxicity that is discussed here.[67,68]

Bleomycin lung damage is clearly dose related, occurring in 3–5% of patients receiving a total cumulative dose of <450 units but in 10% of patients receiving larger cumulative doses. Although risk is increased at cumulative doses over 450 units, no dose is considered absolutely safe. Severe pulmonary toxicity has been documented at cumulative doses of <100 units and in patients who receive high single doses, so individual doses should be limited to a total dose of 30 units. The risk of bleomycin-induced lung toxicity is also increased in the elderly, in patients with emphysema, in patients with previous lung radiation, and in patients exposed to high oxygen concentrations during surgery.[67] Lymphoma may also increase risk.[68] Bleomycin is eliminated renally, so patients with compromised renal function, including patients receiving cisplatin, are at increased risk for pulmonary damage.[69]

The cause of pulmonary toxicity from bleomycin is not defined. The lung may be a target site of toxicity because bleomycin is normally metabolized by hydrolase enzymes that, though widely distributed throughout the body, are present only in low concentrations in the lungs. The low concentration of hydrolases compromises the inactivation of bleomycin in lung tissue, contributing to the damage.[68] Bleomycin induces the formation of oxygen free radicals in lung tissue by forming a complex with iron. These reactive compounds can lead to membrane instability in the lungs by oxidizing fatty acids. Lung fibroblasts are also stimulated to produce large amounts of collagen when exposed to bleomycin; these collagen deposits eventually stiffen the lungs. Cytokines that stimulate fibroblasts to produce collagen have also been implicated in the pathogenesis of bleomycin-induced lung injury.[63,64,67]

Characteristic clinical symptoms of bleomycin lung damage include dry hacking cough and shortness of breath with exertion. Chest X-rays may be normal early in the course of damage, or they may show interstitial markings or, occasionally, nodules that resemble tumors. Later, the X-rays show patches of reticulonodular infiltrates that can merge together to form large areas of air-deprived lung tissue. The most useful pulmonary function test is the carbon monoxide diffusing capacity (DL_{CO}) test. This measurement falls in most patients receiving bleomycin, however, and is therefore not an accurate predictor of serious pulmonary damage. Because chest X-ray findings and pulmonary function tests are nonspecific, lung biopsy is the only definitive method for diagnosing bleomycin-induced lung damage.[67,68]

As with other drug-induced pulmonary toxicity, there is no specific therapy. Symptoms sometimes continue to worsen even when the drug is stopped, reversing partially after several months. Although subclinical damage and mild pulmonary fibrosis gradually resolve over a few years, severe pulmonary fibrosis is not completely reversible. The usefulness of corticosteroids is controversial. High-dose steroids have appeared useful in anecdotal reports and are usually given, but their value has not been objectively proved. No other intervention has yet been documented to be useful in management of this serious toxicity.[67,68]

Cytarabine and Gemcitabine

HDAC regimens are established causes of pulmonary damage. Incidence is as high as one third of patients when doses of 2–3 g/m² are given for several days. Risk is clearly associated with dose and decreases when fewer or lower doses are given. Patients demonstrate sudden onset of respiratory distress syndrome (RDS) and pulmonary edema within a few days to weeks after cytarabine treatment. Damage is believed to be caused by increased capillary permeability in the lungs. Lung damage caused by cytarabine is usually reversible over the course of several days, but it has been fatal in up to one fourth of patients.[63,70]

More recently, gemcitabine (Gemzar), a nucleoside analogue closely related to cytarabine, has been associated with similar pulmonary damage. Shortness of breath occurs within a few hours of the injection in about 8% of patients who receive gemcitabine. It is usually mild and reverses without treatment. However, life-threatening pulmonary damage also occurs. In case reports, patients develop symptoms of RDS distinguished by presence of noncardiogenic pulmonary edema. As with cytarabine, capillary fluid leakage is believed to cause pulmonary edema. Diuretics and corticosteroids have been useful in treating these patients.[71]

Interleukin 2

Capillary leakage is very strongly linked with pulmonary damage from IL-2 administration. Most patients who receive FDA-approved doses of IL-2 develop severe fluid retention during treatment. Although peripheral edema is the most common symptom, many patients show evidence of fluid accumulation in the lungs. Respiratory distress is sometimes severe enough to require mechanical ventilation. Pulmonary damage from IL-2 is reversible within several days when IL-2 is discontinued and does not appear to cause permanent pulmonary compromise. Locally produced cytokines, especially tumor necrosis factor alpha (TNF-α), probably contribute to pulmonary damage. Investigational antagonists of TNF-α may prove to be useful countermeasures.[72,73]

Tretinoin

Tretinoin (Vesanoid) is a vitamin A derivative indicated for the management of acute promyelocytic leukemia. Use of tretinoin is limited by the occurrence of retinoic acid syndrome, an acute complex of fever, respiratory distress, weight gain, edema, effusions, and hypotension that develops 2–21 days after initiation of tretinoin therapy. Corticosteroid treatment early in the course of this syndrome can produce prompt improvement.[74]

NEUROLOGICAL TOXICITY

Neurological toxicity is a common outcome of cancer chemotherapy treatment. It is unusual for neurotoxicity to be life threatening, but symptoms are often debilitating and cause significant chronic discomfort.[75] Chemotherapy agents may cause damage to the central nervous system (CNS), peripheral nervous system, or both. A few drugs produce autonomic neuropathy or damage to sensory organs. Table 8-3 lists agents that are strongly associated with damage to the nervous systems. It is important to recognize that, although many neurotoxic agents produce one characteristic form of neurological toxicity, most may produce other patterns as well.

CNS toxicity has a wide spectrum of manifestations, including somnolence, confusion, delirium, neuropsychiatric symptoms, ataxia, impaired intellect, dizziness, seizures, encephalopathy, cortical blindness, coma, and death. Peripheral neuropathies are much more limited in scope. Patients usually complain of tingling and numbness in their hands and/or their feet, most often in a stocking-and-glove distribution. Severe damage can affect all the extremities and can cause paralysis. Autonomic damage is also fairly limited in

Table 8-3. Selected Cytotoxic Agents Associated with Neurological Toxicity

Central Nervous System

Agent	Toxicity
Interleukin 2	Mental status changes, delirium
Asparaginase	Somnolence, lethargy, or confusion
Busulfan	Seizures in bone marrow transplantation patients
Cladribine	Paralysis in early studies
Cytarabine (high-dose regimens)	Cerebellar or cerebral toxicity
Fludarabine	Somnolence, coma, blindness, paralysis
Ifosfamide	Lethargy, somnolence, encephalopathy
Interferon alfa	Lethargy, depression, cognitive dysfunction
Pentostatin	Lethargy, somnolence, coma, encephalopathy

Peripheral Nervous System

Agent	Toxicity
Cisplatin	Sensory polyneuropathies
Docetaxel	Sensory and motor neuropathies
Fludarabine	Motor neuropathies
Interferon alfa	Peripheral neuropathies
Paclitaxel	Sensory and motor neuropathies
Vincristine	Sensory and motor neuropathies
Vinblastine	Sensory and motor neuropathies
Vinorelbine	Sensory and motor neuropathies

Autonomic Nervous System

Agent	Toxicity
Cisplatin	Orthostatic changes
Vinblastine	Constipation
Vincristine	Constipation
Vinorelbine	Constipation

scope, generally producing constipation or orthostatic instability.[28,76]

The chemotherapy agents that are most commonly implicated in producing CNS damage are HDAC, ifosfamide, IL-2, methotrexate, and several purine analogues.

Cytarabine

Cytarabine enters the CNS when given intravenously. The CNS concentration is about 20–50% of plasma levels and declines more slowly than plasma levels. Neurological toxicity from cytarabine was first noted following intrathecal administration. The most severe and common toxicity, however, has been associated with intravenous HDAC regimens. The incidence of neurological damage is about 10% among HDAC recipients. Most cases of mild neurological toxicity are not reported, so the actual incidence is probably much higher.[28,76,77]

HDAC can produce a variety of neurological syndromes, but the most characteristic and common pattern is cerebellar toxicity. The cerebellum is responsible for coordination, so manifestations of cerebellar damage include ataxia and impaired balance, similar to the manifestations of inebriation. The muscles that control speech may be affected (dysarthria), or position sense (dysmetria) may be altered. Damage may prevent the patient from performing rapidly alternating movements (dysdiadochokinesia). Symptoms usually begin 3–8 days after therapy is begun on the first cycle of HDAC. Ataxia and nystagmus are usually the first indicators of neurological damage. Stopping cytarabine if these signs appear helps limit additional toxicity. A cerebral syndrome of somnolence, altered mentation, headache, or (in rare cases) seizures can occur independently or can accompany the cerebellar toxicity. Either pattern of toxicity can result in death or permanent neurological dysfunction, but damage is reversible in about 70% of patients over several days.[28,76,77]

Patients with cytarabine-induced neurological damage show brain loss of large neurons (Purkinje cells) in the cerebellum. The mechanism of this cell loss is not known, but several risk factors have been suggested in addition to high doses. Risk is increased in the elderly and perhaps in patients with poor liver function, prior CNS dysfunction, or previous cytarabine administration.[28,76,77] Recently, a very strong correlation with decreased renal function has been established. This correlation may account for the association of neurotoxicity with increased age, because creatinine clearance decreases with age.[78] Although cytarabine is metabolized, its main metabolite, Ara-U, is eliminated renally. Ara-U accumulates in the CNS of patients with poor renal function, resulting in higher CNS levels of the phosphorylated form of cytarabine (Ara-CTP) that is believed to be the neurotoxic agent. Use of lower cytarabine doses, longer dose intervals, and most important, dose reduction for patients with impaired renal function, appear to reduce the risk of severe neurological damage without compromising efficacy (Figure 8-4). Prevention of HDAC neurotoxicity is essential because no treatment is known.

Ifosfamide

Ifosfamide neurotoxic damage is more global than that produced by cytarabine. Patients experience hallucinations and vivid dreams, with confusion, anxiety and restlessness or sometimes somnolence occurring. Seizures, coma, and death have occurred. Incidence varies by regimen but averages about 10%.[28,76]

Symptoms of ifosfamide neurotoxicity usually begin 2–5 days after ifosfamide is begun. Diagnosis is often complicated by overlapping side effects of other drugs, such as antiemetics. Diazepam and methylene blue have been used in

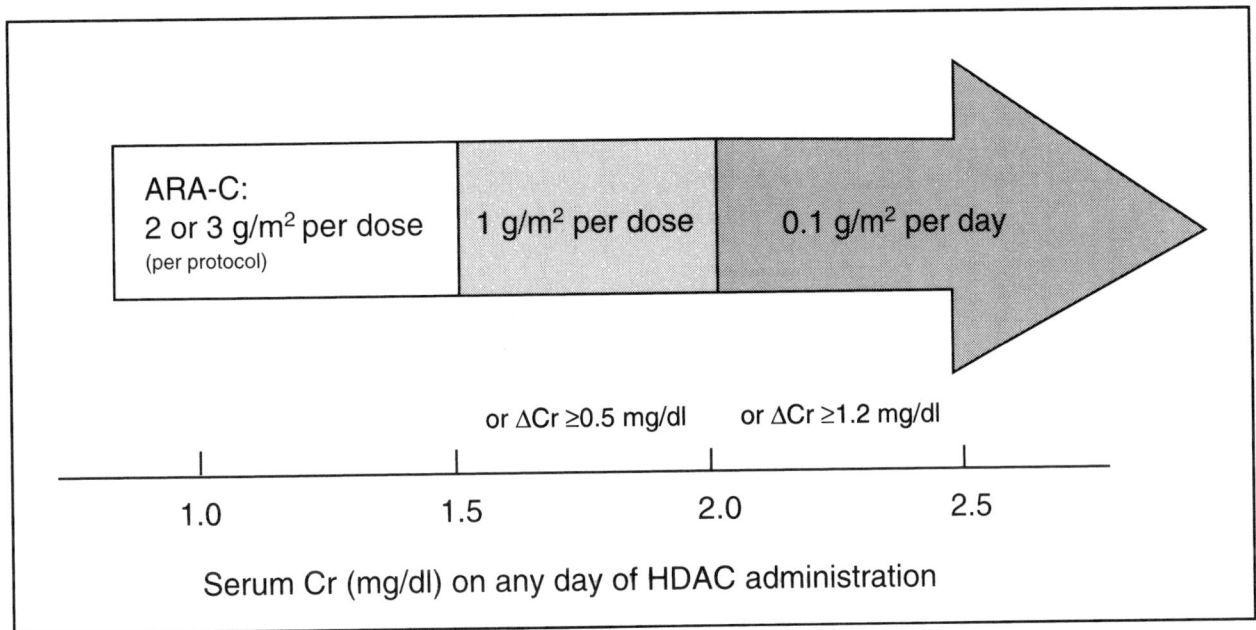

Figure 8-4. High-dose Ara-C (HDAC) dose modification algorithm. Ara-C, cytarabine; Cr, creatinine. Serum creatinine may be a poor reflection of actual renal function, especially in the elderly. Measured creatinine clearances offer the most accurate, readily available indication of renal function.

SOURCE: reprinted with permission from Smith GA, Damon LE, Rugo HS, et al. High-dose cytarabine dose modification reduces the incidence of neurotoxicity in patients with renal insufficiency. *J Clin Oncol* 1997;15:834.

the treatment of neurotoxicity in case reports of patients with severe neurological damage. Methylene blue has also shown prophylactic effects, by functioning as a neuroprotective agent against ifosfamide-induced encephalopathy. Methylene blue inhibits monoamine oxidase, which is needed to convert ifosfamide to chloroacetaldehyde, a potential neurotoxin.[79] Toxicity usually reverses within a few days after ifosfamide is discontinued.

Antimetabolites

The antimetabolites fludarabine (Fludara), cladribine (Leustatin), and pentostatin (Nipent) all produced life-threatening and fatal neurotoxicity as doses were escalated in early dose-finding studies. Cladribine caused paralysis in a dozen patients. Fludarabine was almost discarded after phase I trials because of very serious neurological toxicity. Patients developed blindness and either paralysis or encephalopathy with coma. Pentostatin's neurotoxicity was less dramatic but also important. Somnolence, lethargy, encephalopathy, seizures, and coma were reported.[80]

Each of these drugs produced neurological toxicity in patients receiving relatively high-dose therapy. Development of symptoms was usually delayed for weeks or months after drug administration and was generally irreversible. Neurological damage is clearly dose related. Although about 15% of patients receiving recommended doses of each of these drugs experience neurological toxicity, it is severe in only about 1% of patients. Symptoms typically occur during rather than after the end of therapy and are usually transient, reversible, and not dose limiting.[80]

Methotrexate

Neurotoxicity is a well-recognized adverse effect from high-dose intravenous methotrexate therapy or direct instillation into the CNS. High parenteral doses produce two forms of neurotoxicity. Acute transient cerebral dysfunction occurs in about 15% of patients receiving high-dose regimens. It begins within a few days after methotrexate is begun and also resolves within days. This toxicity is similar to a stroke, with seizures, hemiparesis, confusion, and speech disorders. High-dose methotrexate can also produce a chronic delayed leukoencephalopathy. The onset of this very serious damage usually occurs several months after methotrexate is initiated. Personality changes are the first sign, and progressive dementia, seizures, spasticity, stupor, or delirium follow. Stopping methotrexate results in some improvement, but most patients have permanent neurological deficits.[28,41,76]

Intrathecal or intraventricular administration of methotrexate may also cause neurotoxicity. It occurs in three distinct patterns: acute, subacute, or delayed. The delayed form is the most serious. The acute form, the most common, is a chemical meningitis caused by direct irritation of the meninges by methotrexate. Symptoms begin within a few hours and are similar to meningitis from other causes: headache, nausea, vomiting, fever, back pain, and stiff neck (meningism). These symptoms occur in 5–40% of patients receiving methotrexate directly into the CNS but reverse within 1–2 days. The subacute form is most common among patients receiving frequent intrathecal or intraventricular methotrexate doses. It begins within days or weeks after methotrexate is started and is characterized by stiffness or paralysis, dementia, confusion, ataxia, irritability, and somnolence. It is also reversible. The delayed form of toxicity is leukoencephalopathy, similar to the one caused by high parenteral doses. It is the most serious form and the least likely to be reversible. Patients receiving cranial irradiation have an especially high risk of delayed toxicity. It can be progressive and is sometimes fatal, but some patients do recover.[28,41,76]

Methotrexate, especially when given directly into the CNS and when combined with cranial irradiation, has been implicated as a cause of long-term impaired neuropsychological functioning in childhood survivors of leukemia. Performance on academic achievement tests declines slightly. Careful documentation of long-term effects suggest that chemotherapy alone has relatively modest effects.[81]

Interleukin 2

Neurological damage from IL-2, like cardiac and pulmonary damage, is associated to some degree with the capillary leak syndrome and resulting edema. Fluid retention in the CNS probably contributes to mental status changes, such as confusion, disorientation, and delirium, that are common in patients receiving IL-2, although the precise mechanism of this neurotoxicity is not known. A variety of other CNS abnormalities have also been reported, such as paresthesia, motor weakness, and severe constipation.[82] Edema in peripheral tissues can cause peripheral neuropathic problems, such as carpal tunnel syndrome from compression of the median nerve in the wrist.[83] Most central and peripheral neurological symptoms clear rapidly when IL-2 is discontinued.

Interferon Alfa

Neurological toxicity is also common with interferon alfa (IFN-α). In very high single doses (e.g., 50 million units/m²), IFN-α can cause severe neurological compromise, such as marked somnolence, coma, or seizures. Most cancer chemotherapy regimens include chronic administration of much lower doses, and in these regimens, subacute and chronic neurological toxicity patterns can emerge. The most common are depression and cognitive dysfunction. Distal paresthesias and peripheral neuropathies have been reported. Dose-limiting fatigue may also be a form of neurological toxicity.[84] IFN-α–induced neurological damage may be due to changes in neuroendocrine hormone levels or to immunoregulatory effects of IFN-α. It is managed by decreasing the IFN-α dose or discontinuing treatment.[85]

Vinca Alkaloids

The vinca alkaloids (vincristine [Oncovin], vinblastine [Velban], and vinorelbine [Navelbine]) were the first chemotherapy drugs recognized as neurotoxins. They primarily damage the peripheral nervous system, although autonomic neurotoxicity and cranial nerve toxicity also occur. Vinca alkaloids bind to tubulin in the mitotic spindles and disrupt normal microtubule processes. Tubulin is also a component of neurotubules and the filaments of nerve axons. Tubulin disruption at these sites is believed to be the mechanism of their neurotoxicity. Neurotoxicity is dose related and is most common in patients who receive high individual doses at intervals of <1 week. Age is an important risk factor; children are quite tolerant of the neurotoxic effects, whereas patients >60 years old have an increased risk.[26,28,76,86]

Vincristine, the most commonly used vinca alkaloid, is also the most neurotoxic. Toxicity is a combination of sensory loss and motor weakness, and it is dose limiting for vincristine. Most patients begin to develop symptoms after 2–3 weekly doses of vincristine (a cumulative dose of 5–6 mg), but serious toxicity usually does not occur until the patient has received 7–10 weekly doses (15–20 mg total cumulative dose).[75,86,87] Patients may tolerate higher cumulative doses if the dose interval is >1 week. The first objective sign of peripheral neurotoxicity is loss of the Achilles tendon reflex in the heel cords and other deep tendon reflexes. The first symptom that patients notice is numbness, tingling, or a pins-and-needles sensation (paresthesias) in the fingers and then later in the toes. These symptoms evolve into sensory loss and sometimes muscle weakness. Patients' fingers become clumsy, making patients unable to perform fine motor tasks, such as buttoning their clothing. They develop a wide-based slapping gait to compensate for sensory loss in their feet, and may demonstrate foot drop. The only known treatment is to stop or decrease the vincristine dose, which usually improves the weakness within a few weeks. Paresthesias also subside over several weeks. Sensory and motor losses resolve more slowly and may take many months to resolve.[26,28,76,86,87]

Case-based data suggest that the risk of severe atypical neuropathy consisting of excruciating foot pain with motor weakness is increased when vincristine is given in combination with colony-stimulating factors.[88]

Autonomic neuropathy usually affects the gastrointestinal tract, resulting in constipation and colicky abdominal pain. These symptoms occur within a few days of vincristine administration and resolve over several days. Autonomic neuropathy occurs in up to one third of patients who receive high individual doses (>2 mg). Laxatives and prokinetic agents, such as metoclopramide, are helpful in preventing constipation. In severe cases, gut motility is completely suppressed, resulting in paralytic ileus that manifests clinically as bowel obstruction.[76,86]

Cranial nerve damage most commonly affects the trigeminal nerve, causing jaw pain that begins within a few hours of vincristine administration and persists for several days.[76,86]

Vinblastine and vinorelbine are also neurotoxic, but their potential for producing neurological damage is less than that of vincristine. Their patterns of neurotoxicity are similar to those produced by vincristine but are rarely dose limiting.[26,28,89] Vinorelbine produces peripheral neuropathy in most patients, but it is usually very mild and not clinically significant.[89] However, severe neurotoxicity can occur in patients with pre-existing peripheral neuropathy who receive vinorelbine in combination with paclitaxel, an established microtubule-acting neurotoxin discussed below.[90]

Cisplatin

Neurotoxicity, like renal damage, can be dose limiting for cisplatin patients. The most common form of nerve damage from cisplatin is sensory polyneuropathy, a form of peripheral neuropathy that affects multiple sensory nerves. Motor neurons are not affected. Unlike vincristine neuropathy, which is first noted by patients as numbness and tingling in the fingertips, cisplatin patients first complain of these symptoms in their toes and feet. Later, fingers and hands are also affected, in a stocking-and-glove distribution. The abnormal sensations may also continue to progress further up the legs and arms. Generally, the neuropathy is slowly reversible after cisplatin therapy is stopped. Several months may be required for reversal of symptoms. Electrophysiological evidence of damage may persist for many years or for life.[28,76,91]

The mechanism of cisplatin neurotoxicity is not known. Cisplatin is a heavy-metal compound, and nervous system damage is a well-known sign of poisoning with other heavy metals, such as lead and mercury. Inorganic platinum accumulates within neurons and seems to remain there indefinitely in an actively neurotoxic form.[91]

Dose is the only proven risk factor for cisplatin peripheral neuropathy. Neuropathic symptoms occur in about 50% of patients who have received 300–500 mg/m^2 (three to six doses) of cisplatin, but neuropathy can occur after a single dose. The incidence is 100% in patients receiving high single doses (i.e., ≥200 mg/m^2). Risk does not appear to be associated with patient age, diabetes, alcohol ingestion, renal function, or smoking history, so it is difficult to select patients at high risk for nerve damage. Women may be at slightly higher risk than men.[28,76,91]

The issue of patient risk factors to identify high-risk groups is an important one because chemoprotectant compounds have shown some neuroprotective effects. Amifostine, a chemoprotectant that reduces cisplatin renal toxicity, also appears to decrease cisplatin-induced peripheral neuropathy.[37,92] Other forms of nerve damage from cisplatin include autonomic neuropathies, seizures, encephalopathy, myasthenic syndrome, and cortical blindness.

Paclitaxel and Docetaxel

The taxanes, paclitaxel and docetaxel, interfere with microtubule function in tumor cells. A similar effect in neuronal microtubules is the likely cause of their peripheral neuropathy, which can be dose limiting. The clinical picture is similar to the neurotoxicity caused by the vinca alkaloids. Patients complain of numbness, tingling, or burning pain in a stocking-and-glove distribution or around their mouths. Vibration sense and deep tendon reflexes are lost, and some motor weakness can occur. It is also possible that myalgias, which are common a few days after paclitaxel treatment, are also a manifestation of neurological damage.[26,28]

Peripheral neurotoxicity is related to both high individual paclitaxel and docetaxel doses and cumulative doses, although there is no neurotoxic dose threshold. Symptoms are detectable in up to 50% of patients after three to four taxane cycles but can occur at any dose level.[26,28] The risk of peripheral neuropathy from paclitaxel is greater and occurs at lower cumulative doses for patients who have received previous cisplatin therapy or who are receiving these two neurotoxic agents concurrently.[93] Vinorelbine combination regimens with paclitaxel may also potentiate neurotoxicity.[90]

Chemoprotectants may have a role in preventing neurotoxic damage produced by taxanes, but stopping the drug is the only treatment known to help existing neuropathic damage. Taxane neurotoxicity is slowly reversible after the drug is discontinued.[37]

SPECIAL SENSES

Disorders of vision and hearing can seriously affect patient well-being and quality of life. Loss of either of these sensory capacities can be severely disabling, so these disorders are included in this chapter on major organ toxicity.

Ototoxicity

Ototoxicity is a unique target organ form of neurological toxicity. Cisplatin is the only chemotherapy drug that is commonly and unequivocally responsible for hearing loss in cancer patients. Hearing loss occurs first in high-frequency ranges. Compromise of ability to hear human speech is a relatively late finding. Patients may complain first of being unable to hear voices on the telephone. Tinnitus also occurs. Cisplatin-induced ototoxicity is pathologically similar to the hearing loss caused by aminoglycosides, in which patients lose the outer hair cells in the cochlea that are necessary to detect vibration of sound waves.[30,91]

Ototoxicity is associated with both high individual cisplatin doses and high cumulative doses. Combination of cisplatin therapy with cranial irradiation may increase the risk of ototoxicity. Unfortunately, hearing impairment is usually irreversible, but use of hearing aids can help compensate for the hearing loss. At present, there are no established preventive measures or treatment that can reverse cisplatin-induced hearing loss, although the chemoprotectant amifostine may protect against hearing damage.[37] Patients with pre-existing hearing compromise should be evaluated before receiving cisplatin. The closely related platinum analogue carboplatin has much less potential for producing ototoxicity and should be considered as an alternate therapy for these patients.[30,91]

Ocular Toxicity

Ocular toxicity may be neurologically based or occur by a wide variety of non-neurological mechanisms. Cisplatin can produce optic neuritis, color blindness, and rare cortical blindness that appear to be neurologically based. It can also produce retinal toxicities, primarily blurred vision and altered color perception that may be the result of changes in retinal pigment. A similar spectrum of ocular damage is possible with carboplatin therapy, but as with ototoxicity, ocular toxicity is less common from carboplatin treatment than from cisplatin.[37,94,95]

The vinca alkaloids can also produce cranial nerve palsies, optic neuropathy and atrophy, cortical blindness, and night blindness. Cranial nerve damage is the most common effect, producing ptosis (drooping eyelids) and nerve pain or paresthesias.[94,95]

Most antimetabolites are secreted in tears, and several can cause irritative effects on the conjunctiva, cornea, and eyelids. Cytarabine is the antimetabolite best known for producing ocular damage. The eyes may be a particular target for cytarabine damage because the enzyme responsible for cytarabine's metabolism is present in only very low concentrations in tears. The damage that is produced is often described as chemical conjunctivitis or keratitis. It is quite common. Without preventive measures, 40–100% of patients receiving HDAC experience ocular pain, increased tear production, the sensation of a foreign body in the eye, photophobia, blurred vision, and swelling of the conjunctiva. Symptoms usually last several days, and vision improves within 2 weeks. The risk of cytarabine-induced ocular toxicity can be markedly reduced by prophylactic administration of corticosteroid eye drops throughout the period of HDAC administration.[94,95]

Fluorouracil primarily produces ocular surface problems, such as excessive lacrimation (tearing), blurred vision, photophobia, and eye irritation. The increased tearing can be dramatic, with some patients having to change clothing frequently because of wetness. Applying ice packs to the eyes before, during, and for 30 minutes after fluorouracil injection decreases the ocular toxicity.[96]

Several hormonal agents can produce ocular damage. The most common of these are the corticosteroids, which are used as anticancer drugs in the management of several hematological malignancies. Corticosteroids are a well-established cause of subcapsular cataracts. The cataracts that they produce do not usually affect visual acuity or progress after corticosteroid therapy is stopped.[94,95] Tamoxifen can cause retinopathy with visual impairment and corneal opacities, especially in high-dose regimens. Crystalline retinal deposits and corneal opacities with leakage of pigment can also occur with conventional doses, but they are uncommon and do not usually affect visual acuity.[97] The androgen antagonist nilutamide produces an unusual toxicity pattern of delayed adaptation to dark that may be dose limiting.[98]

SUMMARY

Chemotherapy drugs may affect every organ system of the body. Damage to any major organ (heart, lungs, kidneys, liver, nervous system, or special senses) can be dose limiting. Most can be life threatening. All can be disabling and severely impact a patient's quality of life. Fortunately, many major organ system toxicities can be prevented or ameliorated by careful patient selection or a variety of toxicity-specific and/or drug-specific interventions. Chemoprotectants have established value in preventing cardiac, bladder, and renal damage and may prove useful in preventing peripheral neuropathies and ototoxicity.

REFERENCES

1. Boice JD, Travis LB. Body wars: effect of friendly fire (cancer therapy) [editorial]. *J Natl Cancer Inst* 1995;87:705–6.
2. Allen A. The cardiotoxicity of chemotherapeutic drugs. *Semin Oncol* 1992;19:529–42.
3. Steiherz LJ, Yahalom J. Toxicity. In: DeVita VT Jr, Hellman S, Rosenberg SA, editors. *Cancer: Principles and Practice of Oncology.* 5th ed. Philadelphia, PA: Lippincott-Raven; 1997. p. 2739–56.
4. Doroshow JH. Anthracyclines and anthracenediones. In: Chabner BA, Longo DL, editors. *Cancer Chemotherapy and Biotherapy.* 2nd ed. Philadelphia, PA: Lippincott-Raven; 1996. p. 409–34.
5. Hale JP, Lewis IJ. Anthracyclines: cardiotoxicity and its prevention. *Arch Dis Child* 1994;71:457–62.
6. Lipschultz SE, Colan SD, Gelber RD. Late effects of doxorubicin therapy for acute lymphoblastic leukemia in childhood. *N Engl J Med* 1991;324:808–15.
7. Von Hoff DD, Layard MW, Basa P, et al. Risk factors for doxorubicin-induced congestive heart failure. *Ann Intern Med* 1979;91:710–7.
8. Lipshultz SE, Lipsitz SR, Mone SM, et al. Female sex and higher drug dose as risk factors for late cardiotoxic effects of doxorubicin therapy for childhood cancer. *N Engl J Med* 1995;332:1738–43.
9. Sorensen K, Levitt G, Bull C, et al. Anthracycline dose in childhood acute lymphoblastic leukemia: issues of early survival versus late cardiotoxicity. *J Clin Oncol* 1997;15:61–8.
10. Seifert CF, Nesser ME, Thompson DF. Dexrazoxane in the prevention of doxorubicin-induced cardiotoxicity. *Ann Pharmacother* 1994;28:1063–71.
11. Basser RL, Green MD. Strategies for prevention of anthracycline cardiotoxicity. *Cancer Treat Rev* 1993;19:57–77.
12. Allen A. The cardiotoxicity of chemotherapeutic drugs. *Semin Oncol* 1992;19:529–42.
13. Weiss RB. The anthracyclines: will we ever find a better doxorubicin. *Semin Oncol* 1992;19:670–86.
14. Venturini M, Michelotti A, Del Mastro L, et al. Multicenter randomized controlled clinical trial to evaluate cardioprotection of dexrazoxane versus no cardioprotection in women receiving epirubicin chemotherapy for advanced breast cancer. *J Clin Oncol* 1996;14:3112–20.

15. Linsky KF, Ignoffo RJ. Liposomal doxorubicin. *Cancer Pract* 1996;4:288–90.
16. Swain SM, Whaley FS, Gerber MC, et al. Cardioprotection with dexrazoxane for doxorubicin-containing therapy in advanced breast cancer. *J Clin Oncol* 1997;15:1318–32.
17. Swain SM, Whaley FS, Gerber MC, et al. Delayed administration of dexrazoxane provides cardioprotection for patients with advanced breast cancer treated with doxorubicin-containing therapy. *J Clin Oncol* 1997;15:1333–40.
18. Wexler LH, Andrich MP, Venon D, et al. Randomized trial of the cardioprotective agent ICRF-187 in pediatric sarcoma patients treated with doxorubicin. *J Clin Oncol* 1996;14:901–10.
19. Tew KD, Colvin M, Chabner BA. Alkylating agents. In: Chabner BA, Longo DL, editors. *Cancer Chemotherapy and Biotherapy*. 2nd ed. Philadephia, PA: Lippincott-Raven; 1996. p. 297–332.
20. Roush W. Dana Farber death sends a warning to research hospitals. *Science* 1995;269;295–6.
21. Meyer CC, Calis KA, Burke LB, et al. Symptomatic cardiotoxicity associated with 5-fluorouracil. *Pharmacotherapy* 1997;17:729–36.
22. Anand AJ. Fluorouracil cardiotoxicity. *Ann Pharmacother* 1994;28:374–8.
23. White RL, Schwartzentruber DJ, Guleria A, et al. Cardiopulmonary toxicity of treatment with high dose interleukin-2 in 199 consecutive patients with metastatic melanoma or renal cell carcinoma. *Cancer* 1994;74:3212–22.
24. DuBois JS, Udelson JE, Atkins MB. Severe reversible global and regional ventricular dysfunction associated with high-dose interleukin-2 immunotherapy. *J Immunother* 1995;18:119–23.
25. Rowinsky EK, Mcguire WP, Guarnieri T, et al. Cardiac disturbances during the administration of taxol. *J Clin Oncol* 1991;9:1704–12.
26. Rowinsky EK, Donehower RC. Antimicrotubule agents. In: Chabner BA, Longo DL, editors. *Cancer Chemotherapy and Biotherapy*. 2nd ed. Philadelphia, PA: Lippincott-Raven; 1996. p. 263–96.
27. Patterson WP, Reams GP. Renal toxicities of chemotherapy. *Semin Oncol* 1992;19:521–8.
28. Weiss RB. Miscellaneous toxicities. In: DeVita VT Jr, Hellman S, Rosenberg SA, editors. *Cancer: Principles and Practice of Oncology*. 5th ed. Philadelphia, PA: Lippincott-Raven; 1997. p. 2796–806.
29. Cornelison TL, Reed E. Nephrotoxicity and hydration management for cisplatin, carboplatin, and ormaplatin. *Gyn Oncol* 1993;50:147–58.
30. Reed E, Dabholkar M, Chabner BA. Platinum analogues. In: Chabner BA, Longo DL, editors. *Cancer Chemotherapy and Biotherapy*. 2nd ed. Philadelphia, PA: Lippincott-Raven; 1996. p. 357–78.
31. Pinzani V, Bressolle F, Haug IJ, et al. Cisplatin-induced renal toxicity and toxicity-modulating strategies: a review. *Cancer Chemother Pharmacol* 1994;35:1–9.
32. Anand AJ, Bashey B. Newer insights into cisplatin nephrotoxicity. *Ann Pharmacother* 1993;27:1519–25.
33. Reece PA, Stafford I, Russel J, et al. Reduced ability to clear ultrafilterable platinum with repeated courses of cisplatin. *J Clin Oncol* 1986;4:1392–8.
34. Ariceta G, Rodriguez-Soriano J, Vallo A, et al. Acute and chronic effects of cisplatin therapy on renal magnesium homeostasis. *Med Pediatr Oncol* 1997;28:35–40.
35. Evans TRJ, Harper CL, Beveridge IG, et al. A randomized study to determine whether routine intravenous magnesium supplements are necessary in patients receiving cisplatin chemotherapy with continuous infusion 5-fluorouracil. *Eur J Cancer* 1995;31A:174–8.
36. Kemp G, Rose P, Lurain J, et al. Amifostine pretreatment for protection against cyclophosphamide-induced and cisplatin-induced toxicities: results of a randomized controlled trial in patients with advanced ovarian cancer. *J Clin Oncol* 1996;14:2101–12.
37. Foster-Nora JA, Siden R. Amifostine for protection from antineoplastic drug toxicity. *Am J Health-Syst Pharm* 1997;54:787–800.
38. Berns JS, Haghighat A, Staddon A, et al. Severe, irreversible renal failure after ifosfamide treatment. *Cancer* 1995;76:497–500.
39. Guleria AS, Yang JC, Topalian SL, et al. Renal dysfunction associated with the administration of high-dose interleukin-2 in 199 consecutive patients with metastatic melanoma or renal carcinoma. *J Clin Oncol* 1994;12:2714–22.
40. Memoli B, DeNicola L, Libetta C, et al. Interleukin-2-induced renal dysfunction in cancer patients is reversed by low-dose dopamine infusion. *Am J Kidney Dis* 1995;26:27–33.
41. Chu E, Allegra CJ. Antifolates. In: Chabner BA, Longo DL, editors. *Cancer Chemotherapy and Biotherapy*. 2nd ed. Philadelphia, PA: Lippincott-Raven; 1996. p. 109–48.
42. Widemann BC, Hetherington ML, Murphy RF, et al. Carboxypeptidase-G2 rescue in a patient with high dose methotrexate-induced nephrotoxicity. *Cancer* 1995;76:521–6.
43. Widemann BC, Balis FM, Murphy RF, et al. Carboxypeptidase-G2, thymidine, and leucovorin rescue in cancer patients with methotrexate-induced renal dysfunction. *J Clin Oncol* 1997;15: 2125–34.
44. West NJ. Prevention and treatment of hemorrhagic cystitis. *Pharmacotherapy* 1997;17:696–706.
45. Walther MM. Cystitis. In: DeVita VT Jr, Hellman S, Rosenberg SA, editors. *Cancer: Principles and Practice*. 5th ed. Philadelphia, PA: Lippincott-Raven; 1997. p. 2725–9.
46. Stillwell TJ, Benson RC. Cyclophosphamide-induced hemorrhagic cystitis: a review of 100 patients. *Cancer* 1988;61:451–7.
47. Haselberger MB, Schwinghammer TL. Efficacy of mesna for prevention of hemorrhagic cystitis after high-dose cyclophosphamide therapy. *Ann Pharmacother* 1995;29:918–21.
48. Vose JM, Reed EC, Pippert GC, et al. Mesna compared with continuous bladder irrigation as uroprotection during high-dose chemotherapy and transplantation: a randomized trial. *J Clin Oncol* 1993;11:1306–10.
49. Laszlo D, Bosi A, Guidi S, et al. Prostaglandin E2 bladder instillation for the treatment of hemorrhagic cystitis after allogeneic bone marrow transplantation. *Haematologica* 1995;80:421–5.
50. Miller LJ, Chandler SW, Ippoliti CM. Treatment of cyclophosphamide-induced hemorrhagic cystitis with prostaglandins. *Ann Pharmacother* 1994;28:590–4.

51. Lee WM. Drug-induced hepatotoxicity. *N Engl J Med* 1995; 333:1118–27.
52. Cersosimo RJ. Hepatotoxicity associated with cisplatin chemotherapy. *Ann Pharmacotherapy* 1993;27:438–41.
53. King PD, Perry MC. Hepatotoxicity of chemotherapeutic and oncologic agents. *Gastroenterol Clin N Am* 1995;24:969–90.
54. Hande KR, Garrow GC. Purine antimetabolites. In: Chabner BA, Longo DL, editors. *Cancer Chemotherapy and Biotherapy.* 2nd ed. Philadelphia, PA: Lippincott-Raven; 1996. p. 235–52.
55. Feenstra J, Vermeer RJ, Stricker BH. Fatal hepatic coma attributed to paclitaxel [letter]. *J Natl Cancer Inst* 1997;89:582–4.
56. Whiting-O'Keefe QE, Fye KH, Sack KD. Methotrexate and histologic hepatic abnormalities: a meta-analysis. *Am J Med* 1991;90:711–6.
57. Moertel CG, Fleming TR, Macdonald JS, et al. Hepatic toxicity associated with fluorouracil plus levamisole adjuvant therapy. *J Clin Oncol* 1993;11:236–9.
58. McLeod DG. Tolerability of nonsteroidal antiandrogens in the treatment of advanced prostate cancer. *Oncologist* 1997;2: 18–27.
59. Swain SM. Endocrine therapies of cancer. In: Chabner BA, Longo DL, editors. *Cancer Chemotherapy and Biotherapy.* 2nd ed. Philadelphia, PA: Lippincott-Raven; 1996. p. 59–108.
60. Kirkwood JM, Strawderman MH, Ernstoff MS, et al. Interferon alfa-2b adjuvant therapy of high-risk resected cutaneous melanoma: the Eastern Cooperative Oncology Group trial EST 1684. *J Clin Oncol* 1996;14:7–17.
61. Fisher B, Keenan AM, Garra BS, et al. Interleukin-2 induces profound reversible cholestasis: a detailed analysis in treated cancer patients. *J Clin Oncol* 1989;7:1852–62.
62. Nakagawa K, Miller F, Sims DE, et al. Mechanisms of interleukin-2 induced hepatic toxicity. *Cancer Res* 1996;56:507–10.
63. Kreisman H, Wolkovee N. Pulmonary toxicity of antineoplastic agents. *Semin Oncol* 1992;19:508–20.
64. Stover DE, Kaner RJ. Pulmonary toxicity. In: DeVita VT Jr, Hellman S, Rosenberg SA, editors. *Cancer: Principles and Practice.* 5th ed. Philadelphia, PA: Lippincott-Raven; 1997. p. 2729–939.
65. Wong MK, Bjarnason GA, Hrushesky WJ, et al. Steroid-responsive interstitial lung disease in patients receiving 2'-deoxy-5-fluorouridine-infusion chemotherapy. *Cancer* 1995;75: 2558–64.
66. Crilley P, Topolsky D, Styler MJ, et al. Extramedullary toxicity of a conditioning regimen containing busulfan, cyclophosphamide and etoposide in 84 patients undergoing autologous and allogenic BMT. *Bone Marrow Transplant* 1995;15:361–5.
67. Lazo JS, Chabner BA. Bleomycin. In: Chabner BA, Longo DL, editors. *Cancer Chemotherapy and Biotherapy.* 2nd ed. Philadelphia, PA: Lippincott-Raven; 1996. p. 379–93.
68. Comis RL. Bleomycin pulmonary toxicity: current status and future directions. *Semin Oncol* 1992:19 (*Suppl* 5):64–70.
69. Sleijfer S, van der Mark TW, Koops HS, et al. Enhanced effects of bleomycin on pulmonary function disturbances in patients with decreased renal function due to cisplatin. *Eur J Cancer* 1996;32A:550–2.
70. Shearer P, Katz J, Boseman P, et al. Pulmonary insufficiency complicating therapy with high dose cytosine arabinoside in five pediatric patients with relapsed acute myelogenous leukemia. *Cancer* 1994;74:1953–8.
71. Pavlakis N, Bell DR, Millward MJ, et al. Fatal pulmonary toxicity resulting from treatment with gemcitabine. *Cancer* 1997;80:286–91.
72. Berthiaume Y, Boiteau P, Fick G, et al. Pulmonary edema during IL-2 therapy: combined effect of increased permeability and hydrostatic pressure. *Am J Respir Crit Care Med* 1995: 152:329–35.
73. Rabinovici R, Gfeuerstein G, Abdullah F, et al. Locally produced tumor necrosis factor-alpha mediates interleukin-2-induced lung injury. *Circ Res* 1996;78:329–36.
74. Frankel SR, Eardley A, Lauwers G, et al. The "retinoic acid syndrome" in acute promyelocytic leukemia. *Ann Intern Med* 1992;117:292–6.
75. Markman M. Chemotherapy-associated neurotoxicity: an important side effect impacting on quality, rather than quantity, of life [editorial]. *J Cancer Res Clin Oncol* 1996;122:511–2.
76. Tuxen MK, Hansen SW. Neurotoxicity secondary to antineoplastic drugs. *Cancer Treat Rev* 1994;20:191–214.
77. Baker WJ, Royer GL Jr, Weiss RB. Cytarabine and neurologic toxicity. *J Clin Oncol* 1991;9:679–93.
78. Smith GA, Damon LE, Rugo HS, et al. High-dose cytarabine dose modification reduces the incidence of neurotoxicity in patients with renal insufficiency. *J Clin Oncol* 1997;15:833–9.
79. Aeschlimann C, Cerny T, Kupfer A. Inhibition of monoamine oxidase activity and prevention of ifosfamide encephalopathy by methylene blue. *Drug Metab Dispos* 1996;24:1336–9.
80. Cheson BD, Vena DA, Foss FM, et al. Neurotoxicity of purine analogs: a review. *J Clin Oncol* 1994;12:2216–28.
81. Copeland DR, Moore BD III, Francis DJ, et al. Neuropsychologic effects of chemotherapy on children with cancer: a longitudinal study. *J Clin Oncol* 1996;14:2826–35.
82. Karp BI, Yang JC, Korsand M, et al. Multiple cerebral lesions complicating therapy with interleukin-2. *Neurology* 1996;47:417–24.
83. Puduvalli VK, Sella A, Austin SG, et al. Carpal tunnel syndrome associated with interleukin-2 therapy. *Cancer* 1996; 77:1189–92.
84. Vial T, Descotes J. Clinical toxicity of the interferons. *Drug Safety* 1994;10:115–50.
85. Bender CM, Monti EJ, Kerr ME. Potential mechanisms of interferon neurotoxicity. *Cancer Pract* 1996;4:35–9.
86. Legha SS. Vincristine neurotoxicity: pathophysiology and management. *Med Toxicol* 1986;1:421–7.
87. McCune JS, Lindley C. Appropriateness of maximum-dose guideline for vincristine. *Am J Health-Syst Pharm* 1997;54: 1755–8.
88. Weintraub M, Adde MA, Venzon DJ, et al. Severe atypical neuropathy associated with administration of hematopoietic colony-stimulating factors and vincristine. *J Clin Oncol* 1996;14:935–40.
89. Pace A, Bove L, Nistico C, et al. Vinorelbine neurotoxicity: clinical and neurophysiological findings in 23 patients. *J Neurol Neurosurg Psychiatry* 1996;61:409–11.
90. Parimoo D, Jeffers S, Muggia FM. Severe neurotoxicity from vinorelbine-paclitaxel combinations. *J Natl Cancer Inst* 1996;88:1079–80.
91. Gregg RW, Molepo M, Mopetit VJA, et al. Cisplatin neurotoxicity: the relationship between dosage, time, and platinum concentration in neurologic tissues, and morphologic evidence of toxicity. *J Clin Oncol* 1992;10:795–803.
92. Cavaletti G, Cascinu S, Venturino P, et al. Neuroprotectant

drugs in cisplatin neurotoxicity. *Anticancer Res* 1996;16: 3149–59.
93. Cavaletti G, Bogliun G, Marzorati L, et al. Peripheral neurotoxicity of taxol in patients previously treated with cisplatin. *Cancer* 1995;75;1141–50.
94. Al-Tweigeri T, Nabholtz J-M, Mackey JR. Ocular toxicity and cancer chemotherapy: a review. *Cancer* 1996;78:1359–73.
95. Burns LJ. Ocular toxicities of chemotherapy. *Semin Oncol* 1992;19:492–500.
96. Loprinzi CL, Wender DB, Beeder MH, et al. Inhibition of 5-fluorouracil-induced ocular irritation by ocular ice packs. *Cancer* 1994;74:945–8.
97. Nayfield SG, Gorin MB. Tamoxifen-associated eye diseases: a review. *J Clin Oncol* 1996;14:1018–26.
98. Dole EJ, Holdsworth MT. Nilutamide: an antiandrogen for the treatment of prostate cancer. *Ann Pharmacother* 1997; 31:65–75.

SELF-STUDY QUESTIONS

1. The anticancer agent most commonly implicated in producing cardiac toxicity is:

    a. idarubicin.
    b. doxorubicin.
    c. fluorouracil.
    d. interleukin 2.

2. Which of the following risk factors does NOT increase a patient's risk of developing subacute anthracycline-induced cardiac toxicity?

    a. cumulative dose >550 mg/m^2
    b. mediastinal radiation
    c. very young age
    d. male gender

3. Describe the rationale for the use of dexrazoxane in the prevention of doxorubicin-induced cardiac toxicity.

4. Administration of doxorubicin by infusion rather than bolus injection decreases the risk of developing subacute cardiac toxicity.

    a. true
    b. false

5. Select the true statement:

    a. Acute cardiac rhythm changes produced by anthracyclines lead to subacute and late forms of cardiac toxicity.
    b. Late cardiac toxicity becomes clinically evident within 1 year of initiating anthracycline administration.
    c. Subacute and late forms of anthracycline-induced cardiac toxicity usually produce symptoms of congestive heart failure.
    d. An increase in left ventricular ejection fraction is an indicator of progressive anthracycline cardiac damage.

6. Dose-limiting toxicity of cisplatin is most commonly neurological toxicity or:

    a. nausea and vomiting.
    b. nephrotoxicity.
    c. ototoxicity.
    d. hepatotoxicity.

7. Compared with cisplatin, carboplatin produces less risk of:

    a. nephrotoxicity.
    b. neurological toxicity.
    c. ototoxicity.
    d. all of the above.

8. From the following list, select the most appropriate hydration fluid for patients receiving cisplatin therapy:

    a. sodium chloride 0.9% with magnesium sulfate 8 mEq/L.
    b. sodium chloride 0.9% with sodium bicarbonate 100 mEq/L.
    c. dextrose 5% in water with magnesium sulfate 8 mEq/L.
    d. dextrose 5% in water with sodium bicarbonate 100 mEq/L.

9. From the following list, select a chemoprotectant that can reduce the risk of cisplatin-induced renal damage.

    a. mesna
    b. carboxypeptidase G2
    c. dexrazoxane
    d. amifostine

10. A patient who has received four cycles of cisplatin therapy has had no change in his serum creatinine since beginning therapy. This is proof that he has not incurred any renal damage from his cisplatin therapy.

    a. true
    b. false

11. Methotrexate produces renal damage by precipitating within the renal tubules.

    a. true
    b. false

12. The recommended interventions to decrease the risk of methotrexate-induced nephrotoxicity include hydration and:

    a. amifostine.
    b. magnesium supplementation.
    c. urine alkalinization.
    d. leucovorin.

13. Describe the rationale for the use of carboxypeptidase G2 in the management of methotrexate-induced renal dysfunction.

14. Which of the following factors does NOT increase the risk of methotrexate-induced renal dysfunction?

    a. concomitant cisplatin therapy
    b. concomitant nonsteroidal anti-inflammatory drug therapy
    c. chronic low-dose administration
    d. high-dose therapy

15. Damage to the urinary tract from cyclophosphamide is characterized by:

    a. nephrotoxicity.
    b. hemorrhagic cystitis.
    c. renal cancer.
    d. bladder infection.

16. JG will receive 600 mg/m^2 of cyclophosphamide intravenously every 3 weeks as part of her breast cancer therapy. She has normal renal function and is otherwise healthy. Recommend a treatment plan to minimize JG's risk of cyclophosphamide-induced urinary tract toxicity.

17. What is the rationale for the use of hydration and the use of mesna in the prevention of bladder toxicity secondary to treatment with cyclophosphamide or ifosfamide?

18. RT will receive ifosfamide 2000 mg IV each day for 4 days over 1 hour as treatment of his testicular cancer. What intravenous dose of mesna is appropriate for prevention of ifosfamide bladder damage in this patient?

    a. 2000 mg before ifosfamide
    b. 400 mg before ifosfamide
    c. 2000 mg before ifosfamide and at 4 and 8 hours after ifosfamide
    d. 400 mg before ifosfamide and at 4 and 8 hours after ifosfamide

19. Mesna interferes with the antitumor activity of cyclophosphamide and ifosfamide.

    a. true
    b. false

20. The risk of bladder damage from high-dose cyclophosphamide administered as part of bone marrow transplantation regimens can be effectively decreased by:

    a. hyperhydration regimens.
    b. recommending oral fluid intake of 2 L/day.
    c. mesna administration.
    d. both a and c are correct.

21. Which of the following anticancer agents characteristically produces liver fibrosis during chronic oral administration over several years?

    a. interleukin 2
    b. methotrexate
    c. mercaptopurine
    d. flutamide

22. Hepatic damage is associated with high-dose cytarabine therapy, but rarely if at all with standard (100–200 mg/m^2) doses.

    a. true
    b. false

23. The mechanism of asparaginase hepatotoxicity is believed to be:

    a. interference with protein synthesis in the liver.
    b. a direct toxic effect on hepatocytes.
    c. occlusion of blood vessels in the liver.
    d. none of the above.

24. Which of the following chemotherapy regimens produces the highest risk of hepatic damage?

    a. fluorouracil alone
    b. fluorouracil plus leucovorin
    c. fluorouracil plus levamisole
    d. levamisole alone

25. Select the agent(s) whose safe administration requires routine monitoring of liver function tests.

    a. flutamide
    b. interferon alfa
    c. tamoxifen
    d. both a and b

26. Describe the characteristic signs and symptoms of the most common form of pulmonary damage produced by antineoplastic drugs.

27. The value of corticosteroids in treatment of tretinoin-induced pulmonary damage is not established.

    a. true
    b. false

28. The first anticancer drug that was established as a cause of pulmonary toxicity was:

    a. busulfan.
    b. bleomycin.
    c. interleukin 2.
    d. tretinoin.

29. Select the false statement:

    a. Bleomycin lung damage is related to high cumulative doses.
    b. Bleomycin lung damage is related to high individual doses.
    c. Cisplatin administration may increase the risk of bleomycin lung damage.
    d. None of the above statements is true.

30. What is the proposed mechanism of lung damage in patients receiving interleukin 2?

31. Which of the following anticancer agents produces peripheral neuropathy as their most common pattern of neurological damage?

    a. cytarabine
    b. vincristine
    c. interleukin 2
    d. all of the above

32. Which of the following patients is at greatest risk of neurological toxicity from high-dose cytarabine administration?

    a. 72-year-old patient with rapidly decreasing renal function
    b. 24-year-old patient with rapidly decreasing renal function
    c. 72-year-old patient with rapidly decreasing liver function
    d. 24-year-old patient with rapidly decreasing liver function

33. Which of the following anticancer drugs produces impaired coordination and balance as characteristic symptoms of neurological toxicity?

    a. cytarabine
    b. vincristine
    c. cisplatin
    d. paclitaxel

34. Select the true statement:

    a. Ifosfamide typically produces symptoms of peripheral neuropathy.
    b. Fludarabine and cladribine produce a high incidence of coma and blindness at recommended therapeutic doses.
    c. Neurotoxic damage from paclitaxel can be potentiated by treatment with cisplatin or vinorelbine.
    d. All of the above statements are true.

35. Select the true statement:

    a. Vincristine produces a greater risk of neurological toxicity than vinblastine or vinorelbine.
    b. The vinca alkaloids are believed to cause neurological damage by production of free radicals that destroy nerve tissue.
    c. Neurological damage produced by the vinca alkaloids can be reversed by administration of dexamethasone.
    d. All of the above statements are true.

Chapter 9: Gastrointestinal Complications of Cancer Chemotherapy

Amy Valley, Pharm.D.
Oncology Pharmacy Specialist
South Texas Veterans Health Care System
Audie L. Murphy Division, and
Clinical Assistant Professor
University of Texas Health Science Center at
San Antonio, Texas

Nausea and Vomiting	149
Pathophysiology and Etiology	149
Risk Factors	151
Prevention and Treatment	152
Principles of Antiemetic Therapy	152
Assessment of Response	153
Antiemetic Agents	153
Mechanisms of Action	153
Antiemetic Potency	155
Adverse Effects	156
Dosing and Administration	156
Cost	157
Designing an Antiemetic Regimen	157
Role of the Pharmacist	157
Oral Complications	158
Pathophysiology and Etiology	159
Risk Factors	159
Prevention and Treatment	160
Oral Hygiene	160
Local Protective Agents	161
Oral Cryotherapy	161
Analgesics	161
Antifungal Agents	162
Antiviral Agents	162
Other Agents	162
Role of the Pharmacist	163
Diarrhea	163
Pathophysiology and Etiology	163
Risk Factors	163
Prevention and Treatment	164
General Supportive Care	164
Antidiarrheal Agents	164
Octreotide	164
Role of the Pharmacist	164
Constipation	165
Pathophysiology and Etiology	165

Risk Factors 165
Prevention and Treatment. 165
Role of the Pharmacist. 165
Summary 166
References 166
Self-Study Questions 169

Current anticancer agents have narrow therapeutic indices and may result in severe toxicities affecting multiple organ systems, even when given at standard doses. The gastrointestinal (GI) tract is a common site of toxicity with diverse manifestations, including nausea and vomiting, mucositis, diarrhea, and constipation. The clinical spectrum of these adverse events ranges from mild discomfort and inconvenience to life-threatening toxicity (Table 9-1). GI side effects may affect the ability to deliver curative and palliative cancer chemotherapy by causing treatment delays, reduction of antineoplastic doses, and patient refusal of chemotherapy.

These toxicities also significantly compromise cancer patients' quality of life.

After completing this chapter, the reader should be able to:

1. Describe the clinical significance of chemotherapy-induced GI toxicities, including nausea and vomiting, mucositis, diarrhea, and constipation.
2. List several possible mechanisms of GI toxicity in cancer patients.
3. Identify the phases of emesis and the pathways of vomiting center stimulation and vomiting control.

Table 9-1. Gastrointestinal Toxicity Grading System

Toxicity	Toxicity Grade				
	0	1	2	3	4
Nausea	none	able to eat reasonable intake	intake significantly decreased but can eat	no significant intake	NA
Vomiting	none	1 episode in 24 hr	2–5 episodes in 24 hr	6–10 episodes in 24 hr	>10 episodes in 24 hr or parenteral support required
Mucositis	none	painless ulcers or erythema or mild soreness	painful ulcers, erythema or edema, but can eat	painful ulcers, erythema or edema, and cannot eat	parenteral or enteral support required
Diarrhea	none	increase of 2–3 stools/day over baseline	increase of 4–6 stools/day or nocturnal stools or moderate cramping	increase of 7–9 stools/day or incontinence or severe cramping	increase of ≥10 stools/day or grossly bloody diarrhea or parenteral support required
Constipation	none	stool softener required	laxatives required	obstipation with enema; manual or surgical evacuation required	NA

SOURCE: adapted with permission from Southwest Oncology Group (SWOG) Toxicity Criteria. NA, not applicable.

4. Describe the mechanism of action, emetogenic potency, and usual adverse effects of antiemetic agents.
5. Design an antiemetic plan for a given chemotherapy regimen.
6. Identify chemotherapeutic agents associated with an increased risk of mucositis.
7. Recommend appropriate prevention and treatment plans for a patient with chemotherapy-induced mucositis.
8. List supportive care measures for the management of diarrhea and constipation in cancer patients.

This chapter is divided into four major sections covering nausea and vomiting, mucositis, diarrhea, and constipation. Each section presents an overview of the GI toxicity, including: 1) an introduction; 2) the pathophysiology and etiology of the complication; 3) its risk factors; 4) methods for prevention and treatment of the toxicity, focusing on specific pharmacologic interventions; and 5) potential roles of the pharmacist.

NAUSEA AND VOMITING

Of all the potential side effects of cancer chemotherapy, nausea and vomiting are among the most commonly feared by cancer patients and their families.[1] Uncontrolled nausea and vomiting in these patients can result in serious and potentially life-threatening sequelae, including significant weight loss, malnutrition, dehydration, electrolyte and acid-base imbalances, GI mucosal tears, wound dehiscence, aspiration pneumonia, and pathological fractures.[2,3] Poorly controlled nausea and vomiting are also known to adversely affect cancer patients' quality of life.[4,5] The psychological effects of inadequate emesis control range from mild anxiety and fatigue to the development of refractory anticipatory nausea and vomiting. The current incidence of uncontrolled nausea and vomiting is unclear, but past research has documented that uncontrolled nausea and vomiting cause as many as 25–50% of cancer patients to refuse chemotherapy at some point in their treatment.[2] These figures may be decreasing with better control of nausea and vomiting due to widespread use of combination antiemetic regimens that incorporate serotonin receptor antagonists.

Pathophysiology and Etiology

There are three distinct phases of emesis: nausea, retching, and vomiting.[3,6] Nausea, defined as an awareness of the urge to vomit, is an autonomic process associated with pallor, flushing, and tachycardia. It is accompanied by relaxation of gastric and pyloric tone and diminished or reversed peristalsis. Nausea is a potentially reversible phase of emesis. Retching is characterized by spasmodic, abortive movements of the diaphragm and the thoracic and abdominal muscles. Vomiting occurs as the diaphragm descends, the abdominal muscles contract to increase intragastric pressure, and the lower esophageal sphincter relaxes to permit the expulsion of stomach contents. Although nausea usually precedes retching and vomiting, vomiting may occur in the absence of nausea. Conditions associated with this phenomenon include intracranial metastases and intestinal obstruction.

Despite extensive basic and clinical research, the pathophysiology of chemotherapy-induced nausea and vomiting is still not completely understood. Vomiting is a complex physiological process coordinated by an area in the medulla oblongata known as the vomiting center (Figure 9-1).[3,6] The vomiting center receives afferent (or incoming) impulses from several sites, including the chemoreceptor trigger zone, the GI tract, the brain cortex, and the vestibular apparatus. The vestibular apparatus is not believed to play an important role in chemotherapy-induced emesis and is not pictured in Figure 9-1. The chemoreceptor trigger zone is located in the area postrema of the brainstem, forming part of the floor of the

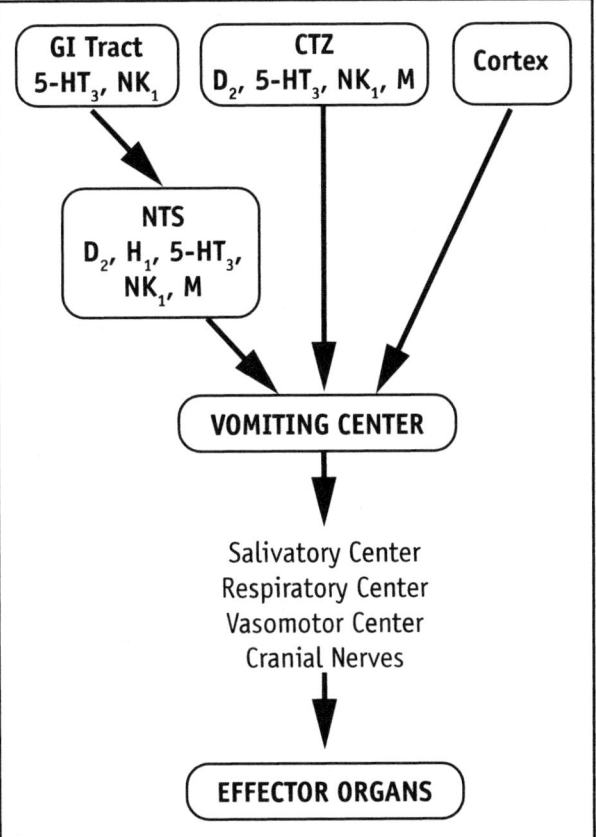

Figure 9-1. Pathways and neurotransmitter receptors in chemotherapy-induced nausea and vomiting. GI, gastrointestinal; CTZ, chemoreceptor trigger zone; NTS, nucleus tractus solitarius; D_2, dopamine type 2 receptor; $5\text{-}HT_3$, serotonin type 3 receptor; M, muscarinic receptor; H_1, histamine 1 receptor; NK_1, tachykinin neurokinin NK_1 receptor.

SOURCE: adapted from references 3 and 6–8.

fourth ventricle. Positioned outside the blood-brain barrier, the chemoreceptor trigger zone is accessible to circulating emetogenic substances in both the blood and cerebrospinal fluid. A variety of drugs, including antineoplastic agents, are known to stimulate the chemoreceptor trigger zone.

The vagal and sympathetic afferent nerves from the GI tract transmit nausea and vomiting stimuli to the vomiting center via the nucleus tractus solitarius and, to a lesser extent, the chemoreceptor trigger zone. The nucleus tractus solitarius, a bundle of afferent nerve fiber endings located in the medulla oblongata, is distinct from the chemoreceptor trigger zone. Higher brainstem and cortical structures receive stimuli from sight, smell, taste, and memory and communicate this information to the vomiting center. This mechanism of input into the vomiting center may be particularly important in the development of anticipatory nausea and vomiting. The cerebellum relays stimuli from the vestibular apparatus to the vomiting center and is believed to be the primary mechanism for nausea and vomiting due to motion sickness. The vomiting center receives and integrates nausea and vomiting stimuli from all of these sources and sends efferent (or outgoing) impulses to the salivary, vasomotor, and respiratory centers and to cranial nerves VIII and X. This results in activation of the many muscles and organs involved in nausea and vomiting (the abdominal muscles, diaphragm, stomach, and esophagus).

Several neurotransmitters are involved in the transmission of information involved in the vomiting process, including dopamine, serotonin, acetylcholine, and histamine.[3,6-8] Receptors for these neurotransmitters are known to be present throughout the nausea and vomiting pathway (Figure 9-1). Dopamine type 2 (D_2) and serotonin type 3 (5-hydroxytryptamine type 3 [$5-HT_3$]) receptors seem to be the most important receptors involved in chemotherapy-induced nausea and vomiting. Antagonism of these neurotransmitters or their receptors interrupts the nausea and vomiting pathway. This is the manner in which currently available antiemetics are believed to prevent and control chemotherapy-related nausea and vomiting. Recently, serotonin type 4 ($5-HT_4$) receptors have also been implicated in vomiting, possibly mediated via GI tract afferent nerve fibers. The neurotransmitter compound substance P may also play an important role in chemotherapy-induced nausea and vomiting. Substance P interacts with the neurokinin (NK_1) receptor. NK_1 receptor antagonists have shown potent antiemetic activity in animal models and are now entering clinical trials in humans.[8] The roles of other substances, such as the prostaglandins, cytokines, endogenous opioids, vasopressin, enkephalin, peptide YY, and catecholamines, in the nausea and vomiting process are not completely defined. Specific mechanisms of action of commonly used antiemetics are discussed further in the sections that follow.

Chemotherapy-induced nausea and vomiting may be subdivided into three types: acute, delayed, and anticipatory.[9] Nausea and vomiting are considered acute when they occur within 24 hours of chemotherapy administration. Acute nausea and vomiting are most easily prevented and treated with currently available antiemetics.

Delayed nausea and vomiting are arbitrarily defined as nausea and vomiting that occur more than 24 hours after chemotherapy. Delayed nausea and vomiting are more refractory to antiemetics than acute nausea and vomiting and may result in significant weight loss, dehydration, and malnutrition. The underlying pathophysiology is not well understood but appears to differ from that of acute nausea and vomiting. Delayed nausea and vomiting are most commonly associated with cisplatin-based chemotherapy and may persist for more than a week after administration. Without prophylactic antiemetics, most patients receiving cisplatin-based therapy experience some degree of delayed nausea or vomiting. In a classic observational study of two consecutive trials of cisplatin-induced emesis, delayed vomiting occurred in 21–61% of patients, and delayed nausea in 24–78%. Overall, 93% of studied patients experienced some degree of delayed nausea and vomiting.[10] The nausea and vomiting usually occurred 2–5 days after cisplatin administration, with a peak incidence at 48–72 hours. The most important risk factor for the development of delayed emesis appears to be uncontrolled nausea and vomiting in the acute phase. The first regimens found to be effective in prevention of delayed nausea and vomiting from cisplatin combined oral metoclopramide and dexamethasone with or without lorazepam and/or diphenhydramine. These regimens prevented significant nausea and vomiting in 70% of patients.[11,12] Similar results have been obtained with regimens using oral prochlorperazine and dexamethasone.[13] Unfortunately, although other antiemetics, including the $5-HT_3$ receptor antagonists, are effective, they have not been found to improve on this response rate.[14-16] Cyclophosphamide-containing regimens[17] may also produce clinically significant delayed nausea and vomiting. However, this type of nausea and vomiting appears to be more responsive to antiemetics than cisplatin-induced delayed emesis.

Anticipatory nausea and vomiting, the third type of chemotherapy-related nausea and vomiting, are defined as nausea and vomiting that occur before the administration of chemotherapy. Anticipatory nausea and vomiting differ from the other types of nausea and vomiting in that they are a conditioned response typically resulting from poor control of nausea and vomiting with previous cycles of chemotherapy. The incidence of anticipatory nausea and vomiting ranges from 18 to 65%, depending on several factors, including the emetogenic potential of the chemotherapy regimen.[18] They are notoriously difficult to manage and are most responsive to nonpharmacologic interventions. The anxiolytic and amnestic effects of the benzodiazepines may also prove useful.

Although chemotherapy is the most common culprit in producing nausea and vomiting in cancer patients, several other causative factors must also be considered. GI causes of nausea and vomiting include gastric outlet obstruction, radiation-induced enteritis, hepatic metastases, and constipation. Within the central nervous system, increased intracranial pressure, anxiety, severe or chronic pain, and other drugs (e.g., narcotics) may induce nausea and vomiting. Metabolic causes of nausea and vomiting include hypercalcemia, uremia, and hypoadrenalism. It is important to thoroughly evaluate each patient for causes of nausea and vomiting other than chemotherapy, so that the underlying etiology may be specifically treated or removed, if possible. This is particularly true for patients with unexplained or protracted nausea and vomiting that are not temporally associated with chemotherapy administration.

Risk Factors

The reported incidence of chemotherapy-induced nausea and vomiting varies markedly. It depends on several factors, including the emetogenic potential of the chemotherapeutic agent(s), dose and method of administration, patient-specific factors, and the use of combination antineoplastic regimens. Of these factors, the emetogenic potential of the antineoplastic agent(s) is believed to be the most important determinant of nausea and vomiting risk (Table 9-2).[19] For most of these drugs, the usual onset of nausea and vomiting is 1–4 hours following drug administration, with a peak incidence at 4–12 hours and resolution by 12–24 hours.[3] There are, however, exceptions to this generalization. The onset of nausea and vomiting with mechlorethamine (nitrogen mustard) may occur within 30 minutes of administration. In contrast, the onset of nausea and vomiting following cyclophosphamide is often delayed by at least 4–10 hours. Perhaps the most notable exception is the two-phase nausea and vomiting pattern seen with cisplatin. Without prophylactic antiemetics, acute nausea and vomiting in the first 24 hours after cisplatin administration are almost universal. Cisplatin also produces delayed nausea and vomiting that peak in incidence at 48–72 hours following administration.[10] Patterns of emesis have significant implications for design of antiemetic regimens.

Many institutions have developed antiemetic guidelines based on the information presented in Table 9-2. However, it is important to note that the data in the table do not reflect the synergistic effects on nausea and vomiting risk that may occur in combination regimens employing agents with varying emetogenic potential. Hesketh et al. recently proposed a method to calculate the emetic risk for multiagent regimens.[19] The emetogenicity of a combination regimen is determined by modifying the emetogenic rating of the most emetogenic agent in the combination (Table 9-2) according to the following rules:

- level 1 agents do not contribute to the emetogenic potential of the regimen,
- adding one or more level 2 agents increases the emetogenicity of the regimen by one level, and
- adding level 3 or 4 agents increases the emetogenicity of the combination by one level per agent.

Although this is the largest report to date that has validated a system for estimating the emetogenicity of combination regimens, most of the patients studied were females with breast cancer. This intriguing proposal requires validation in a large series of male and female cancer chemotherapy patients with other types of tumors.

The potential for nausea and vomiting is also greatly

Table 9-2. Relative Emetogenic Potential of Antineoplastic Agents

Level 1 Low (<10%)	Level 2 Moderately Low (10–30%)	Level 3 Moderate (30–60%)	Level 4 Moderately High (60–90%)	Level 5 High (>90%)

Bleomycin
Busulfan
Chlorambucil
Cladribine
Estramustine*
Fludarabine
Hydroxyurea
Melphalan (oral)
Mercaptopurine*
Methotrexate
  (<50 mg/m²)
Thioguanine
Vinblastine
Vincristine
Vinorelbine
	Cytarabine* (<1 g/m²)
	Docetaxel
	Doxorubicin (<20 mg/m²)
	Etoposide (VP-16)
	Fluorouracil
	Gemcitabine
	Asparaginase*
	Methotrexate
	  (>50 & <250 mg/m²)
	Mitomycin
	Paclitaxel
	Teniposide*
	Thiotepa (<15 mg/m²)*
	Topotecan*
		Altretamine
		Cyclophosphamide
		  (≤750 mg/m²)
		Doxorubicin
		  (20–60 mg/m²)
		Daunorubicin*
		Epirubicin (≤90 mg/m²)
		Idarubicin
		Ifosfamide
		Methotrexate
		  (250–1000 mg/m²)
		Mitoxantrone
		  (<15 mg/m²)
			Carboplatin
			Carmustine
			  (≤250 mg/m²)
			Cisplatin (<50 mg/m²)
			Cyclophosphamide
			  (>750 & ≤1500
			  mg/m²)
			Cytarabine (>1 g/m²)
			Doxorubicin
			  (>60 mg/m²)
			Dactinomycin*
			Irinotecan*
			Methotrexate (>1 g/m²)
			Lomustine (CCNU)*
			Procarbazine
				Carmustine
				  (>250 mg/m²)
				Cisplatin
				  (≥50 mg/m²)
				Cyclophosphamide
				  (>1500 mg/m²)
				Dacarbazine
				Mechlorethamine
				Pentostatin
				Streptozocin

SOURCE: adapted from references 3, 19, and product literature (*). Descriptors and (%) refer to the incidence of moderate to severe nausea and vomiting without antiemetics. The above information pertains to conventional doses of chemotherapy and is not applicable to bone marrow transplantation.

influenced by dose and schedule of the antineoplastic agent. For example, low doses of cytarabine (ara-C) (100–200 mg/m^2 per day) are associated with moderately low risk of nausea and vomiting, whereas larger doses (1–3 g/m^2 per dose) are associated with moderately high risk of severe nausea and vomiting.[3] The emetogenic potential of cyclophosphamide is also very dose dependent. At single doses of <1 g/m^2, cyclophosphamide possesses only moderate emetogenic potential; however, at doses used in bone marrow transplantation (e.g., 60 mg/kg, or approximately 2.4 g/m^2 for 2 days), the drug is very highly emetogenic. The method or schedule of administration also influences nausea and vomiting risk. When agents such as doxorubicin or cisplatin are given as an intravenous (IV) bolus or short infusion, they produce significantly more nausea and vomiting than when infused over 24 hours.[20] The risk of nausea and vomiting may be cumulative with repeated administration of some chemotherapy regimens, especially those containing cisplatin or high doses of cyclophosphamide. It is difficult to distinguish cumulative nausea and vomiting risk from potential loss of antiemetic effects over time. There are some reports of tolerance to the antiemetic effects of 5-HT$_3$ receptor antagonists over time, although not all studies have confirmed these results.[21]

Patient-specific factors also play a role in determining nausea and vomiting risk.[22] Patients with a history of severe or uncontrolled nausea and vomiting from chemotherapy are more likely to have nausea and vomiting with subsequent regimens. A history of chronic heavy alcohol use (defined as more than five mixed drinks [or 100 g of alcohol] per day) decreases the risk of chemotherapy-related nausea and vomiting. Susceptibility to motion sickness appears to be a risk factor for development of anticipatory nausea and vomiting. Although some studies have indicated that nausea and vomiting are more common in women, other factors, such as the type of chemotherapy regimens women receive or higher alcohol intake in men enrolled in these studies, may have influenced the results. There is some evidence that elderly patients may experience less nausea and vomiting from chemotherapy than young adults (<30 years of age) and children. It is not clear whether this observation represents a true difference in incidence of nausea and vomiting or an age-related difference in the response to antiemetic regimens. The most relevant age-related difference may be in the incidence of adverse effects from antiemetics, particularly metoclopramide.

Prevention and Treatment

Principles of Antiemetic Therapy

The general principles of antiemetic therapy are outlined in Table 9-3. Antiemetics are most effective when administered prophylactically. It is much easier to prevent nausea and vomiting from chemotherapy than it is to control them once they occur. Antiemetics should be administered approximately 30 minutes before chemotherapy. Because the onset of nausea and vomiting from most chemotherapeutic agents is 1–4 hours

Table 9-3. General Principles of Antiemetic Therapy

Administer antiemetics prophylactically to prevent N/V

Continue antiemetics on a regular schedule throughout period of N/V risk

Provide *prn* antiemetics for breakthrough N/V between scheduled doses

Match the antiemetic potency to the emetogenic potential of the chemotherapy agent(s)

Take patient history to identify risk factors for N/V and past experience with antiemetics

Use antiemetic combinations with nonoverlapping mechanisms of action and adverse effects, when possible

Re-evaluate patients frequently during and between chemotherapy courses

Individualize antiemetic regimens as indicated by efficacy and adverse effects

Consider nonpharmacologic interventions, especially in patients with anticipatory N/V

N/V, nausea and/or vomiting; *prn*, as needed.

following administration, the 30-minute premedication guideline should be sufficient even with most orally administered antiemetics. Antiemetics should be given regularly (around the clock) throughout the period of emetic risk. For most chemotherapy regimens, the duration of risk is 24 hours, and a single dose of long-acting antiemetic is sufficient. For example, a single dose of a 5-HT$_3$ receptor antagonist and corticosteroids provides adequate protection for the first 24 hours of the cyclophosphamide plus methotrexate plus fluorouracil regimen. In contrast, regularly scheduled antiemetics should be provided for at least 3 days following cisplatin administration. The antiemetic regimen used for prophylaxis of acute nausea and vomiting is not necessarily the same regimen used for prevention of delayed nausea and vomiting. Antiemetics should also be provided on an as-needed basis for breakthrough nausea and vomiting (nausea and vomiting that require additional antiemetics for control). The antiemetic regimen should be explained to the patient, and the patient should be reassured that every effort is being made to prevent nausea and vomiting.

In the selection of specific antiemetic regimens, the antiemetic potency should be matched to the emetogenic potential of the chemotherapeutic agent or regimen. For patients receiving moderately to highly emetogenic chemotherapeutic agents or regimens, combination antiemetic regimens containing a corticosteroid and a 5-HT$_3$ receptor antagonist are considered the mainstay of therapy. When using antiemetics in combination regimens, selection of agents with non-overlapping mechanisms of action and side effect profiles should be attempted, if possible.

Individualization of antiemetic regimens is an ongoing

process in chemotherapy patients. Antiemetic efficacy should be evaluated during chemotherapy and between chemotherapy courses. Patients should be interviewed specifically about control of nausea and vomiting, as well as antiemetic side effects, before each chemotherapy treatment, and antiemetic regimens should be adjusted as indicated. For example, if a patient did well for the first 24 hours after chemotherapy but developed nausea and vomiting after that point, the duration of the antiemetic regimen for delayed emesis should be extended to cover that period. If a patient fails in the acute period, several management strategies may be employed. An antiemetic with a different mechanism of action may be substituted or added to the existing regimen. Alternatively, the doses of the antiemetic used may be maximized. Nonpharmacologic interventions should also be considered, including use of hard candy to mask metallic tastes from chemotherapy and techniques such as diversion, imagery, behavior modification, biofeedback, and hypnosis. These measures are particularly helpful in the management of anticipatory nausea and vomiting.

Assessment of Response

The methods of evaluating nausea, vomiting, and response to antiemetic regimens have varied widely in clinical trials. The Southwest Oncology Group (SWOG) Toxicity Criteria for nausea and vomiting are listed in Table 9-1 and may be useful in describing the magnitude of GI toxicity. The most commonly employed response classification for vomiting in antiemetic trials differs from the SWOG Toxicity Criteria and usually defines complete response as no vomiting, major response as one or two episodes of vomiting, minor response as three to five episodes of vomiting, and failure as six or more episodes. Complete and major responses are commonly combined and presented as overall response rates. Nausea is graded separately as none, mild, moderate, or severe, often using visual analogue or numerical rating scales. These definitions may be useful in objectively assessing patient response to antiemetic therapy.

Antiemetic Agents

Several antiemetic agents are available for the management of chemotherapy-induced nausea and vomiting, including the phenothiazines, butyrophenones, metoclopramide, 5-HT$_3$ receptor antagonists, corticosteroids, benzodiazepines, and cannabinoids. These agents differ in their mechanisms of action, antiemetic potency, adverse effects, dosing, and cost (Table 9-4).

Mechanisms of Action

The mechanisms by which the antiemetic agents interrupt the nausea and vomiting pathway are illustrated in Figure 9-2. The phenothiazines and butyrophenones are believed to exert their antiemetic actions by inhibiting dopamine in the chemoreceptor trigger zone.[2,3,6-8] The phenothiazines were the first agents to be routinely employed as antiemetics in oncology. Piperazine phenothiazine derivatives, such as prochlor-perazine and thiethylperazine, are considered more potent antiemetics than aliphatic derivatives, such as chlorpromazine and promethazine. The anticholinergic actions of the phenothiazines may also add to their effectiveness as antiemetics. The butyrophenones, haloperidol and droperidol, are more potent inhibitors of dopamine receptors in the chemoreceptor trigger zone than the phenothiazines and may be more effective antiemetics.

Inhibition of dopamine receptors was also initially believed to be the principal antiemetic mechanism of metoclopramide. Subsequent research found that, at high doses (1–3 mg/kg per dose), metoclopramide's antiemetic effect was mediated by inhibition of 5-HT$_3$ receptors in the GI tract and chemoreceptor trigger zone.[3,7,8,12] Metoclopramide is also known to have promotility effects on the gut at low doses (10–20 mg/dose), which appear to be independent of dopamine and 5-HT$_3$ receptor inhibition. It is important to note that although low doses produce promotility effects, higher doses are required for antiemetic effects against highly emetogenic chemotherapy.

Antineoplastic agents and radiation therapy increase serotonin release from enterochromaffin cells in the gut, resulting in nausea and vomiting.[6-8,12] Recognition of the role of serotonin in the pathophysiology of chemotherapy-induced nausea and vomiting led to the development of pure serotonin receptor antagonists, such as ondansetron, granisetron, dolasetron, and tropisetron. These agents act by selective inhibition of 5-HT$_3$ receptors in the chemoreceptor trigger zone and the GI tract. They exert minimal or no activity on dopamine, acetylcholine, histamine, and other serotonin (5-HT$_1$, 5-HT$_2$, or 5-HT$_4$) receptors.

The mechanism of antiemetic action of the corticosteroids is less clear. Early studies noted that patients treated with corticosteroids often reported subjective improvement in nausea and vomiting, without accompanying objective evidence of benefit. These results led to the theory that corticosteroids act as antiemetics by inhibition of cortical input into the vomiting center. Other theories have focused on the inhibition of prostaglandin synthesis or interference with cellular permeability.[3,7,9] The most commonly employed corticosteroid agents are dexamethasone and methylprednisolone.

Benzodiazepines are believed to inhibit limbic system and cortical input into the vomiting center. Other benefits of these agents as antiemetics include their anxiolytic and amnestic actions, making them especially useful in the prevention and treatment of anticipatory nausea and vomiting.[3,6,7,23] Because of its short to intermediate duration of action, lorazepam has been the benzodiazepine most commonly employed as an antiemetic.

In the 1970s, patients receiving MOPP (*m*echlorethamine, vincristine [*O*ncovin], *p*rocarbazine, and *p*rednisone) chemotherapy reported that they experienced less nausea and vomiting if they smoked marijuana before treatment.[3,24] The main psychoactive substance in marijuana, tetrahydrocannabinol (THC), was subsequently isolated and

Table 9-4. Comparison of Antiemetic Agents

Class Generic (Brand) Name	Mechanism of Action	Potency[a]	Adverse Effects	Usual Adult Doses	Cost[b]	Comments
Phenothiazines Prochlorperazine (Compazine) Thiethylperazine (Torecan)	Dopamine inhibition at CTZ	Mild to moderate	Mild sedation, anticholinergic effects, EPS	P: 10 mg IV/IM/PO q6hr or 25 mg RS BID or 15–30 mg SR PO q12hr T: 10 mg IM/PO/RS q8hr	+	Side effects minimal, multiple routes of administration (PO/IV/IM/PR)
Butyrophenones Haloperidol (Haldol) Droperidol (Inapsine)	Dopamine inhibition at CTZ	Mild to moderate	Mild sedation, EPS	H: 1–3 mg IV/IM/PO q8hr D: 1.25–2.5 mg IV/IM q6hr	+	Low doses effective, less EPS than with antipsychotic doses
Benzodiazepines Lorazepam (Ativan)	Inhibition of cortical input into VC?	Mild	Sedation, amnesia, respiratory depression (uncommon)	1–2 mg IV/IM/PO/SL q6–8hr	+	Anxiolytic effects useful in some patients, used to prevent/treat anticipatory N/V
Cannabinoids Dronabinol (Marinol)	Inhibition of cortical input into VC?	Mild to moderate	Sedation, anticholinergic effects, euphoria/dysphoria	5–10 mg PO q6hr starting 24 hr before chemotherapy	++	Appetite stimulation may be useful side effect
Corticosteroids Dexamethasone (Decadron) Methylprednisolone (Solu-Medrol)	Inhibition of cortical input into VC?	Moderate to severe	Short-term effects: insomnia, agitation, mild euphoria, perirectal burning with IV use	Dex: 10–20 mg IV/PO × 1 MP: 125–500 mg IV × 1 Delayed N/V: Dex 4–8 mg PO BID × 3–5 days	+	Side effects preclude long-term use.
Serotonin antagonists Ondansetron (Zofran) Granisetron (Kytril) Dolasetron (Anzemet)	5-HT$_3$ inhibition at CTZ and GI tract	Severe	Mild headache, constipation	Ond: 0.15 mg/kg IV q4hr × 3 doses or 8–32 mg IV × 1[c] Gr: 10 µg/kg IV × 1 or 2 mg PO × 1 Dol: 100 mg IV × 1 or 100 mg PO × 1 Delayed N/V: Ond 8 mg PO BID–TID × 3–5 days	+++	Combine with corticosteroids against severe emetogens
Metoclopramide (Reglan)	5-HT$_3$ inhibition at CTZ and GI tract	Severe	Sedation, EPS (premedicate with Benadryl), diarrhea	1–3 mg/kg IV q2–4hr × 2–5 doses Delayed N/V: 0.5 mg/kg or 30 mg PO q4–6hr × 3–5 days	++ (IV) + (PO)	Combine with corticosteroids against severe emetogens

CTZ, chemoreceptor trigger zone; VC, vomiting center; 5-HT$_3$, serotonin type 3 receptors; GI, gastrointestinal; EPS, extrapyramidal side effects (such as pseudo-Parkinsonism, dystonias, and akathisia); RS, rectal suppository; SR, sustained release; IV, intravenous; IM, intramuscular; PO, by mouth; BID, twice a day; TID, three times a day; SL, sublingual; P, prochlorperazine; T, thiethylperazine; H, haloperidol; D, droperidol; Dex, dexamethasone; MP, methylprednisolone; Ond, ondansetron; Gr, granisetron; Dol, dolasetron.
[a]Expressed as efficacy against antineoplastic agents of mild, moderate, or severe emetogenic potential.
[b]Cost per day: +, $0–3 (PO), $0–20 (IV); ++, $4–25 (PO), $21–95 (IV); +++, $26–70 (PO), $96–160 (IV) (source: *Drug Topics Red Book*. Montvale, NJ: Medical Economics Co; 1997).
[c]Lower doses of ondansetron (8–10 mg IV or 8–16 mg PO) have been used for moderately emetogenic chemotherapy.

studied as an antiemetic in cancer patients. Dronabinol, a synthetic form of THC formulated in sesame oil, is available as capsules for oral use. The mechanism of dronabinol has not been well defined. Theories include inhibition of cortical input to the vomiting center or of prostaglandin synthesis and interaction with endogenous opiate receptors in the vomiting center. The latter theory is supported by the observation that naloxone, an opioid antagonist, reverses the antiemetic activity of the cannabinoids.[7,24]

Antiemetic Potency

The effectiveness of antiemetic agents varies significantly from one agent to the next. In general, the antiemetic potency of the agent should be matched to the emetogenic potential of the antineoplastic agent or regimen. The most effective antiemetic agents are not used for all types of chemotherapy because of adverse effects or cost. When given at standard doses as single agents, the phenothiazines and butyrophenones are effective against mild to moderate emetogens. They may also be useful in combination with other, more potent antiemetics for highly emetogenic chemotherapies.

High-dose metoclopramide (1–3 mg/kg per dose) is effective against severe emetogens, and for many years this drug was considered the antiemetic agent of choice for highly emetogenic chemotherapy regimens. It is significantly more effective than the phenothiazines, butyrophenones, and cannabinoids against strong emetogens.[3,6,7,12] As a single agent, metoclopramide produces response rates of approximately 40–60% in cisplatin-based therapies[25–27]; the response rate increases to 60–80% when metoclopramide is used in combination with corticosteroids.[9,28]

Use of high-dose metoclopramide for moderately to highly emetogenic chemotherapies has been replaced in the past few years by use of 5-HT$_3$ receptor antagonists. In cisplatin-based chemotherapy regimens, these agents have shown efficacy rates of 65–80% as single agents.[29–33] In head-

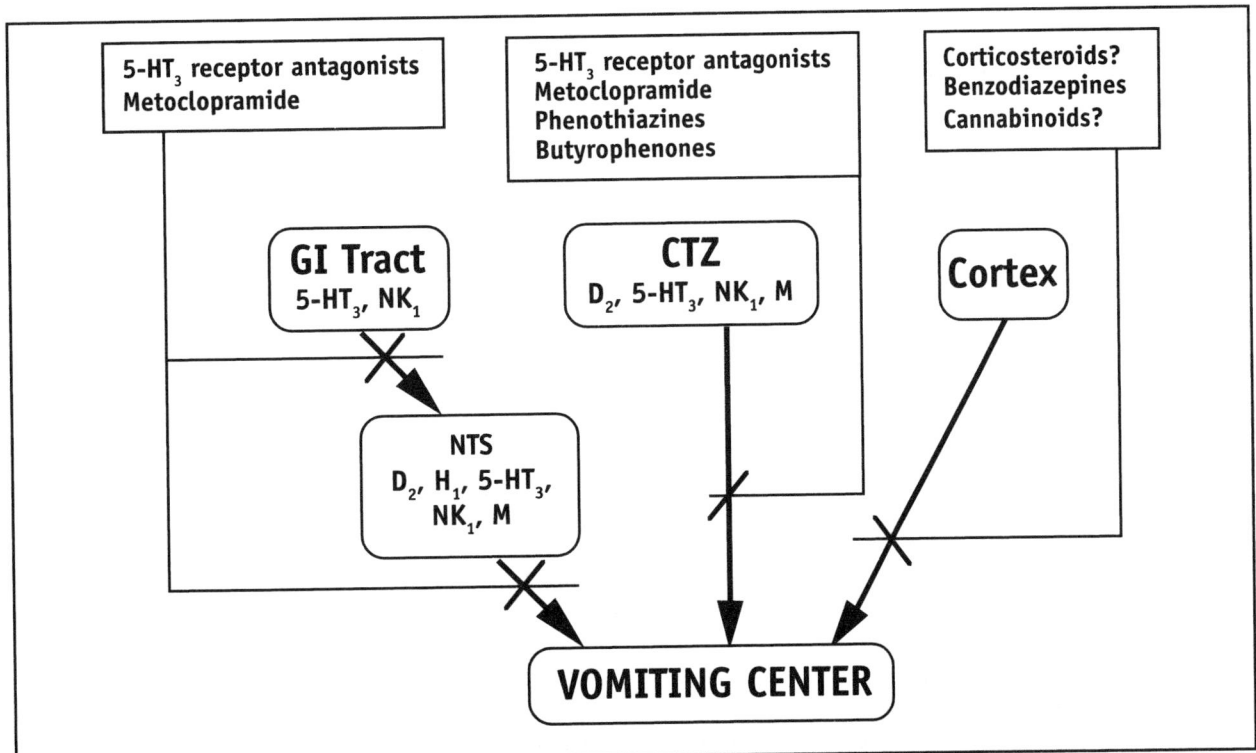

Figure 9-2. Mechanisms of action of antiemetic agents in chemotherapy-induced nausea and vomiting.
SOURCE: adapted from references 3 and 6–8.

to-head comparisons with metoclopramide, ondansetron and granisetron have proved to be equal or superior in control of nausea and vomiting and produce fewer adverse effects than metoclopramide.[29,30] Comparisons among the 5-HT$_3$ receptor antagonists have shown similar efficacy.[29-36] As with metoclopramide, the efficacy against highly emetogenic regimens is enhanced by combining 5-HT$_3$ receptor antagonists with corticosteroids.[31,37,38]

Corticosteroids are highly effective antiemetics against moderately to highly emetogenic chemotherapy.[3,7,39] Benzodiazepines are not very effective antiemetics when given alone. They are most commonly used in combination regimens and may be particularly useful in patients with anticipatory nausea and vomiting or significant anxiety prior to chemotherapy. The cannabinoids are effective against mild to moderate emetogens, with antiemetic efficacy comparable to that of the phenothiazines.[3,7,24]

Adverse Effects

Antagonism of dopamine receptors in the chemoreceptor trigger zone is the mechanism of action for many antiemetic agents. Unfortunately, these antidopamine effects may also lead to extrapyramidal side effects, such as dystonic reactions, pseudo-Parkinsonism, and akathisia (restlessness).[2,3,6,7] Specific dystonic reactions include torticollis (contraction of cervical neck muscles resulting in unnatural twisting of neck and head to one side), trismus (contraction of jaw muscles resulting in lockjaw), and oculogyric crisis (contraction of ocular muscles resulting in fixation of eyeballs in one position). Although not usually life-threatening, these reactions are extremely distressing to patients. Extrapyramidal side effects appear to be most common in younger patients (<30 years of age) and children.[9] Although the piperazine phenothiazines (prochlorperazine and thiethylperazine) possess more potent antiemetic efficacy than other phenothiazines, they also cause a higher incidence of extrapyramidal side effects. Haloperidol doses needed for antiemetic effect are lower than those required to treat psychosis, so extrapyramidal side effects are not common. Dystonic reactions may be effectively treated or prevented with antihistamines, such as diphenhydramine, or with anticholinergic agents, such as benztropine. Unfortunately, akathisia does not often respond to these treatments; lorazepam may be a more effective treatment for patients experiencing akathisia. Other common adverse effects noted with the phenothiazines include sedation, anticholinergic effects, and hypotension.

The risk of extrapyramidal side effects is much higher with metoclopramide than with the phenothiazines and butyrophenones, particularly in younger patients. As a result, diphenhydramine is routinely administered with high-dose metoclopramide to prevent extrapyramidal side effects. Diphenhydramine has not been found to enhance the antiemetic activity of metoclopramide, however. The promotility effects of metoclopramide on the gut may also result in diarrhea. Sedation is another common side effect of this agent, especially when used with diphenhydramine.

Because the 5-HT$_3$ receptor antagonists do not interact with dopamine receptors, they do not produce extrapyramidal side effects. In addition, these agents are not as commonly associated with sedation as are phenothiazines, butyrophenones, or metoclopramide. 5-HT$_3$ antagonists are very well tolerated, with headache, constipation, and diarrhea as the most common side effects.[29-33]

The side effects of chronic corticosteroid administration are numerous and preclude the long-term use of these drugs in the management of chronic nausea and vomiting. These agents are well tolerated in the short term, however. The most common side effects in short-term settings include central nervous system stimulation (agitation, euphoria, mood changes, and insomnia), transient hyperglycemia, increased white blood cell count due to demargination of neutrophils, dyspepsia, and perineal burning after rapid IV administration.

Sedation and amnesia are the most common side effects of benzodiazepines. It is particularly important to provide written instructions to patients taking these drugs. Although these agents may produce respiratory depression, it is not a common occurrence. Physical and psychological dependence is not common with short-term use of benzodiazepines in the oncology population.

The most common adverse effects of the cannabinoids include sedation, euphoria or dysphoria, increased appetite, and anticholinergic effects, especially dry mouth and constipation. Euphoria is not required for antiemetic activity of the cannabinoids. Anecdotal reports suggest that the euphoric effects of the cannabinoids may be blocked by coadministration of phenothiazines, without loss of antiemetic effect.[40] Increased appetite is a desirable side effect in patients also suffering from cancer anorexia or cachexia. The adverse effects profile of dronabinol usually limits its use to patients who have failed other antiemetics.

Dosing and Administration

Common dosing regimens for antiemetic agents are provided in Table 9-4. One advantage of the phenothiazines is that they are available in multiple dosage forms. For oral use, long-acting forms of prochloperazine also improve patient compliance and convenience. Because many patients are not able to take oral medications when they are nauseated, the availability of rectal suppository forms of these agents is also convenient. As mentioned earlier, prochlorperazine is effective against mild to moderate emetogens at standard doses. However, doses of up to 40 mg given intravenously over 20–30 minutes have been studied and found to be effective against highly emetogenic regimens, with minimal adverse effects.[41]

Metoclopramide doses of 1–3 mg/kg (approximately 70–210 mg) are needed for antiemetic effect against strong emetogens. Because of the drug's short half-life, doses need to be repeated every 2–4 hours. Continuous IV infusion is another administration alternative, with equal efficacy and safety. Doses for this method of administration usually include a 1–

3 mg/kg loading dose, followed by 0.5 mg/kg per hour for 10–12 hours.[42,43] Although most of the previously cited clinical trials were conducted with intravenously administered metoclopramide, high-dose oral regimens have also been found to be effective.[41] However, because the largest-dose tablet commercially available is only 10 mg, patients must swallow multiple tablets for each dose, often making this an impractical route of administration.

Ondansetron was originally approved by the FDA to be given as three IV boluses of 0.15 mg/kg (approximately 10 mg) at 30 minutes prior to chemotherapy and 4 and 8 hours after chemotherapy. Equivalent efficacy with a single 32-mg dose has since been proved.[44] Lower doses of ondansetron have been found to be effective for both moderately and highly emetogenic chemotherapy.[36,45] All but one of the studies comparing 8-mg doses of ondansetron with higher doses (24–32 mg) have found equivalent results. Ondansetron is also safe and effective when given as a continuous IV infusion.[46] Doses for this method are usually an 8-mg loading dose followed by an infusion of 1 mg/hr for 8–12 hours. Ondansetron is also available in an oral dosage form with a recommended dose of 8 mg given two to three times daily.[47] Initial results with a rectal suppository dosage form of ondansetron are promising.[48]

Although most studies with granisetron were conducted with doses of 40 μg/kg or 3 mg, the FDA-approved dose for granisetron is a single IV dose of 10 μg/kg (approximately 1 mg). The efficacy of the lower granisetron dose appears to be comparable to higher doses.[30,49] Oral granisetron is available, and the recommended dose for prophylaxis of chemotherapy-induced nausea and vomiting is 2 mg PO prior to chemotherapy or 1 mg PO twice daily during chemotherapy.

Dolasetron has received FDA approval as a single dose of 1.8 mg/kg or 100 mg intravenously for moderately to highly emetogenic chemotherapy or 100 mg PO given before moderately emetogenic chemotherapy. Tropisetron is not available in the United States.

5-HT$_3$ receptor antagonists should not be routinely used for breakthrough nausea and vomiting in patients already receiving these drugs at maximal doses. There is no evidence that exceeding recommended daily doses of the 5-HT$_3$ antagonists increases the chance of response. Patients are more likely to benefit from addition of another agent with a different mechanism of action.

Cost

Phenothiazines, butyrophenones, benzodiazepines, and corticosteroids are the least expensive antiemetic agents currently available. These agents are also widely available in generic formulations. For these reasons, they are the initial agents of choice for mildly emetogenic chemotherapy. For patients receiving moderately to highly emetogenic chemotherapy, a combination regimen of a 5-HT$_3$ receptor antagonist and a corticosteroid is indicated. Although 5-HT$_3$ receptor antagonists represent the most expensive option, they are also the most effective and best-tolerated agents available. For these reasons, they have become the standard of therapy in patients at moderate to high risk for nausea and vomiting or for patients who do not tolerate other antiemetics. The selection of specific 5-HT$_3$ receptor antagonists is based mainly on cost. To use the 5-HT$_3$ receptor antagonists in the most cost-effective manner possible, many institutions have adopted strategies such as standardized dosing, dose adjustment based on emetogenic potential of chemotherapy, and use of oral agents when possible. Standardized doses prevent unnecessary waste of unused doses and may decrease the chance of dosage errors. Lower doses of IV ondansetron (8-mg single doses) have been found to be equally effective as higher doses (24–32 mg) for moderately and highly emetogenic regimens and provide cost savings when compared with the recommended 32-mg dose. By using equivalent oral doses of a 5-HT$_3$ antagonist, costs could be reduced even further. The establishment of institutional antiemetic guidelines based on these principles has been shown to produce significant cost savings while maintaining excellent patient outcomes.[50]

Designing an Antiemetic Regimen

When designing an antiemetic regimen, the emetogenic potential of the chemotherapy regimen should be assessed. An antiemetic regimen that corresponds in potency to the emetogenicity of the antineoplastic agents should then be selected. Patient-specific factors may require modification of the selected antiemetic regimen. The general principles of antiemetic therapy should be followed in this process. As mentioned previously, many institutions develop antiemetic guidelines based on these principles. Both the American Society of Health-System Pharmacists (ASHP) and the American Society of Clinical Oncology (ASCO) have developed evidence-based guidelines, which will soon be published. Table 9-5 provides some examples of commonly used antineoplastic regimens and suggested antiemetic regimens based on the information presented above. Clinical practice guidelines should serve as a common starting point for selection of a regimen for patients, and the antiemetic regimens should be individualized based on patient nausea and vomiting outcomes and adverse effects. For patients who do not achieve adequate nausea and vomiting control, therapeutic options include maximizing doses of current antiemetics, adding other antiemetics to the current regimen, changing the antiemetic dosing schedule, or substituting alternative antiemetics.

Role of the Pharmacist

Pharmacists have established roles in educating patients about their medications. It is important for patients to understand how to take their antiemetic medications to achieve the best results. In particular, pharmacists should explain that every effort is being made to prevent nausea and vomiting and that patients should take their antiemetic agents on a regular basis. The duration of emetic risk should be defined. Patients should be informed that additional antiemetics are available for break-

Table 9-5. Commonly Used Chemotherapy Regimens and Suggested Antiemetic Regimens

Chemotherapy Regimens	Antiemetic Regimens
Emetogenic Potential	
High (>90%)	
Cisplatin-based (50–100 mg/m^2)	Granisetron[a] 2 mg PO or 1 mg IV × 1 before chemotherapy **plus** Dexamethasone 10–20 mg PO or IV × 1 before chemotherapy and 4–8 mg PO BID × 3 days **plus** Prochlorperazine 10 mg PO or IV q6hr × 3 days
ABVD (Hodgkin's disease regimen) MOPP (Hodgkin's disease regimen)	Granisetron[a] 2 mg PO or 1 mg IV × 1 before chemotherapy **plus** Dexamethasone 10–20 mg PO or IV × 1 before chemotherapy **plus** Prochlorperazine 10 mg PO or IV q6hr *prn*
Moderate (30–90%)	
Carboplatin/Cyclophosphamide (ovarian cancer regimen) Doxorubicin/Cyclophosphamide (breast cancer regimen) CHOP (non-Hodgkin's lymphoma regimen)	Ondansetron 8–16 mg PO or 8 mg IV × 1 before chemotherapy **plus** Dexamethasone 10–20 mg PO or IV × 1 before chemotherapy **plus** Prochlorperazine 10 mg PO or IV q6hr *prn*
Low to Moderately Low (0–30%)	
Leucovorin/Fluorouracil (colon cancer regimen) Fludarabine (CLL regimen)	Prochlorperazine 10 mg PO or IV before chemotherapy, then *prn* (Consider using antiemetic on *prn* schedule only)

SOURCE: adapted from the University of Texas Health Science Center at San Antonio Clinical Practice Guidelines for Antiemetic Use in Medical Oncology, 1995. ABVD: Adriamycin (doxorubicin), bleomycin, vinblastine, and dacarbazine; MOPP: mechlorethamine, Oncovin (vincristine), procarbazine, and prednisone; CHOP: cyclophosphamide, Adriamycin (hydroxy-daunorubicin or doxorubicin), Oncovin (vincristine), and prednisone; CLL: chronic lymphocytic leukemia.
[a]Granisetron is listed because the cost at this institution is significantly less than that of ondansetron. Ondansetron 32 mg IV × 1 or dolasetron 100 mg IV × 1 before chemotherapy would be effective alternatives to granisetron.

through nausea and vomiting. Outpatients should be instructed to keep a diary of episodes of nausea and vomiting for accurate assessment of outcomes. Finally, the pharmacist should instill confidence in patients by letting them know that each regimen is selected on the basis of prior success and that it will be individualized to their own experience.

Likewise, pharmacists can ensure that the basic principles of antiemetic use are employed, especially in antiemetic selection, ongoing patient assessment, and individualization of antiemetic regimens. Pharmacists can apply their pharmacologic knowledge of antiemetics in developing, implementing, and evaluating antiemetic guidelines, which can improve patient outcomes and result in significant cost savings. The pharmacist should assess nausea and vomiting control with the previous chemotherapy course before recommending and dispensing antiemetics for subsequent cycles. If the patient achieved the desired therapeutic outcome with minimal or no adverse effects, the same antiemetic regimen should be continued. If the patient experienced adverse effects, the doses of the offending antiemetic agent(s) should be reduced or eliminated, if possible. Alternative agents may be required to maintain nausea and vomiting control. For patients without adequate control, the number of vomiting episodes, degree of nausea, and time course of events should be assessed and documented. This information can then be employed to appropriately adjust the antiemetic regimen.

ORAL COMPLICATIONS

GI mucosa is composed of epithelial cells with a high mitotic index and rapid turnover rate, making it a common site of chemotherapy-induced toxicity. The subsequent inflammation or damage to the mucosa is known as mucositis. Mucositis can occur at any point along the GI tract, most typically in the oral cavity, the esophagus, and the intestines, where it is manifested as diarrhea. Within the oral cavity, mucositis is also known as stomatitis, from *stoma*, the Greek word for mouth. Chemotherapy-induced mucosal damage in the mouth can lead to painful ulcerations, local infection, and inability to eat, drink, speak, and swallow. The disruption of the GI mucosal barrier may also provide an avenue for systemic microbial invasion. It is estimated that up to 40% of all patients receiving chemotherapy develop clinically significant mucositis.[51,52] The SWOG grading system for mucositis is listed in Table 9-1.

Pathophysiology and Etiology

Oral complications are caused by either a direct toxic effect on GI mucosa (direct stomatotoxicity) or by the indirect effects of concomitant myelosuppression and immunosuppression (indirect stomatotoxicity).[51,52] Direct stomatotoxicity is manifested as denudation and ulceration of the GI mucosa. Mucosal epithelial cells lining the GI tract are produced in the underlying basal epithelium (Figure 9-3). These cells mature and migrate to the surface as other superficial epithelial cells are shed. Mucosal cells continuously renew themselves. The normal cellular turnover rate is approximately 7–14 days. Cytotoxic chemotherapy damages rapidly reproducing cells in the basal epithelium. Migration and shedding of the existing mucosal cells continues; however, no new cells are produced to replace them. The end result is mucosal atrophy and ulceration.[53,54] Diminished nutritional intake from mucositis may compound the problem by denying the necessary nutrients to the basal epithelium. The usual onset of mucositis from direct cytotoxic effects is 5–7 days following chemotherapy, and recovery usually occurs within 2–3 weeks.

Indirect stomatotoxicity most commonly manifests as oral infection and hemorrhage secondary to myelosuppression. The onset is 10–14 days after chemotherapy and coincides with the development of neutropenia and thrombocytopenia. The clinical course of the mucositis parallels the course of myelosuppression. Although direct and indirect stomatotoxicity are pathophysiologically distinct, they are often difficult to distinguish in the clinical setting. In many patients with oral mucositis, both processes may be sequentially or simultaneously involved.

Early signs and symptoms of mucositis include mouth tenderness, erythema, and burning or tingling of the lips or oral mucosa. These symptoms may be followed by the development of mucosal ulcers. Initially, these ulcers are usually discrete, but they may rapidly progress to confluent lesions covering most of the oral mucosal surface. The most commonly affected areas are the buccal (cheek) mucosa, lips, soft palate, ventral surface (underside) of the tongue, and floor of the mouth. Similar lesions may be present in the esophagus. These ulcers are extremely sensitive and painful, requiring routine use of topical protective agents and analgesics. Mucosal ulcerations can be aggravated by local irritants, such as jagged teeth, deposits of plaque, defective dental restorations, and dentures.

The mouth, an environment rich in bacteria and fungi, is a common site of infection in cancer patients. Normal flora may become pathogenic in patients with compromised immune function, and the presence of oral ulcers provides direct access to the systemic circulation. The incidence of oral infections ranges from 8% in patients with solid tumors to 34% in patients with leukemia.[55] Fungi are the most common cause of these infections, with *Candida albicans* accounting for almost all cases. Superficial oral fungal infections (also known as oral thrush) are manifested as white mucosal plaques. Infections due to herpes simplex virus and bacteria account for the remainder. Although normal oral flora usually consists of fungi and gram-positive bacteria, flora changes to predominantly gram-negative bacteria in patients receiving chemotherapy.[56]

Risk Factors

One of the most important determinants of mucositis risk is the antineoplastic agent. Agents most commonly associated with direct mucositis are fluorouracil, doxorubicin, and meth-

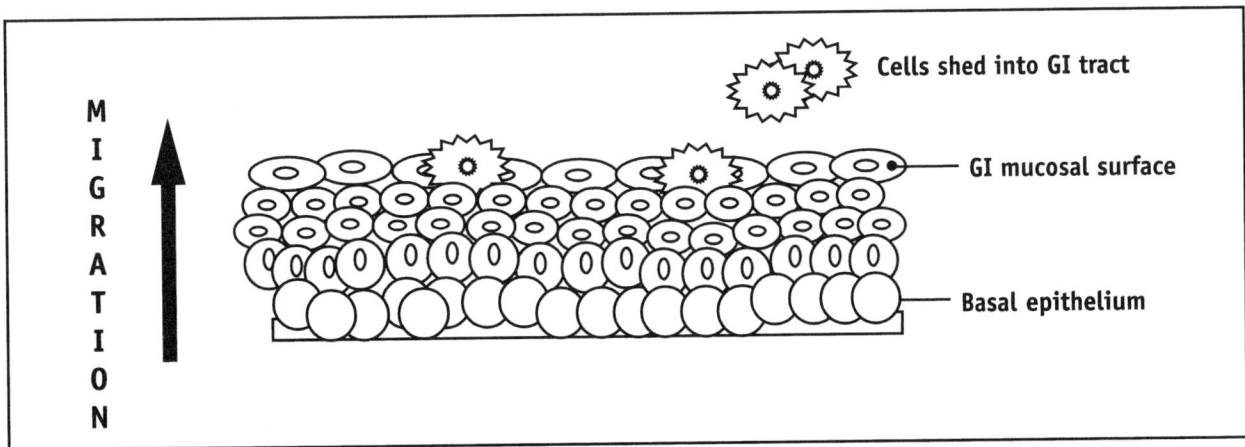

Figure 9-3. Physiology of GI mucosa. Cells are produced in the basement membrane and migrate towards the luminal surface, where they are eventually shed into the GI tract. Chemotherapy damages the basement membrane. Cells continue to migrate upward, but they are not immediately replaced. The result is ulcerations or mucositis.

otrexate. Other agents involved include mechlorethamine, paclitaxel, cytarabine, mercaptopurine, thioguanine, bleomycin, dactinomycin, daunorubicin, mitomycin C, the vinca alkaloids, hydroxyurea, and procarbazine.[51–53,57] Any myelosuppressive agent has the potential to produce indirect stomatotoxicity. The incidence of mucositis with a given agent is also greatly influenced by dose and method of administration. For example, when methotrexate is given in doses of 30 mg/m^2 PO per week, mucositis is rarely observed.[57] In contrast, when methotrexate is given intravenously in doses of >500 mg/m^2, mucositis is universal if leucovorin rescue is not employed. Similarly, the dose-limiting side effect for fluorouracil when given as an IV bolus is myelosuppression, but when the drug is given by continuous IV infusion, the dose-limiting side effect becomes mucositis. Mucositis is also increased when bolus fluorouracil is given in combination with leucovorin. Of all these agents, methotrexate is the only one with a proven pharmacologic method of mucositis prevention. Prophylactic use of leucovorin rescue following administration of methotrexate significantly decreases the incidence of mucositis and myelosuppression, making high-dose regimens possible. However, once mucositis has already occurred, institution of leucovorin does not provide clinical benefit.

Some patient populations are at higher risk for the development of oral complications. The incidence in individuals with hematological malignancies is two to three times higher than in patients with solid tumors. Bone marrow transplantation is associated with the highest risk of mucositis, because of the dose-intensive chemotherapies and radiation administered, as well as profound myelo- and immunosuppression. Patients <20 years of age have significantly more mucositis than those over the age of 60, possibly because of slower mucosal cell replication in the elderly.[51–53] Poor dentition or oral hygiene also increases the risk of mucositis. Although the focus of this chapter is chemotherapy-related GI toxicity, it is important to note that radiation therapy is another significant cause of mucositis in cancer patients. Almost all patients who receive chemotherapy and radiation therapy for the treatment of head and neck malignancies develop serious oral complications.[52]

Prevention and Treatment

In 1989, the National Institutes of Health convened a panel of experts to develop recommendations for the prevention and treatment of oral complications of cancer therapy. For the prevention of oral mucositis, the panel emphasized the importance of comprehensive pretreatment dental evaluations and strict oral hygiene.[58] This recommendation was based on data showing that use of pretreatment dental evaluation, aimed at removal or correction of potential sources of infection and irritation, and institution of preventive oral hygiene measures dramatically reduce the number of patients who suffer from oral complications during chemotherapy.[59] Once mucositis has developed, treatment is mainly supportive, including aggressive oral hygiene programs, use of topical or systemic analgesics, and appropriate antibiotic, antifungal, and antiviral agents. Severe cases may require IV hydration and nutritional support. Patients suffering from moderate to severe mucositis may require reduction of chemotherapy doses for subsequent cycles.

Oral Hygiene

The accumulation of plaque, dehydrated mucus, and mucosal debris that occurs during mucositis creates an environment prone to infection. The importance of good oral hygiene as the cornerstone of mucositis management cannot be overemphasized. Oral hygiene protocols are important in both preventing oral mucositis and treating established lesions. Patients with extensive, painful lesions are often reluctant to comply with these protocols. Education and encouragement are important to ensure compliance and achieve optimal therapeutic outcomes. There are several important elements in achieving and maintaining good oral hygiene in cancer patients (Table 9-6).[60] After dental evaluation, patients should be instructed to routinely perform an oral care regimen consisting of gently brushing their teeth with a soft-bristle toothbrush and fluoride toothpaste. This regimen should be

Table 9-6. Oral Mouth Care Protocols

Oral assessment
  Pretreatment dental evaluation
  Treatment based on findings
  High-risk patients should have oral cavity assessed daily

Routine oral care
  Performed four times each day, usually after meals and at bedtime
  Includes use of fluoride toothpaste, soft toothbrush, dental floss, lip lubricant
  High-risk patients may also use prophylactic mouthwashes
  Patients with dental prostheses should remove and cleanse device and replace it after oral care regimen

Oral care for mild mucositis
  Oral hygiene measures every 2–4 hr while awake, including mouthwashes
  Topical analgesics
  Topical anti-infectives as indicated
  Culture suspicious lesions
  Check complete blood cell and differential counts

Oral care for severe mucositis
  Oral hygiene measures every 1–2 hr while awake, may alternate mouthwashes
  Systemic analgesics
  Topical and systemic anti-infectives as indicated
  Culture suspicious lesions
  Check complete blood cell and differential counts

SOURCE: adapted from reference 60.

performed at least four times a day, usually after meals and at bedtime. For neutropenic or thrombocytopenic patients, a soft foam sponge device (toothette) should be substituted for the toothbrush to prevent additional mucosal damage and introduction of oral bacteria into the blood stream. Dental flossing should also be performed daily, unless platelet counts are <50,000/mm^3 (50 × 10^9/L). Lemon-glycerin swabs may be soothing to damaged mucosa, but when used alone they are not adequate for routine oral care. Smoking should be strongly discouraged, as tobacco may contain fungus or bacteria.

Patients at high risk for the development of mucositis may also be instructed to regularly use cleansing mouthwashes. Normal saline or sodium bicarbonate–saline mouthwashes are most commonly recommended. Patients may be instructed to mix one teaspoonful of baking soda and one-half teaspoonful of salt in a pint (16 oz) of warm water. Sodium bicarbonate increases mouth pH, discouraging bacterial growth, and is very effective at dissolving mucus and loosening debris. Ingredients for these mouthwashes are readily available and very inexpensive. Mouthwashes should be used at least four times a day, especially after meals and at bedtime. Mouthwashes that contain alcohol should be avoided, because they tend to dehydrate the oral mucosa and often cause burning or pain in mucosal ulcerations. Phenol-containing products may promote ulceration and should also be avoided. Hydrogen peroxide solutions are highly effective at removing mucosal debris, but they are not recommended for long-term use, because of their destructive effects on new granulation tissue and the risk of tooth decalcification with chronic exposure. In addition, hydrogen peroxide may cause overgrowth of the white papillae of the tongue, which is an excellent growth medium for fungus.

Chlorhexidine gluconate 0.12% is a commercially available antimicrobial solution that is commonly used to prevent and treat oral mucositis. The most significant benefit has been observed in studies of leukemic and bone marrow transplantation patients, the patient populations with the highest risk of developing mucositis.[52] However, there are at least two clinical trials in these patient populations that have not shown clinical benefit.[52,61] Potential disadvantages of using this product include its astringent properties, teeth staining, alcohol content (11.6%), and cost. Bacterial overgrowth may occur with prolonged use. Usual doses are 15–30 ml swished and spit out at least four times a day.

Local Protective Agents

Direct cytoprotectants have been used in both the prevention and treatment of oral mucositis. Localized lesions can be treated with mucoadherent hydroxypropyl cellulose gels, which form a protective film over discrete ulcers. These products effectively prevent irritation from food and hot beverages and are more durable than other types of topical protectants. These gels are available with or without the local anesthetic benzocaine.[62,63] However, these agents are impractical for diffuse mucositis. Sucralfate slurries are also often employed. Sucralfate acts as a mucosal protectant by forming an ionic bond with exposed proteins in ulcers and creating a protective barrier. Although use of sucralfate suspension has not been effective in treating established mucositis,[64] the results of clinical trials in mucositis prophylaxis have been varied.[65,66] In animal studies, application of sucralfate to mucosal ulcers also increased local production of prostaglandin E_2, a known natural cytoprotectant. Initial uncontrolled studies of topical prostaglandin E_2 (dinoprostone) have also shown encouraging results in the prevention of mucositis.[52] Local protective agents should not be employed until after the patient has completed oral hygiene and topical antifungal treatments.

Oral Cryotherapy

Interventions that diminish access of the antineoplastic agent to the oral mucosa should decrease the incidence of mucositis. Oral cryotherapy, or mouth cooling, is topical application of ice or other frozen products (fruit "slushies" or popsicles) to oral mucosa during chemotherapy. This is an attempt to decrease mucositis by producing local vasoconstriction and decreasing drug delivery to the mucosa. This technique was first investigated in conjunction with fluorouracil-containing regimens and was found to significantly reduce the incidence of mucositis when compared with controls.[67] Patients are instructed to hold ice chips in their mouths for the 5 minutes preceding and the 30 minutes following each administration of their daily fluorouracil and leucovorin bolus chemotherapy regimen. Oral cryotherapy has also been effective for prevention of mucositis from doxorubicin[68] and high-dose melphalan.[69]

Analgesics

The use of analgesics is part of the mainstay in managing mucositis. Commonly used topical agents include viscous lidocaine, dyclonine, and benzocaine.[60] These agents are often combined with diphenhydramine solutions and antacids or kaolin-pectin suspensions to form topical analgesic products. Diphenhydramine is an antihistamine with topical anesthetic properties. When compounding topical analgesic preparations for mucositis, diphenhydramine elixir should be avoided because of the alcohol content. Diphenhydramine syrup or injectable forms should be used instead. Antacids or kaolin-pectin suspensions are incorporated in these products to increase viscosity and promote adherence to oral mucosa. Although these combination products are commonly used, few data are published to support their use. Patients should be counseled to avoid swallowing these preparations, if possible; they numb the gag reflex, increasing the risk of aspiration. For severe cases of mucositis, another alternative is the use of topical 1–5% cocaine solutions. Cocaine is readily absorbed from mucous membranes and should only be used in supervised settings because of the risk of neurotoxicity and abuse. More often, when mucositis is severe or unresponsive to topical agents, systemic analgesics are employed.

Antifungal Agents

As mentioned earlier, local oral infections of *C. albicans* are common in cancer patients. Because these infections are even more common in bone marrow transplant patients, antifungal prophylaxis is routinely employed. Fungal infections are usually easily identified by the presence of white, cottage cheese-like lesions in the oral mucosa. If needed, the diagnosis can be confirmed by performing a potassium hydroxide (KOH) test on scrapings of suspected lesions to identify fungal hyphae.

Antifungal therapy may be delivered topically for mild infections (thrush), using clotrimazole troches (10-mg troche five times a day) or nystatin oral suspension (500,000 units swished and spit out or swallowed five times a day). Prolonged contact (at least 5 minutes) between the topical antifungal agent and oral mucosa is necessary for optimal results. Nystatin vaginal tablets have also been used as oral lozenges to maximize oral contact time. In general, these topical products are well-tolerated, although dental cavities have been observed in pediatric patients. Therapy should be continued for 7–14 days or until the patient is no longer neutropenic. For more severe or refractory oral or esophageal fungal infections, systemic treatment with oral ketoconazole (200 mg PO daily) or fluconazole (100–200 mg PO daily) is indicated. Because of a considerable cost difference, IV fluconazole is only used if patients are not able to take any oral medications. Patients with oral fungal infections unresponsive to these measures may require IV amphotericin B.

Antiviral Agents

The incidence of oral herpes simplex virus (HSV) infection in cancer patients receiving chemotherapy is approximately 50%.[70] In the bone marrow transplantation population, the incidence approaches 90%. Most infections appear to be due to reactivation of latent infection; few seronegative patients develop HSV infections. The presentation of HSV infection in these patients is often atypical, lacking the characteristic vesicles. HSV lesions in these patients most often present as a soft tissue ulceration. Moreover, the clinical course also differs from that seen in immunocompetent patients. Cancer patients tend to have larger, more painful herpetic lesions that are slow to heal. They are also at risk for dissemination of HSV infection. Suspicious lesions should be cultured, and antiviral therapy with acyclovir should be instituted. For outpatients with uncomplicated HSV infections, treatment with oral acyclovir (200 mg PO five times a day for 7 days) is sufficient. For patients with more extensive lesions, use of IV acyclovir (5 mg/kg IV q8hr for 7–14 days) may be required. Dosage reductions of acyclovir are required in patients with impaired renal function. Because the incidence of HSV reactivation is so high in the bone marrow transplantation setting, these patients should receive routine acyclovir prophylaxis. Refer to Chapter 14, Bone Marrow Transplantation, for further discussion.

Other Agents

Initial studies with the colony-stimulating factors (CSFs) unexpectedly found a favorable effect on mucositis. Patients receiving CSFs with myelosuppressive chemotherapy were found to have significantly lower incidences of mucositis.[71] Unfortunately, subsequent studies have not consistently confirmed these results, and the actual impact of CSFs on the incidence and severity of mucositis is still debated.[52] The degree of benefit may depend on the regimen studied. In patients receiving a chemotherapy regimen known to produce high rates of mucositis (e.g., continuous infusion cisplatin, fluorouracil, and leucovorin for head and neck cancers), use of granulocyte-macrophage colony-stimulating factor (GM-CSF) was recently proved to significantly decrease the incidence and severity of mucositis.[72] Cytokine-based mouthwashes containing GM-CSF or transforming growth factor beta (TGF-β), as well as systemically administered keratinocyte growth factor (KGF), are currently under investigation.

The use of systemic allopurinol and allopurinol mouthwashes to prevent fluorouracil-induced mucositis has also received considerable attention.[52,73,74] To exert its cytotoxic action, fluorouracil must be metabolized to its active form, 5-fluoro-2′-deoxyuridine-5′-monophosphate (FdUMP). One of the enzymes that activates fluorouracil is orotate phosphoribosyl transferase (OPRTase). Allopurinol inhibits orotidylate decarboxylase (ODCase), an important enzyme involved in pyrimidine synthesis. Inhibition of this enzyme increases the amount of orotic acid, which competes with fluorouracil for activation by OPRTase. This competition results in lower concentrations of FdUMP in normal tissues and, presumably, less toxicity. Studies of systemically administered allopurinol failed to show a reduction in the incidence of mucositis. Studies of allopurinol mouthwashes have produced conflicting results, and the benefit of allopurinol mouthwashes in preventing fluorouracil-induced mucositis is still unclear.[73,74]

Glutamine is a major source of energy for the intestinal epithelium. Animal studies have shown that glutamine supplementation protects against radiation- and chemotherapy-induced damage to the gut. Initial clinical trials in bone marrow transplantation have not shown substantial benefit,[75] although a pilot study with standard chemotherapy reported considerable benefit in reducing the extent and duration of oral lesions.[76] Glutamine is inexpensive and well tolerated. Further studies are needed to clarify the role of this amino acid.

Xerostomia (dry mouth) due to destruction of the saliva glands is common in patients who have received radiation therapy to the head and neck. Unlike mucositis, which is reversible, xerostomia is often a permanent oral complication. Lack of saliva is uncomfortable for the patient, makes eating and swallowing difficult, and leads to poor nutritional intake. Saliva is also an important factor in control of normal oral flora and in protection from plaque accumulation. Aggressive dental care is recommended. Ice chips and popsicles may be soothing to oral mucosa in these individuals. Artificial saliva and lubricants may also provide symptomatic relief. Use of medications with anticholinergic side effects that may also cause dry mouth should be minimized. Recently, oral pilocarpine has been marketed to increase saliva production in patients with xerostomia. Doses of 5 mg PO three times a day provided relief in 54% of patients, compared with 25% of controls.[77] The most common adverse effect is sweating.

Role of the Pharmacist

The pharmacist can play an important role in the management of mucositis. Patients at risk for mucositis must be educated about the importance of good oral hygiene and encouraged to comply with their mouth care regimen. The pharmacist can also ensure that appropriate preventive measures are employed in high-risk patients, particularly those receiving fluorouracil, doxorubicin, or methotrexate, and in patients undergoing bone marrow transplantation. For patients receiving high doses of methotrexate, the importance of compliance with leucovorin rescue must be emphasized. In patients with already established mucositis, the pharmacist should ensure that oral hygiene is continued, analgesics are provided, and appropriate anti-infectives are employed. Pharmacists may be specifically involved in the pain management of patients with severe mucositis. If nutritional support is required, the pharmacist will have important input into managing the patient's caloric intake and electrolyte balance. The pharmacist can play a critical role in designing and implementing institutional oral care protocols for patients. Finally, the pharmacist can ensure that chemotherapy doses on subsequent cycles are decreased to prevent recurrence of severe mucositis.

DIARRHEA

As mentioned previously, mucosal damage from chemotherapy can occur anywhere along the GI tract. In the lower portion of the GI tract, this damage is usually manifested as diarrhea. The incidence of chemotherapy-induced diarrhea varies widely, ranging from 0 to 40%.[78,79] This type of diarrhea can be very mild and self-limiting, or it can be life-threatening. Toxicity criteria for diarrhea are listed in Table 9-1. Denuded gut mucosa cannot efficiently reabsorb fluids and electrolytes from luminal contents. Uncontrolled diarrhea results in dehydration and electrolyte imbalance. As with oral mucositis, patients are at increased risk for systemic invasion by intestinal bacteria. The disruption of normal gut flora from myelosuppression and mucosal damage also facilitate the development of pseudomembranous colitis from *Clostridia difficile*. Although *C. difficile* infections are most commonly associated with use of antibiotics, cancer patients receiving chemotherapy may develop these infections in the absence of antibiotics.[80]

Pathophysiology and Etiology

The pathophysiology of chemotherapy-induced diarrhea is identical to that of oral mucositis. Although mucosal damage from chemotherapy is a common cause of diarrhea in cancer patients, other potential etiologies must also be investigated and specific treatment provided as indicated.[78,79] Other possible causes in these patients include cancer invading the bowel; graft-versus-host disease in bone marrow transplantation patients; other concomitant medical conditions, such as diverticulitis, lactase deficiency, or diabetes mellitus; or complications from surgery or radiation therapy. Diarrhea may also be caused by local infections of the GI tract. In neutropenic patients, diarrhea may be a harbinger of neutropenic enterocolitis, also known as typhlitis. This is a serious and often life-threatening event in the immunocompromised patient. Several supportive care medications may also produce diarrhea, including antibiotics, laxatives, metoclopramide, cisapride, misoprostol, and enteral nutritional supplements. Diarrhea is also a symptom of opiate withdrawal.

Risk Factors

Any agent known to produce mucositis by direct or indirect means can potentially produce diarrhea. Until recently, the chemotherapeutic agent most commonly associated with diarrhea was fluorouracil.[78,79] Fluorouracil-induced diarrhea occurs in as many as 40% of patients.[81,82] Combinations of leucovorin and fluorouracil have become the standard therapy for patients with advanced GI malignancies. Although leucovorin increases the antitumor effects of fluorouracil, it also unfortunately increases the drug's toxicities, especially mucositis and diarrhea. The diarrhea from leucovorin and fluorouracil combination therapy can become quite severe if unrecognized and has proved fatal. Elderly patients, especially females, appear to be at the highest risk for severe toxicity.[83]

Irinotecan (CPT-11) has even greater potential than fluorouracil to cause life-threatening diarrhea.[84,85] There are two forms of irinotecan-induced diarrhea: early and late. Early diarrhea occurs in up to 50% of patients (8% progress to grade 3 or 4 in severity) and is believed to be a cholinergic process. It is defined as diarrhea that occurs within 24 hours of receiving the drug and most commonly begins during the irinotecan infusion. The onset is often preceded by facial flushing, abdominal cramps, nasal congestion, or diaphoresis. This type of diarrhea responds well to treatment with atropine 0.25–1 mg IV. Patients may be premedicated with atropine before future treatments to prevent recurrence. Ninety percent of patients receiving irinotecan experience late diarrhea, which is grade 3 or 4 in severity in 30% of patients. The etiology is unclear, although it has been speculated to be caused by high levels of carboxylesterase activity in intestinal mucosa, which produce higher than normal levels of irinotecan's active metabolite SN-38 in the colon. The median onset is 11 days following treatment, with a median duration of 3 days. However, the diarrhea can be prolonged, resulting in serious electrolyte imbalance and dehydration. When grade 3 or 4 diarrhea occurs in the presence of severe neutropenia, the toxicity has proved fatal. Patients over the age of 65 years are at increased risk for severe toxicity (40%) when compared with those <65 years old (23%). The late diarrhea has been refractory to most therapeutic interventions, with the exception of a high-dose loperamide regimen, as described in the antidiarrheal section below.

Cisplatin is also known to produce diarrhea; however, the incidence has been difficult to determine because of the past use of metoclopramide-based antiemetic regimens, which can also cause diarrhea.[78,79] High-dose interleukin 2 regimens (600,000 units/kg IV per dose q8hr for 14 doses) produce diarrhea in 76% of patients, which is thought to be a consequence of bowel edema.[86] This diarrhea can be severe, resulting in hypokalemia and hyperchloremic acidosis that require holding scheduled doses of interleukin 2. Bowel hemorrhage, infarction, and intestinal perforation have also been reported.

Prevention and Treatment

General Supportive Care

There is no known method, other than dose reduction, for primary prevention of chemotherapy-induced diarrhea. Patients receiving fluorouracil or irinotecan require close monitoring and early initiation of supportive care. Medications that may exacerbate diarrhea should be discontinued, especially laxatives. Individuals with mild diarrhea can be managed with liberal oral fluid intake. Support with IV fluids and electrolyte supplementation should be initiated promptly in severe cases of diarrhea to prevent complications of dehydration. In patients with protracted courses of intestinal mucotoxicity, bowel rest and support with parenteral nutrition may be required. Patients experiencing moderate to severe toxicity despite pharmacologic treatment should receive reduced doses of chemotherapy on subsequent cycles to prevent recurrence. The exception to this rule is interleukin 2; its doses are held rather than reduced. Patients with documented *C. difficile* infections should receive appropriate antibiotic therapy with oral metronidazole or oral vancomycin.[87]

Antidiarrheal Agents

Diarrhea can be safely treated with systemic antidiarrheals, such as loperamide or diphenoxylate/atropine, if infectious causes (e.g., *C. difficile* or recent antibiotic treatment) are not suspected or identified. Atropine-containing products may produce more anticholinergic side effects than other antidiarrheals. Unlike diphenoxylate/atropine, loperamide does not possess central opioid activity at standard doses. Usual doses for loperamide are two capsules or tablets (2 mg each; total dose 4 mg) at the onset of diarrhea, followed by an additional 2 mg after each loose stool (not to exceed 16 mg/day). Doses for Lomotil (diphenoxylate 2.5 mg/atropine 0.025 mg tablets) are two tablets (5 mg diphenoxylate) at onset of diarrhea, with a maximum dose of 20 mg of diphenoxylate per day. Codeine is another potent antidiarrheal option, with usual doses of 30–60 mg PO q4–6hr. Adsorbent antidiarrheals, such as kaolin-pectin and bismuth subsalicylate, have limited utility in the management of chemotherapy-induced diarrhea.

For patients receiving irinotecan, a high-dose loperamide regimen is recommended. Patients should be instructed to take two capsules (4 mg) at the first episode of loose or frequent bowel movements or diarrhea and to repeat one capsule every 2 hours until 12 hours have passed without a bowel movement. If the diarrhea recurs, they should begin the regimen again. Although this regimen exceeds the recommended daily dose of loperamide, it is well tolerated. The importance of prompt treatment of irinotecan-induced late diarrhea with high-dose loperamide cannot be overemphasized. This regimen has reduced the incidence of grade 4 diarrhea from 17 to 5%.[88] Lower doses of loperamide have failed to produce beneficial results. Other antidiarrheals, including diphenoxylate/atropine, octreotide, scopolamine, and diphenhydramine, have produced equivocal results.[84,85]

Octreotide

The somatostatin analogue octreotide has been used successfully to treat severe cases of fluorouracil-induced diarrhea.[81,82,89] The specific mechanism of octreotide's antisecretory action in the gut is not completely understood, but it is known to promote the absorption of sodium, chloride, and water from luminal contents. In randomized controlled clinical studies, octreotide has proved more effective than loperamide in the treatment of moderate to severe diarrhea from fluorouracil.[82,89] In one study, octreotide doses of 100 μg SQ twice daily produced relief in the majority of patients within 3 days.[82] A recent phase I trial of octreotide in the treatment of fluorouracil-induced diarrhea determined the maximum tolerated dose to be 2000 μg SQ three times daily. Response rates correlated with octreotide dose. The dose-limiting side effects in this setting were allergic reactions and hypoglycemia.[90] One trial has also shown octreotide to be useful in the prevention of cisplatin-induced diarrhea.[91] Although effective, octreotide is considerably more expensive than other antidiarrheal therapy. A recent study comparing a high-dose loperamide regimen with escalating doses of octreotide in bone marrow transplantation or leukemia patients found loperamide to be more effective.[92] Clearly, more studies are needed to determine optimal doses of antidiarrheals and octreotide and the most cost-effective approach to treatment of diarrhea in oncology patients.

Role of the Pharmacist

As a patient educator, the pharmacist has an important role in counseling patients at risk for chemotherapy-related diarrhea. Patients receiving fluorouracil-based regimens should be instructed to seek medical attention at the onset of diarrhea. In addition, patients receiving irinotecan should be provided with loperamide to initiate at the first episode of loose or frequent bowel movements or diarrhea and instructed to continue the loperamide as previously described. Early interventions (e.g., IV fluids and electrolyte supplementation) may have a profound impact on the patient's clinical course. Pharmacists can also use their pharmacology knowledge to identify other medications that may produce diarrhea in these patients, such as metoclopramide or cisapride. In addition, they can recommend appropriate antidiarrheal agents. The pharmacist can also make sure that the patients' chemotherapy doses are reduced appropriately on subsequent cycles to prevent recurrence of severe diarrhea.

CONSTIPATION

Constipation is more common than diarrhea in cancer patients, occurring in 50–78% of all cancer patients.[78,93] Constipation is defined as decreased frequency of stool, with accompanying abdominal discomfort, and is often accompanied by anorexia, nausea, and lethargy. Severe or unrelieved constipation can result in bowel obstruction, with accompanying abdominal pain and vomiting.[78,93,94] Toxicity criteria for constipation are listed in Table 9-1. Constipation may have a significant negative effect on the quality of life of cancer patients.

Pathophysiology and Etiology

There are multiple possible causes of constipation in cancer patients. Successful management of this GI complication requires identification of the underlying cause(s) and institution of specific therapy. In addition to neoplastic agents as a cause, constipation may result from tumor invasion of the bowel, from paraneoplastic syndromes (such as hypercalcemia), or from spinal cord compression. Cancer patients with poor oral intake and dehydration may also become constipated. Patients with limited physical activity are also more prone to constipation. One of the most common causes of constipation in cancer patients is the use of opioid analgesics. All patients receiving chronic opioids require a regular bowel regimen, individualized to produce a bowel movement every 1–2 days. In these patients, the use of other medications that cause constipation should be minimized. Other supportive care medications known to cause constipation include anticholinergic agents, antiemetics (phenothiazines, cannabinoids, and 5-HT$_3$ receptor antagonists), and tricyclic antidepressants, which are employed for management of pain and depression.[78,93]

Risk Factors

The antineoplastic agents most commonly associated with constipation are the vinca alkaloids, including vincristine, vinblastine, and vinorelbine. Neurotoxicity is the dose-limiting side effect of vincristine, whereas myelosuppression is the dose-limiting side effect for vinblastine and vinorelbine. Neurotoxicity occurs to a much lesser extent with vinblastine and vinorelbine than with vincristine. Vincristine neurotoxicity may be manifested as peripheral neuropathy, cranial nerve palsies, central nervous system toxicity, and autonomic neuropathy. Constipation results from neurotoxicity to autonomic nerves supplying the gut. It occurs in approximately 33% of patients treated with vincristine and in only 17% of patients receiving vinorelbine.[95] Elderly patients are at higher risk for vincristine-induced constipation, as are patients receiving individual doses exceeding 2 mg.[96] Patients receiving single doses of vinblastine >10 mg are also more likely to experience constipation. If not recognized early, vinca alkaloid constipation can result in paralytic ileus and bowel obstruction. The autonomic neuropathy from these agents can also produce severe colicky abdominal pain. These symptoms usually appear 3–10 days after administration and resolve in several days. Prophylactic laxative regimens are indicated in high-risk patients.

Prevention and Treatment

The basic approach to the management of constipation is to prevent it when possible, to remove the underlying cause when identified, and to provide specific treatment. Maintaining adequate hydration, exercising, and increasing dietary fiber when feasible, are important strategies in preventing constipation. A variety of laxatives are available to prevent and treat constipation. The reader is directed to other sources for a complete review of stool softeners and other laxatives.[78,93] Most cancer patients with constipation will require a stool softener and a stimulant laxative to maintain regular bowel movements. Doses of these laxatives should be titrated to produce a bowel movement every 1–2 days. Some patients will occasionally require additional stimulant laxatives to achieve results. The sugars lactulose and sorbitol are osmotic laxatives that are very effective in patients refractory to other laxatives. Sorbitol is usually much less expensive than lactulose. Although these agents are effective, many chemotherapy patients have a heightened taste sensitivity to sweets and find lactulose and sorbitol to be unpalatable. Patients with constipation refractory to these measures and patients without bowel sounds should undergo rectal examination to rule out impaction. Promotility agents, such as metoclopramide and cisapride, can also be employed to facilitate normal bowel function.

Role of the Pharmacist

Pharmacists play important roles in informing cancer patients of the risk of constipation with commonly used medications, such as narcotics and certain antineoplastic drugs, especially vinca alkaloids. Patients also depend on their pharmacist to assist them in selection of the most appropriate laxatives. A stool softener and stimulant laxative should be recommended, with instructions to titrate bowel regimen to produce a bowel movement every 1–2 days. Use of other drugs that can cause constipation should be minimized when possible. Nonpharmacologic measures, such as increased dietary fiber and fluid intake and regular exercise, may decrease the need for laxatives. By keeping these common causes of constipation in mind, pharmacists can recommend preventive measures, identify constipation early, and prevent serious complications.

SUMMARY

Nausea and vomiting are serious and potentially life-threatening complications of cancer chemotherapy. Although not completely understood, the pathophysiological process appears to be mediated through the vomiting center in the brain, which receives input from stimuli in the chemoreceptor trigger zone, GI tract, and brain cortex. Antagonism of neurotransmitter receptors (e.g., D_2 and 5-HT_3 receptors) in these areas results in prevention and control of nausea and vomiting. The incidence of nausea and vomiting after chemotherapy depends on several factors, but the emetogenic potential of the chemotherapeutic agent is the most important. Antiemetics should be started before chemotherapy and continued on a regular basis throughout the period of nausea and emesis risk. For most chemotherapy regimens, the duration of risk is 24–36 hours after chemotherapy, with the major exception being the 72 hours or more duration with cisplatin. Additional antiemetics should be provided for breakthrough nausea and vomiting. When selecting antiemetic agents, the antiemetic potency should be matched to the emetogenic potential of the chemotherapeutic agent. Antiemetic regimens should be individualized based on patient outcomes. Although highly effective and well tolerated, the high cost of the 5-HT_3 receptor antagonists limits their use to moderately to highly emetogenic chemotherapy regimens or to those patients unable to tolerate other antiemetics. The combination of a 5-HT_3 receptor antagonist and a corticosteroid is considered first-line therapy for moderately to highly emetogenic chemotherapy regimens. Other antiemetic agents, such as the phenothiazines, butyrophenones, and corticosteroids, given alone or in combination, should be considered first-line therapy for mildly to moderately emetogenic chemotherapy regimens. Pharmacists have important roles in optimal control of chemotherapy-induced nausea and vomiting, especially in design of antiemetic regimens, education of patients, and assessment of therapeutic outcomes.

Mucositis, caused by direct or indirect damage to the GI mucosa, is a common complication of cancer chemotherapy. The onset of mucositis may be as early as 5–7 days after chemotherapy, and the lesions may persist until the patient has recovered from myelosuppression. Oral lesions may become infected with native fungus, bacteria, or viruses; fungal infections are the most common. The most important determinant of mucositis risk is the chemotherapy regimen, with the highest reported incidence in regimens containing fluorouracil, doxorubicin, or methotrexate. Because of the high doses of chemotherapy employed, bone marrow transplantation patients carry the highest risk of all, with or without radiation therapy. The cornerstone of prevention and management of oral mucositis is good oral hygiene, which often involves use of saline or sodium bicarbonate–saline mouthwashes. Oral cryotherapy may prevent lesions associated with some regimens, especially those incorporating fluorouracil. Analgesics should also be provided to control associated mucosal pain. Systemic narcotics may be required in severe cases. Antifungal and antiviral agents should be employed as indicated. In the most severe cases of mucositis, IV fluids and nutritional support may be warranted. Pharmacists have important roles in the prevention and treatment of oral mucositis through educating patients, designing oral care regimens, controlling pain, and providing nutritional support when indicated.

Diarrhea is a manifestation of mucositis from many types of chemotherapy, especially from fluorouracil-based regimens. The damaged mucosa in the gut can no longer absorb fluid and electrolytes, resulting in potentially life-threatening complications from dehydration, acid-base imbalance, and electrolyte disturbances. The denuded gut is also at risk for bacterial invasion into the systemic circulation and superinfection with *C. difficile*. Patients should be advised to seek medical advice if diarrhea occurs, so that treatment may be administered early. Treatment is mainly supportive, consisting of IV fluids, electrolyte replacement, and antidiarrheals after *C. difficile* has been ruled out. Severe cases may require octreotide and parenteral nutritional support. Pharmacists can contribute to the management of chemotherapy-induced diarrhea: identifying other drugs that potentiate diarrhea, educating patients to report diarrhea early, and providing supportive care until the patient recovers.

Constipation is a common and potentially serious GI complication of chemotherapy and supportive care drugs used in cancer patients. The vinca alkaloids are the chemotherapeutic agents most commonly associated with constipation. Supportive care drugs, including narcotic analgesics, some antiemetics, and tricyclic antidepressants, are also common causes of constipation. Patients at risk for constipation should receive stool softeners and stimulant laxatives to produce a bowel movement every 1–2 days. Patients who do not respond to laxatives or who lack active bowel sounds should undergo rectal examination to rule out impaction. Pharmacists participate in patient care in prevention and treatment of constipation through patient education and recommendation of bowel regimens.

REFERENCES

1. Griffin AM, Butow PN, Coates AS, et al. On the receiving end V: Patient perception of the side effects of chemotherapy in 1993. *Ann Oncol* 1996;7:189–95.
2. Laszlo J. Nausea and vomiting as major complications of cancer chemotherapy. *Drugs* 1983;25(*Suppl* 1):1–7.
3. Craig JB, Powell B. The management of nausea and vomiting in clinical oncology. *Am J Med Sci* 1987;30:34–44.
4. Lindley CM, Hirsch JD, O'Neill CV, et al. Quality of life consequences of chemotherapy-induced emesis. *Qual Life Res* 1992;1:331–40.
5. Osoba D, Zee B, Warr D, et al. Quality of life studies in chemotherapy-induced emesis. *Oncology* 1996;53(*Suppl* 1):92–5.
6. Mitchelson F. Pharmacological agents affecting emesis: a review. *Drugs* 1992;43:295–315.

7. Grunberg SM, Hesketh PJ. Control of chemotherapy-induced emesis. *N Engl J Med* 1993;329:1790–6.
8. Veyrat-Follet C, Farinotti R, Palmer J. Physiology of chemotherapy-induced emesis and antiemetic therapy. *Drugs* 1997;53:206–34.
9. Gralla RJ, Tyson LB, Kris MG, et al. The management of chemotherapy-induced nausea and vomiting. *Med Clin North Am* 1987;71:289–301.
10. Kris MG, Gralla RJ, Clark RA, et al. Incidence, course, and severity of delayed nausea and vomiting following the administration of high-dose cisplatin. *J Clin Oncol* 1985;3:1379–84.
11. Kris MG, Gralla RJ, Tyson LB, et al. Controlling delayed vomiting: double-blind, randomized trial comparing placebo, dexamethasone alone, and metoclopramide plus dexamethasone in patients receiving cisplatin. *J Clin Oncol* 1989;7:108–14.
12. Del Favero A, Roila F, Tonato M. Reducing chemotherapy-induced nausea and vomiting. *Drug Safety* 1993;9:410–28.
13. Louvet C, Lorange A, Letendre F, et al. Acute and delayed emesis after cisplatin-based regimen: description and prevention. *Oncology* 1991;48:392–6.
14. Navari RM, Madajewicz S, Anderson N, et al. Oral ondansetron for the control of cisplatin-induced delayed emesis: a large, multicenter, double-blind, randomized comparative trial of ondansetron versus placebo. *J Clin Oncol* 1995;13:2408–16.
15. Gralla RJ, Rittenberg C, Peralta M, et al. Cisplatin and emesis: aspects of treatment and a new trial for delayed emesis using oral dexamethasone plus ondansetron beginning at 16 hours after cisplatin. *Oncology* 1996;53(*Suppl* 1):86–91.
16. Italian Group for Antiemetic Research. Ondansetron versus metoclopramide, both combined with dexamethasone, in the prevention of cisplatin-induced emesis. *J Clin Oncol* 1997;15:124–30.
17. Tavorath R, Heskath PJ. Drug treatment of chemotherapy-induced delayed emesis. *Drugs* 1996;52:639–48.
18. Boakes RA, Tarrier N, Barnes BW, et al. Prevalence of anticipatory nausea and other side effects in cancer patients receiving chemotherapy. *Eur J Cancer* 1993;29A(6):866–70.
19. Hesketh PJ, Kris MG, Grunberg SM, et al. Proposal for classifying the acute emetogenicity of cancer chemotherapy. *J Clin Oncol* 1997;15:103–9.
20. Reece PA, Stafford I, Abbott RL, et al. Two- versus 24-hour infusion of cisplatin: pharmacokinetic considerations. *J Clin Oncol* 1989;7:270–5.
21. de Wit R, Schmitz PIM, Verweij J, et al. Analysis of cumulative probabilities shows that the efficacy of 5-HT$_3$ antagonist prophylaxis is not maintained. *J Clin Oncol* 1996;14:644–51.
22. Gralla RJ, Clark RA, Kris MG, et al. Methodology in antiemetic trials. *Eur J Cancer* 1992;27(*Suppl* 1):S5–S8.
23. Triozzi PL, Goldstein D, Laszlo J. Contributions of benzodiazepines to cancer therapy. *Cancer Invest* 1988;6:103–11.
24. Plasse TF, Gorter RW, Krasnow SH, et al. Recent clinical experience with dronabinol. *Pharmacol Biochem Behav* 1991;40:695–700.
25. Gralla RJ. Metoclopramide: a review of antiemetic trials. *Drugs* 1983;25(*Suppl* 1):63–73.
26. Marty M, Pouillart P, Scholl S, et al. Comparison of the 5-hydroxytryptamine 3 (serotonin) antagonist ondansetron (GR38032F) with high-dose metoclopramide in the control of cisplatin-induced emesis. *N Engl J Med* 1990;322:816–21.
27. Hainsworth J, Harvey W, Pendergrass K, et al. A single-blind comparison of intravenous ondansetron, a selective serotonin antagonist, with intravenous metoclopramide in the prevention of nausea and vomiting associated with high-dose cisplatin chemotherapy. *J Clin Oncol* 1991;9:721–8.
28. Kris MG, Gralla RJ, Tyson LB, et al. Improved control of cisplatin-induced emesis with high-dose metoclopramide and with combinations of metoclopramide, dexamethasone, and diphenhydramine. *Cancer* 1985;55:527–34.
29. Kohler DR, Goldspiel BR. Ondansetron: a serotonin receptor (5-HT$_3$) antagonist for antineoplastic chemotherapy-induced nausea and vomiting. *Ann Pharmacother* 1992;25:367–80.
30. Adams VR, Valley AW. Granisetron: the second serotonin receptor antagonist. *Ann Pharmacother* 1995;29:1240–51.
31. Morrow GR, Hickok JT, Rosenthal SN. Progress in reducing nausea and emesis: comparisons of ondansetron (Zofran), granisetron (Kytril) and tropisetron (Navoban). *Cancer* 1995;76:343–57.
32. Audhuy B, Cappelaere P, Martin M, et al. A double-blind, randomised comparison of the antiemetic efficacy of two intravenous doses of dolasetron mesilate and granisetron in patients receiving high dose cisplatin chemotherapy. *Eur J Cancer* 1996;32A:807–13.
33. Hesketh P, Navari R, Grote T, et al. Double-blind randomized comparison of the antiemetic efficacy of intravenous dolasetron mesylate and intravenous ondansetron in the prevention of acute cisplatin-induced emesis in patients with cancer. Dolasetron Comparative Chemotherapy-induced Emesis Prevention Group. *J Clin Oncol* 1996;14:2242–9.
34. Navari R, Gandara D, Hesketh P, et al. Comparative trial of granisetron and ondansetron in the prophylaxis of cisplatin-induced emesis. *J Clin Oncol* 1995;13:1242–8.
35. Gebbia V, Cannata G, Testa A, et al. Ondansetron versus granisetron in the prevention of chemotherapy-induced nausea and vomiting. *Cancer* 1994;74:11945–52.
36. Perez EA. Review of the preclinical pharmacology and comparative efficacy of 5-hydroxytryptamine-3 receptor antagonists for chemotherapy-induced emesis. *J Clin Oncol* 1995;13:1036–43.
37. Hesketh PJ, Harvey WH, Harker WG, et al. A randomized, double-blind comparison of intravenous ondansetron alone and in combination with intravenous dexamethasone in the prevention of high dose cisplatin-induced emesis. *J Clin Oncol* 1994;12:596–600.
38. Carmichael J, Russel E, Hucheon A. IV granisetron vs IV granisetron plus IV dexamethasone in the prophylaxis of emesis induced by cytotoxic chemotherapy. *Eur J Cancer* 1993;29A(*Suppl* 6):S206.
39. Jones AL, Hill AS, Soukop M, et al. Comparison of dexamethasone and ondansetron in prophylaxis of emesis induced by moderately emetogenic chemotherapy. *Lancet* 1991;338:483–7.
40. Lane M, Vogel CL, Ferguson J, et al. Dronabinol and prochlorperazine in combination for treatment of cancer chemotherapy-induced nausea and vomiting. *J Pain Symptom Manage* 1991;6:352–9.
41. Merrifield KR, Chaffee BJ. Recent advances in the management of nausea and vomiting caused by antineoplastic agents. *Clin Pharm* 1989;8:187–99.
42. Agostinucci WA, Gannon RH, Golub GR, et al. Continuous i.v. infusion versus multiple bolus doses of metoclopramide

for prevention of cisplatin-induced emesis. *Clin Pharm* 1988;7:454–7.
43. Navari RM. Comparison of intermittent versus continuous infusion metoclopramide in control of acute nausea induced by cisplatin chemotherapy. *J Clin Oncol* 1989;7:943–6.
44. Beck TM, Hesketh PJ, Madajewicz S, et al. Stratified, randomized, double-blind comparison of intravenous ondansetron administered as a multiple-dose regimen versus two single-dose regimens in the prevention of cisplatin-induced nausea and vomiting. *J Clin Oncol* 1992;10:1969–75.
45. Hesketh PJ, Beck T, Uhlenhopp M, et al. Adjusting the dose of intravenous ondansetron plus dexamethasone to the emetogenic potential of the chemotherapy regimen. *J Clin Oncol* 1995;13:2117–22.
46. de Mulder PHM, Seynaeve C, Vermoken JB, et al. Ondansetron compared with high-dose metoclopramide in prophylaxis of acute and delayed cisplatin-induced nausea and vomiting. *Ann Intern Med* 1990;113:834–40.
47. Cooke CE, Mehra IV. Oral ondansetron for preventing nausea and vomiting. *Am J Hosp Pharm* 1994;51:762–71.
48. de Wit R, Beijnen JH, van Tellingen O, et al. Pharmacokinetic profile and clinical efficacy of a once daily ondansetron suppository in cyclophosphamide-induced emesis: a double blind comparative study with ondansetron tablets. *Br J Cancer* 1996;74:323–6.
49. Navari RM, Kaplan HG, Gralla RJ, et al. Efficacy and safety of granisetron, a selective 5-hydroxytryptamine-3 receptor antagonist, in the prevention of nausea and vomiting induced by high-dose cisplatin. *J Clin Oncol* 1994;12:2204–10.
50. Berard CM, Mahoney CD. Cost-reducing treatment algorithms for antineoplastic drug-induced nausea and vomiting. *Am J Health-Syst Pharm* 1995;52:1879–85.
51. Sonis ST. Oral complications of cancer therapy. In: DeVita VT Jr, Hellman S, Rosenberg SA, editors. *Cancer: Principles and Practice of Oncology.* 4th ed. Philadelphia, PA: JB Lippincott; 1993. p. 2385–94.
52. Verdi CJ. Cancer therapy and oral mucositis: an appraisal of drug prophylaxis. *Drug Saf* 1993;9:185–95.
53. Sonis S, Clark J. Prevention and management of oral mucositis induced by antineoplastic therapy. *Oncology* 1991;5:11–8.
54. Lockhart PB, Sonis ST. Alterations in the oral mucosa caused by chemotherapeutic agents. *J Dermatol Surg Oncol* 1981;7:1019–25.
55. Driezen S. Description and incidence of oral complications. *NCI Monogr* 1990;9:11–5.
56. Dreizen S, Brown LR. Oral microbial changes and infections during cancer chemotherapy. In: Peterson DE, Sonis ST, editors. *Oral Complications of Cancer Therapy.* Boston, MA: Martinus-Nijhoff; 1983. p. 41–7.
57. Mitchell EP. Gastrointestinal toxicity of chemotherapeutic agents. *Semin Oncol* 1992;19:566–79.
58. National Institutes of Health Consensus Development Conference Statement: Oral Complications of Cancer Therapies: Diagnosis, prevention and treatment. US Department of Health and Human Services, April 17–19, 1989.
59. Sonis ST, Woods PD, White BA. Pretreatment oral assessment. *J Natl Cancer Inst* 1990;9:29–32.
60. Miaskowski C. Management of mucositis during therapy. *NCI Monogr* 1990;9:95–8.
61. Epstein JB, Vickars L, Spinelli J, et al. Efficacy of chlorhexidine and nystatin rinses in prevention of oral complications in leukemia and bone marrow transplantation. *Oral Surg Oral Med Oral Path* 1992;73:682–9.
62. Rodu B, Russell CM. Performance of a hydroxypropylcellulose film former in normal and ulcerated mucosa. *Oral Surg Oral Med Oral Path* 1988;65:699–703.
63. LeVeque FG, Parzuchowski JB, Farinacci GC, et al. Clinical evaluation of MGI 209, an anesthetic, film-forming agent for relief from painful oral ulcers associated with chemotherapy. *J Clin Oncol* 1992;10:1963–8.
64. Loprinzi CL, Ghosh C, Camoriano J, et al. Phase III controlled evaluation of sucralfate to alleviate stomatitis in patients receiving fluorouracil-based chemotherapy. *J Clin Oncol* 1997;15:1235–8.
65. Pfeiffer P, Madsen EL, Hansen O, et al. Effect of prophylactic sucralfate suspension on stomatitis induced by cancer chemotherapy. *Acta Oncol* 1990;29:171–3.
66. Shenep JL, Kalwinsky DK, Hutsone PR, et al. Efficacy of oral sucralfate suspension in prevention and treatment of chemotherapy-induced mucositis. *J Pediatr* 1988;113:758–63.
67. Mahood DJ, Dose AM, Loprinzi CL, et al. Inhibition of fluorouracil-induced stomatitis by oral cryotherapy. *J Clin Oncol* 1991; 9:449–52.
68. Twelves CJ, Seymour AM. Mouth cooling to prevent doxorubicin-induced stomatitis [letter]. *Ann Oncol* 1991;2:695.
69. Dumont C, Sonnet A, Bastion Y, et al. Prevention of high-dose L-PAM induced mucositis by cryotherapy. *Bone Marrow Transplant* 1994;14:492–4.
70. Redding SW. Role of herpes simplex virus reactivation in chemotherapy-induced oral mucositis. *NCI Monogr* 1990;9:103–5.
71. Gabrilove JL, Jakubowski A, Scher H, et al. Effect of granulocyte colony stimulating factor on neutropenia and associated morbidity due to chemotherapy for transitional cell carcinoma of the urothelium. *N Engl J Med* 1988;318:1414–22.
72. Chi KH, Chen CH, Chan WK, et al. Effect of granulocyte-macrophage colony-stimulating factor on oral mucositis in head and neck cancer patients after cisplatin, fluorouracil, and leucovorin chemotherapy. *J Clin Oncol* 1995;13:2620–8.
73. Porta C, Moroni M, Nastasi G. Allopurinol mouthwashes in the treatment of 5-fluorouracil–induced stomatitis. *Am J Clin Oncol* 1994;17:246–7.
74. Loprinzi C, Cianflone S, Dose A, et al. A controlled evaluation of an allopurinol mouthwash as prophylaxis against fluorouracil-induced stomatitis. *Cancer* 1990;65:1879–82.
75. Jebb SA, Marcus R, Elia M. A pilot study of oral glutamine supplementation in patients receiving bone marrow transplants. *Clin Nutrition* 1995;14:162–5.
76. Skubitz KM, Anderson PM. Oral glutamine to prevent chemotherapy induced stomatitis: a pilot study. *J Lab Clin Med* 1996;127:223–8.
77. Johnson JT, Ferretti GA, Nethery WJ, et al. Oral pilocarpine for post-irradiation xerostomia in patients with head and neck cancer. *N Engl J Med* 1993;329:390–5.
78. Levy MH. Constipation and diarrhea in cancer patients. *Cancer Bulletin* 1991;43:412–22.
79. Cascinu S. Drug therapy in diarrheal disease in oncology/hematology patients. *Crit Rev Oncol/Hematol* 1995;18:37–50.
80. Anand A, Glatt AE. *Clostridium difficile* infection associated with antineoplastic chemotherapy: a review. *Clin Infect Dis* 1993;17:109–13.

81. Petrelli NJ, Rodriguez-Bigas M, Rustum Y, et al. Bowel rest, intravenous hydration, and continuous high-dose infusion of octreotide acetate for the treatment of chemotherapy-induced diarrhea in patients with colorectal carcinoma. *Cancer* 1993;72:1543–6.
82. Cascinu S, Fedeli A, Fedeli SL, et al. Octreotide versus loperamide in the treatment of fluorouracil-induced diarrhea: a randomized trial. *J Clin Oncol* 1993;11:148–51.
83. Stein BN, Petrelli NJ, Douglass HO, et al. Age and sex are independent predictors of 5-fluorouracil toxicity. *Cancer* 1995;75:11–7.
84. Rougier P, Bugat R. CPT-11 in the treatment of colorectal cancer: clinical efficacy and safety profile. *Semin Oncol* 1996;23(1 *Suppl* 3): 34–41.
85. Burris HA, Fields SM. Topoisomerase I inhibitors: an overview of the camptothecin analogs. *Hematol/Oncol Clin N Am* 1994;8:333–55.
86. Siegel JP, Puri RK. Interleukin-2 toxicity. *J Clin Oncol* 1991;9:694–704.
87. Kelly CP, Pothoulakis C, LaMont JT. *Clostridium difficile* colitis. *N Engl J Med* 1994;330:257–62.
88. Rothenberg M, Eckardt JR, Kuhn JG, et al. Phase II trial of irinotecan in patients with progressive or rapidly recurrent colorectal cancer. *J Clin Oncol* 1996;14:1128–35.
89. Gebbia V, Carreca I, Testa A, et al. Subcutaneous octreotide versus oral loperamide in the treatment of diarrhea following chemotherapy. *Anticancer Drugs* 1993;4:443–5.
90. Wadler S, Haynes H, Wiernik PH. Phase I trial of the somatostatin analog octreotide acetate in the treatment of fluoropyrimidine-induced diarrhea. *J Clin Oncol* 1995;13:222–6.
91. Cascinu S, Fedeli A, Fedeli SL, et al. Control of chemotherapy-induced diarrhea with octreotide. A randomized trial with placebo in patients receiving cisplatin. *Oncology* 1994;51:70–3.
92. Geller RB, Gilmore CE, Dix SP, et al. Randomized trial of loperamide versus dose escalation of octreotide acetate for chemotherapy-induced diarrhea in bone marrow transplant and leukemia patients. *Am J Hematol* 1995;50:167–72.
93. Sykes NP. Current approaches to the management of constipation. *Cancer Surv* 1994;21:137–46.
94. Camilleri M, Thompson WG, Fleshman JW, et al. Clinical management of intractable constipation. *Ann Intern Med* 1994;121:520–8.
95. Cvitkovic E, Izzo J. The current and future place of vinorelbine in cancer therapy. *Drugs* 1992;44(*Suppl* 4):36–45.
96. Legha SS. Vincristine neurotoxicity: pathophysiology and management. *Medical Toxicol* 1986;1:421–7.

SELF-STUDY QUESTIONS

1. The clinical consequences of uncontrolled nausea and vomiting include dehydration, malnutrition, and:

    a. bowel obstruction.
    b. metabolic acidosis.
    c. hyperkalemia.
    d. aspiration pneumonia.
    e. cerebral edema.

2. The most important determinant of risk for nausea and vomiting from chemotherapy is the:

    a. patient's anxiety level.
    b. emetogenic potential of the chemotherapy.
    c. performance status of the patient.
    d. route and schedule of administration.
    e. patient's history of nausea and vomiting.

3. Common cause(s) of nausea and vomiting in cancer patients other than chemotherapy include:

    a. constipation.
    b. hypercalcemia.
    c. depression.
    d. a and b only.
    e. a, b, and c.

4. The phases of emesis include all of the following, *except*:

    a. nausea.
    b. gagging.
    c. retching.
    d. vomiting.
    e. All of the above are correct.

5. The main pathway(s) of stimulation of the vomiting center include the:

    a. chemoreceptor trigger zone.
    b. cortex.
    c. nucleus tractus solitarius.
    d. a and b only.
    e. a, b, and c.

6. Which of the following neurotransmitter(s) does not play an important role in chemotherapy-induced emesis?

    a. dopamine
    b. serotonin
    c. histamine
    d. neurokinin
    e. All of the above are important.

7. Which of the following antiemetic(s) acts primarily as a dopamine receptor antagonist?

    a. metoclopramide
    b. prochlorperazine
    c. dronabinol
    d. a and b only.
    e. a, b, and c.

8. Ondansetron, granisetron, and dolasetron act by inhibiting serotonin activity at the level of the:

    a. gastrointestinal tract.
    b. chemoreceptor zone.

c. vomiting center.
d. a and b only.
e. a, b, and c.

9. Constipation and headache are the most common side effects of:

   a. haloperidol.
   b. metoclopramide.
   c. ondansetron.
   d. lorazepam.
   e. dronabinol.

10. Tremors, akathisia, and dystonic reactions may result from which of the following antiemetics?

    a. metoclopramide
    b. lorazepam
    c. granisetron
    d. diphenhydramine
    e. dexamethasone

11. Antiemetics with efficacy against strong emetogens include:

    a. dolasetron 100 mg PO.
    b. dexamethasone 20 mg IV.
    c. metoclopramide 10 mg IV.
    d. a and b only.
    e. a, b, and c.

12. PL is a 65-year-old, 70-kg man with non-small cell lung cancer who is to receive his first cycle of chemotherapy. He has no anxiety about starting chemotherapy. He has minimal symptoms from his disease. His regimen will be cisplatin 100 mg/m^2 IV on day 1 and vinorelbine 20 mg/m^2 IV on days 1, 8, 15, and 22. Based on this information, the most appropriate antiemetic regimen for prophylaxis of acute nausea and vomiting on day 1 of chemotherapy is:

    a. granisetron 2 mg PO × 1 and dexamethasone 20 mg PO × 1, both given 30 minutes before chemotherapy.
    b. metoclopramide 140 mg IV plus diphenhydramine 25 mg IV at 0, 3, and 6 hours and dexamethasone 10 mg IV × 1.
    c. ondansetron 32 mg IV × 1 30 minutes before chemotherapy.
    d. dexamethasone 20 mg IV × 1 and prochlorperazine 10 mg IV q6hr beginning 30 minutes before chemotherapy.
    e. dolasetron 100 mg IV × 1, dexamethasone 20 mg IV × 1, prochlorperazine 10 mg PO q6hr, lorazepam 2 mg IV × 1, and haloperidol 2 mg PO q8hr.

13. Based on the patient case in the previous question, which antiemetic regimen is the most appropriate for prophylaxis of delayed emesis?

    a. No antiemetics are needed if the patient does not develop acute emesis.
    b. granisetron 1 mg PO q12hr × 3 days, beginning on day 2 of chemotherapy
    c. prochlorperazine 15 mg SR PO q12hr plus dexamethasone 8 mg PO q12 hr × 3 days, starting day 1 in the evening
    d. lorazepam 1 mg PO q8hr plus dexamethasone 4 mg PO q12hr × 4 days, starting on day 2
    e. prochlorperazine 10 mg PO q6hr *prn* nausea and vomiting, starting on day 1 of chemotherapy.

14. Based on the patient case in question 12, which antiemetic regimen is the most appropriate for days 8, 15, and 22 of the chemotherapy regimen?

    a. The same regimen used on day 1 should be continued if it works.
    b. Ondansetron 8 mg PO × 1 before vinorelbine chemotherapy.
    c. Lorazepam 1 mg PO × 1 before vinorelbine chemotherapy.
    d. Prochlorperazine 10 mg PO × 1 before vinorelbine chemotherapy.
    e. No antiemetics are needed.

15. WD is a 55-year-old woman with early stage breast cancer who is to receive cyclophosphamide 600 mg/m^2 IV, methotrexate 40 mg/m^2 IV, and fluorouracil 600 mg/m^2 IV (CMF) for treatment of her breast cancer. The most effective treatment regimen(s) for prophylaxis of nausea and vomiting is (are):

    a. ondansetron 8 mg PO × 1 plus dexamethasone 20 mg PO × 1 prior to chemotherapy.
    b. dexamethasone 10 mg PO × 1 plus prochlorperazine 10 mg PO × 1 prior to chemotherapy.
    c. thiethylperazine 10 mg PO × 1 plus lorazepam 2 mg PO × 1.
    d. a and b only.
    e. a, b, and c.

16. The most common pathogen(s) responsible for superinfection of oral mucositis lesions is/are:

    a. staphylococcal and streptococcal species.
    b. gram-negative enteric bacterial rods.
    c. herpes simplex virus.
    d. anaerobic nasopharyngeal flora.
    e. fungi, especially *Candida* species.

17. For most chemotherapeutic agents, the onset and duration of nausea and vomiting are:

a. 1–4 hr and 24 hours, respectively.
b. 30 minutes and 72 hours, respectively.
c. 6–10 hours and 48 hours, respectively.
d. 4–24 hours and 7 days, respectively.
e. unpredictable. No pattern can be identified.

18. Which of the following agents is associated with the highest risk of developing mucositis at standard doses?

    a. irinotecan
    b. cyclophosphamide
    c. etoposide
    d. fluorouracil
    e. vincristine

19. The most critical component in any regimen for prevention and treatment of oral mucositis is:

    a. leucovorin.
    b. oral hygiene.
    c. analgesics.
    d. fluconazole.
    e. soft toothbrushes.

20. Antineoplastic agents most commonly associated with diarrhea include:

    a. irinotecan.
    b. fluorouracil.
    c. interleukin 2.
    d. a and b only.
    e. a, b, and c.

21. For prevention of late diarrhea from irinotecan, patients should receive:

    a. high-dose loperamide beginning at the onset of diarrhea.
    b. octreotide 200 mg SQ twice daily starting at the onset of diarrhea.
    c. NS 100 ml/hr IV for 24 hours after two episodes of diarrhea.
    d. filgrastim 300 µg SQ once daily beginning 24 hours after treatment.
    e. kaopectate 30 ml q4–6hr *prn* for loose stools.

22. The antineoplastic agents most commonly associated with constipation include the:

    a. vinca alkaloids.
    b. taxanes.
    c. topoisomerase I inhibitors.
    d. a and b only.
    e. a, b, and c.

23. Treatments found to be effective in prevention of mucositis include:

    a. oral cryotherapy.
    b. sucralfate slurries.
    c. allopurinol mouthwashes.
    d. a and b only.
    e. a, b, and c.

True or False:

24. _____ Before effective antiemetics were available, 25–50% of patients refused chemotherapy because of fears of nausea and vomiting.

25. _____ Systemic infections in patients with mucositis are due to overuse of broad spectrum antibiotics.

26. _____ Lorazepam's mechanism of antiemetic action is believed to be inhibition of histamine activity in the vestibular apparatus.

27. _____ Dronabinol is a potent antiemetic with activity equivalent to ondansetron against cisplatin-based regimens.

28. _____ Cisplatin is the antineoplastic agent most likely to produce clinically significant delayed nausea and vomiting.

29. _____ Antiemetic agents for prevention and treatment of chemotherapy-induced nausea and vomiting should be administered on an as-needed basis rather than scheduled in order to minimize adverse effects and cost.

30. _____ Early diarrhea from irinotecan is a cholinergic process that responds well to administration of atropine.

Chapter 10

Administration of Cancer Chemotherapy

Rebecca S. Finley, Pharm.D., M.S.
Chair and Associate Professor
Department of Pharmacy Practice and Pharmacy Administration
Philadelphia College of Pharmacy
Philadelphia, Pennsylvania

Systemic Chemotherapy Administration 174
   Oral Administration 174
   Intravenous Administration 175
      Peripheral Venous Access and Administration 175
         Complications 177
            Extravasation 177
            Venous Sclerosis and Thrombosis 178
      Central Venous Access and Administration 178
         Percutaneous (Nontunneled) Central Venous Access 178
         Peripherally Inserted Central Venous Catheters 179
         Tunneled Central Venous Catheters 179
         Totally Implantable Intravascular Devices 180
         Complications 181
            Intravascular Thrombosis and Occlusion of Catheter Lumens 181
            Catheter-Related Infections 182
      Intravenous Infusion Devices 182
   Intramuscular and Subcutaneous Administration 184
Local and Regional Chemotherapy Administration 184
   Intraperitoneal Administration 184
   Intrathecal and Intraventricular Administration 185
   Intravesical Administration 186
   Intra-arterial Administration 186
      Hepatic Arterial Infusions 187
      Regional Limb Perfusion 187
Other Routes of Administration 188
Summary 188
References 188
Appendix 10-A 192
Appendix 10-B 193
Appendix 10-C 194
Self-Study Questions 195

Optimizing the safety and effectiveness of chemotherapy administration is an important component of pharmaceutical care for patients with cancer. Pharmacists must be able to identify the potential advantages and complications that may be associated with methods of drug administration for individual patients. When doses and routes of administration are outside the labeling approved by the Food and Drug Administration—as they often are—the pharmacist must carefully review professional and manufacturer's literature, as well as institutional guidelines, while exercising sound professional judgment to ensure optimal patient outcomes. The pharmacist often plays an integral role in designing drug administration protocols and selecting drug delivery systems for individual patients.

This chapter is organized according to the methods of drug administration. The discussion of systemic therapy covers infusion and vascular access devices and the potential advantages and hazards of oral, intravenous, intramuscular, and subcutaneous administration. The discussion of local and regional methods of chemotherapy administration includes the uses, benefits, and hazards of intraperitoneal, intrathecal, intravesical, and intra-arterial (e.g., hepatic arterial infusions and limb perfusion) administration. The types of cancer most often treated with these alternative methods of administration are discussed as well.

After completing this chapter, the reader should be able to:

1. Discuss the potential advantages and disadvantages of oral and intravenous administration of anticancer drugs.
2. Identify cytotoxic drugs likely to cause the most serious reactions when extravasated and discuss methods for reducing patient risk.
3. Describe the uses and potential complications of vascular access devices.
4. Discuss the features of infusion devices that influence product selection and describe their applications in caring for patients with cancer.
5. Discuss the types, advantages, and potential complications of local and regional chemotherapy administration.

SYSTEMIC CHEMOTHERAPY ADMINISTRATION

An unfortunate characteristic of neoplastic cells is their lack of adhesion, which gives them the ability to break off from the original clone and disseminate throughout the body. Some of these cells eventually adhere to other tissue and begin a new tumor clone, a process known as metastasis. As these new tumors grow, they develop new blood vessels (angiogenesis), which carry oxygen, nutrients, endogenous growth factors, and drugs to the tumor cells. Chemotherapy was developed to systemically treat malignancies that spread beyond the regional applications of surgery and radiation therapy by delivering cytotoxic drugs to all the tumor sites in the body simultaneously.

Oral and intravenous administration are the most common routes for the systemic administration of chemotherapy, although intramuscular and subcutaneous methods are occasionally used. Techniques designed to concentrate the distribution and antitumor effects of chemotherapy drugs at a specific site or within a defined region of the body include intraventricular, intrathecal, intravesical, and intra-arterial administration. When these local or regional routes of administration are used, some systemic distribution of drug may occur, depending on the route and characteristics of the drug.

For cytotoxic drugs to be effective, they must reach the target site (i.e., the tumor cell) in sufficient concentrations. Factors that aid in determining the most appropriate route of administration for chemotherapy agents include bioavailability, pharmacokinetics, stability in solution, pH of the drug, tumor site, presence or absence of metastasis, general condition of the patient, and availability of vascular access. Many of these factors were explained in more depth in chapter 6. Whichever route is selected, it is imperative that the individual who administers the medication be proficient in that method of drug delivery as well as knowledgeable about the acute and chronic toxicities of the drug. All aspects of drug administration should be discussed with the patient before therapy begins, including what the patient will feel during the process, how long administration will last, anticipated as well as unlikely toxicities, and possible complications.

Oral Administration

A number of cytotoxic drugs are well absorbed from the gastrointestinal tract and are available in oral dosage forms (Table 10-1). In addition, many orally administered hormonal and steroidal drugs are used to treat various malignancies. Under most circumstances, oral administration is the safest, most economical, and most convenient route for the patient.

However, careful attention must be given to factors that could interfere with or limit absorption and consequently compromise the cytotoxic activity of the drug. These may include drug-related factors, such as active transport–mediated absorption, as in the case of methotrexate. Bioavailability of methotrexate decreases with increasing oral dose (see chapter 4).[1] Doses of ≥25 mg are erratically absorbed in most patients, and some patients demonstrate erratic absorption even at doses of <15 mg. In the case of oral melphalan, it appears that absorption varies widely among patients. Some absorb <50% of the administered dose, but others absorb more. The presence

Table 10-1. Orally Administered Cytotoxic Drugs[a]

Generic Name	Trade Name	Strength and Form
Altretamine	Hexalen	50-mg tablets
Busulfan	Myleran	2-mg tablets
Chlorambucil	Leukeran	2-mg tablets
Cyclophosphamide	Cytoxan	25- and 50-mg tablets
Etoposide	VePesid	50-mg capsules
Hydroxyurea	Hydrea	500-mg capsules
Lomustine	CeeNU	10-, 40-, and 100-mg capsules
Melphalan	Alkeran	2-mg tablets
Mercaptopurine	Purinethol	50-mg tablets
Methotrexate		2.5-mg tablets
Mitotane	Lysodren	500-mg tablets
Procarbazine	Matulane	50-mg tablets
Thioguanine	Thioguanine Tabloid	40-mg tablets

[a] Many oral hormonal and steroidal drugs are also used in the treatment of cancer; they are not included in this table.

of food or other drugs in the gut also may affect absorption characteristics. The presence of a large meal appears to enhance melphalan degradation at alkaline pH in the upper small bowel before absorption,[2,3] and cimetidine has been reported to decrease bioavailability. Therefore, oral doses of melphalan must be titrated based on the toxicity the patient experiences.

Oral etoposide also has variable bioavailability, with a range of 25–74% and a mean of about 50%.[4] For this reason, the recommended oral dose is usually twice that of the intravenous dose. Although neither food nor other chemotherapy appears to alter absorption, the bioavailability appears to be dose dependent. Hande et al.[5] reported that oral bioavailability following a 100-mg dose was 76 ± 22%, whereas it decreased to 48 ± 18% following a 400-mg dose. This has led some clinicians to recommend that larger daily doses be divided.

Tumors in the gastrointestinal tract may also adversely affect a patient's ability to absorb oral medications. In addition, patients who experience vomiting due to the emetogenic effects of chemotherapy or the underlying malignancy may be unable to tolerate or comply with oral therapy. There are also circumstances in which the dose of chemotherapy is too high to administer conveniently by the oral route. For example, although 2000 mg of cyclophosphamide can easily be administered intravenously, to take this dose orally the patient would need to swallow 40 tablets (50 mg each). For high-dose oral busulfan used in preparation for allogeneic bone marrow transplantation, various cancer centers have placed several tablets in gelatin capsules to facilitate easier ingestion.

Although the oral route of administration is generally considered the safest and most convenient method of drug administration, most cancer chemotherapy is administered intravenously.

Intravenous Administration

Intravenous (IV) administration of chemotherapy presents advantages over oral administration, but it also presents potential hazards. IV administration allows drugs to be delivered immediately to the systemic circulation, but it may also be associated with greater toxicity because of the high serum levels that may be attained. In addition, the same risks or complications (e.g., extravasation, phlebitis, and embolization) that are associated with any IV drug administration exist for chemotherapy drugs. In many instances, the antitumor efficacy of the drug depends on high serum concentrations—and the subsequent greater concentrations of drug delivered to the site of the tumor. IV cancer chemotherapy may be given via short bolus injections (generally <15 minutes), short infusions (15 minutes to several hours), or prolonged infusions (several hours to weeks). The pharmacokinetic characteristics, solubility, stability, and rate-related toxicities are predominantly used to determine the most appropriate infusion technique.

When patients receive multiple IV chemotherapy drugs either concurrently or sequentially, many dilemmas are raised by the lack of compatibility information for most of these products. Therefore, when drugs are administered sequentially through the same IV line, the line should be flushed with saline between injections (provided the drugs are compatible with saline). Separate IV lines must be used if drugs are infused concurrently, unless acceptable compatibility data exist.

Many cytotoxic drugs may cause local reactions at the site of administration (Table 10-2[6–13]). Irritants include drugs that produce a local inflammatory reaction (e.g., pain, erythema, or swelling) when extravasated from the vein. Vesicant agents may destroy tissue around the site of extravasation. Local hypersensitivity reactions (e.g., flare reactions—erythema or rash along the vein track) occur in response to local histamine release and typically subside within 45 minutes. Each of these properties may significantly complicate the administration of such drugs. Therefore, many vesicant drugs are commonly given by central venous administration rather than via peripheral veins, and drugs known to cause local hypersensitivity reactions may require premedication with antihistamines or corticosteroids in some patients. The problems associated with vesicant extravasations are further discussed in more detail later in this chapter.

Peripheral Venous Access and Administration

In most circumstances, peripheral venous administration is

Table 10-2. Locally Reactive Cytotoxic Drugs and Suggested Interventions

Drug	Local Toxicity	Suggested Intervention(s)	Comments	References
Carmustine	Irritant	Unknown	May also cause phlebitis	6
Cisplatin	Irritant Vesicant when >20 ml of 0.5 mg/ml	$1/6$ M sodium thiosulfate IV and SC Same as above		6–8
Dacarbazine	Irritant	Unknown		8
Dactinomycin	Vesicant	Unknown	May also cause phlebitis	6, 8
Daunorubicin	Vesicant Hypersensitivity	Apply cold; topical DMSO q6hr and allow to air dry Diphenhydramine 25–50 mg and hydrocortisone 25–50 mg IV		6, 8, 9 10
Doxorubicin	Vesicant Hypersensitivity	Same as daunorubicin Same as daunorubicin		6, 7
Etoposide	Irritant	If severe, hyaluronidase 150 units in 3 ml of saline and apply heat	May also cause phlebitis, urticaria, and erythema	
Idarubicin	Vesicant Hypersensitivity	Same as daunorubicin Same as daunorubicin		
Mechlorethamine	Vesicant Hypersensitivity	$1/6$ M sodium thiosulfate IV and SC Unknown		7, 11
Mitomycin	Vesicant	Same as daunorubicin		6
Mitoxantrone	Irritant	Unknown	Ulcerations are rare	
Paclitaxel	Vesicant	Hyaluronidase 300 units in 3 ml saline IV and SC and apply cold	Some have suggested hyaluronidase impaired healing	6, 12, 13
Plicamycin	Vesicant	Unknown		
Streptozocin	Vesicant	Unknown		
Teniposide	Irritant	Same as etoposide		
Vinblastine	Vesicant	Apply heat; hyaluronidase 150 units in 3 ml saline and IV and SC		6, 7
Vincristine	Vesicant	Same as vinblastine		
Vinorelbine	Vesicant	Same as vinblastine		

IV, intravenous; SC, subcutaneous; DMSO, dimethyl sulfoxide.

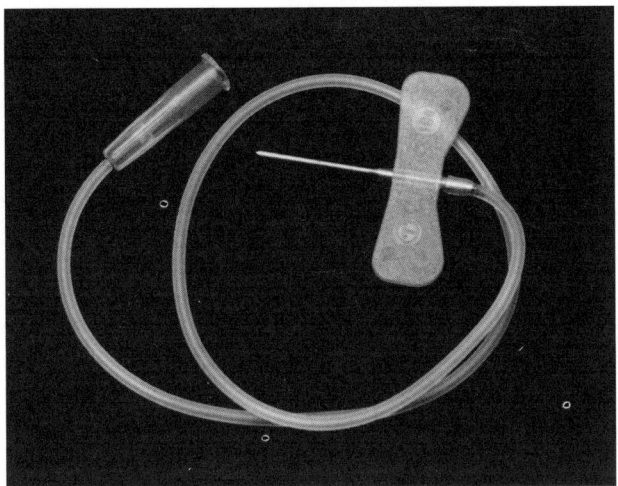

Figure 10-1. Small vein needle with Luer-Lok adapter
SOURCE: reprinted with permission from Lindley CM, Deloatch KH. *Infusion Technology Manual: A Self-Instructional Approach.* Bethesda, MD: American Society of Hospital Pharmacists; 1993. Chapter 5, Vascular access devices. p. 43.

the simplest and safest method of IV chemotherapy delivery, but selecting an appropriate vein is important for patient comfort and safety. Several factors must be considered. First, the purpose and duration of the injection or infusion influence vein selection. For long-term infusions, it is best to avoid the veins overlying joints such as the antecubital fossa, because the needle may become dislodged if the extremity is flexed. When reaccessing a vein within 24 hours, a site should be selected that is proximal to the earlier site to avoid extravasation of drug through the previous venipuncture.

Second, the type of venous access device must be selected. Stainless steel scalp vein needles (also called wing-tipped butterfly needles) are frequently used for peripheral short-term (i.e., ≤60 minutes) administration of chemotherapy drugs, although other types of cannulas or catheters may be used for longer infusions.[14,15] Scalp vein needles range in diameter from 25 to 16 gauge and have plastic wings (Figure 10-1), which provide stability and maximum needle control during insertion. The appropriate needle gauge and length is determined by the size of the vein and the type of drug and fluid to be administered. Steel needles are associated with a low incidence of infection and phlebitis. Stability provided by the wings further reduces mechanical irritation of the vein after insertion.[16] These devices are manufactured with a short length of plastic tubing and a female Luer-Lok adapter that will connect securely to any commercial IV tubing or syringe. After insertion, the needle is anchored to the patient with a short strip of tape over each wing, allowing visualization of the insertion site; the tubing is then looped and taped independently to prevent tension on the tubing from dislodging the needle.

A third factor is the age, general physical condition, and level of activity of the patient. Venous circulation may be compromised significantly in patients who have had an axillary lymph node dissection (e.g., patients with breast cancer), and venipuncture should always be avoided in the affected extremity. Another common problem that complicates peripheral administration is venous fragility in elderly patients. In general, the veins of the forearm are the most suitable for administering chemotherapy because the underlying bones provide a natural splint. If possible, veins in the legs should be avoided because this increases the risk of phlebitis and embolism. The risk of phlebitis is also reduced by using larger veins to administer drugs that cause pain or irritation to the lining of the vein.

Complications

Extravasation—A potential hazard associated with the peripheral administration of chemotherapy is that the needle or cannula can dislodge from the vein and result in extravasation or leakage of the chemotherapy drug into the surrounding soft tissue. Because both irritant and vesicant drugs may produce severe local tissue damage when extravasation occurs, special precautions must be taken when administering these drugs. Table 10-2 suggests some antidotes that have been recommended for vesicant or irritant extravasations. Infiltration of cytotoxic agents into subcutaneous tissues may result in symptoms ranging from localized, self-resolving inflammation (irritants) to full-thickness destruction and sloughing of the skin and underlying vital structures, including tendons and nerves (vesicants). Other signs and symptoms of vesicant extravasation may include hyperpigmentation, induration, and burning. Table 10-2 and similar tables found in many review articles and textbooks classify agents according to whether they are irritants or vesicants. It should be noted, however, that the severity of the reaction is influenced by factors other than just the drug, such as the site of extravasation, condition of the surrounding tissue, the concentration of the drug in solution, the volume of extravasate, the diluent that the drug was reconstituted and/or admixed with, and, of course, early recognition of the complication and the expediency of appropriate interventions.

These potentially devastating reactions have caused attention to focus on factors that may increase the risk of extravasation. Several oncology groups, including the Oncology Nurses Society, have published recommendations for administering vesicant and irritant cytotoxic drugs safely (Appendix 10-A, *Recommended Vesicant and Irritant Administration Procedures to Minimize Risk of Extravasation*). Among the agents reported to cause the most serious reactions are doxorubicin, daunorubicin, idarubicin, dactinomycin, mechlorethamine, vincristine, vinorelbine, and vinblastine. Several reports have suggested that paclitaxel may also cause serious tissue injury if extravasated.[13,17] Some drugs may only produce irritation under some circumstances but produce severe tissue damage under different circumstances. The distinction between irritant and vesicant is often unclear, and when an extravasation occurs, appropriate steps should be implemented to minimize tissue damage. Health care employers should provide special training for individuals administering these drugs and implement explicit policies and procedures for administering antineoplastics and managing extravasation (see chapter 20). Factors that may increase the risk of extravasation include:

- generalized vascular disease, such as venous fragility or decreased local blood flow, often observed in elderly or debilitated patients;
- elevated venous pressure, as seen in patients with superior vena cava syndrome or obstructed venous drainage after axillary surgery;
- previous radiation therapy to the site of drug injection;
- less desirable injection site (lower extremity, antecubital fossa, wrist, and dorsum of the hand should be avoided); and
- recent venipuncture in the same vein, which may allow drug leakage.[18–20]

When multiple chemotherapy drugs are to be administered, there is controversy regarding whether the vesicant drug should be administered first or last. Some clinicians feel that the vesicant should be administered after the nonvesicant drugs, so that the nonvesicants can test the patency of the IV line. Others, however, feel that the patency and reliability of an IV line are best when the line is first started. Therefore, vesicant drugs should be administered immediately after the line has been started with a saline solution and before multiple manipulations that could dislodge the needle or jeopardize the integrity of the line.

Before any drug is administered, the patient should be asked to remember how the IV site feels so that the discomfort of the IV device can be differentiated from an extravasation. All patients must be instructed to report unusual discomfort immediately during or after receiving drugs, because extravasations may be difficult to visualize until a substantial amount of drug has escaped into the tissue. Often, the first sign of extravasation is the patient's complaint of pain, burning, or stinging at the injection site. The injection should be stopped at the first suspicion of an extravasation, because the degree of tissue damage appears to correlate directly with the amount of drug extravasated and the duration of exposure.[8,10,21]

Despite careful adherence to the recommended administration procedures, extravasations of antineoplastic drugs do occur. Controlled studies to determine the most effective procedure for treating vesicant extravasations are lacking. In any case, it is usually wise to have a plastic surgeon examine the site as soon as possible to determine whether the area should be excised. Although various antidotes have been suggested for specific agents, most of these recommendations are based on anecdotal information (Table 10-2).

One of the most promising approaches to the management of anthracycline and mitomycin extravasations is the application of topical dimethyl sulfoxide (DMSO). It is believed that serious ulcers caused by anthracycline extravasations are related to the formation of toxic free radicals of oxygen (see chapter 3 for an explanation of free radicals). DMSO penetrates along all tissue planes and prevents tissue damage by scavenging the free radicals. Animal studies initially confirmed that ulcers were prevented by DMSO, and a subsequent clinical trial reported that no ulcerations occurred in 16 patients followed for 3 months after presumed extravasations when DMSO was applied to an area approximately twice the affected area every 6 hours for 14 days.[9,22–24] It is important to allow DMSO to air dry following application because occlusive dressings may cause DMSO-related local inflammation. Several additional reports have also substantiated the apparent activity of DMSO, either alone or combined with cold or α-tocopherol, in ameliorating tissue damage caused by anthracycline or mitomycin extravasations.[25–29]

Suggested procedures for minimizing the toxic effects of extravasations (Appendix 10-B, *Suggested Procedures for Minimizing Toxic Effects of Vesicant Extravasation*) should be initiated promptly whenever vesicant extravasations are suspected or documented. Considerable controversy exists about whether warm or cold compresses should be applied after extravasations. Some experts advocate heat to produce vasodilation, facilitate fluid absorption, and decrease local drug concentration[8]; others advocate the use of cold to limit dispersement in the tissue and limit the site of potential damage.[30] Currently, heat is generally recommended for vinca alkaloid extravasations and cold for anthracyclines and mitomycin.

Venous Sclerosis and Thrombosis—In addition to the risk of extravasation, other complications associated with administration via peripheral veins include sclerosis and thrombosis.[31] Many patients also may have unsatisfactory peripheral venous access due to obesity, prior therapy with sclerosing or irritating agents, or fragility (usually in the elderly). For these reasons, or if the patient is considered to be at high risk for extravasation or other complications, various methods of central venous access are often used to administer chemotherapy.

Central Venous Access and Administration

A central venous access device may be used for blood sampling as well as drug administration. Semipermanent devices, such as those placed in the vein, dramatically decrease the number of times that veins must be painfully repunctured for drug administration and laboratory tests, because they can be reused for long periods of time (often weeks to months). These devices are commonly used in cancer patients for administering chemotherapy, antiemetics, parenteral nutrition, analgesics, and antimicrobials.

Percutaneous (Nontunneled) Central Venous Access

Central venous lines or catheters have been widely used for many years. Although percutaneously inserted central venous catheters (nontunneled) are commonly used in intensive care and emergency situations, they are not typically used for che-

Table 10-3. Potential Complications of Central Venous Catheters

Complication	Percutaneous Catheter	PICC	Tunneled Catheter	Implanted Port
Occlusion	Yes	Yes	Yes	Yes
Thrombosis	Yes	Yes	Yes	Yes
Leakage	Yes	Yes	Yes	Yes
Infection sites	Skin exits, sepsis	Skin exit, sepsis,	Skin exit, tunnel, sepsis	Port pocket, sepsis
Extravasation	Uncommon	Uncommon	Uncommon	Dislodged needle
Bleeding	Uncommon	After insertion in thrombocytopenic patients	After insertion in thrombocytopenic patients	After insertion in thrombocytopenic patients
Other	Inadvertent removal due to trauma or tension on line	Inadvertent removal due to trauma or tension on line	Inadvertent removal due to trauma or tension on line Line migration into other vessels (e.g., carotid)	Port inversion or migration in pocket

PICC, peripherally inserted central catheter.

motherapy administration. Instead, other devices (including those discussed in the following sections) are preferred because they may be left in place for longer periods and facilitate prolonged or multiple courses of chemotherapy. These catheters are typically inserted into the subclavian vein, the external jugular vein, or the internal jugular vein and threaded into the central venous system; they are then usually sutured to the skin to avoid displacement. These catheters are made of either soft Silastic (e.g., Intracil or Centrasil) or a stiffer plastic (polyethylene or polyurethane). Potential complications associated with the placement and use of other central venous catheters are listed in Table 10-3.[32–35]

Peripherally Inserted Central Venous Catheters

Although peripherally inserted central venous catheters (PICCs) are inserted into a forearm vein (i.e., the antecubital fossa), they are advanced to the superior vena cava and are technically considered central venous catheters. They are also referred to as long-arm or long-line catheters. These catheters are often inserted in the clinic, at the bedside, or even in the home by specially trained nurses (most other types of central venous lines require physician placement). Because the catheter tip is placed in the superior vena cava, it is safe to administer hyperosmolar solutions (including total parenteral nutrition solutions), vesicants, and irritants without substantial risk of phlebitis, sclerosis, or extravasation. PICCs are available in sizes (length and diameter) appropriate for both pediatric and adult patients as well as single and double lumen designs. The catheters are made of very pliable material and are very comfortable for patients following placement. Many reports show that PICCs have been left in place for weeks to months with fewer and less severe complications than those reported for the tunneled catheters described below, and their use appears to be associated with a lower rate of infection than other nontunneled catheters.[36–38] Blood pressure should always be measured in the contralateral arm while the PICC is in place to avoid occlusion or damage to the catheter. Potential complications include phlebitis at the insertion site or along the vein, infection, sepsis, cellulitis, withdrawal occlusion, thrombosis, catheter occlusion due to obstruction or kinking, and catheter tip migration (Table 10-3). Between uses, many catheters (including PICCs and tunneled central venous catheters) require filling with a heparinized (100 units/ml) saline solution and occasional flushing with saline to prevent clot formation, along with care of the skin exit site to prevent infection. When costs of insertion and maintenance are considered, PICCs appear to be a cost-effective alternative to the tunneled catheters.[37] PICCs are well-accepted by patients because of the ease of placement, comfort, and low risk of serious complications.

Tunneled Central Venous Catheters

Development of the tunneled Silastic Broviac[39] and Hickman[40] catheters during the 1970s permitted parenteral nutrition solutions to be administered over longer periods of time with fewer complications. These devices are an extension of the nontunneled devices with the catheter tip carefully placed in a free-floating position in the right atrium of the heart so that infused drugs are diluted rapidly and blood samples are withdrawn easily. If the patency of the catheter is maintained, it may be left in place for the duration of the patient's therapy. In fact, many catheters have been left in place for several years.

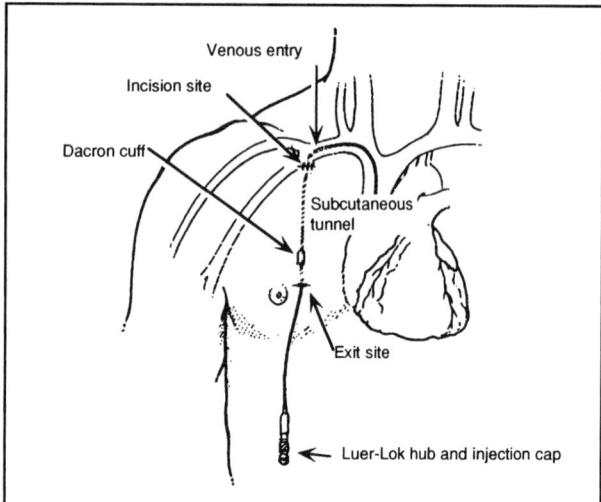

Figure 10-2. Tunneled central venous catheter, such as a Hickman or Broviac catheter

SOURCE: reprinted with permission from Wickham R. Techniques for long-term venous access. Presented at Fifth National Conference on Cancer Nursing, September 1987. Reprinted with permission from the American Cancer Society, Inc., Atlanta, GA.

Once placed in the vein, the catheter is tunneled subcutaneously for a short distance (usually across the chest) to provide a barrier between the skin exit site and the vascular entrance site (Figure 10-2). A Dacron cuff surrounds the catheter under the skin, just proximal to the exit site. This cuff promotes the growth of fibrous tissue that creates an additional barrier to microorganisms and also holds the catheter securely in place. These catheters are usually inserted in the operating room by a surgeon. Double and triple lumen catheters are also available for patients who require multiple lines. Catheters are also now available (VitaCuff) that have cuffs impregnated with silver ion to prevent microbial colonization from the skin exit site and further minimize risk of infection.[41,42]

One design of the tunneled catheters (Groshong) has a pressure-sensitive distal slit valve at the tip or on the side of the catheter (Figure 10-3). When the valve is closed, blood does not flow back into the catheter, minimizing the possibility of clot occlusion of the lumen. One study has, however, documented the aspiration of clots from the lumens of these catheters, thus demonstrating the need for occasional flushing.[43] The manufacturer has recommended that these types of catheters be flushed weekly with saline.

Totally Implantable Intravascular Devices

These systems, also called subcutaneous vascular access ports, are widely used for venous access in patients with cancer. They contain a small-volume reservoir (port) that is constructed of stainless steel, titanium, or plastic and has a Silastic septum. The port is connected to a right atrial catheter (Figure 10-4). A subcutaneous pocket is created surgically for the port, usually in the anterior chest wall. Once the incision is healed, there is little more evidence than a small bump under the skin that the system is in place. These systems are well accepted by patients because of their convenience and obvious cosmetic advantage over the tunneled catheters, which exit through the skin. Access to the device is obtained with a specially designed noncoring, Huber needle placed through the skin and into the Silastic septum. The needle may be left in place for several days. When the subcutaneous port system is not in use, it is flushed with heparinized saline, usually at monthly intervals. Single- and double-lumen ports are available. The implantable access devices have a lower rate of catheter-related

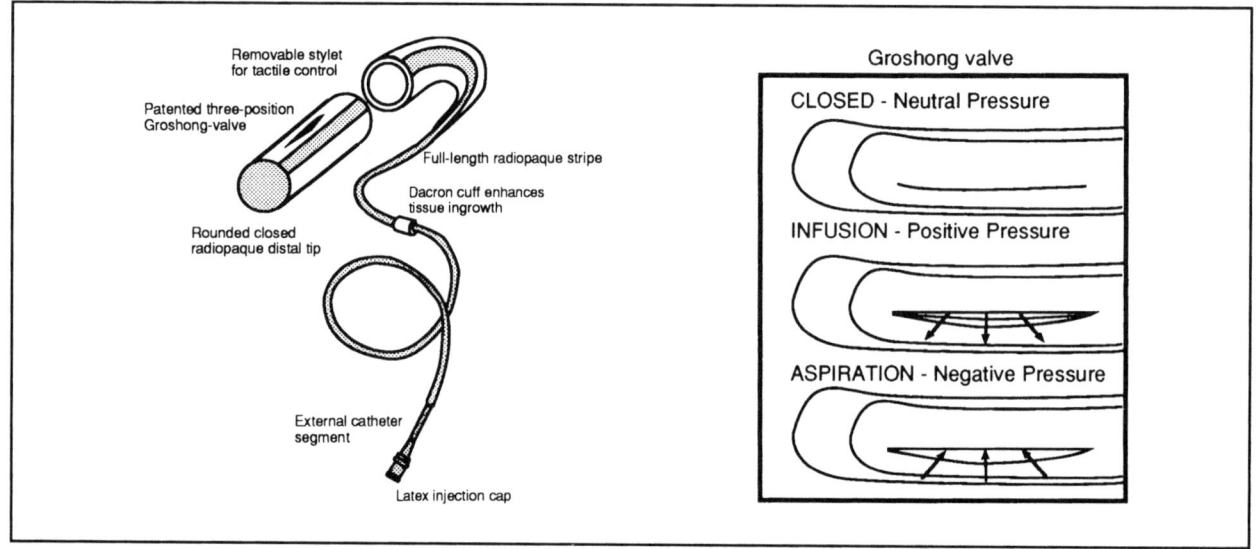

Figure 10-3. Single-lumen Groshong or slit-tip catheter

SOURCE: reprinted with permission from McCauley E. *Medical Illustrations and Photography*, School of Medicine, University of North Carolina at Chapel Hill.

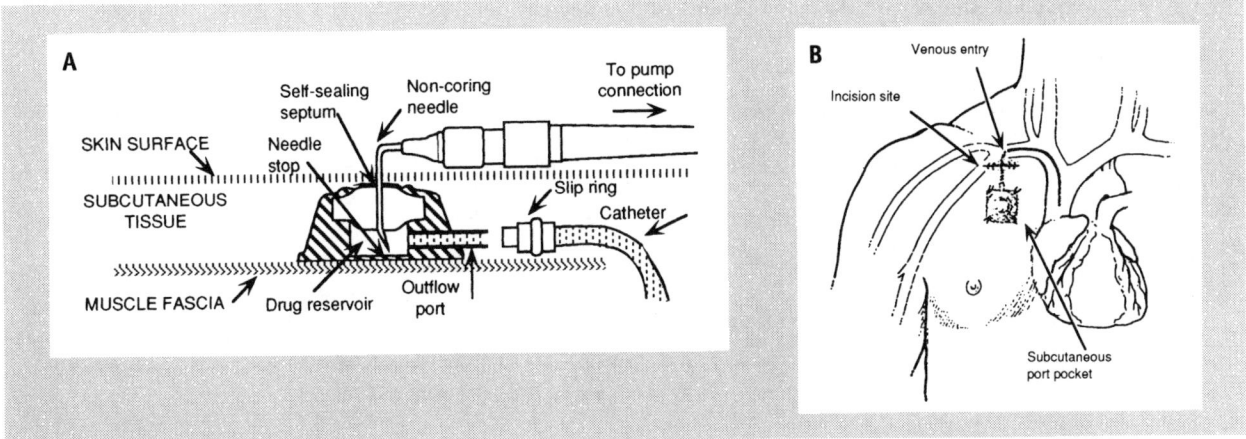

Figure 10-4. Implantable vascular access port. A: cross-section. B: anatomy of insertion into chest wall.
SOURCE: A: reprinted with permission from Pharmacia Deltec, Inc., St. Paul, MN. B: Wickham R. Techniques for long-term venous access. Presented at Fifth National Conference on Cancer Nursing, September 1987. Reprinted with permission from the American Cancer Society, Inc., Atlanta, GA.

bacteremias than the other devices, possibly because they are located beneath the skin, without an opening for microorganism introduction.[44]

Complications

Because serious complications are rare and the devices may be left in place for extended periods, avoiding the need for repeated venipunctures, the net effect is usually very positive for both patient comfort and convenience.

The use of tunneled catheters, subcutaneous ports, soft Silastic percutaneous catheters, and PICCs has greatly reduced the incidence of complications associated with central venous access and allowed the devices to be used for longer periods. The most commonly reported complication is infection; other complications include venous thrombosis, catheter occlusion, incorrect positioning of the catheter, and dislodgement of needles from the subcutaneous ports (Table 10-3).

Intravascular Thrombosis and Occlusion of Catheter Lumens—Venous thrombosis may develop any time a catheter is in place. These thrombi form at any site around the body of the catheter, including around the catheter tip.[44] Thrombosis is usually characterized by a dull ache in the shoulder, arm, or neck; supraclavicular fullness or swelling; venous distension in the neck or chest; and arm swelling.[44] If a thrombus occludes the tip, the function of the catheter may be impaired. Patients who have other underlying risk factors for developing venous thrombosis may also have an increased risk of catheter-related thrombosis.[45]

Documented intravascular thrombosis associated with an indwelling catheter usually requires removal of the device. In rare cases, the catheter has been preserved. IV heparin therapy alleviates symptoms and prevents further clot formation and may be followed by lower doses of subcutaneous heparin or oral anticoagulant therapy to prevent recurrences. Lytic therapy with streptokinase or urokinase has also been used, but its safety and efficacy have been debated.[45–48]

The catheter or port lumen may also become occluded when a clot forms within the lumen or at the catheter tip or when a drug or electrolyte solution precipitates within the lumen. Clotting may result if the flow through the catheter is interrupted without flushing with heparin. Interruption of flow may be caused by infusion pump failure, occlusion or kinking of the catheter or IV tubing, or human error. Catheter patency can often be restored by instilling a small volume of streptokinase or urokinase (Table 10-4). The solution should be allowed to remain in contact with the clot for 5–60 minutes, followed by aspiration of the catheter to restore patency. The outcomes resulting from these techniques suggest that the risk of embolizing such clots is very small. Furthermore, there have not been any hemorrhagic complications associated with thrombolytic therapy in this setting.[49] Because occlusion of a catheter caused by precipitation of a drug is extremely difficult to dissolve, precautions should be taken against this consequence (e.g., avoid incompatible drugs and cold temperatures). Various strategies have been suggested to solubilize drug precipitates within the lumens of catheters; however, none can be routinely recommended.[50,51] Pharmacists should consult with manufacturers of both the drug and the catheter for specific recommendations. Whatever the cause of the occlusion, the catheter must be removed if patency cannot be restored.

As mentioned above, most institutions recommend filling the catheter lumen with a saline solution containing a low concentration of heparin (100 units/ml) between uses. This process is referred to as "locking" the catheter, and it is believed to reduce the likelihood of clot formation at the catheter tip. Before the next use of the catheter, this heparinized saline solution is withdrawn rather than pushed into the patient. Because the volume of the catheter depends on both

Table 10-4. Thrombolytic Therapy for Occluded Venous Access Devices

Thrombolytic Agent	Dose	Duration of Treatment	Outcome of Occlusions	Reference
Urokinase	5000 units/hr	16–72 hr	22 of 25 resolved	32
Urokinase	250,000 units in 250 ml D5W	90 min	10 of 11 cleared	33
Urokinase	0.3–0.4 ml of 5000 units/ml	5–60 min (repeat q5min)	98.6% success (most were Silastic catheters)	34
Urokinase	0.3–0.6 ml of 5000 units/ml	30 min	77% cleared within 22 min	35
Streptokinase	0.3–0.6 ml of 250 units/ml	30 min	100% overall	35

SOURCE: adapted from Alexander HR. Thrombotic and occlusive complications of long-term venous access: diagnosis, management, and prophylaxis. In: Alexander RH, editor. *Vascular Access in the Cancer Patient*. Philadelphia, PA: JB Lippincott; 1994. p. 94. D5W, 5% dextrose in water.

the diameter of the lumen and the length of the device, the volume necessary to lock the catheter differs for each brand and model. Clinicians should consult the manufacturer's information for the appropriate volume. Many institutions also recommend periodic flushing of the catheter with saline between uses to dislodge small clots or precipitates before they evolve into significant occlusions. Some institutions recommend daily flushing, others only flush weekly. As mentioned above, the slit-tip, or Groshong, catheters may alleviate the need for this process.

Sometimes withdrawing blood through the catheter to determine patency becomes difficult, although fluids may still be injected or infused through the device. This problem may be caused by tip migration or abutment against the vein wall or right atrium. A chest X-ray may rule out kinking and tip migration. This problem can occasionally be alleviated by changing the patient's position. If the catheter tip has migrated or the catheter is kinked, the surgeon or radiologist also may be able to reposition the catheter.

Catheter-Related Infections—Infections are probably the most common complication associated with central venous catheter use. They may include skin exit site infections, infections along the subcutaneous catheter tunnel, or pocket infections around the ports. Systemic catheter-related infections or sepsis also may be associated with any of the devices. In 1996, the U.S. Public Health Service Centers for Disease Control and Prevention issued guidelines for prevention of infections related to intravascular devices.[52]

Exit site infections are manifested as either an abscess or cellulitis around the skin exit site. Blood cultures, drawn from both the catheter and a peripheral vein, and exit site cultures, with expression of any discharge around the site, should be done to document local infection and rule out other systemic infections. Many of these infections can be managed with local care, such as topical antibiotics or drainage, but neutropenic patients require systemic antibiotics. Oral antibiotics may suffice in some cases, but the most common pathogen is *Staphylococcus epidermidis*, which is unlikely to respond to available oral antibiotics. Other common pathogens include *Candida* species, enterococci, and *S. aureus*. Infections involving the catheter tunnel or port pocket require systemic antibiotic therapy and, in some cases, removal of the device. Comprehensive patient education regarding the appropriate care of the device may reduce the incidence of these infections.[53]

If bacteremia or other signs of systemic infection occur in a patient with a central venous access device, then the device must be excluded as the source of the infection. If both the central catheter and peripheral vein blood cultures are positive with the same organism, there is a strong likelihood that the device is involved. The patient should receive a full course of IV antibiotic therapy, and usually the catheter must be removed.[53-55] Another device should not be placed until all signs and symptoms of infection have been resolved and repeat blood cultures are negative.

For each patient, the risk of complications must be carefully weighed against the benefits of the device. To minimize complications, only trained persons should care for a central venous device. Patients with long-term devices (tunneled catheters or ports) must be instructed in proper care and maintenance.

Intravenous Infusion Devices

In many circumstances, cytotoxic drugs must be administered at a constant rate over a period of time ranging from an hour to several weeks. The purpose is usually either to avoid specific toxicities associated with too-rapid infusion (e.g., hypotension with etoposide) or to ensure optimal exposure of the tumor cells to the agent. Therefore, it is often desirable to use a mechanical infusion device to maintain a constant rate of infusion. If vesicant agents are to be infused over a sustained period, most experts advise that they be administered only through a central line to avoid the potential for extravasation. If vesicants are given by bolus injection, they can safely be administered via peripheral vein, provided the person administering the drug follows recommended guidelines to minimize risk of extravasation (Appendix 10-A). If nonvesicants are given as prolonged infusions via peripheral lines, infusion devices should be selected that are sensitive enough to detect extravasations and therefore optimize drug delivery.

Many chemotherapy regimens administer drugs via prolonged continuous infusions. This method of administration, in combination with rising health care costs and increasing concern about patient comfort and convenience, has led to the use of many ambulatory (home) infusions. To facilitate long-term outpatient infusions, many small, self-contained ambulatory infusion devices have been marketed that allow safe and efficient delivery of various drugs. The features and specifications of several of these devices are listed in Table 10-5. Features available in ambulatory infusion devices range from the disposable, elastomeric devices with no alarms and a single, preset rate of infusion to the sophisticated multichannel devices that may administer several drugs simultaneously and that have numerous alarms and safety features. Other small infusion pumps can be implanted into surgically constructed pockets in the subcutaneous tissue. Because of the obvious size constraints, these devices are designed to administer small volumes over prolonged periods of time. The implantable devices are expensive and, with the cost of the surgery for placement, must be used for a longer period of time than other devices to be cost efficient. The selection of the most appropriate infusion device should be based on consideration of the capacity of the pump's drug reservoir, the range of infusion rates, the type of infusion (e.g., intermittent, continuous, or on-demand, such as that for patient-controlled analgesia), the alarms and other safety features, the drug or drugs to be administered (and the need for specific safety features and number of delivery channels), the power source (e.g., disposable or rechargeable battery), the size, and ease of use.

Today, there are several hundred infusion devices available. Each of these devices has a variety of features, and the user must carefully study the device specifications before choosing the devices for a particular practice setting. Some pumps are particularly well-designed for home infusions because they are small, light-weight, and easy for the patient or their family to change the drug cassettes in, or to trouble-shoot if an alarm sounds. Other devices are designed primarily for inpatient units because they can administer a large range of infusion rates (e.g., 10–1000 ml/hr) and are larger (generally suspended on a pole with wheels), with large print screens that are convenient for nurses to program. Some of the disposable elastomeric devices have been designed for short-term (e.g., 30- or 60-minute) infusions and are well-suited for ambulatory clinics or infusion centers. Several other references provide more in-depth descriptions of infusion technology and the advantages and disadvantages of the various designs.[56-58]

Table 10-5. Features and Specifications of Ambulatory Infusion Devices

Features	Baxter Infusor Systems	SIMS Deltec CADD Series	ITI Vector MTI	Creative Medical Development EZ Flow Model 80-2
Reservoir	65–275 ml[a]	50-, 100-, and 250-ml custom cassettes or any IV bag	Any IV bag	100-ml cassette
Infusion range	0.5–10 ml/hr[a]	0–400 ml/hr[a]	0.1–400 ml/hr	0.6–250 ml/hr
Power source	Elastomeric	Disposable 9-volt battery or rechargeable pack with AC adapter	Two disposable 9-volt alkaline batteries	Rechargeable nickel-cadmium battery pack
Program modes	Continuous	Continuous, intermittent, on-demand, taper[a]	Continuous, intermittent, taper, on-demand	Continuous
Alarms and safety features	Built-in flow restrictor	Audible and visible low volume in reservoir, infusion complete, low battery, occlusion, stop mode, system error, lock-out	Reservoir empty or low, low battery, infusion end, air-in-line, system malfunction, occlusion	Infusion complete, occlusion, low battery

[a]Depends on model.

Table 10-6. Anticancer Drugs Administered by IM or SC Injection

Drug	IM	SC	Maximum Concentration
Asparaginase (Elspar)	Yes	Yes	5000 IU/ml
Asparaginase (Erwinia)	Yes	No	5000 IU/ml
Bleomycin	Yes	Yes	15 units/ml
Cytarabine (Cytosar-U)	No	Yes	50–100 mg/ml
Interferon alfa-2a (Roferon-A)	Yes	Yes	50 million IU/ml
Methotrexate	Yes	No	25 mg/ml
Pegaspargase (Oncaspar)	Yes	No	750 IU/ml

IM, intramuscular; IU, international units.

Intramuscular and Subcutaneous Administration

Chemotherapy agents are occasionally given by either intramuscular (IM) or subcutaneous (SC) injections (Table 10-6). Cytotoxic agents that are known vesicants or irritants should never be given by these methods. IM and SC administration may pose particular problems in some situations. For example, IM injections may produce severe hematomas in a thrombocytopenic patient and must therefore be avoided. In addition, single IM injections should be limited to 2.0–2.5 ml per site, and SC injections should be limited to 0.5 ml per site. Sometimes, the product may have to be reconstituted to a higher concentration than that indicated in the package insert. Before doing so, the pharmacist should consult the manufacturer and the professional literature to ensure that this manipulation does not increase the risk to the patient or compromise the integrity of the product.

LOCAL AND REGIONAL CHEMOTHERAPY ADMINISTRATION

The rationale for local and regional chemotherapy arose from the recognition that the dose-response curve of both antitumor and toxic effects is steep for most cytotoxic agents. If a systemic route of administration is used, curative concentrations of drug at the tumor site may be prohibited by dose-related toxicities to normal tissues. Local and regional methods deliver high drug concentrations to the predominant tumor site, usually with far less systemic exposure. The ideal indication for these therapies, therefore, is a tumor that has a prolonged period of only regional spread.

Intraperitoneal Administration

Direct instillation of chemotherapy agents into the peritoneal cavity of patients with intra-abdominal malignancies is intended to increase drug levels at the predominant site of disease. This method of therapy has been used most extensively to treat ovarian carcinoma, a disease that remains largely confined to the abdominal cavity. In addition, it has been used to treat gastrointestinal tumors (tumors of the colon or rectum), mesotheliomas, and melanomas that are confined to this cavity. Overall, patients with microscopic tumors or very small nodular disease are most likely to respond, because many drugs may not penetrate large tumor masses well.[59-61]

Technologically, access to the peritoneal cavity for drug delivery is established with a Tenckhoff catheter connected to an implantable port. These systems are surgically implanted and allow for repeated access to the peritoneal cavity. The Tenckhoff catheter (like those used for peritoneal dialysis) is a Silastic tube that is passed into the cavity and then tunneled through the subcutaneous tissue. The catheter is connected to a subcutaneous port in a manner analogous to the venous systems.[62] Complications associated with intraperitoneal catheters include bacterial and chemical peritonitis, abdominal pain, bleeding, bowel perforation, ileus, and fluid leakage. The implantable systems require less maintenance and have met with better patient acceptance and fewer complications than externalized Tenckhoff catheters.[59,62-64] In approximately half of the patients with intraperitoneal catheters, an outflow obstruction of the system develops. This obstruction is caused by the formation of a fibrinous sheath around the tip of the catheter.[64,65] It may be related to adhesion formation; the result is fluid retention in the peritoneal cavity after drug administration.

Ideally, drugs that are selected for intraperitoneal use should have a low clearance from the peritoneum and a rapid clearance from the plasma to keep drug concentration high at the site of the tumor and systemic concentrations low, minimizing systemic side effects. Drugs with a high molecular weight and low lipid solubility meet these specifications. Other factors that may influence peritoneal permeability are particle size and charge, disease state, and tonicity of carrier solution. In addition, drugs should be selected that can kill tumor cells either directly or by metabolic activation within the tumor tissue (e.g., they do not require activation by the liver).[66]

The efficacy of intraperitoneal chemotherapy also depends on the ability of the drug solution to distribute throughout the entire peritoneum. Patients who have had previous abdominal surgery or who have large tumor masses may have uneven flow of fluid in the peritoneum. Diluting the drug in large volumes of fluid (usually 1.5–2 L) results in optimum distribution. To ensure uniformity of fluid distribution, patients who receive intraperitoneal chemotherapy should have radiological studies of fluid distribution after the catheter is placed and before therapy begins.[67] This can be accomplished by instilling 50–75 ml of diatrizoate (Hypaque, Winthrop Labs) diluted in 2 L of saline through the catheter, followed by visualization by a computed tomography (CT) scan.[68] Additional suggestions for intraperitoneal catheter care and drug administration are listed in Appendix 10-C.

Cisplatin, one of the most effective drugs available for ovarian cancer treatment, is by far the most common cytotoxic agent administered intraperitoneally. Initial pharmacologic studies indicated a large difference between peritoneal clearance and plasma clearance. In addition, systemic IV cisplatin therapy is limited by its dose-related nephrotoxicity to single doses of about 100 mg/m^2. Doses as high as 270 mg/m^2 have been given intraperitoneally when sodium thiosulfate is administered concurrently. The thiosulfate neutralizes cisplatin in the kidney and protects against nephrotoxicity.[69] This technique allows for peritoneal concentrations 10–100 times greater than the plasma free cisplatin levels.

Other cytotoxic agents that have been given intraperitoneally include carboplatin, fluorouracil, melphalan, methotrexate, cisplatin, doxorubicin, mitomycin, etoposide, bleomycin, cytarabine, and aldesleukin (IL-2). Combination intraperitoneal therapy has also been used.

Intrathecal and Intraventricular Administration

Several malignancies, including acute leukemias, breast and lung carcinomas, and lymphomas, have the propensity to spread to the meninges. Treatment of meningeal tumor involvement is complicated because many cytotoxic agents do not distribute in the cerebrospinal fluid (CSF) sufficiently to reach cytotoxic concentrations. Therefore, intrathecal (IT) injections via lumbar puncture or intraventricular injection are required. Drugs are usually injected directly into the CSF by lumbar puncture between the L4 and L5 vertebrae; however, drug distribution from the injection site often does not allow effective quantities to distribute to the cisterns or ventricles.[70,71]

Surgically placed small subcutaneous reservoirs (e.g., Ommaya reservoirs) connected to a small catheter leading to the lateral ventricle of the brain are used for direct intraventricular injection. Figure 10-5 shows how the drug is injected and how the reservoir is gently pumped. Shapiro et al.[71] have demonstrated that methotrexate administered via an intraventricular reservoir is distributed rapidly and evenly throughout the CSF in patients with meningeal leukemia and meningeal carcinomatosis. The reservoir also makes it possible to withdraw samples of CSF for cytologic, biochemical, and bacteriological testing.

The volume in which an IT dose is diluted may affect its distribution in the CSF.[70] In adults, volumes of 5–15 ml are well tolerated if an equivalent volume of CSF is first

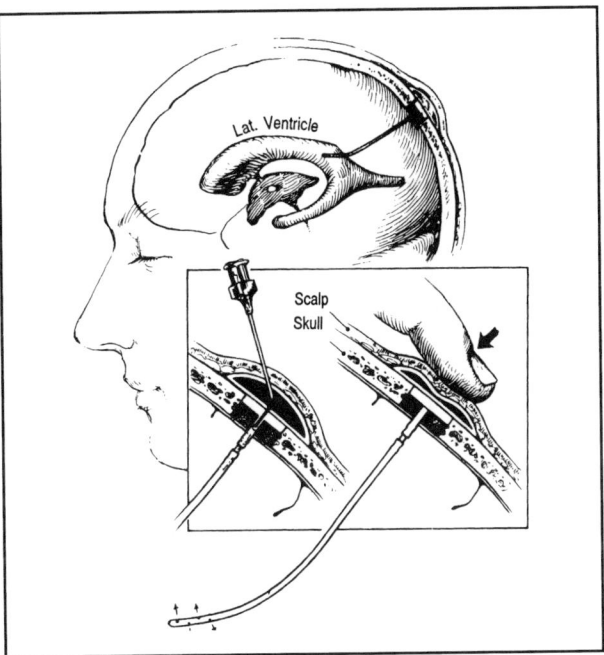

Figure 10-5. Diagrammatic view of subcutaneous reservoir and pump device with an intraventricular catheter. Lat, lateral. *Inset*: pumping of the reservoir.

SOURCE: reprinted with permission from Ratcheson RA, Ommaya, AK. Experience with the use of the subcutaneous cerebrospinal-fluid reservoir: preliminary report of 60 cases. *N Engl J Med* 1968;279:1026. Copyright © 1968 Massachusetts Medical Society. All rights reserved.

removed or used as the diluent. Volumes of ≤2 ml are well tolerated without removing CSF. The diluent used for IT chemotherapy appears to influence toxicity. Enhanced neurotoxicity has been suggested when nonphysiological diluents or commercial products with preservatives are used. Lactated Ringer's injection USP or sodium chloride for injection USP may be used safely in most cases; however, sterile water for injection USP should be used for IT thiotepa. Elliott's B solution (distributed by Orphan Medical) is a buffered electrolyte and dextrose injection available for dilution of IT methotrexate and cytarabine. It is a sterile, nonpyrogenic, isotonic solution without antibacterial preservatives.

Methotrexate, cytarabine, and thiotepa have been the most widely used cytotoxic agents for IT administration. For treating adult meningeal leukemia, methotrexate is usually given in doses of 6–15 mg every 2–4 days until no more leukemic cells are detected in the CSF.[72,73] Typically, 12 or 15 mg are administered to adults. The dose in younger children should be scaled downward in proportion to the CSF volume rather than the body surface area.[74] Bleyer[75] has recommended an IT methotrexate dose of 6 mg for children ≤1 year old, 8 mg for ages 1–2, 10 mg for ages 2–3, and 12 mg for children over 3 years old.

The most common toxicity associated with the IT use

of methotrexate is an arachnoiditis that usually presents with stiff neck, headache, nausea, vomiting, fever, lethargy, and an increased number of white blood cells in the CSF beginning 2–4 hours after injection and lasting 12–72 hours. The frequency of this reaction varies, but it has been reported in up to 61% of patients.[72,76–78] The concomitant use of cranial irradiation seems to decrease the frequency of this reaction, presumably by suppressing the inflammatory response.[77] A much more severe syndrome characterized by transient or permanent paraplegia, leg pains, and neurogenic bladder has been reported to occur between 30 minutes and 48 hours after an IT injection of methotrexate or cytarabine. Improvement may occur as early as 48 hours or be delayed 2–5 months.[78]

Encephalopathy characterized by a variety of neurological symptoms, including confusion, somnolence or irritability, ataxia, dementia, tremor, seizures, spasticity, quadraparesis, visual disturbances, slurred speech, coma, and occasional death, may also occur following IT methotrexate. Partial recovery or stabilization may occur in some patients. The incidence of this reaction increases in frequency as IT and IV methotrexate and cranial irradiation are combined.[78,79] The sequence of administration of radiation therapy and methotrexate seems to be important. There are no reports of delayed encephalopathy in patients whose methotrexate was terminated before radiation and not resumed.[78] The combination is particularly toxic when radiation is given before the methotrexate or along with it.[80] Methotrexate encephalopathy usually begins insidiously in the first year after the radiation; however, it may begin as soon as a few weeks following radiation.[78,79] Other toxic effects of IT methotrexate are mineralizing microangiopathy, cerebral atrophy, and delayed somnolence.[78]

IT dosages of cytarabine range from 5 to 70 mg/m^2 (mean, 50 mg/m^2). Transient or permanent paraplegia similar to that described with methotrexate has also been reported following cytarabine.[80] Neurotoxicity may also be enhanced when IT cytarabine and methotrexate are given together.[81]

Thiotepa is also occasionally used intrathecally in doses of 1–10 mg/m^2 twice weekly. Reported toxicities are generally mild, but fatal paraplegias have been reported.[82,83]

Intravesical Administration

Chemotherapy instilled into the urinary bladder is used to manage superficial bladder cancer, either as an adjuvant to surgery to delay or prevent tumor recurrence or as definitive therapy for widespread disease that is difficult to control surgically. Preventing progression from superficial bladder tumor to muscle invasion is particularly important because the treatment of advanced disease by total cystectomy or radiation therapy or both produces substantial morbidity and cures no more than 50% of patients with locally advanced bladder cancer.[84]

Ideally, agents used intravesically should be poorly absorbed through the bladder mucosa, thereby preventing systemic toxicity while exposing local lesions to a high drug concentration. Agents that are commonly used in this manner include mitomycin, thiotepa, doxorubicin, and Bacillus Calmette-Guérin (BCG) vaccine. Treatment usually consists of diluting the drug in 30–60 ml of sterile water or saline and instilling it into the urinary bladder. Patients are asked to change positions several times to distribute the drug throughout the bladder; they are allowed to void after 1–2 hr.

Thiotepa is absorbed to some extent, and myelosuppression has been seen in 18–40% of cases.[85] Myelosuppression with mitomycin and doxorubicin is rare because the high molecular weight of each molecule prevents absorption through the bladder mucosa. Irritation (chemical cystitis) of the bladder may be caused by any of these drugs. BCG produces a particularly intense local inflammatory reaction in most patients, manifested as dysuria, frequency, urgency, hematuria, and passing of shreds of tissue, lasting from 6 to 24 hours after instillation. Although isoniazid can ameliorate these local effects, it is rarely necessary.[86] Local symptoms generally do not require dose reduction or cessation of therapy. Patients who have active tuberculosis or who are severely immunosuppressed should not receive BCG.

Overall, it appears that patients at the greatest risk for tumor recurrence and progression will benefit from intravesical therapy. Data are still inconclusive on which therapy is the best. However, it is encouraging that BCG use has been demonstrated to delay disease progression and the need for subsequent cystectomy.[87] BCG also appeared to have a significantly greater prophylactic and therapeutic effect than thiotepa or doxorubicin.[88,89] Thiotepa, doxorubicin, and mitomycin appear to be equally effective when used as prophylaxis. When used to treat active disease, mitomycin and doxorubicin appear superior to thiotepa.[90] Mitomycin has also been shown to produce complete remissions in patients who have failed thiotepa therapy.[91,92]

Intra-arterial Administration

Intra-arterial (IA) administrations of chemotherapy are used for treating localized malignancies. In this administration method, the artery that is the primary blood supply for the tumor is cannulated and the drug is infused. In theory, a significant amount of the drug is extracted during the first pass through the capillary bed of the tumor. This technique is believed to increase the drug delivery to the tumor area and simultaneously reduce the amount of drug going into systemic circulation. As a result, tumor kill is enhanced, and toxicity to the rest of the body is minimized (Figure 10-6).[92] Increase in local drug concentration depends largely on the blood flow rate of the infusing artery and the rate of elimination by the rest of the body. This drug administration method is most often used as hepatic arterial infusions for the treatment of liver metastases and as limb perfusion for managing tumors, such as sarcomas or melanomas, that are limited to one extremity. In both situations, the artery must be isolated and cannulated surgically. Techniques have been developed for arterial perfusion of most regions of the body.[93]

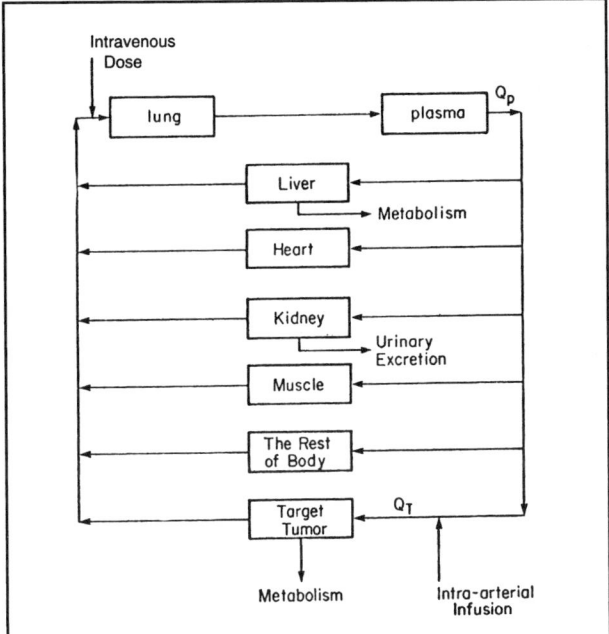

Figure 10-6. Theoretical aspect of intra-arterial infusion of drugs. Q_p, pulmonary blood flow; Q_t, tissue blood flow.
SOURCE: reprinted with permission from Chen HSG, Gross JF. Intra-arterial infusion of anticancer drugs: theoretic aspects of drug delivery and review of responses. *Cancer Treat Rep* 1980;64:31–40.

Hepatic Arterial Infusions

Hepatic arterial infusions of chemotherapy agents are most commonly used to treat metastases of colorectal cancer. The liver is the most frequent site of metastases of colorectal cancer (approximately two thirds of patients with recurrent or advanced disease develop them), and such disease is usually resistant to radiation therapy. Systemic chemotherapy produces responses in only 10–30% of patients, and there are few long-term responders. Malignant lesions in the liver derive most of their blood supply from the hepatic artery, whereas normal hepatocytes are supplied from the portal circulation.[94,95] Therefore, selective infusion of a drug into the hepatic artery should deliver a higher drug concentration to the tumor than an IV infusion.[94]

In the past, most hepatic arterial chemotherapy was administered by an external infusion pump connected to a transcutaneous hepatic arterial catheter. These systems were associated with a high incidence of complications, including arterial thrombosis; catheter displacement, clotting, or damage; infection; and upper gastrointestinal hemorrhage.[94,96,97] This technique of administration has been largely replaced by the use of a totally implantable drug infusion pump (e.g., Infusaid or SynchroMed), which allows for the ambulatory administration of hepatic infusions. The pump is implanted in a subcutaneous pocket in the abdominal wall, and the catheter is placed in the gastroduodenal artery.[94] Mechanical failure of these systems has been rare. Overall, they have been associated with far fewer complications than the externalized systems. In general, however, the advantages of this method remain controversial. The initial cost of the pump and the cost of placing it are high, but maintenance is minimal and patients can avoid multiple hospital admissions for chemotherapy administration.[94]

Fluorouracil, floxuridine, and mitomycin are the most common chemotherapy agents administered in this manner. Numerous studies have suggested encouraging results, but few randomized studies have compared IA with IV chemotherapy. Likewise, most studies have not considered many prognostic variables that may influence outcome in this disease, such as performance status, size of tumor, presence of extrahepatic disease, and the extent of prior radiation and chemotherapy. Two studies have confirmed higher response rates when floxuridine is administered intra-arterially rather than intravenously at maximum tolerated doses. Chang and colleagues[98] at the National Cancer Institute reported response rates of 62% in the IA group and 17% in the IV group; however, no significant difference in survival was reported. In a similar study, Hohn and colleagues[99] of the Northern California Oncology Group reported response rates of 37% in the IA group and 10% in the IV group. Survival information was not available. Significant toxicities were reported in both trials. Although initial results of these studies look promising, further work is required to determine whether IA therapy has significant impact on quality of life and survival. Subgroups of patients who are most likely to respond need to be identified as well. At least three other trials have also reported that IA floxuridine consistently produces higher response rates than IV floxuridine; however, survival was not improved in two of three of these trials.[100–102]

Regional Limb Perfusion

Isolated limb perfusion with chemotherapy has been used for many years.[103] Figure 10-7 illustrates the technique that is generally used. Venous blood is collected by gravity drainage, pumped through an oxygenator, and passed through a heat exchanger. An arterial pump is used to pump the blood back into the major artery supplying the treatment area. (This technique is very similar to the one used during coronary bypass surgery.) A cytotoxic drug is usually administered in three aliquots into the arterial line. Arm perfusions are usually carried out through the first portion of the axillary vessels, and leg perfusions are administered through the common femoral vessel or the external iliac artery.[104,105]

Limb perfusions are most commonly used to treat melanomas and sarcomas. Cytotoxic agents used for this technique include cisplatin, melphalan, mechlorethamine, thiotepa, and dactinomycin. The doses used in isolation perfusion are much higher than doses administered systemically. Limb perfusion has been used both as adjuvant therapy and to manage documented tumors. Toxicities to the limb may be substantial, ranging from discrete erythema (with or without edema) to epidermolysis (with or without damage to deep tissue structures).

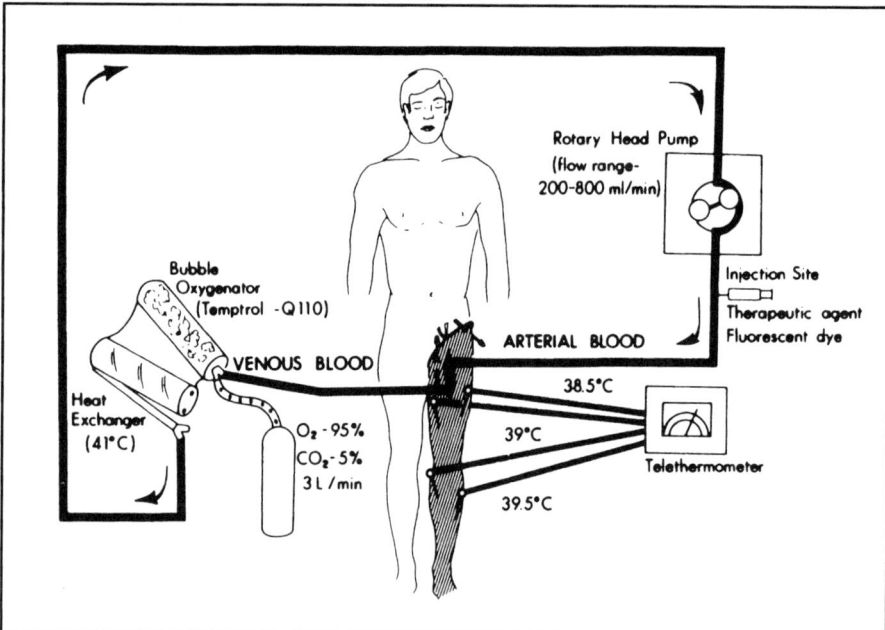

Figure 10-7. Schematic diagram of isolated limb perfusion with heart-lung machine

SOURCE: reprinted with permission from Krementz ET. Chemotherapy by isolated regional perfusion for melanoma of the limbs. In: Schwemmeck AK, editor. *Vascular Perfusion in Cancer Therapy*. Berlin: Springer-Verlag; 1983. p. 196.

Occasionally, amputation has been required because of drug toxicity.

Many studies have reported encouraging results, and most have demonstrated local tumor control and preservation of the limb. However, the overall effects on patient survival are uncertain because patients often succumb to other metastatic disease. More randomized trials are therefore necessary to define the optimal use of limb perfusion.

OTHER ROUTES OF ADMINISTRATION

Other routes are occasionally used for chemotherapy administration. These routes include intralesional injections, topical applications, drug-impregnated implants, intrapleural infusions, pericardial infusions, and targeting methods, such as the attachment of a drug molecule to a monoclonal antibody (see chapter 5). With the exception of topical fluorouracil for treatment of actinic keratoses (a noninvasive skin disorder) and bleomycin for malignant pleural effusions, these methods of drug administration are outside the Food and Drug Administration–recommended indications and are most appropriate within the context of an approved clinical trial. In many cases, the effectiveness of these preparations has not yet been proved. Pharmacists may be requested to make extemporaneous preparations of these dosage forms. Before doing so, they should confirm the safety and stability of the formulation. It is appropriate to request that the prescriber provide applicable references, and the primary literature may be searched for additional information (see chapter 20). Pharmacists may wish to discuss the liability issues regarding the use of unconventional dosage forms and routes of administration with the risk management and legal counsel at their places of practice.

SUMMARY

The effectiveness of chemotherapy depends on achieving sufficient drug concentration at the tumor site to produce cell death. At first, cancer chemotherapy was developed as a modality to treat systemic or advanced malignancies that were not amenable to localized or regional treatments, such as surgery or radiation. Most chemotherapy is still used for systemic therapy and is given either orally or intravenously. However, additional routes of administration are now used to deliver chemotherapy drugs to localized tumors. The most appropriate method of administration depends on a variety of drug-, tumor-, and patient-related factors. In some situations, systemic therapy may be combined with localized therapy. Regardless of the method selected, it is important that individuals preparing and administering the agents be familiar with the acute and chronic toxicities of the agents as well as the safest and most efficient techniques and procedures for administration.

REFERENCES

1. Crom WR, Evans WE. Methotrexate. In: Evans WE, Schentag JJ, Jusko WJ, editors. *Applied Pharmacokinetics: Principles of Therapeutic Drug Monitoring*. 3rd ed. Spokane, WA: Applied Therapeutics; 1992. p. 29-41–29-42.
2. Alberts DS, Peng YM, Fisher B. Minimal melphalan (L-PAM) systemic availability (SA): a potential cause for failure of adjuvant breast cancer trials [abstract]. *Proc Am Soc Clin Oncol* 1984;3:38.

3. Bosanquet AG, Gilby ED. Comparison of the fed and fasting states on the absorption of melphalan in multiple myeloma. *Cancer Chemother Pharmacol* 1984;12:183–6.
4. Smyth RD, Pfeffer M, Scalzo A, et al. Bioavailability and pharmacokinetics of etoposide (VP-16). *Semin Oncol* 1985;12:48–51.
5. Hande KR, Krozely MG, Greco A, et al. Bioavailability of low-dose oral etoposide. *J Clin Oncol* 1993;11:374–7.
6. Oncology Nursing Society. *Cancer Chemotherapy Guidelines and Recommendations for Practice.* Pittsburgh, PA: Oncol Nursing Pr; 1996. p. 1–87.
7. Howell SB, Taetle R. Effect of sodium thiosulfate on *cis*-dichlorodiammineplatinum (II) toxicity and antitumor activity in L1210 leukemia. *Cancer Treat Rep* 1980;64:611–6.
8. Dorr RT. Pharmacologic management of vesicant chemotherapy extravasations. In: Dorr RT, Von Hoff DD, editors. *Cancer Chemotherapy Handbook.* 2nd ed. Norwalk, CT: Appleton & Lange; 1994. p. 109–18.
9. Olver IN, Aisner J, Hament A, et al. A prospective study of topical dimethyl sulfoxide for treating anthracycline extravasation. *J Clin Oncol* 1988;6:1732–5.
10. [Anonymous]. Doxorubicin. In: Dorr RT, Von Hoff DD, editors. *Cancer Chemotherapy Handbook.* 2nd ed. Norwalk, CT: Appleton & Lange; 1994. p. 395–416.
11. Dorr RT, Soble M, Liddil JD, et al. Mitomycin-C skin toxicity studies in mice: reduced ulceration and altered pharmacokinetics with topical dimethyl sulfoxide. *J Clin Oncol* 1986; 4:1399–404.
12. Dorr RT, Snead K, Liddil JD. Skin ulceration potential of paclitaxel in a mouse skin model in vivo. *Cancer* 1996;78:152–6.
13. DuBois A, Fehr MK, Bochtler H, et al. Clinical course and management of paclitaxel extravasation. *Oncol Rep* 1996; 3:973–4.
14. Holmes BC. Administration of chemotherapy. In: Dorr RT, Von Hoff DD, editors. *Cancer Chemotherapy Handbook.* 2nd ed. Norwalk, CT: Appleton & Lange; 1994. p. 57–94.
15. Galassi A, Hubbard SM, Alexander HR, et al. Chemotherapy administration: practical guidelines. In: Chabner BA, Longo DL, editors. *Cancer Chemotherapy and Biotherapy.* 2nd ed. Philadelphia, PA: Lippincott-Raven, 1996. p. 529–51.
16. Tully JL, Friedam GH, Baldini LM, et al. Complications of intravenous therapy with steel needles and Teflon catheters. *Am J Med* 1981;70:702–6.
17. Herrington JD, Figueroa JA. Severe necrosis due to paclitaxel extravasation. *Pharmacotherapy* 1997;17:163–5.
18. Ignoffo RJ, Friedman MA. Therapy of local toxicities caused by extravasation of cancer chemotherapeutic drugs. *Cancer Treat Rev* 1980;7:17–27.
19. Bowers DG, Lynch JB. Adriamycin extravasation. *Plast Reconstr Surg* 1978;61:86–92.
20. Reilly JJ, Neilfeld JP, Rosenberg SA. Clinical course and management of accidental Adriamycin extravasation. *Cancer* 1977;40:2053–6.
21. Rudolph R, Stein RS, Pattillo RA. Skin ulcers due to Adriamycin. *Cancer* 1976;38:1087–94.
22. Desai MH, Teres D. Prevention of doxorubicin-induced skin ulceration in the rat and pig with dimethyl sulfoxide (DMSO). *Cancer Treat Rep* 1982;66:1371–4.
23. Dorr RT, Soble MJ, Liddil JD, et al. Mitomycin C skin toxicity studies in mice: reduced ulceration and altered pharmacokinetics with topical dimethyl sulfoxide. *J Clin Oncol* 1986;4:1399–404.
24. Olver IN, Schwartz MA. Use of dimethyl sulfoxide in limiting tissue damage caused by extravasation of doxorubicin. *Cancer Treat Rep* 1983;67:407–8.
25. Ludwig CU, Stoll HR, Obrist R, et al. Prevention of cytotoxic drug induced skin ulcers with dimethyl sulfoxide (DMSO) and α-tocopherol. *Eur J Cancer Clin Oncol* 1987;23:327–9.
26. Herera D, Burnham N. DMSO and extravasation of mitomycin [letter]. *Oncol Nurs Forum* 1989;16:155.
27. Bertelli G, Dini D, Forno G, et al. Dimethylsulphoxide and cooling after extravasation of antitumour agents. *Lancet* 1993;341:1098–9.
28. Lawrence HJ, Goodhight SH. Dimethyl sulfoxide and extravasation of anthracycline agents [letter]. *Ann Intern Med* 1983;98:1025.
29. Lawrence HJ, Walsh D, Zapotowski KA, et al. Topical dimethylsulfoxide may prevent tissue damage from anthracycline extravasation. *Cancer Chemother Pharmacol* 1989;23:316–8.
30. Harwood KV, Aisner J. Treatment of chemotherapy extravasation: current status. *Cancer Treat Rep* 1984;68:939–45.
31. Wilson SE, Stabile BE, Williams RA, et al. Current status of vascular access techniques. *Surg Clin North Am* 1982;62: 531–51.
32. Kersen C, DiStetano A, Blumenschein G, et al. Treatment of vascular access catheter occlusion with urokinase infusion [abstract]. *Proc Am Assoc Cancer Res* 1988;29:228.
33. Tschirhart JM, Rao MK. Mechanism and management of persistent withdrawal occlusion. *Am Surg* 1988;54:326–8.
34. Lawson M, Bottino JC, Hurtubise MR, et al. The use of urokinase to restore the patency of occluded central venous catheters. *Am J Intraven Ther Clin Nutr* 1982;5:29–32.
35. Hurtubise MR, Bottino JC, Lawson M, et al. Restoring patency of occluded central venous catheters. *Arch Surg* 1980;115:212–3.
36. Masoorii S, Angeles T. PICC lines: the latest home care challenge. *RN* 1990;44–51.
37. James L, Bledsoe L, Hadaway LC. A retrospective look at tip location and complications of peripherally inserted central catheter lines. *J Intraven Nurs* 1993;16:104–9.
38. Raad I, Davis S, Becker M, et al. Low infection rate and long durability of nontunneled Silastic catheters. *Arch Intern Med* 1993;153:1791–6.
39. Broviac JW, Cole JJ, Schribner BH. A silicone rubber atrial catheter for prolonged parenteral alimentation. *Surg Gynecol Obstet* 1973;136:602–6.
40. Hickman RO, Buckner CD, Clift RA, et al. A modified right atrial catheter for access to the venous system in marrow transplant recipients. *Surg Gynecol Obstet* 1979;148:871–5.
41. Maki DG, Cobb L, Garman JK, et al. An attachable silver-impregnated cuff for prevention of infection with central venous catheters: a prospective randomized multicenter trial. *Am J Med* 1988;85:307–14.
42. Groeger JS, Lucas AB, Coit D, et al. A prospective randomized evaluation of the effect of silver impregnated subcutaneous cuffs for preventing tunneled chronic venous access catheter infections in cancer patients. *Ann Surg* 1993;218: 206–10.

43. Anderson AJ, Krasnow SH, Boyer MW, et al. Clots can frequently be aspirated from Groshong catheters [abstract]. *Proc Am Assoc Cancer Res* 1988;29:228.
44. Moore CL. Nursing management of infusion catheters. In: Lokich JJ, editor. *Cancer Chemotherapy by Infusion*. Chicago, IL: Precept Pr; 1987. p. 74–99.
45. Lokich JJ, Bothe A, Benotti P, et al. Complications and management of implanted venous access catheters. *J Clin Oncol* 1985;3:710–7.
46. Bern MM, Lokich JJ, Wallach SR, et al. Very low doses of warfarin can prevent thrombosis in central venous catheters. *Ann Intern Med* 1990;112:423–8.
47. Lewis JA, LaFrance R, Bower RH. Treatment of an infected silicone right atrial catheter with combined fibrinolytic and antibiotic therapy: case report and review of the literature. *J Parenter Enteral Nutr* 1989;13:92–8.
48. Fraschini G, Jadeja J, Lawson M, et al. Local infusion of urokinase for the lysis of thrombosis associated with permanent central venous catheters in cancer patients. *J Clin Oncol* 1987;5:672–8.
49. Alexander HR. Thrombotic and occlusive complications of long-term venous access: diagnosis, management, and prophylaxis. In: Alexander RH, editor. *Vascular Access in the Cancer Patient*. Philadelphia, PA: Lippincott; 1994. p. 91–109.
50. Pennington CR, Pithie AD. Ethanol lock in the management of catheter occlusion. *J Parenter Enteral Nutr* 1987;11:507–8.
51. Duffy L, Kerzner B, Gebus V, et al. Treatment of central venous catheter occlusions with hydrochloric acid. *J Pediatr* 1989;114:1002–4.
52. Centers for Disease Control. Guideline for prevention of intravascular device-related infections. *Am J Infect Control* 1996;24:262–93.
53. Reed WP, Newman KA, DeJongh CA, et al. Prolonged venous access for chemotherapy by means of the Hickman catheter. *Cancer* 1983;52:185–92.
54. Lazarus HM, Lowder JN, Herzig RH. Occlusion and infection in Broviac catheters during intensive cancer therapy. *Cancer* 1983;52:2342–8.
55. Abrahm J, Mullen JL, Jacobson N, et al. Continuous central venous access in patients with acute leukemia. *Cancer Treat Rep* 1979;63:2099–100.
56. Lindley CM, Deloatch KH, editors. *Infusion Technology Manual*. Bethesda, MD: American Society of Health-System Pharmacists; 1993. p. 1–109.
57. Finley RS, Van Echo DA. Drug delivery systems: infusion and access devices. In: Klastersky J, Schimpff SC, Senn H-J, editors. *Handbook of Supportive Care in Cancer*. New York: Marcel Dekker; 1995. p. 459–90.
58. Kwan JW. High-technology i.v. infusion devices. *AJHP* 1991;48(Suppl 1):S36–51.
59. Brenner DE. Intraperitoneal chemotherapy: a review. *J Clin Oncol* 1986;4:1135–47.
60. Dedrick R, Myers C, Bungay P, et al. Pharmacokinetic rationale for peritoneal drug administration in the treatment of ovarian cancer. *Cancer Treat Rep* 1978;62:1–11.
61. McVie JG, Ten Bokkel Huinink W, Dubbelman R, et al. Phase I study and pharmacokinetics of intraperitoneal cisplatin administration in patients [abstract]. *Proc Am Assoc Cancer Res* 1985;25:162.
62. Pfeifle CE, Howell SB, Markman M, et al. Totally implantable system for peritoneal access. *J Clin Oncol* 1984;2:1277–80.
63. Jenkins J, Sugarbaker P, Gianola F, et al. Technical considerations in the use of the intraperitoneal chemotherapy administered by Tenckhoff catheter. *Surg Gynecol Obstet* 1982;154:858–64.
64. Piccart MJ, Speyer JL, Markman M, et al. Intraperitoneal chemotherapy: technical experience at five institutions. *Semin Oncol* 1985;12(Suppl 4):90–6.
65. Van Groeningen CJ. New technical developments in antineoplastic drug delivery and their role in cancer treatment. In: Domelloff L, editor. *Drug Delivery in Cancer Treatment*. New York: Springer-Verlag; 1987. p. 39–52.
66. Markman M. Intraperitoneal antineoplastic agents for tumors principally confined to the peritoneal cavity. *Cancer Treat Rev* 1986;13:219–42.
67. Myers C. The use of intraperitoneal chemotherapy in the treatment of ovarian cancer. *Semin Oncol* 1984;11:275–84.
68. Dunnick NR, Jones RB, Doppman JL, et al. Intraperitoneal contrast infusion for assessment of intraperitoneal fluid dynamics. *Am J Radiol* 1979;133:221–3.
69. Howell SB, Pfeifle CE, Wung WE, et al. Intraperitoneal cisplatin with systemic thiosulfate protection. *Ann Intern Med* 1982;97:845–51.
70. Rieselbach RE, Giovanni DC, Freireich EJ, et al. Subarachnoid distribution of drugs after lumbar injection. *N Engl J Med* 1962;267:161–6.
71. Shapiro WR, Young DF, Mehta BM. Methotrexate distribution in cerebrospinal fluid after intravenous ventricular and lumbar injections. *N Engl J Med* 1975;293:161–6.
72. Duttera MJ, Bleyer WA, Pomeroy TC, et al. Irradiation, methotrexate toxicity, and the treatment of meningeal leukemia. *Lancet* 1973;2:703–7.
73. Posner JB. Central nervous system metastases. *Semin Oncol* 1977;4:81–92.
74. Bleyer WA, Dedrick RL. Clinical pharmacology of intrathecal methotrexate: 1. Pharmacokinetics in nontoxic patients after lumbar injection. *Cancer Treat Rep* 1977;61:703–8.
75. Bleyer WA. The clinical pharmacology of methotrexate. *Cancer* 1978;41:36–44.
76. Naiman JL, Rupprecht LM, Tanyeri G, et al. Intrathecal methotrexate [letter]. *Lancet* 1970;1:571.
77. Geiser CF, Bishop Y, Jaffe N, et al. Adverse effects of intrathecal methotrexate in children with acute leukemia in remission. *Blood* 1975;45:189–95.
78. Kaplan R, Bleyer WA, Griffin TW. White matter necrosis, mineralizing microangiopathy, and intellectual abilities in survivors of childhood leukemia: associations with central nervous system irradiation and methotrexate therapy. In: Gilbert HA, Kagan AR, editors. *Radiation Damage to the Nervous System*. New York: Raven; 1980. p. 155–74.
79. Price RA, Jamieson PA. The central nervous system in childhood leukemia: II. Subacute leukoencephalopathy. *Cancer* 1975;35:306–18.
80. Saiki JH, Thompson S, Smith F, et al. Paraplegia following intrathecal chemotherapy. *Cancer* 1972;29:370–4.
81. Rubinstein LJ, Herman MM, Long TG, et al. Disseminated necrotizing leukoencephalopathy: a complication of treated central nervous system leukemia and lymphoma. *Cancer* 1975;35:291–305.

82. Gutin PH, Weiss HD, Wiernik PH, et al. Intrathecal *N,N',N'*-triethylenethiophosphoramide (Thio-TEPA) [NSC 6396]) in the treatment of malignant meningeal disease. *Cancer* 1976;38:1471–5.
83. Gutin PH, Levi JA, Wiernik PH, et al. Treatment of malignant meningeal disease with intrathecal thio-TEPA: a phase II study. *Cancer Treat Rep* 1977;61:885–7.
84. Whitmore WF. Integrated irradiation and cystectomy for bladder cancer. *Br J Urol* 1980;52:1–9.
85. Hollister D, Coleman M. Hematologic effects of intravesical thiotepa therapy for bladder cancer. *JAMA* 1980;244:2065–7.
86. Orihuela E, Herr HW, Pinsky CM, et al. Toxicity of intravesical BCG and its management in patients with superficial bladder tumors. *Cancer* 1987;60;326–33.
87. Herr HW, Laudone VP, Badalament RA, et al. Bacillus Calmette-Guerin therapy alters the progression of superficial bladder cancer. *J Clin Oncol* 1988;6:1450–5.
88. Brosman SA. Experience with BCG in patients with superficial bladder carcinoma. *J Urol* 1982;128:27–30.
89. Mori K, Lamm DL, Crawford ED. A trial of BCG versus Adriamycin in superficial bladder cancer. *Urol Int* 1986;41:254–9.
90. Herr HW, Laudone VP. Intravesical therapy for superficial bladder cancer. Updates. *Cancer: Principles and Practice of Oncology.* 2nd ed. Philadelphia, PA: JB Lippincott; 1992. p. 1–10.
91. Scher HI, Shipley WU, Herr HW. Cancer of the bladder. In: DeVita VT, Hellman S, Rosenberg SA, editors. *Cancer: Principles and Practice of Oncology.* 5th ed. Philadelphia, PA: JB Lippincott; 1997. p. 1300–22.
92. Chen HSG, Gross JF. Intra-arterial infusion of anticancer drugs: theoretic aspects of drug delivery and review of responses. *Cancer Treat Rep* 1980;64:31–40.
93. Krementz ET. Regional perfusion: current sophistication, what next? *Cancer* 1986;57:416–32.
94. Bierman HR, Byron RL, Kelley KH, et al. Studies on the blood supply of tumors in man: III. Vascular patterns of the liver by hepatic arteriography in vivo. *J Natl Cancer Inst* 1951;12:107–17.
95. Stagg RJ, Lewis BJ, Friedman MA, et al. Hepatic arterial chemotherapy for colorectal cancer metastatic to the liver. *Ann Intern Med* 1984;100:736–43.
96. Ansfield FJ, Ramirez G. The clinical results of 5-fluorouracil intrahepatic arterial infusion in 528 patients with metastatic cancer to the liver. *Prog Clin Cancer* 1978;7:201–6.
97. Oberfield RA, McCaffrey JA, Polio J, et al. Prolonged and continuous percutaneous intra-arterial hepatic infusion chemotherapy in advanced metastatic liver adenocarcinoma from the colorectal primary. *Cancer* 1984;44:414–23.
98. Chang AE, Schneider PD, Sugarbaker PH, et al. A prospective randomized trial of regional versus systemic continuous 5-fluorodeoxyuridine chemotherapy in the treatment of colorectal liver metastases. *Ann Surg* 1987;206:685–93.
99. Hohn D, Stagg R, Friedman M, et al. The NCOG randomized trial of intravenous (IV) vs. hepatic arterial (IA) FUDR for colorectal cancer metastatic to the liver [abstract]. *Semin Clin Oncol* 1987;6:85.
100. Kemeny N, Daly J, Reichman B, et al. Intrahepatic or systemic infusion of fluorodeoxyuridine in patients with liver metastases from colorectal carcinoma. *Ann Intern Med* 1987;107:459.
101. Weiss GR, Garnick MB, Osteen RT, et al. Long-term hepatic arterial infusion of 5-fluorodeoxyuridine for liver metastases using an implantable infusion pump. *J Clin Oncol* 1983;1:337.
102. Rougier P, Laplanche A, Huguier M, et al. Hepatic arterial infusion of floxuridine in patients with liver metastases from colorectal carcinoma: long-term results of a prospective randomized trial. *J Clin Oncol* 1992;10:1112–8.
103. Creech O, Krementz ET, Ryan RF, et al. Chemotherapy of cancer: regional perfusion utilizing an extracorporeal circuit. *Ann Surg* 1958;148:616–32.
104. Nachbur B, Vogt W, Goldhirsch A. Treatment of soft tissue malignancies of the extremities by regional perfusion. *Antibiot Chemother* 1988;40:77–93.
105. Israels SP. Loco-regional drug delivery in cancer treatment, with special reference to isolation perfusion. In: Domellof L, editor. *Drug Delivery in Cancer Treatment.* New York: Springer-Verlag; 1987. p. 53–76.

Appendix 10-A Recommended Vesicant and Irritant Administration Procedures to Minimize Risk of Extravasation

1. Chemotherapy should be administered only by individuals familiar with its toxic effects.

2. Dilute the drug in the appropriate amount of diluent and avoid high concentrations whenever possible.

3. Select an infusion site in the following order of preference: (1) forearm, (2) dorsum of the hand, (3) wrist, (4) antecubital fossa. Sites distal to venipunctures <24 hours old should not be used because of the risk of vesicant leakage.

    a. When selecting the site of administration, consider the ability to clearly visualize the site during administration, the vessel size, and potential tissue damage if extravasation occurs.
    b. Limbs with compromised circulation should not be used. For example, the arm on the same side as a prior axillary dissection and sites with immobilized fracture, edema, invading neoplasm, phlebitis, bruising, or varicosity should be avoided. The lower extremities should not be used.
    c. A new IV site (line) is preferred for the administration of vesicants. Pre-existing lines may already have occult vein or tissue irritation, infection, or phlebitis, and the risk of extravasation increases with the length of time the site has been in use.

4. Insert a 23- or 25-gauge scalp vein needle (also called a butterfly or wing-tipped needle) into the vein.

5. Lightly tape the wings of the needle. Do not obscure the injection site from view during injection.

6. Test the flow by running a small volume of saline solution. Withdraw a small amount of blood to test vein integrity. Observe for extravasation. If extravasation of the saline is obvious, select another site (the other arm, or lateral or proximal to initial site). Avoid a distal point on the same vein because of the potential for extravasation through venipuncture site.

7. Administer the drug at the recommended rate through the tubing of the saline IV line, using gravity to assess for back pressure. During administration, question the patient about discomfort and check blood return, flow rate of the running IV, and IV site frequently. If the patency of the line is doubtful at any time, stop the injection and choose another site.

8. After administering the drug, flush the line with at least 10 ml of IV fluid before removing line to prevent backspill.

9. If multiple drugs are to be given, flush the IV line between drugs.

10. Apply pressure with a sterile gauze for 3–4 minutes after the needle is removed. Inspect the site before applying a bandage.

Source: adapted from references 6, 14, 15, and 18.

Appendix 10-B   Suggested Procedures for Minimizing Toxic Effects of Vesicant Extravasation

1. Stop the injection immediately but do not remove the needle. Remove any drug remaining in the tubing.
2. Aspirate as much of the infiltrated drug as possible.
3. With a 27- or 25-gauge needle, aspirate the subcutaneous bleb to withdraw as much of the remaining drug solution as possible.
4. Contact physician as soon as possible.
5. If deemed appropriate, inject an antidote through the IV needle.
6. Remove the needle.
7. Administer recommended intervention as described in Table 10-2.
8. In the patient's medical record, record the drug and the amount that was suspected to have extravasated, and document any treatment.
9. Check the site regularly for at least 5–7 days.
10. A surgical consultation may be indicated, depending on the severity of tissue damage or drugs involved.

Source: adapted from references 6, 8, 14, 15, and 18.

Appendix 10-C Intraperitoneal Catheter Care and Recommendations for Drug Administration

Intraperitoneal Catheter Care

1. Guidelines range from no flushing between uses to intermittent peritoneal dialysis exchanges. Most clinicians recommend flushing with 20 ml of heparin 100 units/ml.
2. A 100-ml dose of 32% dextran solution may be administered into the peritoneal cavity periodically via the catheter in an effort to decrease fibrous tissue formation around the catheter. Patients may also be placed on a nonsteroidal anti-inflammatory drug to decrease this reaction.

Intraperitoneal Drug Administration

1. Dilute all drugs in a large volume (1–2 L).
2. Warm the solution to body temperature to prevent abdominal cramping.
3. Assure the patency of the catheter with 20 ml of saline flush before administering chemotherapy.
4. Infuse the solution in and out of the peritoneal cavity via gravity; allow 30–45 minutes if using an implanted port (infusion time may be related to the size of the Huber needle).
5. Allow the drug solution to dwell in the peritoneum for 1–4 hours or as specified in the protocol.
6. Change the patient's position periodically during dwell to permit optimal distribution.
7. Drain the drug solution; if the gravity technique is unsuccessful, irrigating forcefully with normal saline or changing the patient's position may help. If the solution cannot be drained, it will take about 2 days/L to be reabsorbed.

Complications of Intraperitoneal Chemotherapy Administration

The following complications may occur after the catheter has been placed:
- intestinal perforation,
- bleeding,
- ileus, or
- incisional discomfort.

The following complications are associated with catheter use and drug administration:
- bacterial peritonitis,
- chemical peritonitis,
- abdominal cramping,
- anorexia, nausea, and vomiting,
- esophageal reflux,
- leakage of infusate, and
- outflow obstruction due to misposition of catheter, fibrin sheath formation at the tip, or kinking of the catheter.

Source: adapted from references 59 and 62–68.

SELF-STUDY QUESTIONS

1. The recommended oral dose of etoposide is _____ that of the corresponding intravenous (IV) dose.

2. List complications that may be associated with the IV administration of any drug that would not be associated with oral administration.

3. What factors must be considered when selecting an appropriate vein for the peripheral IV administration of a chemotherapy drug?

4. Which of the following drugs are likely to produce severe tissue damage if extravasated?
   a. doxorubicin
   b. fludarabine
   c. fluorouracil
   d. carboplatin

5. Describe the reactions caused by irritant and vesicant drugs if they are extravasated during administration and differentiate these reactions from a local hypersensitivity reaction.

6. Which of the following interventions is recommended for anthracycline extravasations?
   a. heat plus hyaluronidase
   b. cold plus sodium bicarbonate
   c. topical DMSO with or without cold
   d. $\frac{1}{6}$ M sodium thiosulfate subcutaneously (SC)

7. List at least three factors that increase the risk of extravasation.

8. Formation of a thrombus around the catheter lumen is usually characterized by _____.

9. "Locking" the catheter with heparinized saline between uses will help to prevent the formation of thrombi around the body of the catheter.
   a. true
   b. false

10. The most common pathogen responsible for venous access device infections is _____.

11. If a blood clot occludes the lumen of the catheter, instillation of _____ may help to restore patency.
    a. heparin
    b. saline
    c. urokinase
    d. warfarin

12. If a patient with a central venous catheter develops bacteremia, what indications may assist in determining whether the access device is involved in the etiology?

13. The major limitations of the disposable elastomeric infusion devices are _____.

14. Potential disadvantages of the implantable infusion devices include _____.

15. Intraperitoneal administration of chemotherapy is most commonly used for which malignancies?

16. What are the most common complications associated with intraperitoneal chemotherapy administration?

17. Which chemotherapy drugs may be administered intrathecally?

18. The Ommaya reservoir may only be used for administering chemotherapy to the upper portion of the spinal column.
    a. true
    b. false

19. List at least three prognostic variables that may influence response to intrahepatic arterial infusions of floxuridine.

Chapter 11

Management of Lung and Colorectal Cancers

Jane Pruemer, Pharm.D.
Oncology Clinical Pharmacy Specialist
University Hospital Health Alliance of Greater Cincinnati
Adjunct Assistant Professor of Pharmacy Practice
University of Cincinnati College of Pharmacy
Cincinnati, Ohio

Lung Cancer	198
Etiology	198
Screening	198
Pathophysiology	198
Clinical Presentation	198
Diagnosis	199
Staging	199
Treatment	200
Non-Small Cell Lung Cancer	200
Early-Stage Disease (Stages I and II)	200
Locally Advanced Resectable Disease (Stage IIIa)	200
Locally Advanced Unresectable Disease (Stage IIIb)	201
Metastatic Disease (Stage IV)	201
Radiation Therapy	201
Small Cell Lung Cancer	202
Chemotherapy	202
Radiation Therapy	202
Prognosis	202
Colorectal Cancer	203
Etiology	203
Screening	204
Pathophysiology	204
Clinical Presentation	204
Diagnosis	204
Staging	204
Treatment	205
Primary Surgery	205
Adjuvant Therapy (Stages II and III)	205
Chemotherapy for Advanced or Metastatic Disease (Stage IV)	205
Intrahepatic Arterial Infusion for Liver Metastases	206
Prognosis	206
Summary	206
References	207
Self-Study Questions	208

Solid tumors account for the vast majority of malignancies in the United States. Lung cancer is the nation's leading cause of cancer-related deaths, and colorectal cancer is the third most common cancer in men and women.[1] Lung and colorectal cancers have a serious impact on society, as a significant proportion of health care dollars is spent treating these diseases. This chapter reviews the etiology, diagnosis, and management of lung and colorectal cancers, with a focus on the pharmacotherapeutic interventions used in the treatments of these diseases.

The first section of this chapter focuses on lung cancer and the treatment of both small cell and non-small cell lung cancers. The focus of the second section is colorectal cancer and the treatment of both colon and rectal cancers.

After completing this chapter, the reader should be able to:

1. Identify risk factors for the development of lung and colorectal cancers.
2. Given a patient history, identify signs and symptoms of lung and colorectal cancers.
3. Compare the disease progression, staging, curative potential with surgery, response to chemotherapy, and drug regimens used to treat small cell lung cancer and non-small cell lung cancer.
4. Give examples of paraneoplastic syndromes associated with lung cancer.
5. Outline potential regimens and their benefits for adjuvant treatment of colon cancer.

LUNG CANCER

The American Cancer Society estimates that approximately 171,500 cases of lung cancer will be diagnosed in the United States in 1998.[1] Although it is the second most common cancer in men and women, second to prostate cancer in men and breast cancer in women, lung cancer is the leading cause of cancer deaths. In 1998, there will be an estimated 160,100 deaths from lung cancer.[1] This disease has a significant impact on society, causing loss of productive work years, as well as a major expense to the nation's health care system. Although a decrease in cigarette smoking began to produce an age-adjusted reduction in the incidence of lung cancer in men in 1988, the incidence among women is increasing.[2] Lung cancer death rates rose 440% between 1957–59 and 1987–89.[3] Even if all cigarette smokers were to quit today, it would take about 20 years before the resultant decrease in deaths due to lung cancer would be realized.

Etiology

All types of lung cancer are thought to originate from the cells of the bronchial epithelium.[4] Carcinogenesis occurs when a chemical initiator damages cellular DNA. There is usually a long latent period from the time of carcinogenic exposure to the development of detectable cancer. The most significant risk factor for lung cancer is tobacco smoking. The American Cancer Society estimates that smoking is responsible for about 85% of all lung cancer cases. The risk is increased by the number of years a person has smoked, the number of cigarettes smoked per day, and the tar and nicotine content of the cigarettes.[5,6] There is now evidence that exposure to environmental tobacco smoke (involuntary or passive smoking) increases the risk of lung cancer.[7,8] If smoking cessation occurs, there is a gradual decrease in the risk of developing lung cancer. The role of the health care professional in motivating patients to stop smoking and in preventing initiation of smoking has received increased attention over the past few years. The development of programs that employ nicotine patches or nicotine gum in combination with behavioral modification may offer hope to those who wish to quit smoking.

Screening

Currently, there are no effective screening methods to detect lung cancer at an early stage. Periodic chest X-rays and sputum samples for cytology have not proved to alter survival when used to screen a large population for lung cancer.[9,10]

Pathophysiology

Lung cancer is generally divided into two major categories: small cell and non-small cell lung cancers, which together account for >90% of all lung cancers. These categories are differentiated by both prognosis and treatment. Non-small cell lung cancer (NSCLC) comprises several histological types: squamous cell carcinoma, adenocarcinoma, and large cell carcinoma. NSCLC accounts for approximately 75% of lung cancers, and small cell lung carcinoma (SCLC) makes up <20%. Squamous cell carcinoma, which is closely related to smoking, is the lung cancer most commonly found in men. The incidence of adenocarcinoma, most commonly found in women, is increasing and now accounts for about 40% of all lung cancers. This increase probably reflects greater numbers of women being diagnosed with lung cancer. In general, NSCLC grows at a slower rate than SCLC, which accounts for differences in the prognosis of untreated disease. SCLC, which is also related to smoking, is distinguished from the other subtypes by its rapid growth rate and usually fatal course. Histological verification of SCLC is essential, since treatment for SCLC is significantly different from that for NSCLC. Table 11-1 compares many of the features of NSCLC with those of SCLC.

Clinical Presentation

Many of the symptoms of lung cancer (e.g., cough, dyspnea, and hoarseness) are common in smokers who do not have lung cancer, which may cause patients to overlook symptoms.

Table 11-1. Comparison of NSCLC and SCLC

Comparisons	NSCLC	SCLC
Cell types	Squamous cell Adenocarcinoma Large cell	Small cell
Percent of total lung cancer	Approximately 75%	<20%
Cancer growth rate	Slow	Rapid
Staging/Prognosis for 5-yr survival	Stage I: 70% Stage II: 30% Stage III: 10–20% Stage IV: <5%	Limited stage: 5–10% Extensive stage: <5%

NSCLC, non-small cell lung cancer; SCLC, small-cell lung cancer.

Other symptoms are included in Table 11-2. The majority of patients with lung cancer have symptoms caused by the primary tumor, intrathoracic extension of the tumor, or distant metastatic disease (i.e., disease spread beyond the lungs and regional lymph nodes).

Paraneoplastic (or endocrine) syndromes are caused by secretion of hormone-like substances by tumors. Lung cancer patients may present with signs and symptoms of a paraneoplastic syndrome before a diagnosis of lung cancer is made. NSCLC and SCLC are often associated with various paraneoplastic syndromes, including hypercalcemia, the syndrome of inappropriate secretion of antidiuretic hormone (SIADH), and Cushing's syndrome (see chapter 19). Squamous cell carcinoma secretes a polypeptide similar to parathyroid hormone and is especially associated with hypercalcemia. This hormone may be responsible for stimulating osteoclasts to break down bone and release excess amounts of calcium. Eradication of the tumor will often cause paraneoplastic syndromes to disappear.

Diagnosis

Several procedures are useful in the diagnosis of lung cancer. Although a chest X-ray is the simplest way to detect a primary lung cancer, tissue diagnosis is needed before treatment is initiated. Methods of obtaining tissue samples include sputum cytology, bronchoscopy with brushings and biopsy, and needle biopsy or aspiration. To correctly stage patients with confirmed lung cancer, additional tests, including computed tomography (CT) scans or magnetic resonance imaging (MRI) to detect lymph node involvement or metastatic disease, should be performed. For patients with SCLC, a bone marrow biopsy is indicated, since this disease often presents with bone marrow metastases. Additional tests, such as a brain CT scan, may be indicated, based on the patient's symptoms.

Table 11-2. Common Signs and Symptoms of Lung Cancer

Chest pain	Pleural effusions
Cough	Rust-tinged or purulent sputum
Dyspnea	
Hemoptysis	Shoulder or arm pain
Hoarseness	Weight loss
Neck vein distention	Wheezing

Staging

Staging is necessary for lung cancer patients to determine treatment for the disease. Staging of lung cancer differs for NSCLC and SCLC. NSCLC is staged by the TNM classification system, in which T describes the size and extent of tumor, N indicates regional lymph node involvement, and M reflects the presence or absence of distant metastasis (Table 11-3). The American Joint Committee on Cancer (AJCC) has divided NSCLC into several stages (stages I–IV), with stage IV indicating the most advanced form of the disease and the presence of metastases.[11] Figure 11-1 illustrates the New International Staging System for NSCLC.

SCLC has a separate staging system that consists of two categories: limited disease and extensive disease.[12] Limited disease is confined to one hemithorax and to the regional

Table 11-3. TNM Staging System Definitions for Lung Cancer

Primary Tumor
- TX Positive malignant cell; no lesion seen
- T1 <3 cm diameter
- T2 >3 cm diameter
- T3 Extension to pleura, chest wall, diaphragm, or pericardium <2 cm from carina, or total atelectasis
- T4 Invasion of mediastinal organs; malignant pleural effusion

Regional Lymph Node Involvement
- N0 No involvement
- N1 Ipsilateral bronchopulmonary or hilar nodes
- N2 Ipsilateral or subcarinal mediastinal; Ipsilateral supraclavicular nodes
- N3 Contralateral mediastinal hilar or supraclavicular nodes

Metastatic Involvement
- M0 None
- M1 Metastases present

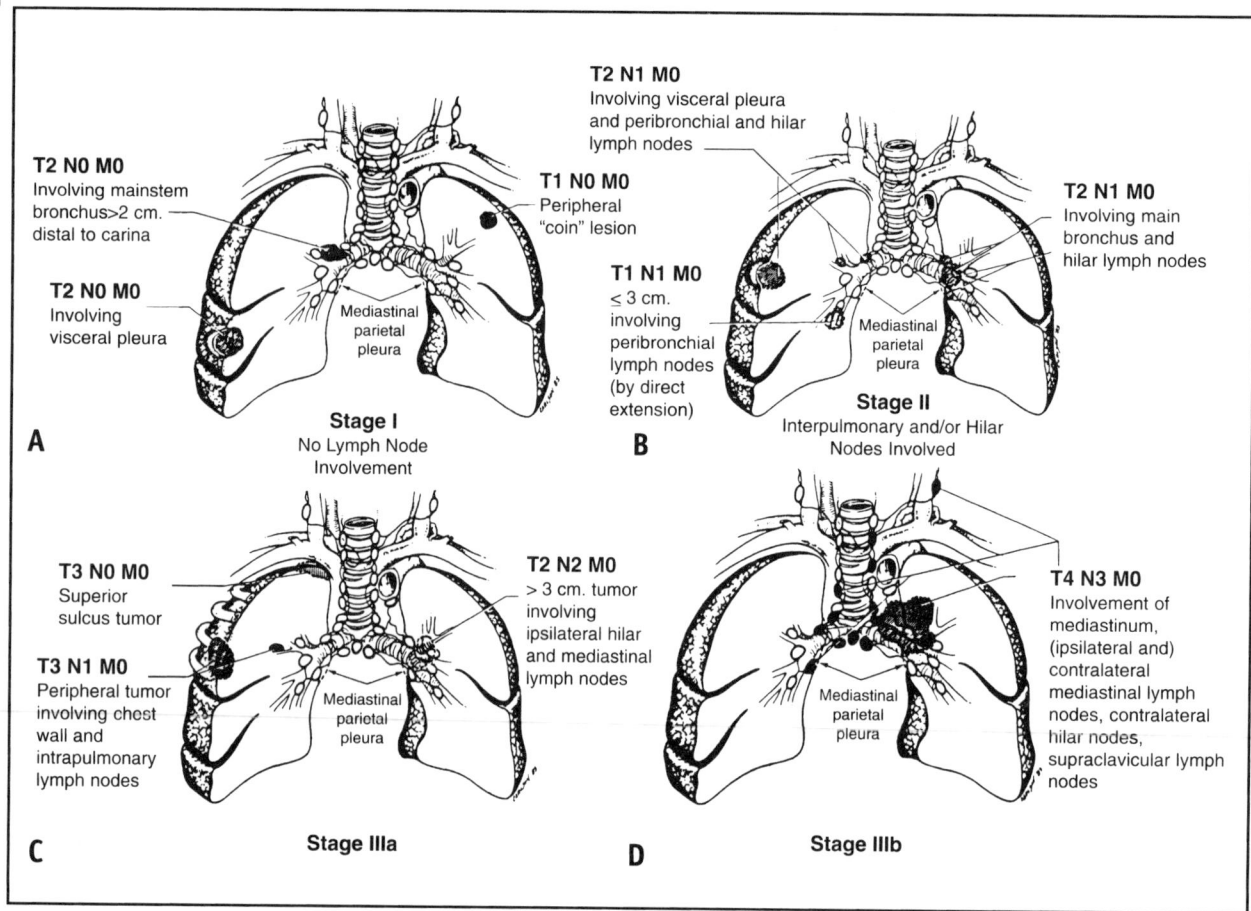

Figure 11-1. New International Staging System for lung cancer (the "TNM staging system") A: categories of stage I disease. B: categories of stage II disease. C: categories of stage IIIa disease. D: categories of stage IIIb disease.
SOURCE: reprinted with permission from Mountain CF. A new international staging system for lung cancer. *Chest* 1986;89:225S.

lymph nodes, which can usually be encompassed in one radiation field. All other disease is considered extensive stage.

Treatment

The primary management of NSCLC differs from that of SCLC. Surgical resection is the primary therapeutic intervention for NSCLC, whereas chemotherapy is the chief treatment for SCLC.

Non-Small Cell Lung Cancer

Early-Stage Disease (Stages I and II)

Surgical resection is the treatment of choice for all stage I and II NSCLC patients. Clinical staging and the patient's ability to withstand a surgical resection are the main determining factors for surgical therapy of NSCLC. It is important to remember that smoking often causes significant chronic obstructive pulmonary disease, which may compromise the patient's ability to survive without a lung or portion of a lung. Newer surgical techniques and improvements in supportive care have reduced postoperative morbidity and mortality in patients with early-stage NSCLC. However, most patients with clinically resectable disease have micrometastases at presentation that cannot be cured with surgery alone. A metanalysis of 52 randomized clinical trials suggests that adjuvant chemotherapy consisting of a cisplatin-based regimen improves 5-year survival by 5%.[13] Adjuvant chemotherapy was associated with a 13% reduction in the overall risk of death.[13]

Locally Advanced Resectable Disease (Stage IIIa)

The most significant development for many years in the management of NSCLC has been the use of preoperative chemotherapy for locally advanced disease. Theoretical benefits from preoperative chemotherapy include control of systemic disease before resistance can develop, improved delivery of drug to tumor before blood flow to tumor is compromised by surgery, evidence of tumor response that may not be seen after surgery, and improved ability to completely resect the tumor if response occurs. Preoperative chemotherapy regimens have included mitomycin with ifosfamide and cisplatin, cyclophosphamide with etoposide and cisplatin, and etoposide with cisplatin. Interim analysis showed significant survival benefits in the use of preoperative chemotherapy in two studies, and the third trial showed a trend toward improved median survival.[14-16]

Locally Advanced Unresectable Disease (Stage IIIb)
Traditionally, locally advanced NSCLC has been treated solely with radiation therapy. For many years, chemotherapy had not been used as a primary form of treatment for NSCLC; it was recommended only as palliative therapy for metastatic disease. However, a recent metanalysis of 14 randomized clinical trials compared chemotherapy plus radiation therapy with radiation therapy alone in patients with locally advanced unresectable (stage IIIb) NSCLC and found that combination therapy benefited patients more than radiation alone.[17] Most of these clinical trials utilized a cisplatin-based regimen. Compared with radiotherapy, combination chemotherapy plus radiation therapy reduced the relative risk of death by 12% at 1 year, 13% at 2 years, and 17% at 3 years. This corresponded to a mean gain in life expectancy of about 2 months. It did not seem to matter whether chemotherapy and radiation were given concurrently or sequentially.[17]

Metastatic Disease (Stage IV)
For the 40–50% of NSCLC patients with stage IV disease, chemotherapy is the primary treatment option. There is no group of patients with NSCLC in which chemotherapy is unequivocally effective.[18] There are, however, increased rates of response and possible improvement in survival for some patients with NSCLC who receive chemotherapy.[19] A variety of chemotherapy agents have been used in the treatment of NSCLC (Table 11-4). Cisplatin is one of the most important agents in combination chemotherapy regimens. Response rates in NSCLC are higher with combination chemotherapy than with single-agent treatment.[20] Table 11-5 includes some chemotherapy regimens commonly used to treat NSCLC.

Table 11-4. Chemotherapy Agents with Activity Against NSCLC

Carboplatin	Ifosfamide
Cisplatin	Irinotecan
Cyclophosphamide	Methotrexate
Docetaxel	Mitomycin
Doxorubicin	Paclitaxel
Etoposide	Vinblastine
Fluorouracil	Vindesine
Gemcitabine	Vinorelbine

Radiation Therapy
Radiation therapy can be given either to attempt to cure NSCLC patients or to palliate symptoms when cure is not possible. Radiation therapy is recommended for patients who are considered inoperable because of more advanced stages of disease or who have medical reasons for not being able to un-

Table 11-5. Combination Chemotherapy Regimens for NSCLC[12,19,20]

Drug Regimen	Dose	Route	Schedule
Paclitaxel/Carboplatin			
Paclitaxel	150–250 mg/m²	IV	Day 1
Carboplatin[a]	AUC = 5–7.5	IV	Day 1
Paclitaxel/Cisplatin			
Paclitaxel	135–250 mg/m²	IV	Day 1
Cisplatin	75–80 mg/m²	IV	Day 1
EP			
Etoposide	80–100 mg/m²	IV	Days 1,2,3
Cisplatin (Platinol)	80–100 mg/m²	IV	Day 1
CE			
Carboplatin	300–375 mg/m²	IV	Day 1
Etoposide	100–120 mg/m²	IV	Days 1,2,3
Cisplatin/Vinorelbine			
Cisplatin	100 mg/m²	IV	Days 1,29
Vinorelbine	30 mg/m²	IV	Weekly until toxicity
Vinorelbine	30 mg/m²	IV	Weekly until toxicity

IV, intravenous; AUC, area under the plasma drug concentration versus time curve. Day 1 is the first day that chemotherapy is administered.
[a]Dose by Calvert formula.

dergo surgery. Radiation therapy is also recommended when surgery has not been successful in removing all of the tumor. Palliative radiation is useful to treat hemoptysis, bronchial obstructions (which can cause pneumonias), and bone and brain metastases.

Small Cell Lung Cancer

Chemotherapy

SCLC rapidly spreads and is always considered a systemic disease, even if metastases cannot be documented. Local treatments are of minimal use with metastatic disease; therefore, systemic chemotherapy is necessary but has varying degrees of success. A number of antineoplastic agents have activity against SCLC (Table 11-6).

As with NSCLC, combination chemotherapy is more effective against SCLC than single-agent therapy. The best results are usually seen when two or more agents are used in combination. Table 11-7 lists some of the regimens commonly used to treat SCLC.

Response rates and survival durations are greater in patients with limited-stage disease than in those with extensive-stage disease. In addition, maintaining the dose intensity with as few interruptions in therapy as possible improves the likelihood of a more favorable outcome. Unfortunately, only a small percentage of patients with limited-stage disease treated with combination chemotherapy will survive >5 years.

Radiation Therapy

The role of radiation therapy in the management of SCLC remains unclear. There is evidence that it may be used in combination with chemotherapy to treat tumors confined to the chest. A significant number of patients with SCLC will develop central nervous system involvement, and radiation to brain metastases is used for palliation. However, the use of prophylactic whole-brain irradiation remains controversial.

Table 11-6. Chemotherapy Agents with Activity Against SCLC

Carboplatin	Ifosfamide
Cisplatin	Methotrexate
Cyclophosphamide	Paclitaxel
Docetaxel	Topotecan
Doxorubicin	Vincristine
Etoposide	

Prognosis

The most significant prognostic factors for patients with lung cancer are the stage of disease and the performance status of the patient. Patients with early-stage NSCLC and a good performance status (e.g., no weight loss and ability to carry out normal daily activities) are more likely to receive potentially curative surgical resection than patients with more advanced disease and poor performance status. Figure 11-2 illustrates actuarial survival curves for patients with the various stages of NSCLC.

Unfortunately, SCLC has a relatively poor prognosis for most patients. The actual 5-year survival rate for limited-stage patients is 7%, and for extensive-stage patients it is 1%. Even though the original SCLC may be eliminated in a small fraction of patients, the risk of death from other causes in these survivors is higher than in the normal population because of other smoking-related cancers, especially NSCLC.

Table 11-7. Combination Chemotherapy Regimens for SCLC[12]

Regimen	Dose	Route	Schedule
CAE			
Cyclophosphamide	1000 mg/m^2	IV	Day 1
Doxorubicin (Adriamycin)	45 mg/m^2	IV	Day 1
Etoposide	80 mg/m^2	IV	Days 1,2,3
	or		
	50 mg/m^2	IV	Days 1,2,3,4,5
CAV			
Cyclophosphamide	750–1500 mg/m^2	IV	Day 1
Doxorubicin (Adriamycin)	45–50 mg/m^2	IV	Day 1
Vincristine	2 mg	IV	Day 1
CE			
Cisplatin	80–100 mg/m^2	IV	Day 1
Etoposide	100–120 mg/m^2	IV	Days 1,2,3
	or		
	150 mg/m^2	IV	Days 3,4,5

Day 1 is the first day that chemotherapy is administered.

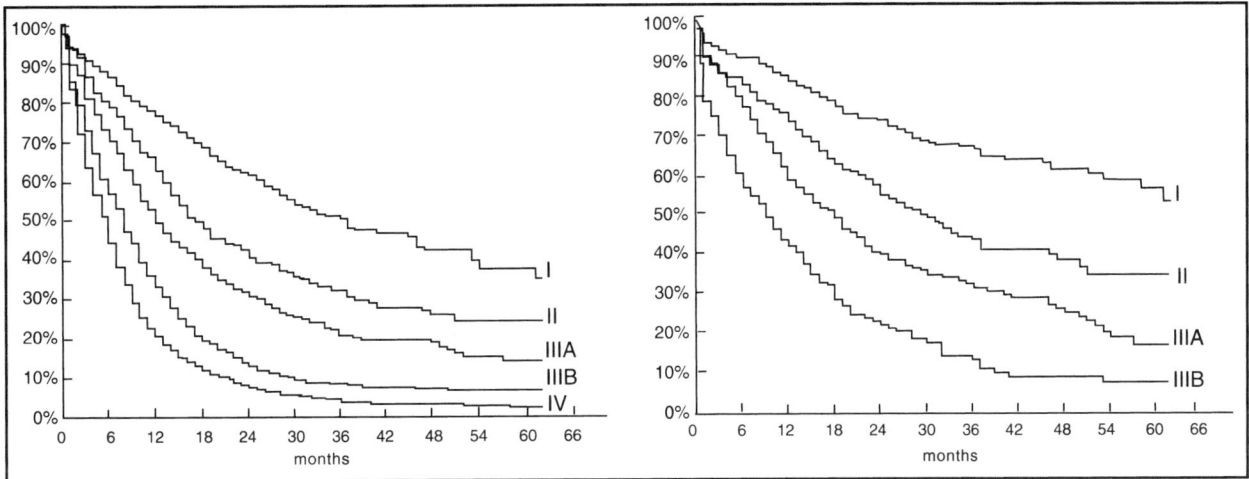

Figure 11-2. Actuarial survival curves for different stages of non-small cell lung cancer. *Left*: clinical staging. *Right*: final pathological staging.
SOURCE: reprinted with permission from Mountain CF. A new international staging system for lung cancer. *Chest* 1986;89:225S.

COLORECTAL CANCER

As the third leading cause of cancer-related mortality for men and women in the United States, colorectal cancer is a major public health problem. Estimated new cancer cases for 1998 rank colorectal cancer behind only prostate and lung cancers in men, and after breast cancer and lung cancer in women.[1] Colorectal cancer accounts for 10% of all cancers in men and 12% of all cancers in women.[1] The annual incidence of colorectal cancer is >150,000, with about 110,000 new cases of colon cancer and 45,000 new cases of rectal cancer diagnosed each year.[1] Over the past 30 years, the population-adjusted incidence has remained constant, but the number of cases has increased because of population growth. Western and highly developed cultures have a higher incidence of colorectal cancer than the rest of the world.[21] However, as people from less-developed countries migrate to Western societies, their chance of developing colorectal cancer increases.[22] The median age at diagnosis is 69 years. About 75% of individuals with these cancers will have a primary surgical resection with the hope of complete tumor eradication. Recently, despite little change in the incidence of colorectal cancer, mortality from colorectal cancer has decreased overall. The decrease is greater for rectal than for colon cancer.

Etiology

The causes of colorectal cancer have not been fully identified. Diet and other environmentally related factors are thought to most significantly affect the development of colorectal cancer. There is also a genetic component to its occurrence. Evidence from epidemiological, experimental, and genetic studies suggest that colorectal cancer may be the product of many interactions of various factors. An increase in dietary fiber intake has been shown to decrease the dose-response risk of the development of colorectal cancer in women.[23] Specifically, cruciferous vegetables may have a protective effect in this disease. In addition, there is a strong correlation between dietary fat consumption and the incidence of colorectal cancer.[23,24] The American Cancer Society has established guidelines for dietary intake to reduce the risk of colorectal cancer (Table 11-8).

A number of genetic disorders can predispose an individual to the development of colorectal cancer. Familial polyposis syndrome, or multiple intestinal polyposis syndrome, an autosomal dominant trait, results in the development of hundreds or thousands of intestinal adenomatous polyps, with a propensity to undergo malignant change. This change usually occurs at around 30 years of age.[25] All patients with untreated multiple intestinal polyposis will develop colorectal cancer by the fourth decade of life. Patients with ulcerative colitis throughout the entire colon have an increased risk of developing colorectal cancer.[26] Crohn's disease is also a risk factor for the development of colorectal cancer; however, the relative risk depends on the length of bowel involved and is slightly lower than the risk associated with ulcerative colitis. Lynch and colleagues[27] described a familial cancer syndrome in which there is an extremely high incidence of colon cancer, as well as breast and uterine cancers.

Table 11-8. American Cancer Society Guidelines to Reduce Risk of Colorectal Cancer

Avoid obesity

Decrease overall fat intake

Increase intake of high-fiber foods

Include foods high in vitamins A and C in the diet

Decrease intake of salt-cured, smoked, and nitrate-cured foods

Maintain only moderate intake of alcohol

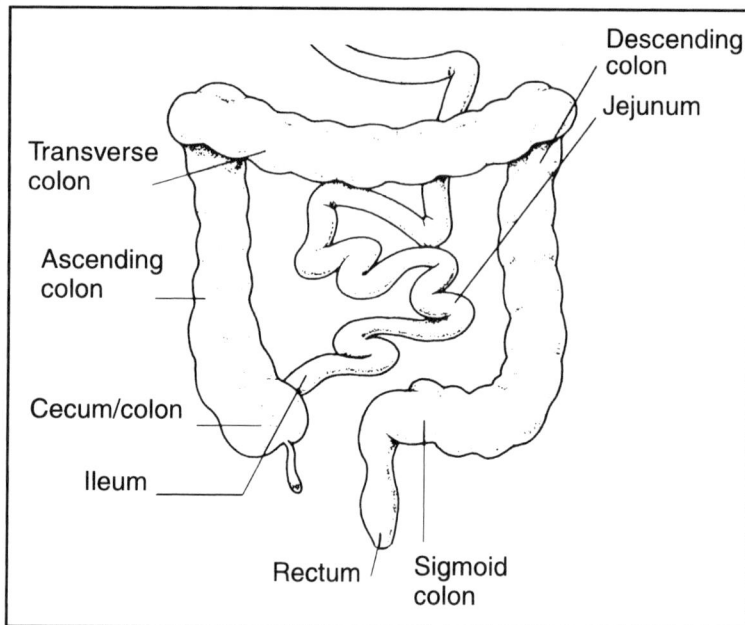

Figure 11-3. Anatomy of the colon and rectum

ing over the last two decades. The sigmoid colon is involved in about 30% of colorectal cancers, and the rectum is involved in about 50%. (The incidence for all areas combined is >100% because of overlap in disease areas.) The incidence of cancer of the rectum appears to be decreasing as an overall portion of colorectal cancer, perhaps as a result of improved screening techniques of the lower bowel.[31] The most common histological type is adenocarcinoma, which is found in >90% of all colorectal cancers. Other subtypes include mucinous adenocarcinoma, signet-ring cell carcinoma, and carcinoma simplex.

Clinical Presentation

The signs and symptoms of colorectal cancer may include changes in bowel habits, rectal bleeding, abdominal pain, abdominal mass, or iron deficiency anemia. These symptoms may be more or less prevalent, depending on the location of the tumor. Rectal bleeding and abdominal pain are the most common presenting symptoms. More advanced stages of the disease may result in additional symptoms, such as nausea and vomiting, especially when associated with liver metastases. The liver is the most common site of distant spread, because of the drainage of blood from the large bowel via the portal vein.

There have been reports of the potential protective effects of aspirin or nonsteroidal anti-inflammatory drugs (NSAIDs) against the development of colorectal cancer. Regular aspirin use at low doses was associated with a decreased risk of fatal colon cancer.[28] The proposed mechanism of protection is inhibited synthesis of prostaglandins, which may play a role in cell proliferation. An overall reduction in the risk of colorectal cancer was seen in men and women who regularly used NSAIDs.[29]

Screening

The American Cancer Society has established recommendations for screening asymptomatic people for colorectal cancer. Persons >50 years of age should have an annual digital rectal examination and fecal occult blood test. Also beginning at age 50, people should have a sigmoidoscopy, repeated after 1 year, and then every 3–5 years if the first two are negative.[30]

Pathophysiology

The anatomy of the large bowel includes the cecum; the appendix; the ascending, transverse, descending, and sigmoid colons; the rectum; and the anus. Figure 11-3 provides an illustration of the anatomy of the colon and rectum. There are four tissue layers of the large intestine: the mucosa, submucosa, muscularis externa, and serosa. Cancer of the large bowel can occur at any of the above sites and may include one or more layers of the intestine. The cecum and the ascending, transverse, and descending colons are involved in about 40% of all colorectal cancers, and this incidence has been increas-

Diagnosis

Several procedures are used in the diagnosis and staging of colorectal cancer. A personal history of polyps and a complete family history of cancer incidence should be included in the patient's medical history. A digital rectal exam, sigmoidoscopy, and barium enema are required to evaluate colorectal cancer. Further evaluation by abdominal CT scan or colonoscopy may be required. Laboratory tests, including a complete blood count, INR (International Normalized Ratio), aPTT (activated partial thromboplastin time), and liver function tests are beneficial. A measure of the plasma carcinoembryonic antigen (CEA) may reflect the extent of spread of disease and prognosis. Patients having a higher CEA plasma concentration are believed to have a higher tumor burden. Although CEA is not useful in screening for colorectal cancer,[32] serial CEA assays are useful in following patients with more advanced disease.[33]

Staging

There are several staging systems for colorectal cancer. The Dukes' staging system depends on the depth of tumor invasion into and through the bowel wall. This classification has been modified several times and is, therefore, confusing when referred to in the literature. The AJCC classification is based

Table 11-9. American Joint Committee on Cancer (AJCC) Classification of Colon and Rectal Cancer

T1	Involves mucosa or submucosa only
T2	Involves muscle or serosa
T3	Extension to contiguous structures with no fistula
T4	Extension to contiguous structures with fistula
T5	Extension beyond contiguous structures
N0	No regional node involvement
N1	Regional node involvement
N2	Juxtaregional node involvement
M0	No distant metastases
M1	Distant metastases present

Table 11-10. AJCC Staging of Colorectal Cancer

Stage Ia	T1	N0	M0
Stage Ib	T2	N0	M0
Stage II	T3, T4	N0	M0
Stage III	Any T	N1	M0
Stage IV	Any T	N2	M0
	Any T	Any N	M1

on similar pathological evaluation but also includes the familiar TNM classification. Tables 11-9 and 11-10 further define this staging system. Currently, both staging systems are used by oncologists. The treatment section of this chapter will refer to the AJCC staging system.

Treatment

Primary Surgery

The main treatment for colorectal cancer is surgery. Cancers of the colon must be removed by wide resection of the lesion together with the surrounding lymph nodes. If the tumor involves adjacent organs, such as the small bowel or bladder, these should also be resected. The bowel can be rejoined after most colon cancer resections, making the need for colostomy uncommon. Complications of bowel surgery may include the development of adhesions and malabsorption syndromes.

Adjuvant Therapy (Stages II and III)

Adjuvant therapy is administered after surgical treatment of the primary colorectal cancer with the intent to improve outcome. Adjuvant therapy options include chemotherapy, radiation therapy, and immunotherapy. In stage I disease, there is at least a 90% probability of cure with surgery alone. This probability drops to 75% with stage II disease and <50% with stage III disease.

Table 11-11. Adjuvant Therapy for Patients with Stage III Colon Cancer[34]

3–5 weeks after surgery, begin:
Fluorouracil: 450 mg/m^2 IVP daily × 5 days, off for 4 weeks, then 450 mg/m^2 IVP weekly × 48 weeks
Levamisole: 50 mg PO TID × 3 days, every 2 weeks × 1 year

IVP, intravenous push; PO, orally; TID, three times daily.

Moertel and colleagues[34] demonstrated the benefit of adjuvant chemotherapy in their study of levamisole and fluorouracil. Patients with stage II or III disease showed a lower recurrence rate than those who received no adjuvant therapy.[35] However, survival was significantly increased only in patients with stage III disease. Levamisole has several pharmacologic activities, including immune stimulation and activation of macrophages, and synergistic effects have been reported with fluorouracil.[36] The National Institutes of Health consensus conference developed the following recommendations: (1) patients with stage II colon cancer or stage II/III rectal cancer are at high risk for recurrence and warrant adjuvant therapy, and (2) stage III colon cancer patients unable to enter a clinical trial should be offered adjuvant fluorouracil and levamisole as administered in the Intergroup Trial (Table 11-11) unless medical or psychosocial contraindications exist.[37]

Because the combination of fluorouracil and leucovorin has activity in advanced disease,[38] it is being studied as adjuvant therapy in patients with stage II or III colorectal cancer. Various dosage regimens, including low- and high-dose (50–200 mg/m^2) leucovorin in combination with fluorouracil are being studied. Whether the efficacy of fluorouracil plus leucovorin is comparable to that of fluorouracil plus levamisole will not be known until long-term follow-up has been accomplished.

The combination of fluorouracil with radiation therapy is being studied as adjuvant therapy for the treatment of rectal carcinoma. Because radiation therapy is also palliative and may be curative for locally unresectable or recurrent rectal cancer, it seems reasonable that it may have efficacy as adjuvant therapy in this disease.

Chemotherapy for Advanced or Metastatic Disease (Stage IV)

Single-agent fluorouracil and fluorouracil in combination with leucovorin are the mainstays of advanced colorectal cancer treatment. The toxicity of fluorouracil is influenced by alterations in the duration or schedule of administration, but administering fluorouracil by rapid injection has proved superior to continuous-infusion fluorouracil at prolonging survival.[39] Several combination regimens have shown improved activity over fluorouracil alone in the treatment of advanced colorectal cancer (Table 11-12).[38,40]

Weekly high-dose (i.e., 500 mg/m^2) leucovorin versus low-dose (i.e., 20 mg/m^2) leucovorin plus fluorouracil has been studied in patients with advanced colorectal cancer.[41] Response rates and survival were comparable. Toxicities of leucovorin plus fluorouracil combination therapy include severe diarrhea, mucositis, and myelosuppression.

Another fluorouracil-modulating agent undergoing investigation for the treatment of advanced colorectal cancer is interferon alfa (IFN-α). There is both laboratory and clinical data to support its use in this setting.[42,43] Typically, doses of 5–10 million units of IFN-α are given subcutaneously three times weekly in combination with fluorouracil 750 mg/m^2 IV push weekly. The dose-limiting toxicity of IFN-α is a flu-like syndrome. Response rates range from 26 to 76%.[43,44] Common toxicities of this regimen include both gastrointestinal (mucositis, nausea, and diarrhea) and neurological (fatigue, gait disturbance, dizziness, memory disturbance, and sensory neuropathy) symptoms.[44]

IFN-α has also been studied in combination with fluorouracil and high-dose leucovorin.[45] When given as 3 MU subcutaneously, three times weekly, combined with leucovorin 200 mg/m^2 and fluorouracil 370 mg/m^2, IFN-α added no benefit to the standard leucovorin plus fluorouracil regimen.

Most recently, the use of irinotecan, a topoisomerase I inhibitor, has demonstrated activity in the management of metastatic colorectal cancer.[46,47] It has activity in both previously untreated patients (32% partial response, 8.1 months median response duration)[46] as well as in patients whose cancers have recurred or progressed following fluorouracil-based chemotherapy.[47] The median response rate in previously treated and untreated patients is approximately 25%.

Intrahepatic Arterial Infusion for Liver Metastases

Approximately 20–25% of patients with colorectal cancer present with or will develop metastases confined to the liver during the course of their disease.[48] Left untreated, hepatic colorectal metastases carry a dismal prognosis; <3% of patients who develop them survive for 5 years.[49] The response rate of hepatic colorectal metastases to conventional systemic chemotherapy is only 18–28%.[44,50]

The primary blood supply of hepatic metastases is the hepatic artery, whereas normal hepatocytes derive most of their blood from the portal circulation. Hepatic arterial infusion of chemotherapy results in high drug concentrations to liver metastases with less systemic exposure. This method of administration requires the surgical placement of an arterial catheter into the hepatic artery and use of an implanted or external infusion pump. Agents most commonly used are fluorouracil and floxuridine. It should be stressed that this method should be reserved for patients with disease only metastatic to the liver. The benefit of intra-arterial administration of chemotherapy is controversial, and the procedure is associated with severe toxicities, such as injury to the liver and bile ducts, which is sometimes irreversible.[51]

Prognosis

The survival rate of patients with colorectal cancer depends on the stage at diagnosis. When detected at stage I and confined to the bowel mucosa, the 5-year survival rate is >70%. However, if patients present with distant metastases (stage IV), <12% will survive beyond 5 years. Today, oncologists understand the prognostic importance of the presence of muscularis mucosae invasion and the spread to lymph nodes (stage II and III disease), in that these predict the development of recurrent disease. The use of adjuvant chemotherapy in these patients has been the most significant change in clinical practice in the past two decades.

SUMMARY

The search for new approaches to treating patients with non-small cell and small cell lung cancers has led to many clinical trials to answer questions and evaluate the interaction of mul-

Table 11-12. Regimens Established as Superior to Fluorouracil Alone in Advanced Colorectal Cancer

Regimen	Reference
Fluorouracil 425 mg/m^2 + leucovorin 20 mg/m^2, both given by rapid IV injection daily for 5 days every 4–5 weeks	40
Fluorouracil 370 mg/m^2 + leucovorin 200 mg/m^2, both given by rapid IV injection daily for 5 days every 4–5 weeks	40
Fluorouracil 600 mg/m^2 + leucovorin 500 mg/m^2, both given by rapid IV injection weekly for 6 weeks, followed by 2-week rest and then repeated	38
Methotrexate 200 mg/m^2 given in a 4-hour infusion + fluorouracil 1100 mg/m^2 given by rapid IV injection at hour 7 + leucovorin 14 mg/m^2 orally beginning at hour 24 and repeated every 6 hours for 8 doses, repeated every 3–4 weeks	40

SOURCE: adapted from Moertel CG. Chemotherapy for colorectal cancer. *N Engl J Med* 1994;330:1136–42.

tiple treatment modalities. However, lung cancer remains the number one cause of cancer deaths in the United States, and efforts to prevent the disease, such as smoking cessation, should have the highest priority among health professionals.

Colorectal cancer remains the third leading cancer in incidence in the United States. Although earlier screening procedures are being performed and the public has become more aware of the impact of diet on the development of this disease, most patients still present with advanced stages of the disease. The overall prognosis of these patients who are unable to undergo curative surgical resection remains poor despite advances in chemotherapy regimens used to treat the disease.

REFERENCES

1. American Cancer Society [ACS]. Cancer Statistics–1998. Atlanta, GA: ACS; 1998.
2. Ries LAB, Hankey BF, Miller BA, et al. Cancer statistics review for 1973–1988. Bethesda, MD: National Cancer Institute; 1991.
3. American Cancer Society [ACS]. Cancer Facts & Figures–1993. Atlanta, GA: ACS; 1993.
4. Linnoila I. Pathology of non-small cell lung cancer. *Hematol Oncol Clin North Am* 1990;4:1027–51.
5. Loeg LA, Ernst VL, Warner KE, et al. Smoking and lung cancer: an overview. *Cancer Res* 1984;44:5940–58.
6. Stellman SD, Garfinkel L. Smoking habits and tar levels in a new American Cancer Society prospective study of 1.2 million men and women. *J Natl Cancer Inst* 1986;76:1057–63.
7. U.S. Department of Health and Human Services [US DHHS]. The health consequences of involuntary smoking. A report of the Surgeon General. US DHHS, Public Health Service, Office of the Assistant Secretary for Health, Office of Smoking and Health, Washington, DC; 1986.
8. National Research Council Committee on Passive Smoking. Environmental tobacco smoke: measuring exposures and assessing health effects. Washington, DC: Natl Acad Pr; 1986.
9. Melamed MR, Flehinger BN, Zaman MD. Impact of early detection on the clinical course of lung cancer. *Surg Clin North Am* 1987;67:909–24.
10. Tochman MS. Survival and mortality from lung cancer in a screened population: the Johns Hopkins study. *Chest* 1986; 89(*Suppl* 4):324S-5S.
11. Mountain CF. A new international staging system for lung cancer. *Chest* 1986(*Suppl*):225S–33S.
12. Ihde DC, Pars HI, Glatstein EJ. Cancer of the lung. Section 2. Small cell lung cancer. In: DeVita VT, Hellman S, Rosenberg SA, editors. *Cancer: Principles and Practice of Oncology*, 4th ed. Philadelphia, PA: JB Lippincott; 1993. p. 723–58.
13. Non-Small Cell Lung Cancer Collaborative Group. Chemotherapy in non-small cell lung cancer: a meta-analysis using updated data on individual patients from 52 randomized trials. *Br Med J* 1995;311:899–909.
14. Rosell R, Gomez-Codina J, Camps C, et al. A randomized trial comparing preoperative chemotherapy plus surgery with surgery alone in patients with non-small cell lung cancer. *N Engl J Med* 1994;330:153–8.
15. Roth J, Fossella F, Kamaki R, et al. A randomized trial comparing preoperative chemotherapy and surgery with surgery alone in resectable stage III non-small cell lung cancer. *J Natl Cancer Inst* 1994;86:673–80.
16. Pass H, Pogrebniak H, Steinberg S, et al. Randomized trial of neoadjuvant therapy for lung cancer: interim analysis. *Ann Thorac Surg* 1992;53:992–8.
17. Pritchard RS, Anthony SP. Chemotherapy plus radiotherapy compared with radiotherapy alone in the treatment of locally advanced, unresectable, non-small-cell lung cancer: a meta-analysis. *Ann Intern Med* 1996;125:123–9.
18. Ihde DC. Chemotherapy of lung cancer. *N Engl J Med* 1992;327:1434–41.
19. Ihde DC, Minna JD. Non-small cell lung cancer. II. Treatment. *Curr Probl Cancer* 1991;15:105–54.
20. Donnadieu N, Paesmans M, Schulier JP. Chemotherapy of non-small cell lung cancer according to disease extent: a meta-analysis of the literature. *Lung Cancer* 1991;7:243–52.
21. Vogel V, McPherson RS. Dietary epidemiology of colon cancer. *Hematol Oncol Clin North Am* 1989;3:35–63.
22. Whittemore AJ, Wu-Williams AH, Lee M, et al. Diet, physical activity and colorectal cancer among Chinese in North America and China. *J Natl Cancer Inst* 1991;83:359–61.
23. Willett WC, Stampfer MJ, Colditz GA, et al. Relation of meat, fat and fiber intake to the risk of colon cancer in a prospective study. *N Engl J Med* 1990;323:1664–72.
24. Graham S, Marshall J, Haughey B, et al. Dietary epidemiology of cancer of the colon in Western New York. *Am J Epidemiol* 1988;128:490–503.
25. Muto T, Bussey HJR, Morson BC. The evolution of cancer of the colon and rectum. *Cancer* 1975;36:2251–79.
26. Ekbon A, Helmick C, Zack M, et al. Ulcerative colitis and colorectal cancer. *N Engl J Med* 1990;323:1228–33.
27. Lynch HT, Guergis H, Swartz M, et al. Genetics and colon cancer. *Arch Surg* 1973;106:669–75.
28. Thun MJ, Naboodiri MM, Heath CW. Aspirin use and reduced risk of fatal colon cancer. *N Engl J Med* 1991; 325:1593–6.
29. Muscat JE, Stellman SC, Wynder EL. Nonsteroidal anti-inflammatory drugs and colorectal cancer. *Cancer* 1994;74:1847–54.
30. Beart RW. Colorectal cancer. In: Holleg AI, Fink DJ, Murphy GP, editors. *American Cancer Society Textbook of Clinical Oncology*. Atlanta, GA: American Cancer Society; 1991. p. 213–8.
31. Vobecky J, Leduc C, Deverode G. Sex differences in the changing anatomic distribution of colorectal carcinoma. *Cancer* 1984;54:3065–9.
32. Anderson HA, Rosenman KD, Snyder J. Carcinoembryonic antigen (CEA) plasma levels in Michigan and Wisconsin dairy farmers. *Environ Health Perspect* 1978;23:193.
33. National Institutes of Health Consensus Committee on Carcinoembryonic Antigens. Its role as a marker in the management of cancer. *Ann Intern Med* 1981;94:407.
34. Moertel CG, Fleming TR, MacDonald JS, et al. Levamisole and fluorouracil for adjuvant therapy of resected colon carcinoma. *N Engl J Med* 1990;322:352–8.
35. Laurie JA, Moertel CG, Fleming TR, et al. Surgical adjuvant therapy of large-bowel carcinoma: an evaluation of levamisole and the combination of levamisole and fluorouracil: the North Central Cancer Treatment Group and the Mayo Clinic. *J Clin Oncol* 1989;7:1447–56.

36. Kovach JS, Svingen PA, Schaid DJ. Levamisole potentiation of fluorouracil antiproliferative activity mimicked by orthovanadate, an inhibitor of tyrosine phosphatase. *J Natl Cancer Inst* 1989;89:1431–7.
37. National Institutes of Health Consensus Conference. Adjuvant therapy for patients with colon and rectal cancer. *JAMA* 1990;264:1444–50.
38. Gastrointestinal Tumor Study Group. The modulation of fluorouracil with leucovorin in metastatic colorectal carcinoma: a prospective randomized phase III trial. *J Clin Oncol* 1989;7:1419–26.
39. Lokich JJ, Ahlgren JD, Gullo JJ, et al. A prospective randomized comparison of continuous infusion fluorouracil with a conventional bolus schedule in metastatic colorectal carcinoma: a Mid-Atlantic Oncology Program study. *J Clin Oncol* 1989;7:425–32.
40. Poon MA, O'Connell JM, Wieand HS, et al. Biochemical modulation of fluorouracil with leucovorin: confirmatory evidence of improved therapeutic efficacy in advanced colorectal cancer. *J Clin Oncol* 1991;9:1967–72.
41. Jager E, Heike M, Bernhard H, et al. Weekly high-dose leucovorin versus low-dose leucovorin combined with fluorouracil in advanced colorectal cancer: results of a randomized multicenter trial. *J Clin Oncol* 1996;14:2274–9.
42. Wadler S, Schwartz EL, Wersto R, et al. Interferon (IFN) modulates the activity of 5-fluorouracil (5-FU) against two human colon cancer cell lines. *Proc Am Assoc Cancer Res* 1989;30:569.
43. Wadler S, Schwartz EL, Goldman M, et al. 5-Fluorouracil and recombinant alpha-2a-interferon: an active regimen against advanced colorectal carcinoma. *J Clin Oncol* 1989;7:1769–75.
44. Kemeny N, Younes A, Seiter K, et al. Interferon alpha-2a and fluorouracil for advanced colorectal carcinoma: assessment of activity and toxicity. *Cancer* 1990;66:2470–5.
45. Recchia F, Nuzzo A, Lalli A, et al. Randomized trial of 5-fluorouracil and high-dose folinic acid with or without alpha-2B interferon in advanced colorectal cancer. *Am J Clin Oncol* 1996;19:301–4.
46. Conti JA, Kemeny NE, Saltz LB, et al. Irinotecan is an active agent in untreated patients with metastatic colorectal cancer. *J Clin Oncol* 1996;14:709–15.
47. Rothenberg ML, Eckardt JR, Kuhn JG, et al. Phase II trial of irinotecan in patients with progressive or rapidly recurrent colorectal cancer. *J Clin Oncol* 1996;14:1128–35.
48. Kemeny N, Niedzwiecki D, Shurgot B, et al. Prognostic variables in patients with hepatic metastases from colorectal cancer: importance of medical assessment of liver involvement. *Cancer* 1989;63:742–7.
49. Stangl R, Altendorf-Hofmann A, Charnely RM, et al. Factors influencing the natural history of colorectal liver metastases. *Lancet* 1994;343:1405–10.
50. Nordic Gastrointestinal Tumor Adjuvant Therapy Group. Superiority of sequential methotrexate, fluorouracil and leucovorin to fluorouracil alone in advanced symptomatic colorectal carcinoma: a randomized trial. *J Clin Oncol* 1989;7:1437–46.
51. Hohn D, Melnick J, Stagg R, et al. Biliary sclerosis in patients receiving hepatic arterial infusions of floxuridine. *J Clin Oncol* 1985;3:98–102.

SELF-STUDY QUESTIONS

1. Which of the following are risk factors for the development of lung cancer?
    a. male sex, tobacco smoking, age >50
    b. female sex, tobacco smoking, age >60
    c. number of years of cigarette smoking, number of cigarettes smoked per day, tar and nicotine content of cigarettes smoked
    d. family history of lung cancer, cigarette smoking, age >50
    e. history of colon cancer, male sex, age >50

2. Which of the following are risk factors for the development of colorectal cancer?
    a. diet low in fiber, familial polyposis, history of ulcerative colitis
    b. diet high in fiber, familial polyposis, history of ulcerative colitis
    c. diet high in fiber, history of ulcerative colitis, history of Crohn's disease
    d. diet high in fat, male sex, age >30
    e. diet low in fiber, female sex, age >30

3. Which of the following is NOT a sign or symptom of lung cancer?
    a. weight loss
    b. hoarseness
    c. shoulder and/or arm pain
    d. hemoptysis
    e. increased heart rate

4. What are the most common signs and symptoms of colorectal cancer?
    a. changes in bowel habits
    b. rectal bleeding
    c. abdominal pain
    d. all of the above
    e. none of the above

5. Small cell lung cancer (SCLC) has a tendency to be more rapidly proliferating than non-small cell lung cancer (NSCLC).
    a. true
    b. false

6. The staging system for SCLC:
    a. is the same as the staging system for non-small cell lung cancer.
    b. utilizes the T, N, and M system.

c. includes four stages: I, II, III, and IV.
d. is based on the cell cycling time of the tumor.
e. consists of two stages: limited stage and extensive stage.

7. Colorectal cancer staging using the TNM system is also known as the "Dukes' staging system."

    a. true
    b. false

8. The type of lung cancer most likely to be cured by surgery is:

    a. stage I NSCLC.
    b. limited-stage SCLC.
    c. stage IIIb NSCLC.
    d. extensive-stage SCLC.
    e. No lung cancer is ever cured by surgery.

9. The most active agents used to treat lung cancer include:

    a. cisplatin, etoposide, and cytarabine.
    b. cisplatin, cytarabine, and paclitaxel.
    c. carboplatin, paclitaxel, and pentostatin.
    d. cisplatin, etoposide, and paclitaxel.
    e. carboplatin, etoposide, and chlorambucil.

10. The NIH Consensus Conference recommendation for the treatment of stage III colon cancer is to use adjuvant therapy with:

    a. fluorouracil alone.
    b. fluorouracil plus levamisole.
    c. fluorouracil plus leucovorin.
    d. flourouracil plus interferon.
    e. No adjuvant therapy is recommended outside of a clinical trial.

11. Which of the following paraneoplastic syndromes is not commonly found in patients with advanced lung cancer?

    a. hypercalcemia
    b. syndrome of inappropriate secretion of antidiuretic hormone (SIADH)
    c. hyperkalemia
    d. Cushing's syndrome
    e. none of the above

12. The toxicities of combination leucovorin with fluorouracil for the adjuvant treatment of colorectal cancer can include:

    a. severe diarrhea.
    b. mucositis.
    c. myelosuppression.
    d. renal failure.
    e. a, b, and c.

Chapter 12
Management of Breast and Prostate Cancers

Carol Balmer, Pharm.D.
Associate Professor
University of Colorado School of Pharmacy
Denver, Colorado

Marianne Irani, Pharm.D.
Clinical Oncology Specialist
University of Pennsylvania Health System
Philadelphia, Pennsylvania

Breast Cancer 212
    Anatomy, Pathophysiology, and Etiology 212
    Pathology 213
    Clinical Presentation and Natural History 213
    Screening and Diagnosis 214
    Staging and Prognosis 214
    Treatment 215
        Local and Regional Breast Cancer 215
        Advanced Disease 217
    Prevention 218
Prostate Cancer 219
    Anatomy, Pathophysiology, and Etiology 219
    Clinical Presentation and Natural History 220
    Screening and Diagnosis 220
    Staging and Prognosis 221
    Treatment 222
        Localized Disease 222
        Locally Advanced Disease 223
        Metastatic Disease 223
    Prevention 226
Summary 226
References 227
Self-Study Questions 228

Breast and prostate cancers are the two most common cancers in the United States. Together, these cancers account for more than one quarter of all new cancer diagnoses each year. Each of these cancers arises from hormone-dependent tissue, and in most cases the malignant tissue retains that hormonal dependence. Because of this dependence, hormonal manipulation becomes an important treatment option for patients with these diseases. Their hormonal dependence also opens new avenues for prevention of these common cancers.

After completing this chapter, the reader will be able to:

1. Identify populations at high risk for developing breast or prostate cancers.
2. Discuss the pathophysiology and natural history of breast and prostate cancers.
3. Outline the clinical staging of breast and prostate cancers and describe how the clinical stage of disease affects management choices.
4. Compare the risks and benefits of adjuvant treatment in the management of breast cancer.
5. Outline a management plan for a patient with metastatic breast cancer who is hormone receptor positive or hormone receptor negative.
6. Outline a treatment plan for a patient with metastatic prostate cancer that includes first-line hormonal therapy, second-line hormonal interventions, and management of hormone-refractory disease.

BREAST CANCER

Breast cancer is the most common malignancy in North American women, representing about 30% of reported cancers. The American Cancer Society (ACS) estimates that approximately 180,000 women will be diagnosed with breast cancer in 1998. About 25% of these women (43,500) will die of the disease. Only lung cancer causes more cancer-related deaths among women.[1] The odds of developing breast cancer have increased steadily in the last two decades. In 1975 it was estimated that 1 in 14 women in the United States would develop breast cancer in her lifetime. Estimates in 1998 state that 1 in 8 women will develop breast cancer.[1-4] Despite the increase in incidence, age-adjusted mortality has decreased only slightly in the United States, perhaps because of earlier detection, advances in treatment, or increased detection of more benign forms of the disease.[2-4] Breast cancer is rare in males, with approximately 1600 cases diagnosed per year in the United States.[1]

Anatomy, Pathophysiology, and Etiology

Adult female breast tissue is mainly composed of milk-producing epithelial ducts, which terminate in secretory alveoli or lobules. These ducts are embedded in a framework of fibrous tissue and fat (Figure 12-1).

Normal breast growth and development are regulated by a complex interaction of hormones and growth factors. Some of these include estrogens, progesterone, androgens, glucocorticoids, prolactin, thyroid hormone, insulin and the insulin-like growth factors, epidermal growth factors, transforming growth factor alpha (TGF-α), and other more recently identified polypeptides. Both normal breast tissue growth and cancerous growth are regulated by these hormones and growth factors.[2,3,6]

Although the cause of most breast cancers is unknown, many risk factors have been identified. Some factors associated with an increased risk of breast cancer include personal or family history of breast cancer, reproductive and menstrual histories, age, diet, geographic factors, and radiation exposure. The impact of chronic hormonal administration in the form of oral contraceptives or hormone replacement therapy has been evaluated in many studies, and it has proved to be a very small risk factor for women without other factors that increase their risk of breast cancer. Table 12-1 indicates the impact of a variety of environmental factors on a woman's risk of de-

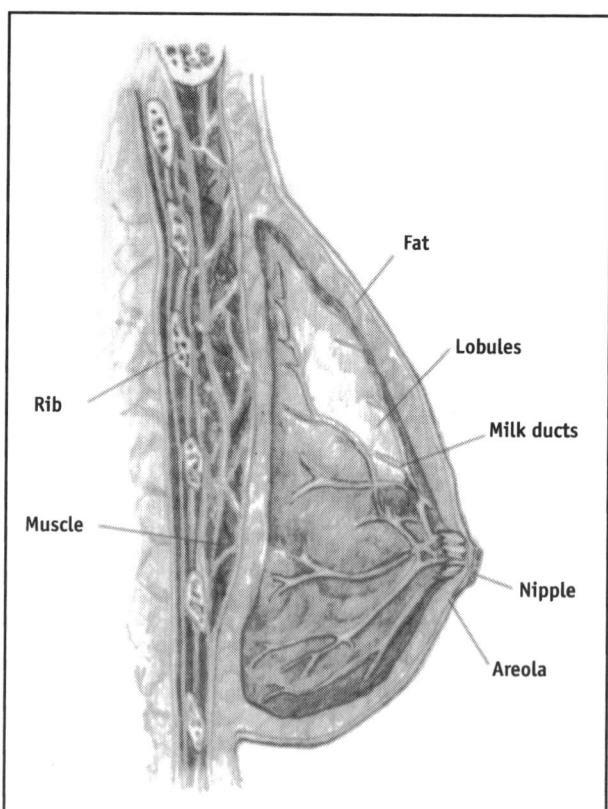

Figure 12-1. Anatomy of the female breast

SOURCE: reprinted with permission from Singletary SE, Judkins AF. *Breast Cancer: Myths and Facts*. Huntington, NY: PRR Inc.; 1997. p. 4.

Table 12-1. Summary of Environmental Risk Factors for Breast Cancer[a]

Factors Influencing Risk	Estimated Relative Risk
ESTABLISHED RISK FACTORS	
Older ages (65–69 versus 30–34 y.o.)	17
Residency in North America or Europe versus Asia	4–5
Residency in urban areas	1.5
Higher educational status or family income	1.5
Mother or sister with breast cancer	2–3
Nulliparity or late age at first birth (≥30 versus <20 y.o.)	2–3
Absence of breast-feeding for long durations	1.5
Early age at menarche (<12 versus ≥15 y.o.)	1.5
Late age at menopause (≥55 versus natural menopause at <45 y.o. or removal of ovaries at a comparable age)	2
Biopsy-confirmed proliferative breast disease	2–4
Mammographically dense breasts	2–4
Obesity (postmenopausal only) (≥200 versus <125 lb)	2
Tallness (≥68 versus <62 in.)	1.5–2
Radiation to chest in moderate to high doses	2–4
History of breast cancer in one breast	2–4
History of primary cancer in endometrium or ovary	1.5–2
SPECULATIVE RISK FACTORS	
Induced abortions or miscarriages	?
Infertility and associated treatment	?
Prenatal conditions involving high in utero estrogen levels	?
Postnatal exposures (breast-feeding)	?
Electromagnetic fields	?
Excessive light exposure	?
Restricted solar or vitamin D exposure	?
Organochlorines	?

SOURCE: reprinted with permission from Brinton LA, Devesa SS. Etiology and pathogenesis of breast cancer. Epidemiologic factors. Incidence, demographics, and environmental factors. In: Harris JR, Lippman ME, Morrow M, et al., editors. *Diseases of the Breast*. Philadelphia, PA: Lippincott-Raven; 1996. p. 166.
[a]Hormonal and dietary factors are not included in this table.

veloping breast cancer. Data is presented as relative risk, a figure that compares the risk of breast cancer in women who demonstrate that factor with average breast cancer risk, which is considered a risk of one. A relative risk of 1.5, for example, indicates that the woman's risk of breast cancer is 1.5 times higher than that of the average female. This can also be viewed as a 50% increase in risk compared with the average woman. Despite the many known risk factors for breast cancer, most women who are diagnosed with breast cancer have no identifiable risk factors other than the fact that they are from developed countries.[2,3]

Recently, genetic abnormalities associated with hereditary breast cancer risk have been identified. *BRCA1* and *BRCA2*, named after the first letters of *br*east *ca*ncer, are breast cancer susceptibility genes. *BRCA1* was identified in 1994. Women with inherited mutations in *BRCA1* have an 85% lifetime risk of breast cancer (and a 40–50% risk of ovarian cancer), compared with a 12% risk in the general female population. *BRCA2* mutations also increase risk. Both genes appear to be tumor suppressor genes. Mutations in either gene interfere with the normal ability of tumor suppressor genes to block the development of breast cancer.[5]

Pathology

Breast cancers can be classified as noninvasive (confined to the lumen of the breast ducts) or invasive (extending beyond the lumen of the breast ducts). Noninvasive breast cancers are referred to as *carcinoma in situ*. Ductal cancer (*ductal carcinoma in situ* or DCIS) is the most common form of noninvasive breast cancer. The most common form of invasive breast cancer is infiltrating ductal (also called intraductal) carcinoma, which accounts for about 75% of breast cancers. Infiltrating lobular carcinoma accounts for about 10% of invasive breast cancers. Other unusual forms of breast cancer include Paget's disease, inflammatory breast carcinoma, and a variety of other pathological forms.[2,3]

Clinical Presentation and Natural History

Breast cancers are typically noted as a mass or lump in one breast, discovered by the patient or by a health care practitioner. The lump is usually painless and hard. It feels solid, is often an irregular shape, and is not easily movable. Signs of more advanced disease include nipple retraction, nipple discharge, and skin changes (such as dimpling). Breast cancer can spread locally by direct infiltration into the breast tissue, along the mammary ducts, and through the lymphatic vessels. Regional spread most commonly involves axillary, internal mammary, and supraclavicular lymph nodes. About half of patients have evidence of spread to nearby axillary lymph nodes at the time of diagnosis.

The most common sites of metastasis are lymph nodes, lungs, liver, bone, and brain.[3] Patients with metastatic disease at the time of diagnosis may present with symptoms relating to the organ affected, such as bone pain, dyspnea as a symptom of lung involvement, abdominal pain from liver involvement, or nausea and vomiting, which may indicate the presence of brain metastases.[2] Less common forms of breast cancer may present very differently. Inflammatory changes of the breast skin, such as redness, warmth, edema and erythema, and induration of the underlying tissue, characterize inflammatory breast cancer. It may be misdiagnosed as a breast infection. Paget's disease of the breast usually presents with a long history of eczematous changes in the nipple area that included itching, redness, burning, and/or bleeding.[2,3]

Screening and Diagnosis

The purpose of screening is earlier detection of breast cancer, with the goal of decreased mortality from the disease. The main methods for early detection are monthly breast self-exam, physical examination by a health care professional experienced in breast exam, and mammography.[5] Monthly breast self-examination is strongly encouraged for all women over the age of 20.[7] However, there is much debate about the age at which mammographic screening should begin. Currently, ACS and the National Cancer Institute (NCI) recommend screening with mammography and clinical breast examination every year for women 40 years of age and older, even though the value of routine screening mammography for women 40–49 years of age continues to be debated.[8]

Diagnostic work-up of a breast lump includes several components. A careful patient history is taken to assess risk factors. Detailed physical examination of the breast and axillary and supraclavicular lymph nodes is performed. A mammogram is obtained to investigate any clinical abnormalities. Breast ultrasound may be useful to distinguish solid from fluid-filled masses. Fluid-filled masses are usually benign cysts. Fine needle aspiration biopsy of the mass is a minimally invasive procedure that can confirm the diagnosis of breast cancer in 95% of malignant lumps. Its usefulness, however, is limited by sampling error, since only a small portion of the tissue is evaluated. The definitive diagnostic test is excisional biopsy, in which the mass is removed surgically and sent for histopathological evaluation.[2,3]

Staging and Prognosis

The natural history of breast cancer varies considerably from patient to patient. Some patients are initially diagnosed with very indolent or slowly growing disease, and others may present with aggressive, rapidly growing breast cancer. A prognostic factor is a measurement available at the time of diagnosis or surgical treatment of the breast cancer that can help predict the natural history of the tumor for that individual patient.

Several pathological tests that provide prognostic information can be performed on the biopsy tissue sample. Tissue is assayed for the presence or absence of estrogen receptors (ERs) and progesterone receptors (PgRs). Tumors that are ER and/or PgR positive tend to be slower growing, less aggressive tumors than those that are ER and/or PgR negative. Other tissue assessments include histological subtype (type of tissue) and histological grade (degree of differentiation of the cancer cells). Well-differentiated or low-grade tumors generally grow more slowly and are less likely to spread than poorly differentiated or high-grade tumors. The proliferation rate of malignant cells is extrapolated from the S-phase fraction—the percentage of breast cancer cells in the active synthesis, or S phase, of growth—or from the mitotic index, an indicator of the proportion of cells that are actively dividing. A high S-phase fraction or mitotic index indicates that tumor growth rate is rapid. Prognosis also depends on tumor size. Small tumors have better prognoses than large tumors, with tumors <1 cm in diameter having the best prognosis. Perhaps the most important assessments are whether the cancer has spread to axillary lymph nodes and the number of lymph nodes involved. Five-year disease-free survival decreases dramatically as the number of lymph nodes involved with breast cancer increases (Figure 12-2).[9] Some other important prognostic factors include ploidy (whether the number of chromosomes in the tumor cells is normal or abnormal); the degree of angiogenesis (new blood vessel growth); *HER2/neu* gene (an oncogene related to epidermal growth factor) amplification; and mutations of tumor suppressor genes, such as *p53*.[3,9]

Staging refers to the grouping of patients according to the extent of their disease. In breast cancer, two staging systems are used: the first classifies disease as stages I–IV; the second is a TNM staging system. The TNM system classifies cancers based on tumor size (T), lymph node involvement (N), and presence or absence of metastatic disease (M). Table 12-2 combines these two staging systems. The patient's stage is an important prognostic factor. Five-year survival decreases from 90% for patients with stage I breast cancer to 70, 50, and 15% for patients with stage II, III, and IV disease, respectively.[10] Staging is also used to help determine the most appropriate treatment.

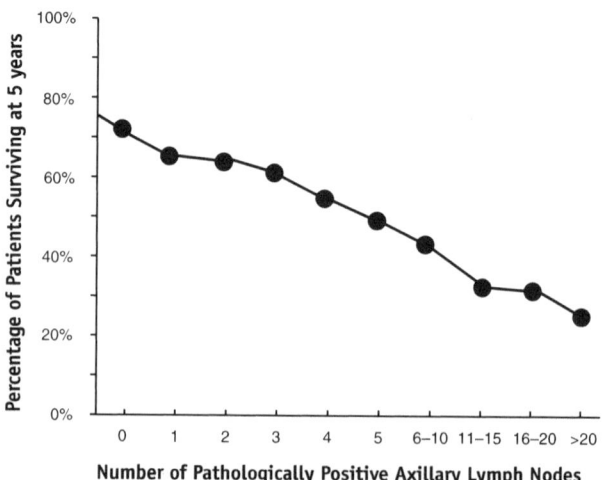

Figure 12-2. Five-year disease-free survival versus the number of pathologically positive axillary lymph nodes in breast cancer patients

SOURCE: data from reference 3.

Table 12-2. Stage Grouping for Breast Cancer

Stage	
Stage I	Tumor ≤2 cm in diameter (T1) No evident involvement of lymph nodes (N0) No distant metastases (M0)
Stage II$_A$	Tumor ≤5 cm in diameter (T0, 1, or 2) May be evidence of axillary lymph node involvement (N0 or 1) No distant metastases (M0)
Stage II$_B$	Tumor 2–5 cm in diameter (T2) Evidence of axillary lymph node involvement (N1) or tumor >5 cm in diameter with no evidence of lymph node involvement (N0) No distant metastases (M0)
Stage III$_A$	Tumor >5 cm in diameter (T1, 2, or 3) Evidence of axillary lymph node involvement (N1 or 2) No distant metastases (M0)
Stage III$_B$	Tumor of any size (T1–4) with mammary lymph node involvement (N3) or tumor directly extended to chest wall and skin (T4) Any lymph node involvement (N1, 2, or 3) No distant metastases (M0)
Stage IV	Tumor of any size (T1–4) Evidence of lymph node involvement (any N) Evidence of distant metastases (M1)

SOURCE: adapted from reference 3.

Treatment

Current treatment modalities for breast cancer include surgery, radiation therapy, systemic therapy with antineoplastic or hormonal agents, or combinations of these modalities. Treatment is divided into two types, treatment of local and/or regional breast cancer, and treatment of advanced disease.

Local and Regional Breast Cancer

Modified radical mastectomy and lumpectomy followed by radiation therapy are the primary treatment modalities for early-stage breast cancer (stages I and II). Radical mastectomy involves the removal of the whole breast, the skin overlying the tumor, the pectoralis major and minor muscles (which underlie the breast), and all the axillary contents. This invasive surgery produces a high incidence of arm swelling, shoulder dysfunction, and cosmetic defect. Radical mastectomy has been replaced by modified radical mastectomy. This procedure involves removal of the entire breast and some or all of the axillary lymph nodes. The pectoralis major muscle is preserved. Modified radical mastectomy is associated with a much lower risk of complications.

Lumpectomy involves excision of the entire tumor with a margin of surrounding normal tissue. This procedure allows breast conservation, provided the tumor is not large relative to the size of the breast.[2,3] Because of a high risk of local recurrence associated with lumpectomy alone, it must be followed by radiation therapy to the remaining breast tissue, to destroy any undetected residual cancer cells.[11] Randomized clinical trials with large numbers of patients and long follow-up have shown that total mastectomy and lumpectomy with radiation therapy result in identical survival rates.[11–13] An investigational treatment involves administering chemotherapy prior to lumpectomy to decrease the size of breast masses and permit more conservative surgery.[3]

Despite mastectomy or lumpectomy plus radiation, about 30% of women with stage I breast cancer and 60% of women with stage II disease will eventually have clinical recurrence of breast cancer. Because metastatic breast cancer remains incurable, these women will eventually die of the disease. Adjuvant systemic therapy can reduce the recurrence rate and increase both disease-free and overall survival in patients with early-stage breast cancer by destroying or controlling the growth of micrometastases (Figure 12-3).

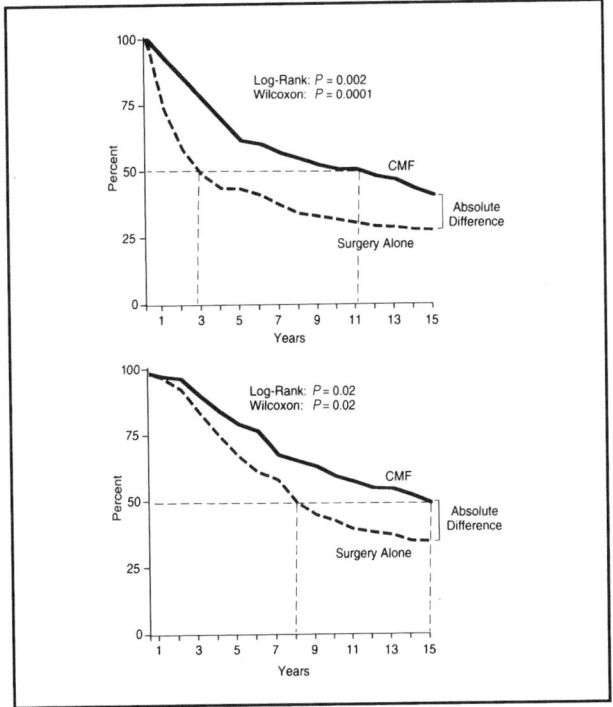

Figure 12-3. Kaplan-Meier plot of relapse-free survival (*top*) and overall survival (*bottom*) in premenopausal patients in the first Milan study of adjuvant cyclophosphamide + methotrexate + fluorouracil (CMF) therapy.

SOURCE: reprinted with permission from Osborne KC, Clark GM, Ravdin PM. Adjuvant systemic therapy of primary breast cancer. In: Harris JR, Lippman ME, Morrow M, et al., editors. *Diseases of the Breast*. Philadelphia, PA: Lippincott-Raven; 1996. p. 549.

Adjuvant therapy reduces but does not eliminate the risk of breast cancer recurrence. In general, the recurrence rate is decreased by 20–30% in either stage I (node negative) or stage II (node positive) disease. Breast cancer patients with very small tumors (<1 cm) and good prognostic factors have a very low chance of recurrence and may not be offered systemic adjuvant therapy, except as part of a clinical trial.[14]

Combination chemotherapy, hormonal therapy, or both may be administered for adjuvant breast cancer therapy. Combination chemotherapy is most effective in hormone-receptor-negative patients, who are usually premenopausal. Hormonal therapy has a greater effect in hormone-receptor-positive women, who are usually postmenopausal.[15,16]

The ER antagonist tamoxifen is the most widely used hormonal adjuvant therapy. The benefits of tamoxifen are greater for patients with ER-positive tumors than for those with ER-negative tumors. It is well tolerated and has positive effects on bone density[17] and blood lipid levels.[18] The most frequently reported side effects are menopausal symptoms, such as hot flashes and irregular menses. Chronic tamoxifen therapy has been clearly associated with an increased incidence of endometrial cancer. The risk rises with each year of treatment, which indicates the need for regular gynecological examination. Although the clinical benefits of tamoxifen

Table 12-3. Chemotherapy Regimens Used in the Adjuvant Therapy of Breast Cancer

Regimen	Dose and Schedule	Frequency (days)	Number of Cycles
CMF (STANDARD)			
Cyclophosphamide	100 mg/m² per day PO × 14 days	28	6
Methotrexate	40 mg/m² IV days 1 and 8	28	6
Fluorouracil	600 mg/m² IV days 1 and 8	28	6
CMF (IV; TESTED IN NODE-NEGATIVE PATIENTS ONLY)			
Cyclophosphamide	600 mg/m² IV	21	12
Methotrexate	40 mg/m² IV	21	12
Fluorouracil	600 mg/m² IV	21	12
CMFVP			
Cyclophosphamide	60 mg/m² per day PO	1	1 yr
Fluorouracil	400 mg/m² IV	7	1 yr
Methotrexate	15 mg/m²	7	1 yr
Vincristine	0.625 mg/m²	weekly × 10 doses	
Prednisone	30 mg/m² tapering over 10 wk		
CAF			
Cyclophosphamide	100 mg/m² per day PO × 14 days	28	6
Doxorubicin	30 mg/m² IV days 1 and 8	28	6
Fluorouracil	500 mg/m² IV days 1 and 8	28	6
CAF			
Cyclophosphamide	600 mg/m² per day IV day 1	21–28	4–6
Doxorubicin	60 mg/m² IV day 1	21–28	4–6
Fluorouracil	600 mg/m² IV days 1 and 8	21–28	4–6
AC			
Doxorubicin	60 mg/m² IV day 1	21	4
Cyclophosphamide	600 mg/m² day 1	21	4
A→CMF (TESTED IN NODE-POSITIVE PATIENTS ONLY)			
Doxorubicin	75 mg/m² IV day 1	21	4 (cycles 1–4)
Cyclophosphamide	600 mg/m² IV	21	8 (cycles 5–12)
Methotrexate	40 mg/m² IV	21	8 (cycles 5–12)
Fluorouracil	600 mg/m² IV	21	8 (cycles 5–12)

SOURCE: reprinted with permission from Osborne KC, Clark GM, Ravdin PM. Adjuvant systemic therapy of primary breast cancer. In: Harris JR, Lippman ME, Morrow M, et al., editors. *Diseases of the Breast*. Philadelphia, PA: Lippincott-Raven; 1996. p. 562. PO, orally; IV, intravenous.

continue to outweigh its adverse effects, its potentially serious carcinogenic effects raise caution for long-term therapy (>5 years) or use for noncancerous conditions (such as breast cancer prevention).[15] A variety of more selective estrogen receptor modulators (SERMs) are under evaluation.

The most common chemotherapy regimens for adjuvant breast cancer treatment are outlined in Table 12-3. Several useful guidelines for administration of adjuvant chemotherapy have evolved. Combination regimens are more effective than single agents. Administration of full doses of chemotherapy is associated with greater decreases in breast cancer recurrence rates and improved overall survival, compared with compromised drug doses. Six months of chemotherapy is as useful as 12 months, and newer regimens are exploring shorter durations of therapy.[14,15]

The toxic effects of adjuvant chemotherapy are greater than those of hormonal therapy and must be weighed against the potential benefits. In general, most patients maintain a reasonable quality of life. The most common short-term adverse effects include nausea and vomiting, alopecia, neutropenia, weight gain, and fatigue. Chemotherapy-induced secondary leukemias occur at a rate of 5 in 10,000 patients who are treated for 6 months with a cyclophosphamide-containing regimen.[15]

Combinations of hormonal therapy and chemotherapy have been evaluated. The advantage of adding tamoxifen to adjuvant chemotherapy in ER-positive patients is well established. Although the incremental benefit varies by hormone receptor status and presence or absence of positive lymph nodes, recent evidence suggests that all ER-negative patients with stage I or II breast cancer can derive some benefit from combined therapy with chemotherapy and tamoxifen.[19]

High-dose chemotherapy with autologous stem cell rescue is under investigation as a form of very aggressive adjuvant chemotherapy for patients with a high risk of experiencing recurrence of their disease (usually patients with >10 positive nodes).

Stage III breast cancer is classified as an extensive local-regional disease. Stage III disease is treated with mastectomy, primary radiation, chemotherapy, or a combination of these modalities. Systemic chemotherapy may be administered prior to mastectomy or radiation to shrink the tumor mass. This use of chemotherapy is called primary chemotherapy, neoadjuvant therapy, or preoperative chemotherapy. Successful neoadjuvant chemotherapy may shrink the tumor mass enough to make it possible to perform lumpectomy and radiation rather than mastectomy, conserving the breast.

Advanced Disease

The goal in treating metastatic breast cancer (stage IV disease) is palliation of symptoms, since current medical practice cannot cure this condition. Median survival following diagnosis of metastatic disease is 2–3 years. Treatment interventions may involve surgery, hormonal manipulations, radiation therapy, and/or chemotherapy. Hormonal manipulation

Table 12-4. Relationship Between Estrogen and Progesterone Receptor Status of Breast Tumor and the Patient's Objective Response to Endocrine Therapy

Hormone Receptor Status	Chance of Response (%)
ER + / PgR +	78
ER − / PgR +	45
ER + / PgR −	34
ER − / PgR −	10

SOURCE: reprinted with permission from Flamm HS. Treatment of metastatic disease: hormonal therapy and chemotherapy. In: Harris JR, Lippman ME, Morrow M, et al., editors. *Diseases of the Breast*. Philadelphia, PA: Lippincott-Raven; 1996. p. 675. ER, estrogen receptor; PgR, progesterone receptor.

and chemotherapy are the major treatment modalities for the management of metastatic breast cancer. Their use can prolong symptom-free intervals and improve quality of life.[2,3] Weighing potential drug toxicities against potential benefits and documenting continued response to treatment is of utmost importance to ensure that benefit exceeds the risks of adverse effects from ineffective therapy.

Hormonal therapy is the first-line treatment for women whose tumors express ERs and/or PgRs, because it is less toxic than chemotherapy. Women whose breast tumors express high levels of both receptors have the best chance of response to hormonal therapy (Table 12-4). Note that a few patients who do not express hormone receptors may respond to hormonal intervention.

The best candidates for hormonal therapy are patients with slow-growing disease in bone or soft tissue metastatic sites who had a long (>2 years) disease-free interval following surgical removal of their primary breast cancer (Table 12-5).

A variety of endocrine manipulations can be used to treat breast cancer. The choice of initial hormonal therapy depends somewhat on the patient's age and menopausal status. Tamoxifen is the most commonly used first-line agent in postmenopausal patients. Women who have received tamoxifen as adjuvant hormonal therapy are unlikely to respond to tamoxifen for management of metastatic disease, although its use may be attempted in women who have not received tamoxifen for more than 1 year. For premenopausal women, surgical removal of the ovaries (ovariectomy or oophorectomy) is sometimes recommended as first-line endocrine treatment. Pharmacologic ovariectomy with gonadotropin-releasing hormone agonists, such as leuprolide or goserelin, is an alternative to ovariectomy.[3]

There are many choices for second- and third-line hormonal therapy in ER- and PgR-positive patients who respond to, and then later fail, first-line endocrine therapy. Progestins, such as megestrol acetate or medroxyprogesterone acetate, have traditionally been used as second-line therapy. The selective aromatase inhibitors, such as anastrozole and letrozole, have recently been approved by the FDA. Aromatase mediates the

Table 12-5. General Criteria to Select Patients for Endocrine Manipulations or Chemotherapy for Management of Metastatic Breast Cancer

Hormone Therapy	Chemotherapy
Slow-growing disease	Rapidly growing disease
Soft tissue and/or bone metastases	Massive liver involvement or lung or skin involvement with lymphangitic metastases
Disease-free interval of >2 years following mastectomy or lumpectomy	Disease-free interval of <2 years
Age >35 years	Any age group
ER-positive tumor	ER-negative tumor
Objective response to prior hormonal manipulations	Negative response to first hormonal manipulations

SOURCE: adapted from reference 2.

conversion of androgen substrates to estrogens. By inhibiting estrogen production, these agents provide another treatment option for patients who have become resistant to tamoxifen. Unlike aminoglutethimide, a nonspecific aromatase inhibitor, anastrozole does not lead to secondary reductions of adrenal steroids or aldosterone, so corticosteroid replacement therapy is not required.[20] Other hormonal alternatives are the SERMs toremifene and raloxifene, androgen therapy (such as fluoxymesterone), and high doses of estrogens.

Hormonal therapies usually produce slow responses, over ≥1 month. Although hormonal therapy is usually the treatment of choice for most patients with receptor-positive disease, the slow response time makes it inappropriate for women with rapidly growing, aggressive cancer. For these patients, chemotherapy should be considered as initial treatment, regardless of their receptor status (Table 12-5). All the agents that are useful as adjuvant chemotherapy are effective in management of metastatic disease. Doxorubicin had traditionally been accepted as the most effective single agent in this setting, with an objective response rate of about 40%. Paclitaxel,[21,22] docetaxel,[23] and vinorelbine[3] are the newest agents with proven effectiveness in the treatment of metastatic breast cancer. These agents have been shown to produce response rates similar to (and in the case of docetaxel, greater than) those of doxorubicin and are considered good second-line chemotherapy choices for patients who have failed doxorubicin. An increasing body of literature supports use of paclitaxel or docetaxel as first-line therapy of metastatic breast cancer patients.[22,23]

Although it is currently used widely in the United States, high-dose therapy with autologous bone marrow transplantation or stem cell support continues to be under investigation in comparative trials against standard regimens for the management of advanced disease. Evidence from these studies suggests that a small percentage of patients are long-term survivors following bone marrow transplantation and may prove to be cured of disease as follow-up of these studies matures.[3]

Radiation therapy and surgery are used to palliate localized areas of metastatic disease. For example, breast cancer that has destroyed a weight-bearing bone, such as a femur, may be managed surgically with a prosthetic implant to reduce pain and the risk of fracture. Radiation therapy is used for patients with brain metastases or compression from spinal metastases. It should also be considered for patients with severe bone pain unresponsive to standard analgesic therapy. Radioactive bone-seeking agents, such as strontium-89, can be of benefit as an alternative to external-beam radiation therapy. However, the onset of pain relief may be delayed. The predominant toxicity of strontium-89 is hematological damage, with thrombocytopenia occurring in 20% of patients.[24]

Pamidronate, a bisphosphonate originally approved for the management of hypercalcemia, given as monthly infusions, has been shown to delay further development of skeletal complications and alleviate bone pain in women with breast cancer that has metastasized to bones. Benefits are seen in patients receiving either chemotherapy or hormonal therapy. Adverse effects most commonly reported include fever and generalized pain.[25]

Prevention

Women at very high risk of breast cancer, such as those with a strong family history of breast cancer or those with genetic markers, may consider prophylactic mastectomy with reconstruction as an alternative to living with the prospect of developing breast cancer. Prophylactic mastectomies dramatically decrease but do not completely eliminate the risk of breast cancer. Small amounts of breast tissue may remain, or breast cancer cells may have shed from undetected cancers before the breasts were removed.[26] Chemoprevention, the use of drugs to prevent the development of the cancer, is being studied for high-risk patients. The two main agents being evaluated are tamoxifen and raloxifene. A large randomized controlled trial comparing tamoxifen and placebo for breast cancer prevention in women at increased risk indicated a 45% reduction in risk of invasive breast cancer among women receiving tamoxifen.[27] The SERM raloxifene also significantly reduced the risk of breast cancer for postmenopausal women, with less risk of secondary endometrial cancer than tamoxifen.[28] A chemoprevention trial comparing tamoxifen and raloxifene in women at risk for breast cancer is under way.

PROSTATE CANCER

Prostate cancer is the most common neoplasm in American males. In 1998, about 184,500 men will be diagnosed with prostate cancer, and about 39,200 men will die of the disease.[1] The incidence of prostate cancer increased rapidly between 1993 and 1996; 165,000 new cases were diagnosed in 1993, 244,000 in 1994, and 317,000 in 1996.[1,29] Much of the increase is explained by improved methods of detection. Prostate cancer can now be diagnosed in patients without clinical evidence of disease who would previously have remained undiagnosed. In 1997, a downward adjustment was made in the annual estimate of prostate cancer to account for plateauing of the rapid rise in prostate cancer diagnoses attributable to better detection methods.[29] This factor accounts for only part of the increase in incidence; some of the remainder is explained by the increasing age of the male population.

Anatomy, Pathophysiology, and Etiology

The prostate is a small, encapsulated gland located just below the neck of the bladder, surrounding the urethra (Figure 12-4). Its posterior lobe lies slightly above the rectum. The prostate produces prostatic fluid, a milky liquid that contributes to the volume of ejaculate.

Both normal and cancerous prostate growths are stimulated by androgens. Testosterone accounts for 90–95% of circulating androgens in males and is produced primarily by the testes. Testosterone is converted to dihydrotestosterone (DHT) within prostate tissue by the enzyme 5-alpha reductase. DHT is the primary androgen affecting both normal and cancerous prostate cells. A small proportion of androgens is produced by the adrenal glands.

Most prostate cancers arise in the posterior lobe of the prostate, nearest to the rectum, and are classified as adenocarcinomas. They are graded pathologically based on the degree of differentiation of the cancer cells. Cells closely resembling normal prostate tissue are classified as well differentiated. Those with little resemblance are classified as poorly differentiated. The most widely accepted histological grading system for prostate cancer is the Gleason grading system (Figure 12-5). Tumor samples each receive two scores of 1 to 5 that are added to make the total Gleason score. A Gleason score of 2 indicates a very well-differentiated tumor; the most poorly differentiated tumors receive a 10.[30]

Both normal and cancerous prostate tissues produce a glycoprotein called prostate-specific antigen (PSA). PSA is produced exclusively by prostate tissue and circulates in the blood. It has many useful roles in the screening, diagnosis, monitoring, and management of prostate disorders.[31,32]

The cause of prostate cancer is not known. Androgens appear to be necessary for the development of prostate cancer, since it is not known to occur in eunuchs. Prostate cancer

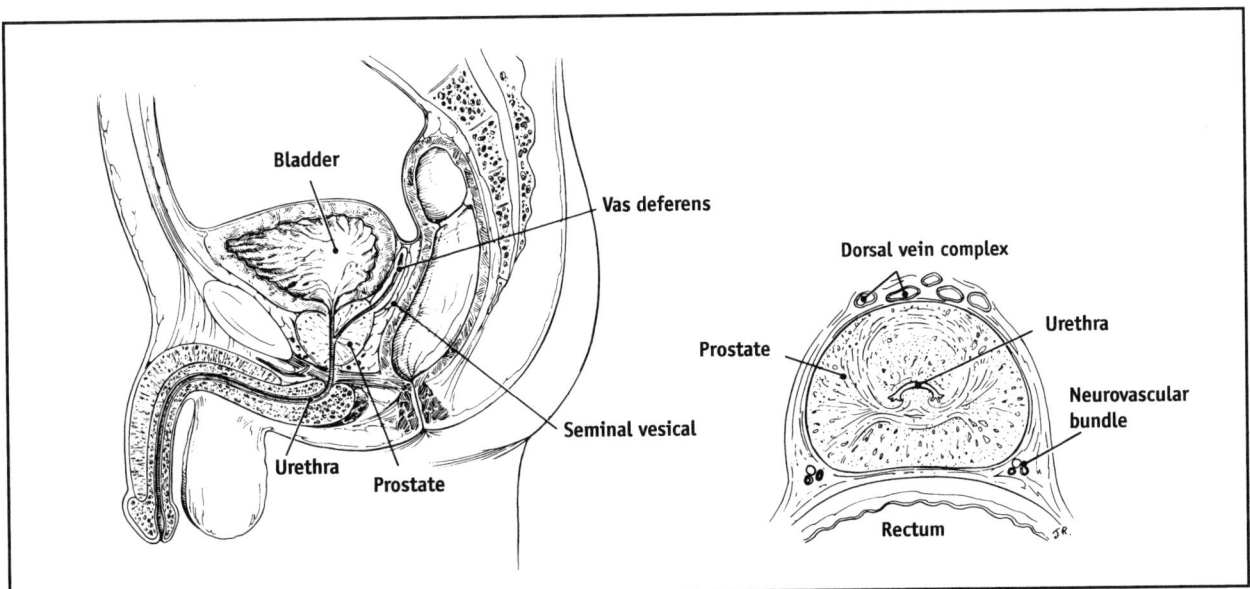

Figure 12-4. Male anatomy of the pelvis (*left*) and transverse section through the midportion of the prostate gland (*right*).
SOURCE: reprinted with permission from Hanks GE, Myers CE, Scardino PT. Cancer of the prostate. In: DeVita VT, Hellman S, Rosenberg SA, editors. *Cancer: Principles and Practice of Oncology.* Philadelphia, PA: JB Lippincott; 1997. p. 1078.

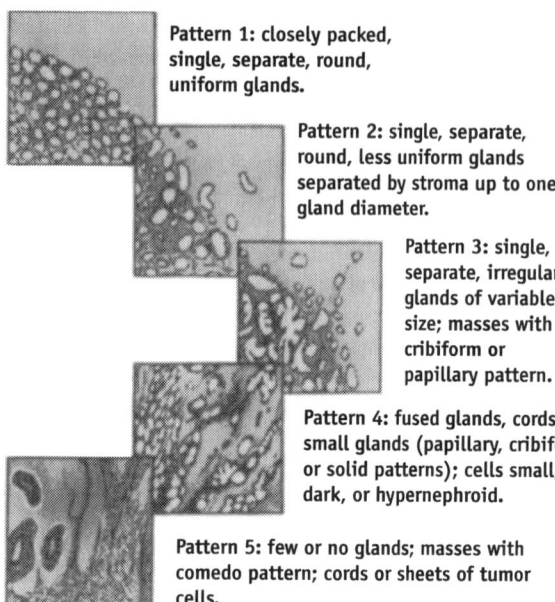

Figure 12-5. Gleason grading system

SOURCE: reprinted with permission from Trump DL, Shipley WU, Dilloglugil O, et al. Neoplasms of the prostate. In: Holland JF, Frei E III, Bast RC Jr, et al., editors. *Cancer Medicine*. 4th ed. Baltimore, MD: Williams & Wilkins; 1997. p. 2129.

incidence increases with age; the disease is most common in men over 50 years old. It is primarily a disease of the Western world, and it is more common in black men. African-American males in the United States have the highest incidence of prostate cancer in the world. Their incidence is about double that of white males. Asian-American males have a much lower incidence of prostate cancer than white males. Differences in androgen levels or in androgen regulation may account for some of the racial differences.[33] Benign overgrowth of prostate tissue (benign prostatic hypertrophy [BPH]) is not known to increase the risk of prostate cancer. Vasectomy may increase risk, although it is not well established whether the link between vasectomy and prostate cancer is causation or only association.[30,34]

Genetic factors are important in defining individual risk. Prostate cancer incidence is increased in males with a strong family history of this disease. A specific prostate cancer gene, the hereditary prostate cancer (HPC) gene, has been identified and is believed to be causative in a small proportion of prostate cancer patients. Other genetically related changes that increase risk include the loss of tumor suppressor genes. Risk factors include diets high in animal fats, especially red meats and dairy products. Occupational exposures have not been strongly linked with prostate cancer, although slightly higher rates of prostate cancer have been reported among workers exposed to cadmium, farmers, and rubber tire workers.[30,34]

Clinical Presentation and Natural History

The natural history of prostate cancer is usually a slow continuum from a borderline malignant form (prostatic intraepithelial neoplasm [PIN]) to widespread metastatic disease. Some prostate cancers remain latent for many years and may never progress to clinically evident disease during the patient's lifetime. In general, prostate cancer growth is slow, with a doubling time that may be 2 years or longer. The usual time course from diagnosis of localized disease to death from metastatic prostate cancer is several years.[30]

Prostate cancer always begins in the prostate, but it may then spread by any combination of direct extensions through the prostate capsule into nearby structures or by circulation in the lymph system or blood. Blood-borne spread of cancer cells usually carries prostate cancer to the bones, which are overwhelmingly the most common sites of metastases. Bones that are nearest to the prostate (lower spine, pelvis, and femurs) are usually the first to be affected. Metastases also occur in other sites, such as lungs, soft tissue, and liver, but these are much less common than bone metastases.[32]

Presenting signs and symptoms of prostate cancer depend on both the location and extent of disease. Patients with disease confined to the prostate are often asymptomatic. They may experience some symptoms of lower urinary tract obstruction, as the growing prostate partially compresses the urethra. These symptoms are similar to those of BPH and include urinary frequency, nocturia, difficulty initiating the urinary stream, dribbling, and urgency. Locally advanced disease may present with bladder outlet obstructive symptoms such as urinary retention, with possible anuria and uremia. Bone pain, especially in the lower back, pelvis, or femur, is the most common presenting complaint in patients with metastatic disease. Anemia and weight loss may be signs of advanced prostate cancer.[32]

Screening and Diagnosis

Several simple tests are available for prostate cancer screening in asymptomatic males. Many of the same tests are also used for diagnostic work-up in males who have symptoms attributable to the prostate or who have shown an abnormality on screening exams.[32]

PSA is measured by a simple blood test. It is the single most accurate screening test for prostate cancer, but it has serious limitations. Normal and cancerous prostate tissues both produce PSA. The normal range overlaps with cancerous values, so an elevated PSA is not specific for prostate cancer (Table 12-6). Patients with PSA levels higher than the recommended age-specific normal values should be evaluated further. PSA levels >10 ng/ml are most likely to be indicative of prostate cancer.[31,32]

Digital rectal exam (DRE) consists of palpation of the posterior lobe of the prostate by a trained health care profes-

Table 12-6. Guide to Interpretation of Prostate-Specific Antigen Values

Value (ng/ml)	Interpretation
0–4	Normal range, age non-specific
0–2.5	Age-specific normal range, ages 40–49
0–3.5	Age-specific normal range, ages 50–59
0–4.5	Age-specific normal range, ages 60–69
0–6.5	Age-specific normal range, ages 70–79
4–10	Overlap area of BPH and prostate cancer
>10	High likelihood of prostate cancer
<0.2	Expected level after radical prostatectomy

SOURCE: reprinted with permission from Balmer CM. Prostate cancer. In: Herfindal ET, Gourley DR, editors. *Textbook of Therapeutics: Drug and Disease Management*. 6th ed. Baltimore, MD: Williams & Wilkins; 1996. p. 1608. Values were determined by Hybritech Tandem assay. BPH, benign prostatic hypertrophy.

sional who inserts a gloved finger (digit) into the rectum. The purpose is to evaluate the size, configuration, and consistency of the gland. Nodules can be felt as hard masses within a usually rubbery gland.

Transrectal ultrasound (TRUS) uses ultrasound images produced by means of a probe inserted into the rectum to visualize prostate size, nodules, and invasion of surrounding tissues. This test is approximately twice as sensitive as DRE.[32]

Prostate biopsy is the removal of a small amount of suspicious prostate tissue to evaluate it for the presence of cancer cells. It is usually performed by needle biopsy through the wall of the rectum using a high-speed, gun-like biopsy device. This procedure is usually very well tolerated and does not require any anesthesia. The high speed and small needle size minimize patient discomfort.

ACS currently recommends annual screening with PSA and DRE for males >50 years old. Screening should begin at age 40 for high-risk patients.[35,36] However, widespread screening for prostate cancer is controversial. The basis for the controversy lies in the natural history of prostate cancer. Autopsy data from males who have died from unrelated causes demonstrate a high incidence of pathologically detectable prostate cancer, >30% in males over 50 and >67% in males over 80 years old. Most of these cancers never become clinically active throughout the patient's lifetime. These are called clinically unimportant cancers. Those who oppose widespread screening argue that most cancers never cause clinical symptoms, or progress so slowly that patients die of unrelated causes. They also argue that treatments for prostate cancer are expensive and produce unpleasant side effects.[37]

Proponents of screening counter that cancers detected by PSA and DRE testing are usually clinically important rather than latent cancers. Screening permits early diagnosis of prostate cancers, when the patient has the best chance of cure and when treatment is less costly than treatment of advanced disease. Screening is viewed as particularly valuable in young, otherwise healthy patients, who could most benefit from early treatment.[37]

Research is under way to find more specific screening tests, which could distinguish latent cancers from clinically important ones.

Staging and Prognosis

The most commonly used prostate cancer staging system is that of the American Urologic Association (AUA), proposed by Whitmore and modified by Jewett (Figure 12-6). Stage A indicates a nonpalpable tumor, which is often found inciden-

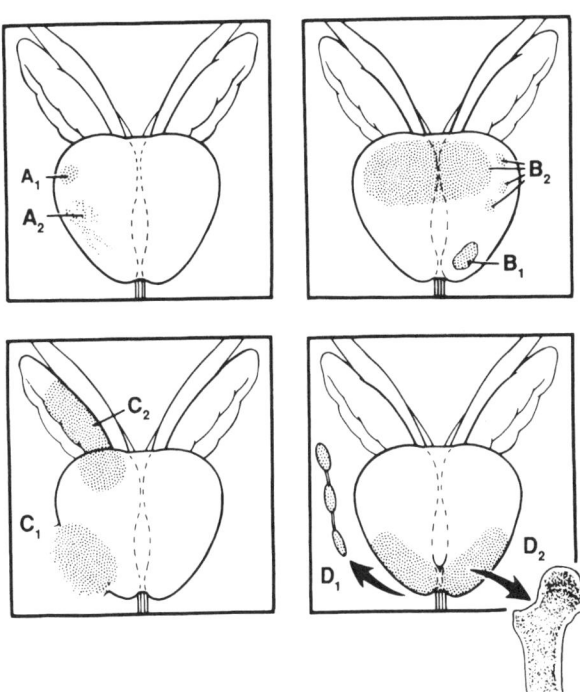

Figure 12-6. Modified Whitmore-Jewett or American Urologic Association (AUA) staging system for prostate cancer. A_1, focal; A_2, diffuse; B_1, single nodule in one lobe (<1.5 cm); B_2, diffuse involvement of whole gland (>1.5 cm); C_1, no seminal vesicle involvement (<70 g); C_2, seminal vesicle involvement (>70 g); D_1, pelvic lymph nodes or urethral obstruction; D_2, distant lymph node, bone, or soft tissue metastases.

SOURCE: reprinted with permission from Trump DL, Shipley WU, Dillioglugil O, et al. Neoplasms of the prostate. In: Holland JF, Frei E III, Bast RC Jr, et al., editors. *Cancer Medicine*. 4th ed. Baltimore, MD: Williams & Wilkins; 1997. p. 2133.

Table 12-7. Risk of Death and Cure Rates by Stage of Prostate Cancer

Stage of Disease	Percentage of Patients (%)	10-Year Survival (%)[a]	Estimated Cure Rate (%)	Prognosis
All stages	100	51	32	
A	10	95	85	Treatment may not be necessary
B	30	80	65	Often curable
C	10	60	25	Occasionally curable
D_1	20	40	<5	Rarely curable
D_2	30	10	<1	Incurable

SOURCE: reprinted with permission from Balmer CM. Prostate cancer. In: Herfindal ET, Gourley DR, editors. *Textbook of Therapeutics: Drug and Disease Management*. 6th ed. Baltimore, MD: Williams & Wilkins; 1996. p. 1611. Stage is based on clinical stage plus pelvic lymph node dissection, bone scan, and acid phosphatase.
[a] Cancer-specific survival rates.

tally during surgery for treatment of BPH. Stage B describes a palpable nodule or nodules confined to the prostate. Stage C disease extends outside the prostate capsule to nearby structures. Prostate cancer staging is unusual, in that lymph node involvement and distant metastases are both rated as stage D (D_1 and D_2, respectively). D_3 is sometimes used to indicate advanced, hormone-refractory disease. The TNM system is also used in the staging of prostate cancer.[30]

Stage of disease is the most important predictor of survival for patients with prostate cancer (Table 12-7). In addition, the degree of differentiation of the cancer cells inversely correlates with prognosis. The higher the Gleason score (Figure 12-5), the higher the mortality rate from prostate cancer.

Treatment

Localized Disease

Prostate cancer is classified as localized disease when the cancer is confined to the prostate gland (stages A and B, Figure 12-6). There are three primary treatment options for localized disease: surgery, radiation therapy, or close observation without treatment. The standard of treatment is radical prostatectomy, or surgical removal of the prostate gland. This procedure offers the overall best chance of cure. PSA levels decline rapidly to near zero after successful surgery (Table 12-6). Radical prostatectomy has been technically improved in recent years but remains major surgery, with a mortality risk of up to 2%. The most common complications are impotence and urinary incontinence.[38]

Impotence occurs because the neurovascular bundles that carry enervation for erectile control run in channels along each side of the prostate gland (Figure 12-4). In the past, these bundles were always removed with the prostate. Newer "nerve-sparing" surgical techniques leave at least one neurovascular bundle intact. This makes erections possible in about one third of patients, although erections are usually weaker than before surgery. Erectile ability that is lost from the effects of surgery may be restored artificially with vacuum erection devices, penile injections, urethral insertion or oral administration of vasodilators, or penile prostheses.[38,39]

Urinary incontinence is less common than impotence but may have a serious impact on quality of life. About 85% of men recover normal urinary continence or report only stress-induced spotting. The remainder require pads to keep their outer garments dry or are totally incontinent.[38]

Radiation therapy can be used to destroy localized prostate cancers in patients who are not good surgical candidates because of advanced age or other health problems. External-beam radiation is the most commonly used method of radiation therapy. It is a slow process, usually taking 6–8 weeks, and results in a much slower decrease in the PSA than surgery. Overall, the PSA is less likely to decrease to zero than it is with radical prostatectomy, but if it does, the cure rate from radiation therapy is as good as with surgery. Although overall long-term survival rates are lower with radiation therapy than with surgery, the differences may not be clinically important in an elderly population.[40] Radiation may also be administered from within the prostate tissue by means of implanted seeds of radioisotopes, a method called brachytherapy.

Although the techniques of radiation therapy have improved in accuracy, it is still not possible to irradiate all the prostate tissue with cytotoxic doses without delivering some radiation to nearby normal tissues as well. The rectum and urinary bladder, the tissues closest to the prostate gland, are the tissues most likely to be damaged by radiation therapy. Rectal or bladder irritation and bleeding are therefore the most common acute complications. These symptoms persist for many years in 3–8% of patients. Impotence is common but develops more slowly than after prostatectomy. Urinary incontinence is substantially less frequent than with radical prostatectomy.[38,39]

Observation (or "watchful waiting") is an alternative but highly controversial approach to managing localized prostate cancer. The rationale for observation is based on the slow-growing natural history of prostate cancer and the advanced age of patients with this disease. Observation may be an appropriate choice for elderly men with short life expectancy (<10 years) who have early-stage tumors with a low Gleason score; these men are likely to die of causes unrelated to prostate cancer. Younger, healthy men have a greater chance of prostate cancer affecting their life span and should be offered active treatment.[35,38,41]

Cryotherapy, or freezing of prostate tissue, is being studied as an alternative to radical prostatectomy and radiation therapy.[30]

Locally Advanced Disease

Once prostate cancer has penetrated the prostate capsule (stage C), the chances of cure with local treatment are much lower, because there is a high likelihood that micrometastases are already present at the time of diagnosis. Growth of micrometastases will eventually result in disease recurrence. Locally extensive prostate cancer is treated with radiation therapy to control local symptoms related to urinary obstruction.[30,38] Hormonal therapy given before and during radiation therapy acts to shrink the tumor mass and make radiation more effective. This treatment is sometimes referred to as "down-staging," because a stage C prostate cancer may become clinical stage B disease after hormonal therapy.[42]

Metastatic Disease

The mainstay of therapy for metastatic prostate cancer is hormonal or endocrine therapy. It is aimed at androgen ablation—the elimination of the growth-stimulating effects of androgens on prostate cancer cells. Androgen ablation can be accomplished in two ways, by interfering either with androgen production or with the interaction of androgens within prostate cancer cells.

Normal regulation of male hormone secretion is outlined in Figure 12-7. Testosterone is the main circulating androgen. Its production is regulated by a negative feedback system that includes the hypothalamus, pituitary, testes, and the adrenal glands. Secretion of testosterone by the testes is controlled within the brain. When low levels of testosterone are detected by the hypothalamus, it secretes luteinizing hormone–releasing hormone (LHRH), which is also called gonadotropin-releasing hormone (GnRH). LHRH stimulates the pituitary to secrete luteinizing hormone (LH), a gonadotropin, which stimulates the testes to secrete testosterone. A similar feedback loop controls steroid hormone production in the adrenal glands. The adrenals produce androgenic precursors that can be enzymatically converted to testosterone in peripheral tissues. DHT, formed from testosterone within prostate cells, is the main androgen affecting the cells' growth. DHT, like other hormones, stimulates protein production. In prostate cells, this results in cell division and growth. DHT

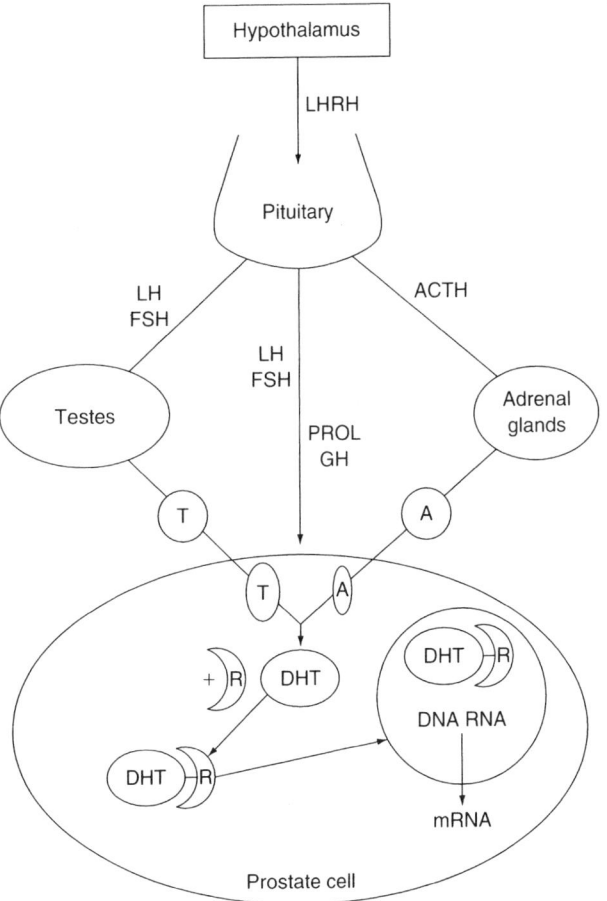

Figure 12-7. Hormonal regulation of the prostate gland LH, luteinizing hormone; LHRH, LH-releasing hormone; FSH, follicle-stimulating hormone; ACTH, adrenocorticotropic hormone; PROL, prolactin; GH, growth hormone; T, testosterone; A, androgens; R, receptor; DHT, dihydrotestosterone.
SOURCE: reprinted with permission from Goldspiel BR, Kuhn JG. Prostate cancer. In: DiPiro JT, Talbert RL, Yee GC, et al., editors. *Pharmacotherapy: A Pathophysiologic Approach*. 3rd ed. Stamford, CN: Appleton & Lange, 1997. p. 2542.

also inhibits normal programmed cell death (apoptosis).[32,43] Hormonal interventions for control of prostate cancer growth can be made at any point in the schema outlined in Figure 12-7.

Several general guidelines apply to the use of hormonal therapy in the management of prostate cancer patients.[35,43] First-line hormonal therapy produces objective responses (shrinking of measurable tumor) or subjective response (relief of symptoms) in about 85% of prostate cancer patients. This response generally persists for about 18 months. Hormonal therapy does not cure prostate cancer and usually does not prolong the patient's life, but it provides valuable palliation of symptoms and may increase disease-free survival. Second-line hormonal therapies have a much lower response rate and a shorter duration of response. Choice of hormonal therapy depends on patient and

Table 12-8. Hormonal Interventions for Management of Advanced Prostate Cancer

Intervention	Mechanism	Advantages	Disadvantages
Orchiectomy	Surgical removal of both testes; surgical castration	Outpatient procedure; inexpensive; low morbidity; very rapid onset of effect; avoids compliance issues	Psychological issues; lack of acceptance; irreversibility; impotence and loss of libido; hot flashes
Leuprolide	LHRH analogue; increases then decreases LH production to shut off testosterone production in the testes	Avoids psychological issues of surgical castration; reversible; subcutaneous depot delivery system	Tumor flare; very costly; monthly or every-3-month intramuscular injections required; impotence, loss of libido; hot flashes
Goserelin	LHRH analogue; same mechanism as leuprolide	Same as leuprolide; less costly than leuprolide	Same as leuprolide; subcutaneous depot delivery system
Flutamide	Antiandrogen	Oral medication; prevents tumor flare from LHRH analogues	Diarrhea; hepatotoxicity; costly; dosing every 8 hours; not approved as single agent; preserves potency and libido
Bicalutamide	Antiandrogen	Oral; once-daily dosing; less diarrhea-inducing than flutamide	Similar to flutamide; long half-life produces slow onset of effect and delayed withdrawal syndrome
Nilutamide	Antiandrogen	Less diarrhea and liver damage than flutamide; oral; once-daily dosing	Similar to flutamide; delayed adaptation to dark; disulfram-like reaction; interstitial pneumonitis; three tablets per dose
Estrogens	Interfere with LH secretion, which shuts off testosterone production; may also interfere with apoptosis	Inexpensive; simple oral therapy; reversible; does not cause hot flashes	Thromboembolic side effects (blood clots, myocardial infarctions, strokes); gynecomastia; fluid retention; nausea; impotence; loss of libido
Megestrol acetate	Progestin, which inhibits LH secretion; acts as steroidal antiandrogen	Oral medication; low toxicity; reduces hot flashes from LHRH analogues or orchiectomy	Short duration of effect (Megace escape); weight gain may be undesirable; impaired glucose control in diabetics
Ketoconazole	Inhibits adrenal and testicular hormone synthesis	Very rapid onset of action; useful salvage therapy; oral	Requires high doses; emetogenic; hepatotoxic; causes hypoadrenalism, which may require steroid replacement
Aminoglutethimide	Inhibits adrenal hormone synthesis	Useful salvage therapy; oral	Rash; sedation; nausea; drug interactions; requires supplementation with hydrocortisone
Corticosteroids	Suppress adrenal hormone production; anti-inflammatory effect decreases bone pain	Low dose required (prednisone 5–10 mg daily); few steroid side effects; improved sense of well-being	Chronic steroid side effects are possible; impaired glucose control in diabetics

LH, luteinizing hormone; LHRH, LH-releasing hormone.

physician preference, costs, concomitant medical conditions, and rapidity of response required. Most share common side effects of impotence and loss of sexual desire.

Table 12-8 outlines available hormonal interventions for treatment of advanced prostate cancer. First-line choices generally include surgical or medical castration. Antiandrogens may be added to either method of testicular suppression.

Surgical removal of the testes (bilateral orchiectomy or surgical castration) has been recognized as effective treatment of patients with advanced prostate cancer since the early 1940s and is still widely used.[44] Orchiectomy is an inexpensive outpatient surgical procedure with very low surgical risk, but many patients find it an unacceptable form of therapy.

In the 1960s, pharmacologic methods of castration became available in the form of estrogen therapy. Estrogens interfere with pituitary release of LH, which in turn stops testosterone production in the testes. Estrogens may also interfere with prostate cancer cell growth by mechanisms unrelated to their hormonal activity. Diethylstilbestrol (DES) has been the most widely used estrogen in prostate cancer patients. It was proved to be as effective as orchiectomy in a landmark Veterans Administration trial[45] using 5-mg doses, but it was also found to be very toxic. The study was closed early because of a high incidence of cardiovascular deaths in the diethylstilbestrol group. Doses of 1 mg produced response rates similar to 5 mg but did not maintain castration testosterone levels consistently, and testosterone levels often began to rise within 6–12 months of treatment. With little objective data, a compromise dose of 3 mg became widely used. Even at this dose, thromboembolic side effects occur in 5–10% of patients, and myocardial infarctions, angina, or congestive heart failure occur in about 5%. Because of these side effects, use of diethylstilbestrol has declined dramatically during the past decade, as less toxic pharmacologic therapies have become available. Diethylstilbestrol production was discontinued by the manufacturer in 1997. Although experience with other estrogens is limited, it is likely that other estrogens will share similar efficacy and toxicity with diethylstilbestrol. Recently, interest in the use of low-dose estrogen has increased because it is the least expensive hormonal therapy for prostate cancer management. Estrogen therapy should not be used in patients at high risk for thromboembolic disorders, such as patients with a history of stroke.[32,43,46]

The pharmacologic alternatives that displaced estrogens in the 1980s were the LHRH (or GnRH) analogues, leuprolide and goserelin. LHRH begins the cascade of signals that results in testosterone production, so administration of an LHRH analogue should increase testosterone and stimulate the growth of prostate cancer. This growth does occur during the first weeks of leuprolide or goserelin administration and is called the "flare" phenomenon. With continued administration, the receptors for LHRH in the pituitary are downregulated. LH production is suppressed, and testosterone production decreases within 4 weeks to levels comparable with those achieved with orchiectomy.[43,47]

Tumor flare caused by LHRH analogues can be prevented by antiandrogens, androgen receptor antagonists that competitively block the uptake of androgens in prostate tissues. Flutamide was the first nonsteroidal antiandrogen. Recently, bicalutamide and nilutamide have also been approved by the FDA. These agents do not interfere with testosterone production, so they do not cause impotence or hot flashes. They are not indicated as single agents for the management of metastatic prostate cancer, because the androgen blockade is competitive and may be overridden by increases in androgen production.[32,43,46]

Because antiandrogens interfere with the effects of any androgens on prostate cells, they have been widely used in combination with LHRH analogues or orchiectomy to counteract the effects of adrenal androgens and produce so-called "combined androgen blockade" (CAB). Because orchiectomy or LHRH analogues eliminate testicular androgen production and the antiandrogen prevents adrenal androgens from interacting with androgen receptors, CAB theoretically eliminates the effects of all androgens in the body. In one study, CAB increased survival in prostate cancer patients when compared with LHRH analogues alone. The survival benefit was limited to a few months, except in the small subgroup of patients with good performance status and minimal disease. These patients gained >2 years of increased survival with CAB therapy.[48] Although some subsequent studies confirmed these results, others have not. Most recently, a large trial that compared orchiectomy plus flutamide or placebo did not show benefit from CAB therapy.[49] Unless the results of LHRH analogue studies differ from combination trials with orchiectomy, or subsets of patients who clearly benefit from CAB therapy can be identified, the additional costs and toxicities of CAB therapy cannot be justified.

If a patient's prostate cancer progresses while receiving first-line hormonal therapy, or if the patient's cancer never responds to first-line hormonal intervention, his cancer is classified as hormone-refractory prostate cancer (HRPC).[50] It is helpful to think of these patients as only relatively refractory, since many will still respond to hormonal interventions, although the response rate and duration of response are lower than with first-line therapy. Several hormonal interventions are usually tried in succession before conventional chemotherapy treatments are attempted.

The choice of second-line and subsequent hormonal therapies is not well defined. Choice depends somewhat on the therapy the patient has received previously. If the patient has been receiving antiandrogens in combination with LHRH analogues or after orchiectomy, the simplest and recommended intervention is to stop the antiandrogen. A well-established phenomenon of antiandrogen withdrawal occurs in 20–30% of patients, with a duration of response of 4–5 months. It has been suggested that antiandrogens may begin to act as androgens, especially in patients who have received them for several years. More specifically, mutations in the androgen receptor over time may permit the antiandrogen to have androgenic effects by activating the androgen receptor. Withdrawal of the antiandrogen then becomes a form of androgen ablation. If a patient has not been receiving antiandrogens, many physicians add antiandrogens to testicular suppression, although the objective benefit of this intervention is not well defined.[43,46,50] Other hormonal intervention choices are outlined in Table 12-8.

Cytotoxic agents are usually reserved for patients with advanced prostate cancer who are symptomatic from their disease and no longer responding to hormone interventions. The value of chemotherapy in management of prostate cancer patients has long been questioned, because chemotherapy has not been proved to increase survival.[51] During the past decade, however, it has become firmly established that selected chemotherapy regimens effectively relieve symptoms of advanced prostate cancer and sometimes prolong disease-free intervals. This contributes to improved quality of life. Several regimens that appear to have value in management of patients with advanced prostate cancer are listed in Table 12-9.

The only chemotherapy regimen currently approved for these patients is the combination of mitoxantrone plus prednisone. The combination of these two drugs provides pain relief and improves performance status compared with prednisone alone in patients with pain caused by advanced prostate cancer. The response is classified as a clinical benefit rather than an objective tumor response.[52] Several regimens include estramustine, an oral agent that structurally combines an alkylating agent with an estrogen. Although it was first thought to work as an estrogen, it is now known to be an antimitotic agent. Combinations of estramustine with other chemotherapy agents that affect mitosis, such as the vinca alkaloids, etoposide, or taxanes, may lead to additive or synergistic effects in prostate cancer cells.[46]

Other approaches to managing HRPC are under investigation. Liarozole can slow the growth of prostate cancer cells by increasing serum levels of retinoic acid, which acts as a differentiating agent.[53,54] Suramin is an antitrypanosomal agent, previously used for treatment of African sleeping sickness. It interferes with several growth factors required by prostate cancer cells and has significant activity in patients with HRPC.[30,46] Genes linked to HRPC may some day provide useful targets for new genetic treatments of this challenging disorder.

Prevention

At present, no definitive method for preventing prostate cancer is known. A large trial is under way to evaluate the effects of the 5-alpha reductase inhibitor finasteride on the incidence of prostate cancer in males at high risk for developing this disease. Testosterone is converted to DHT, the androgen with greatest effect on prostate cancer cells, by 5-alpha reductase. Reducing DHT production could potentially reduce the development of this androgen-dependent tumor.[55] Retinoids and selenium are also being evaluated for prostate cancer prevention. Because prostate cancer risk is increased in patients who eat high-fat diets, especially those containing a lot of red meat, a diet low in fats and red meat products may be protective.

SUMMARY

Breast cancer and prostate cancer are the most common cancers in females and males, respectively. Together they account for >350,000 new cases of cancer each year in the United States, more than a fourth of the cancers diagnosed. Both cancers arise from hormone-dependent tissue, and because of this dependence, both cancers may often be managed by manipulation of the tumor's hormonal environment.

Both breast and prostate cancers are curable when detected in their early stages. Effective screening methods are available and are recommended to improve early detection. The use of screening for prostate cancer is somewhat controversial, because some prostate cancers remain latent for many years and may never develop into clinically important cancers. Localized breast and prostate cancers can be managed by surgery or radiation therapy. Extensive local disease is managed with radiation therapy combined with systemic treatments.

One important difference between breast and prostate cancers is the role of adjuvant therapy. Systemic adjuvant therapy is recommended for patients with stage I and II breast cancer to destroy micrometastases and increase the chance of cure. Adjuvant therapy has not proved to benefit prostate cancer patients.

Metastatic breast cancer is managed with hormonal therapy in women whose tumors express hormone receptors. Tamoxifen is the most widely used agent. Successive hormonal therapies may be used for women who have responded to hormonal interventions. Chemotherapy is used as first-line therapy for breast cancer patients who are hormone receptor negative. A wide range of chemotherapy drugs have established efficacy in advanced breast cancer.

Table 12-9. Representative Chemotherapy Regimens for Management of Patients with HRPC

Mitoxantrone plus prednisone
Estramustine plus vinblastine
Estramustine plus oral etoposide
Estramustine plus paclitaxel
Doxorubicin plus ketoconazole
Doxorubicin plus IV cyclophosphamide
Oral cyclophosphamide
Oral cyclophosphamide plus oral etoposide

SOURCE: adapted from references 30, 45, 51, and 52. HRPC, hormone-refractory prostate cancer.

In contrast, hormone receptor status is not a useful determinant of therapy in males with prostate cancer. Hormonal therapy is given to all patients with metastatic prostate cancer as first-line therapy, because about 85% of these patients will respond to androgen-ablative therapies. Orchiectomy and luteinizing hormone–releasing hormone analogues are considered first-line hormonal therapies for advanced prostate cancer. Successive hormonal interventions are used as the cornerstone of hormone-refractive prostate cancer management. The role of cytotoxic chemotherapy is less well established in the management of prostate cancer patients than in the treatment of breast cancer patients, and cytotoxic agents have less efficacy. Chemotherapy is used primarily for pain management. Objective responses are rare.

Chemoprevention trials are under way for males and females at high risk for developing prostate and breast cancers. The largest prostate cancer prevention trial is studying the effects of finasteride, which prevents the formation of dihydrotestosterone. The antiestrogens tamoxifen and raloxifene have been shown to reduce the risk of breast cancer. Retinoids may also have a role in prevention of these cancers.

REFERENCES

1. Parker SL, Tong T, Bolden S, et al. Cancer statistics, 1997. *CA Cancer J Clin* 1997;47:5–27.
2. Fisher B, Osborne CK, Margolese R, et al. Neoplasms of the breast. In: Holland JF, Frei E III, Bast RC, et al., editors. *Cancer Medicine.* Baltimore, MD: Williams & Wilkins; 1997. p. 2349–2429.
3. Harris JR, Morrow M, Norton L. Malignant tumors of the breast. In: DeVita VT, Hellman S, Rosenberg SA, editors. *Cancer: Principles and Practice of Oncology.* Philadelphia, PA: JB Lippincott; 1997. p. 1557–616.
4. Brinton LA, Devesa SS. Etiology and pathogenesis of breast cancer. Epidemiologic factors. Incidence, demographics, and environmental factors. In: Harris JR, Lippman ME, Morrow M, et al., editors. *Diseases of the Breast.* Philadelphia, PA: Lippincott-Raven; 1996. p. 159–68.
5. Healy B. BRCA genes—bookmaking, fortune telling, and medical care [editorial]. *N Engl J Med* 1997;336:1448–9.
6. Harris JR, Lippman ME, Veronesi U, et al. Breast cancer [first of three parts]. *N Engl J Med* 1992;327:319–28.
7. Morrison AS. Is self-examination effective in screening for breast cancer? *J Natl Cancer Inst* 1991;83:226–7.
8. American Cancer Society [ACS]. New guidelines for early detection of breast cancer. Publication number 97-750M–Number 3304-BCN. Atlanta, GA: ACS; 1997.
9. Clark GM. Prognostic and predictive factors. In: Harris JR, Lippman ME, Morrow M, et al., editors. *Diseases of the Breast.* Philadelphia, PA: Lippincott-Raven; 1996. p. 461–85.
10. Fields KK, Goldstein SC, Clark RA, et al. Breast cancer. In: Djulbigovic B, Sullivan DM, editors. *Decision Making in Oncology: Evidence-Based Management.* New York: Churchill-Livingston; 1997. p. 253–65.
11. Fisher B, Redmond C, Poisson R, et al. Eight-year results of a randomized clinical trial comparing total mastectomy and lumpectomy with or without irradiation in the treatment of breast cancer. *N Engl J Med* 1989;320:822–8.
12. Veronesi U, Banfi A, Salvadori B, et al. Breast conservation is the treatment of choice in small breast cancer: long-term results of a randomized trial. *Eur J Cancer* 1990;26:668–70.
13. NIH Consensus Conference. Treatment of early-stage breast cancer. *JAMA* 1991;265:391–5.
14. Hortobagyi GN, Buzdar AU. Current status of adjuvant systemic toxicity for primary breast cancer: progress and controversy. *CA Cancer J Clin* 1995;45:199–226.
15. Osborne KC, Clark GM, Ravdin PM. Adjuvant systemic therapy of primary breast cancer. In: Harris JR, Lippman ME, Morrow M, et al., editors. *Diseases of the Breast.* Philadelphia, PA: Lippincott-Raven; 1996. p. 548–78.
16. Harris JR, Lippman ME, Veronesi U, et al. Breast cancer [third of three parts]. *N Engl J Med* 1992;327:473–80.
17. Fornander T, Rutqvist LE, Sjoberg HE, et al. Long-term adjuvant tamoxifen in early breast cancer: effect on bone mineral density in postmenopausal women. *J Clin Oncol* 1990;8:1019–24.
18. Bagdade JD, Wolter J, Subbaiah PV, et al. Effects of tamoxifen treatment on plasma lipids and lipoprotein lipid composition. *J Clin Endocrinol Metab* 1990;70:1132–5.
19. Fisher B, Dignam J, DeCills A, et al. The worth of chemotherapy and tamoxifen over tamoxifen alone in node negative patients with ER positive invasive breast cancer; first results of NSABP B-20 [abstract]. *Proc Amer Soc Clin Oncol* 1997;16:1A.
20. Buzdar AU, Plourde PV, Hortobagyi GN. Aromatase inhibitors in metastatic breast cancer. *Semin Oncol* 1996;23(4 *Suppl* 9):21–7.
21. Holmes F, Walters R, Thenault R, et al. Phase II trial of Taxol, an active drug in the treatment of metastatic breast cancer. *J Natl Cancer Inst* 1991;83:1797–805.
22. Reichman B, Seidman A, Crown J, et al. Paclitaxel and recombinant human granulocyte colony-stimulating factor as initial chemotherapy for metastatic breast cancer. *J Clin Oncol* 1993;11:1943–51.
23. Fulton B, Spencer CM. Docetaxel: a review of its pharmacodynamic and pharmacokinetic properties and therapeutic efficacy in the management of metastatic breast cancer. *Drugs* 1996;51:1075–92.
24. Theriault RL. Specific sites and emergencies: medical treatment of bone metastasis. In: Harris JR, Lippman ME, Morrow M, et al., editors. *Diseases of the Breast.* Philadelphia, PA: Lippincott-Raven; 1996. p. 819–26.
25. Hortobagyi GN, Theriault RL, Porter L, et al. Efficacy of pamidronate in reducing skeletal complications in patients with breast cancer and lytic bone metastases. *N Engl J Med* 1996;335:1785–91.
26. Schrag D, Kuntz KM, Garber JE, et al. Decision analysis—effects of prophylactic mastectomy and oophorectomy on life expectancy among women with BRCA1 or BRCA2 mutations. *N Engl J Med* 1997;336:1465–72.
27. Constantino JC, Fisher B, Kavanagh M, et al. The initial results from NABP protocol P-1: a clinical trial to determine the worth of tamoxifen for preventing breast cancer in women at increased risk [abstract]. *Proc Am Soc Clin Oncol Ann Mtg* 1998;17:3A.

28. Cummings SR, Norton L, Eckert S, et al. Raloxifene reduces the risk of breast cancer and may decrease the risk of endometrial cancer in postmenopausal women. Two-year findings from the multiple outcomes of raloxifene evaluation (MORE) trial [abstract]. *Proc Am Soc Clin Oncol Ann Mtg* 1998;17:3A.
29. Wingo PA, Landis S, Ries LAG. An adjustment to the 1997 estimate for new prostate cancer cases. *CA Cancer J Clin* 1997;47:239–42.
30. Oesterling J, Fuks Z, Lee CT, et al. Cancer of the prostate. In: DeVita VT, Hellman S, Rosenberg SA, editors. *Cancer: Principles and Practice of Oncology.* 5th ed. Philadelphia, PA: Lippincott-Raven; 1997. p. 1322–86.
31. Brawer MK. How to use prostate-specific antigen in the early detection or screening for prostatic carcinoma. *CA Cancer J Clin* 1995;45:48–164.
32. Goldspiel BR, Kuhn JG. Prostate cancer. In: DiPiro JT, Talbert RL, Yee GC, et al., editors. *Pharmacotherapy: A Pathophysiologic Approach.* 3rd ed. Stamford, CN: Appleton & Lange; 1997. p. 2539–57.
33. Ross RK, Coetzee GA, Reichardt J, et al. Does the racial-ethnic variation in prostate cancer risk have a hormonal basis? *Cancer* 1995;75:1778–82.
34. Giovannucci E. Epidemiologic characteristics of prostate cancer. *Cancer* 1995;75:1766–77.
35. Balmer CM. Prostate cancer. In: Herfindal ET, Gourley DR, editors. *Textbook of Therapeutics: Drug and Disease Management.* 6th ed. Baltimore, MD: Williams & Wilkins, 1996. p. 1607–17.
36. Hamblin J, Connor PD. An overview of the American Cancer Society screening guidelines. *J Tenn Med Assoc* 1995;88:10–6.
37. Slawin KM, Ohori M, Dillioglugil O, et al. Screening for prostate cancer: an analysis of the early experience. *CA Cancer J Clin* 1995;45:134–47.
38. Catalona WJ. Management of cancer of the prostate. *N Engl J Med* 1994;331:996–1004.
39. Beard CJ, Popert KJ, Rieker PP, et al. Complications after treatment with external beam irradiation in early-stage prostate cancer patients: a prospective multi-institutional outcomes study. *J Clin Oncol* 1997;15:223–9.
40. Lee WR, Hanks GE, Schultheiss TE, et al. Localized prostate cancer treated by external-beam radiotherapy alone: serum prostate-specific antigen-driven outcome analysis. *J Clin Oncol* 1995;13:464–9.
41. Chodak GW. The role of watchful waiting in the management of localized prostate cancer. *J Urol* 1994;152:1766–8.
42. Pilepich MV, Krall JM, Al-Sarraf M, et al. Androgen deprivation with radiation therapy compared with radiation therapy alone for locally advanced prostate carcinoma: a randomized comparative trial of the radiation therapy oncology group. *Urology* 1995;45:616–23.
43. Garnick MB. Hormonal therapy in the management of prostate cancer: from Huggins to the present. *Urology* 1997;49(*Suppl* 3A):5–15.
44. Huggins C, Stevens R, Hodges C. The effect of castration on advanced carcinoma of the prostate gland. *Arch Surg* 1941;43:209–23.
45. The Veterans Administration Cooperative Urological Research Group. Carcinoma of the prostate: treatment comparisons. *J Urol* 1967;98:516–22.
46. Goethuys H, Baert L, Poppel HV, et al. Treatment of metastatic carcinoma of the prostate. *Am J Clin Oncol* 1997;20:40–45.
47. The Leuprolide Study Group. Leuprolide versus diethylstilbestrol for metastatic prostate cancer. *N Engl J Med* 1984;311:1281–6.
48. Crawford ED, Eisenberger MA, McLeod DG, et al. A controlled trial of leuprolide with and without flutamide in prostatic carcinoma. *N Engl J Med* 1989;321:419–24.
49. Eisenberger M, Crawford ED, McLeod D, et al. A comparison of bilateral orchiectomy with or without flutamide in stage D2 prostate cancer (NCI INT-0105 SWOG/ECOG) [abstract]. *Proc Am Soc Clin Oncol* 1997;16:2a.
50. Small EJ, Vogelzang NJ. Second-line hormonal therapy for advanced prostate cancer: a shifting paradigm. *J Clin Oncol* 1997;15:382–8.
51. Tannock IF. Is there evidence that chemotherapy is of benefit to patients with carcinoma of the prostate? *J Clin Oncol* 1985;3:1013–21.
52. Tannock IF, Osaba D, Stockler MR, et al. Chemotherapy with mitoxantrone plus prednisone or prednisone alone for symptomatic hormone-resistant prostate cancer: a Canadian randomized trial with palliative end points. *J Clin Oncol* 1996;14:1756–64.
53. Vogelzang NJ. One hundred thirteen men with hormone-refractory prostate cancer died today [editorial]. *J Clin Oncol* 1996;14:1753–5.
54. Kreis W. Current chemotherapy and future directions in research for the treatment of advanced hormone-refractory prostate cancer. *Cancer Invest* 1995;13:296–312.
55. Brawley OW, Thompson IM. Chemoprevention of prostate cancer. *Urology* 1994;43:594–9.

SELF-STUDY QUESTIONS

1. Which of the following is *not* an established risk factor for breast cancer?

    a. chronic hormonal administration
    b. family history of breast cancer
    c. age 20–30 years
    d. residence in North America

2. *BRCA1* is used in the treatment of breast cancer.

    a. true
    b. false

3. The symptom(s) of locally advanced prostate cancer include:

    a. bone pain.
    b. anemia.
    c. urinary retention.
    d. a and b only.
    e. all of the above.

4. Infiltrating lobular carcinoma makes up the majority of breast cancer cases.

    a. true
    b. false

5. Hormonal therapy is the first-line treatment for, and has the best chance of response in, women whose tumors have which of the following receptor profiles?

    a. ER–/PgR–
    b. ER+/PgR–
    c. ER–/PgR+
    d. ER+/PgR+

6. The risk of prostate cancer is increased in patients who are:

    a. African-American males.
    b. Asian-American males.
    c. over 50 years old.
    d. a and c only.
    e. all of the above.

7. Benign prostatic hypertrophy (BPH) is known to increase the risk of prostate cancer.

    a. true
    b. false

8. Recommended screening for women <40 years of age with no known risk factors for breast cancer includes:

    a. mammography.
    b. clinical breast examination every 6 months.
    c. monthly breast self-examination.
    d. all of the above.

9. Chronic tamoxifen therapy has not been associated with an increased incidence of:

    a. endometrial cancer.
    b. cervical cancers.
    c. bone cancer.
    d. leukemia.

10. Adjuvant breast cancer therapy includes only chemotherapy.

    a. true
    b. false

11. Adjuvant systemic therapy in stage II breast cancer decreases recurrence.

    a. true
    b. false

12. Breast cancer staging helps determine the most appropriate treatment.

    a. true
    b. false

13. Chemotherapy in metastatic prostate cancer includes the combination of:

    a. cyclophosphamide plus vincristine.
    b. methotrexate plus leucovorin.
    c. mitoxantrone plus prednisone.
    d. leuprolide plus mitoxantrone.

14. First-line radiation therapy in prostate cancer for localized disease may include hormonal therapy with leuprolide.

    a. true
    b. false

15. Chemotherapy regimens that are effective in the first-line management of breast cancer include:

    a. doxorubicin plus cyclophosphamide
    b. busulfan plus hydroxyurea
    c. streptozotocin plus fluorouracil
    d. cisplatin plus mitomycin

16. Prostate-specific antigen (PSA) is produced only by cancerous prostate tissues.

    a. true
    b. false

Chapter 13
Management of Hematological Malignancies

Andrea Iannucci, Pharm.D.
Assistant Professor/Oncology Clinical Pharmacist
School of Pharmacy
University of Colorado School of Pharmacy
Denver, Colorado

Normal Hematopoiesis	232
Leukemias	233
Pathophysiology	233
Etiology	233
Acute Leukemias	233
Acute Myelogenous Leukemia	234
Clinical Presentation	234
Diagnosis and Classification	234
Treatment	235
Treatment-Related Toxicities and Complications	236
Prognosis	236
Acute Lymphocytic Leukemia	236
Clinical Presentation	236
Diagnosis and Classification	236
Treatment	237
Treatment-Related Toxicities and Complications	238
Prognosis	238
The Role of Colony-Stimulating Factors in Acute Leukemias	238
Chronic Leukemias	239
Chronic Myelogenous Leukemia	239
Clinical Presentation	239
Diagnosis and Classification	239
Treatment	239
Chronic Phase	239
Accelerated Phase and Blast Crisis	240
Treatment-Related Toxicities and Complications	240
Prognosis	240
Chronic Lymphocytic Leukemia	241
Clinical Presentation	241
Diagnosis and Classification	241
Treatment	241
Treatment-Related Toxicities and Complications	242
Prognosis	242
Lymphomas	242
Clinical Presentation	242
Diagnosis	244
Classification	244
Treatment	245
Hodgkin's Disease	245

Non-Hodgkin's Lymphomas 246
Bone Marrow Transplantation 246
Treatment-Related Toxicities and Complications 246
Summary 246
References 247
Self-Study Questions 248

Leukemias and lymphomas are hematological malignancies, cancers of the blood and lymphatic systems. In 1997, hematological malignancies accounted for approximately 8% of all new cancers and approximately 10% of all cancer deaths in the United States.[1] The spectrum of hematological malignancies includes some of the deadliest, as well as some of the malignancies most responsive to aggressive chemotherapy.

Chemotherapy is the primary curative treatment modality used in the management of leukemias and lymphomas. Pharmacists play a critical role by anticipating and managing chemotherapy-related toxicities and helping optimize supportive care for patients being treated for hematological malignancies. However, to best be suited to assist in the multidisciplinary care of these patients, pharmacists must first become familiar with the various aspects of the common hematological malignancies.

After completing this chapter, the reader should be able to:

1. Describe the classification of leukemias (acute, chronic, myeloid, and lymphoid).
2. Describe the natural history (e.g., populations affected, risk factors, clinical features, signs and symptoms, and prognosis) of each type of leukemia discussed.
3. Describe a typical treatment plan for each type of leukemia discussed (induction, intensification/consolidation, maintenance, and central nervous system treatments).
4. Identify common chemotherapy agents and regimens used to treat patients with each type of leukemia discussed.
5. Describe common treatment-related toxicities and complications associated with each type of leukemia discussed.
6. Differentiate between Hodgkin's disease and non-Hodgkin's lymphoma with respect to risk factors, tissue pathology, clinical features, prognosis, and treatment.
7. Identify common chemotherapy agents and regimens used to treat patients with Hodgkin's and non-Hodgkin's lymphomas.
8. Describe common treatment-related toxicities and complications associated with Hodgkin's and non-Hodgkin's lymphomas.
9. Describe the role of bone marrow transplantation in treatment of hematological malignancies.

This chapter begins with a brief review of the normal hematopoietic process, to provide a basis for understanding the abnormal processes of hematological malignancies. A discussion of leukemias follows, beginning with classification of the various leukemias by pathophysiology and etiology. The four major types of leukemia are then reviewed separately. A discussion of lymphomas compares and contrasts the clinical presentation, classification, diagnosis, and treatment of Hodgkin's disease and non-Hodgkin's lymphomas.

NORMAL HEMATOPOIESIS

The normal hematopoietic process begins in the bone marrow (Figure 13-1). A pluripotent stem cell is the precursor of both lymphoid and myeloid cell lines. As the pluripotent stem cell matures, it becomes committed to differentiate into cells of either the lymphoid or myeloid lineage. Lymphoid stem cells further differentiate into B and T lymphocytes. Myeloid stem cells ultimately differentiate into red blood cells, neutrophils and other granulocytes, macrophages, and platelets. When fully differentiated, mature blood cells leave the bone marrow and enter the circulating blood. Regulation of hematopoiesis depends on a variety of growth factors, such as erythropoietin, granulocyte colony-stimulating factor, and granulocyte-macrophage colony-stimulating factor.

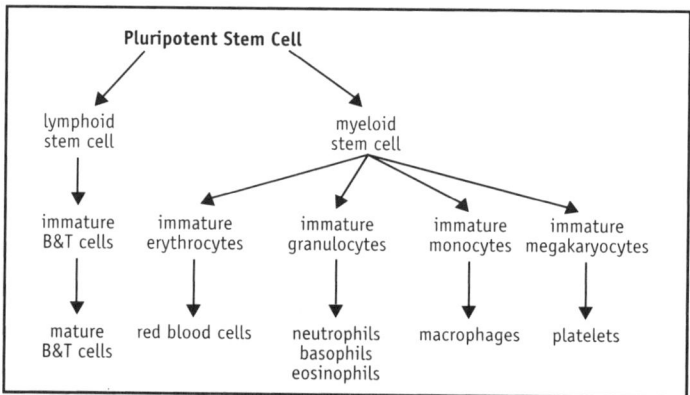

Figure 13-1. Normal hematopoiesis and differentiation in the bone marrow

LEUKEMIAS

Pathophysiology

Leukemias are a group of malignancies of the blood and bone marrow that affect either myeloid or lymphoid cell lines. In 1998, approximately 28,600 new cases of leukemia were diagnosed in the United States, and leukemias caused approximately 21,600 deaths.[1] Leukemias are characterized by uncontrolled proliferation, incomplete maturation, and accumulation of blood cells and their immature precursors (blast cells).[2] The word *leukemia* actually means "white blood." When leukemia was first described, it was named for the white or light pinkish color of the blood, visible to the naked eye, that was observed in patients who had high white blood cell (WBC) counts associated with their disease.

Leukemias are classified as myeloid or lymphoid, depending on which cell line is affected. They are also divided into broad categories of acute or chronic, based on their clinical courses (Table 13-1). Acute leukemias are characterized by the presence of very immature cells, a rapid onset of symptoms, and progression over weeks to months. Chronic leukemias are characterized by more mature cells, a gradual onset of symptoms, and a natural history measured in years. Although acute leukemias display a more aggressive course, they are more frequently curable than chronic leukemias; thus, the goal in treatment of acute leukemias is cure. Chronic leukemias are less often curable, so the goals in their treatment are to delay disease progression and to manage symptoms.

Etiology

The etiology of leukemias is largely unknown. Occupational and environmental factors may increase the risk of developing acute leukemia. Chemical exposure to carcinogens, such as benzene, is linked with the development of leukemia.[3] Petroleum and rubber industry workers have a notably increased risk of developing acute leukemia.[4] Cigarette smoking has also been associated with the development of leukemias,[4] although the link is much weaker than with lung cancer. Genetic factors may also be involved; the incidence of acute leukemias is high in Eastern European Jews, whereas the incidence in Asians is very low.[4] Patients with certain hereditary and congenital chromosomal abnormalities, including Down's syndrome, have an increased incidence of leukemia.[4] Finally, viruses, such as human T-cell leukemia virus 1 (HTLV-1), have also been associated with development of leukemia.[4]

De novo acute leukemia is an acute leukemia without a clearly identifiable causative factor. De novo leukemias account for the majority of cases of acute leukemia. Secondary leukemias are acquired leukemias that can be traced to a causative factor. Secondary leukemias are typically more resistant to chemotherapy agents than de novo leukemias. Chemotherapy agents—particularly alkylating agents (e.g., cyclophosphamide, procarbazine, and mechlorethamine), nitrosoureas, and, more recently, topoisomerase inhibitors, such as etoposide—have been implicated as causative agents of secondary leukemias.[3,5] Secondary leukemias resulting from exposure to chemotherapy agents are typically a late complication of chemotherapy and may occur anywhere from 2 to 9 years following treatment.[5] Exposure to ionizing radiation is also a significant risk factor for the development of secondary leukemia, as has been well documented in survivors of the atomic bombings of Hiroshima and Nagasaki.[3,4] Radiotherapy can also predispose patients to secondary leukemias.

Myelodysplastic syndromes are bone marrow disorders associated with impaired maturation of blood cells, which ultimately results in anemia and/or neutropenia. Myelodysplasia poses a significant risk for the development of secondary acute myelogenous leukemia.

ACUTE LEUKEMIAS

Left untreated, acute leukemias are universally fatal. Although the incidence of acute leukemias is lower than that of solid tumors (such as breast and prostate cancers), acute leukemia is the leading cause of cancer death in persons under 35 years of age.[1]

The primary goal of treating patients with acute leukemia is cure. Treatment for acute leukemias typically involves

Table 13-1. Classification and Epidemiology of Leukemias

	Median Age at Onset (Years)	Incidence per Year in U.S.	Estimated 5-Year Survival (%)
Acute Leukemias			
Acute myelogenous leukemia (AML)	65[5]	9200[5]	15–50[6]
Acute lymphocytic leukemia (ALL)	10[5]	3000[5]	20–30[19]*
Chronic Leukemias			
Chronic myelogenous leukemia (CML)	53[30]	4300[30]	50–60[31]
Chronic lymphocytic leukemia (CLL)	65[34]	7400[32]	80–90[33]

*adult ALL

multiple courses of chemotherapy. The following definitions describe the various phases of treatment. *Induction* refers to initial chemotherapy administered to induce or produce a complete remission, that is, elimination of all clinically detectable evidence of disease. *Clinically detectable disease* refers to leukemia that is measurable under the microscope. At the time of diagnosis, most patients with acute leukemia have approximately 10^{12} leukemic cells.[5] Effective chemotherapy produces a reduction to approximately 10^9 cells, the lower limit of detection for leukemia by conventional methods. Because large numbers of cancer cells, although not clinically detectable, may still be present after one course of chemotherapy, complete remission is not synonymous with cure. *Consolidation* describes chemotherapy administered after induction therapy in an attempt to destroy any residual leukemic cells. *Intensification* refers to consolidation therapy administered in significantly higher doses than those used in induction. The rationale for higher doses is that residual cells may be resistant to the original doses of chemotherapy agents. The term *postremission therapy* may be used to describe consolidation or intensification. *Maintenance therapy* describes low doses of chemotherapy administered daily or weekly to maintain remission. *Central nervous system (CNS) prophylaxis* describes chemotherapy and/or radiotherapy administered to prevent development of CNS leukemia.

Acute Myelogenous Leukemia

Clinical Presentation

Acute myelogenous leukemia (AML), also termed acute nonlymphocytic leukemia (ANLL), accounts for 80–90% of adult acute leukemias.[2,3] Approximately 9200 new cases are diagnosed each year.[5] Although the average age at onset is 65 years (Table 13-1), AML can occur at any age.[5] The onset of symptoms with AML is abrupt, usually occurring over a period of a few weeks to a few months. Presenting symptoms of AML are frequently related to bone marrow suppression, resulting from crowding out of the bone marrow by leukemic cells.[2] Production of normal cells (such as red blood cells, neutrophils, and/or platelets) may be impaired, resulting in anemia, neutropenia, and/or thrombocytopenia. Deficiencies in these cell lines produce characteristic signs and symptoms. Shortness of breath and pallor, which may be associated with anemia, are often present. Patients may present with infection, recurrent colds, flu, sore throat, or fevers associated with neutropenia. They most commonly complain of extreme fatigue and general malaise. Signs of bruising or bleeding related to thrombocytopenia may also be present. Patients with certain subtypes of AML—i.e., M4, M5 (Table 13-2, and see discussion under *Diagnosis and Classification* below)—may exhibit signs of leukemic infiltrates into tissue in the form of skin nodules, chloromas, or gum hypertrophy.

Laboratory findings in AML are usually consistent with bone marrow failure. Patients are frequently anemic and thrombocytopenic. WBC counts may be high, low, or normal. The differential count may show a high percentage of leukemic blast cells, although blast cells do not always appear in the peripheral smear. Very high WBC counts, or hyperleukocytosis, may make the blood too thick to circulate freely through small capillaries. Patients with WBC counts >100,000 cells/mm^3 are at greatest risk for symptoms related to decreased blood flow, or leukostasis. They must be treated emergently with chemotherapy and/or leukapheresis to decrease WBC levels and prevent damage to the lungs and brain.

Diagnosis and Classification

Clinical presentation and laboratory findings are the foundation for further work-up and evaluation of AML. However, definitive diagnosis depends on bone marrow biopsy. In this procedure, a large-bore needle is inserted through the bone of the posterior iliac crest, into the bone marrow. A core of solid bone tissue and an aspirate of liquid bone marrow fluid are removed. Aspirated bone marrow with >30% leukemic blast cells is diagnostic of acute leukemia. The cells from the bone marrow aspirate are then stained with a variety of diagnostic stains to determine the type of acute leukemia. Myeloperoxidase and Sudan black stains detect the presence of myeloperoxidase (an enzyme present in cells of the myeloid line) and confirm the diagnosis of AML.[5]

AML is then subclassified pathologically on the basis of the type of cell involved. Table 13-2 describes the French-American-British (FAB) morphological classification of AML. After myeloperoxidase staining, AML is further differentiated by the presence of certain antigens or immune markers (clusters of differentiation [CDs]) present on the cell surface (e.g., CD13 or CD33) and chromosomal abnormalities (e.g., trans-

Table 13-2. FAB Classification of AML

FAB Type	Subtype	Frequency (%)
M0	Undifferentiated AML	5
M1	Acute myeloblastic leukemia	15
M2	AML, with differentiation	25
M3	Acute promyelocytic leukemia	10
M4	Acute myelomonocytic leukemia	30
M5	Acute monocytic leukemia	10
M6	Acute erythrocytic leukemia	4
M7	Acute megakaryocytic leukemia	1

SOURCE: adapted from references 2 and 4. FAB, French-American-British.

location of chromosomes 8 and 21). Table 13-3 lists common stains, immune markers, and chromosomal abnormalities in acute leukemias.

Certain chromosomal abnormalities and morphological subtypes are associated with a better or worse prognosis. For example, chromosomal aberrations associated with secondary leukemias [e.g., the deletions del(5) or del(7)] and trisomy 8 are typically associated with a poor prognosis (Table 13-3).[5] Inversion inv(16) and translocation t(8,21) are associated with a more favorable prognosis. The chromosomal abnormality associated with the M3 (or acute promyelocytic leukemia [APL]) subtype of AML [t(15,17)] affects the retinoic acid (vitamin A) receptor and prevents proper maturation of those cells. When recognized and appropriately treated, this variant of AML is associated with a highly favorable prognosis.

With the exception of the M3 subtype, FAB classification of the disease does not currently have an impact on treatment (see *Treatment* below). The treatment implications of AML's different morphologies are under extensive investigation.

Treatment

Unlike solid tumor malignancies, leukemias are generally not staged according to extent of disease; they are always widespread. Because truly localized leukemia does not occur, there is no role for surgery or, with a few exceptions, radiation therapy in the primary treatment of AML. Systemic chemotherapy is the cornerstone of treatment. Treatment of AML is divided into induction and postremission therapy. CNS involvement is uncommon in AML, so routine CNS prophylaxis is not typically included in AML treatment regimens.

The goal in induction treatment of AML is bone marrow ablation, in an attempt to kill the most leukemic cells in the bone marrow. Combinations of cytarabine (ara-C) with an anthracycline (e.g., daunorubicin or idarubicin) or mitoxantrone, a closely related anthracene analogue, are standard for induction therapy in AML. Typical induction regimens with cytarabine and an anthracycline employ a 7-day course of cytarabine administered as a continuous infusion and a 3-day course of the anthracycline (a "7 + 3 regimen").[6] Doses of cytarabine used for induction are usually 100–200 mg/m^2 per day. The choice of daunorubicin, idarubicin, or mitoxantrone varies, depending on institutional protocols. However, there are data to suggest significant improvements in response rates, response duration, and survival with the use of idarubicin[7-9] in comparison with daunorubicin. These 7 + 3 regimens are the gold standard for induction treatment of AML and produce complete remission in 65–70% of patients.[6] A second induction course with the same chemotherapy regimen is sometimes necessary to achieve a complete remission.

One exception to the use of the standard 7 + 3 induction chemotherapy regimen is in the treatment of patients with APL, the M3 subtype of AML. In APL, a defect in the retinoic acid receptor results in inhibition of normal promyelocyte differentiation.[1] Tretinoin, or all-*trans*-retinoic acid (ATRA, Vesanoid), a vitamin A derivative, causes the immature APL cells to differentiate. Induction chemotherapy consists of a 45- to 90-day course of treatment with ATRA.[10,11] Induction therapy must be followed by conventional chemotherapy to produce a lasting remission.[11,12]

Once AML patients achieve a complete remission and recover from the adverse effects of induction therapy, postremission chemotherapy begins. In contrast to induction treatment, there is no gold standard for postremission therapy. Consolidation or intensification regimens often involve variations of the remission induction regimen. The same drugs and doses may be administered in a modified schedule (e.g., in a "5 + 2" regimen: 5 days of cytarabine and 2 days of anthracycline) or in significantly higher doses (e.g., high-dose cytarabine, often abbreviated "HDAC" [high-dose ara-C], 1–3 g/m^2 per dose). A recent multicenter study conducted by the Cancer and Leukemia Group B (CALGB) supports the use of HDAC over standard- to moderate-dose cytarabine for postremission therapy of AML.[13] This study demonstrated a significant improvement in continued complete remission after 4 years with HDAC (3 g/m^2 q12hr for six doses, administered on days 1, 3, and 5) compared with lower doses of

Table 13-3. Differentiating Between AML and ALL

	AML	ALL
Stains	Myeloperoxidase + Sudan black +	TdT +
Immune markers	CD13, CD14, CD33, CD34	CD2, CD7, CD10, CD19, CD20
Common chromosomal abnormalities	+8; del(5), del(7) (M1) t(8,21) (M2) t(15,17) (M3) inv(16) (M4) t(9,11) (M5)	t(9,22) (Philadelphia chromosome) t(8,14) (Burkitt's)

SOURCE: adapted from references 2 and 5. +, positive; TdT, terminal deoxynucleotidyl transferase; CD, clusters of differentiation; del, deletion; t, translocation; inv, inversion.

cytarabine (100 and 400 mg/m² per day, continuous infusion) in patients under 60 years of age. Increased morbidity and mortality related to infection and CNS toxicity make HDAC unsuitable for elderly patients.[13]

Duration of postremission therapy for AML is generally several months following complete remission. Longer courses of postremission therapy or maintenance therapy have not been shown to improve survival in AML.[6] For patients with a suitable donor, bone marrow transplantation (BMT) is a viable option for postremission treatment of AML. (See chapter 14 for discussion of BMT.)

Treatment-Related Toxicities and Complications

Patients with a high WBC count at the time of diagnosis (>50,000 cells/mm³) are at high risk for developing tumor lysis syndrome (TLS) during induction treatment. These patients should receive prophylactic treatment for TLS (as discussed in chapter 19). Because it is necessary to ablate the bone marrow with chemotherapy agents to achieve a complete remission, patients develop many toxicities related to prolonged bone marrow suppression. They are typically anemic and thrombocytopenic, requiring blood and platelet support, often for several weeks following induction treatment. Patients also become severely neutropenic and are predisposed to infections. Most patients require hospitalization for 3–4 weeks following treatment for AML. The majority of patients who die during induction therapy for AML die from complications related to infection or bleeding.[14]

Nausea and vomiting are potentially low or moderate with the most common AML treatment regimen, the 7 + 3 regimen. Diarrhea is very common after AML induction therapy. Mucositis may be severe, and alopecia is almost universal, following therapy for AML.

Prognosis

There are many factors that influence a patient's chance of long-term survival with AML. The impact of chromosomal abnormalities has already been discussed. Secondary leukemias carry a poor prognosis. Advanced age (>60 years) is an adverse factor, as are poor performance status and underlying major organ dysfunction prior to treatment.[5] In addition, the number of induction treatment courses required to achieve a remission is inversely related to the chance of long-term survival. In other words, the longer it takes to achieve a remission, the less the chance of cure.

Although most patients achieve complete remission following induction therapy, the median duration of complete remission is only 1–2 years and the response to chemotherapy following relapse is usually poor. Long-term survival rates (continuous complete remission >5 years) have been reported in the range of 15–50% (Table 13-1).[6] These rates vary, depending on the postremission treatment and a number of prognostic factors, particularly patient age.

Prognosis for APL is more favorable than other subtypes of AML. Complete remission rates exceeding 90% are reported with chemotherapy programs incorporating ATRA followed by consolidation chemotherapy.[10–12] Fenaux and colleagues[15] recently reported data from a trial of ATRA and chemotherapy in which the disease-free survival at 3 years was 76%.

Acute Lymphocytic Leukemia

Clinical Presentation

Acute lymphocytic leukemia (ALL) is the most common malignancy in childhood but represents only about 10–20% of adult acute leukemias.[2,3] Adult ALL is the focus of this discussion. Presentation of adult ALL closely resembles that of AML. Symptoms (bleeding, bruising, pallor, and infection) are often related to bone marrow failure, and their onset is usually abrupt. Patients commonly complain of extreme fatigue and malaise. Hepatomegaly, splenomegaly, and lymph node enlargement may be present. CNS involvement is also more common in ALL than in AML, being present at the time of diagnosis in approximately 5–10% of adult ALL patients.[16]

Laboratory findings in patients with ALL are usually consistent with bone marrow failure (i.e., anemia, thrombocytopenia, and neutropenia). High WBC counts (>50,000 cells/mm³) are more common in ALL than in AML patients. As with AML, WBC counts >100,000 cells/mm³ require emergent treatment. In addition, because of high cell turnover, serum lactate dehydrogenase (LDH) and uric acid levels may be elevated in ALL patients.

Diagnosis and Classification

As with AML, clinical and laboratory findings are highly suggestive of the diagnosis, but definitive diagnosis of ALL depends on results of the bone marrow biopsy. The presence of >30% leukemic blast cells in the bone marrow is diagnostic of acute leukemia. The bone marrow is then stained to differentiate ALL from AML. If the bone marrow specimen is myeloperoxidase negative, it is tested for terminal deoxynucleotidyl transferase (TdT), an enzyme found in T- and B-cell precursors. Bone marrow that is myeloperoxidase negative and TdT positive is highly suggestive of ALL. In addition, immunophenotyping is done to identify immune markers commonly associated with ALL, and cytogenetic studies are conducted to detect chromosomal abnormalities that further distinguish ALL from AML (Table 13-3).

The FAB system categorizes ALL into L1, L2, and L3 subtypes, based on cell size, number of nucleoli, amount of cytoplasm, and other morphological features (Table 13-4).[2] In adult ALL patients, approximately 33% are L1 subtype, <5% are L3 subtype, and the remaining are L2 subtype.[5] Morphological classification of ALL does not affect treatment choices but is associated with prognosis. L1 subtypes are

Table 13-4. FAB Classification of ALL

FAB Subtype	Frequency of Occurrence (%)	Lineage	Comments
L1	30	B cell or T cell	Most common subtype in children
L2	65	B cell or T cell	Most common subtype in adults
L3	5	B cell	Burkitt's subtype; poor prognosis

SOURCE: adapted from references 2 and 5.

associated with the best prognosis; L3 subtypes, with the worst (Table 13-5).[4]

Immunologic classification of ALL by expression of surface CD antigens permits assessment of B- or T-cell lineage. CD19 and CD20 are B-cell antigens, designating B-cell lineage; CD2 and CD7 are T-cell antigens, designating T-cell lineage; and CD10 is the common ALL antigen (CALLA), associated with pediatric ALL.[2] CALLA indicates neither B- nor T-cell lineage; such cells were formerly called "null cells." Approximately 75% of adult ALLs are of the pre-B-cell and B-cell lineage, and 25% are of T-cell origin (Table 13-5).[17] Adult T-cell ALL, sometimes called adult T-cell lymphoma, is a very aggressive type of ALL, but it is associated with a more favorable prognosis than B-cell ALL.[5]

The significance of chromosomal abnormalities associated with ALL (Table 13-3) in prognosis and treatment is not well established. The exception is the presence of the Philadelphia chromosome [t(9,22); see discussion under *Chronic Myelogenous Leukemia*, below]. Philadelphia chromosome–positive ALL is associated with a very poor prognosis despite aggressive treatment.[5]

Treatment

Treatment of adult ALL traditionally involves four phases: induction, CNS prophylaxis, consolidation, and maintenance. Experience with treatment of adult ALL is limited by its low incidence. Because most experience with ALL treatment has been gained in the pediatric population, the majority of adult ALL treatment protocols are modeled after pediatric regimens. In pediatric ALL, approximately 95% of patients achieve complete remission following induction chemotherapy and as many as 80% are ultimately cured of their disease.[18] The use of pediatric protocols for treatment of adult ALL has not met with such success, so a standard regimen for treatment of adult ALL has yet to be established.

Most induction regimens for adult ALL include an anthracycline (doxorubicin or daunorubicin) with vincristine and dexamethasone or prednisone.[19] Asparaginase is also often included. Although asparaginase has been shown to improve remission rates in pediatric populations, its role in treatment of adult ALL is uncertain.[19] Cyclophosphamide, often included in adult ALL induction regimens, may improve overall response rates and long-term survival in adult ALL patients.[16] A list of common chemotherapy regimens for remission induction in ALL are listed in Table 13-6.

Because chemotherapy agents do not readily penetrate the blood-brain barrier, the CNS is a sanctuary site for residual leukemic cells in ALL. Without prophylactic CNS treatment, approximately one third of adult ALL patients will eventually relapse with CNS disease, despite induction treatment.[5] Routine CNS prophylaxis reduces the rate of CNS relapse to <10%,[16] so all patients should receive some type of prophylactic CNS treatment. Cranial irradiation combined with intrathecal methotrexate has traditionally been used for CNS prophylaxis. However, because of the neurotoxicity associated with cranial irradiation, its use in CNS prophylaxis has fallen out of favor. Combinations of intrathecal methotrexate and cytarabine are also effective, and they are more commonly used today.[16] Intrathecal hydrocortisone may also be administered, for its lymphotoxic effects as well as to decrease local

Table 13-5. Immunologic Classification of ALL

Subtype	FAB Subtype	Frequency (%)	CD Antigens	Prognosis
Pre-B cell	L1, L2	70	CD10 (CALLA), CD19, CD20	Intermediate
B cell (Burkitt's)	L3	5	CD10, CD19, CD20	Poor
T cell (lymphoblastic lymphoma)	L1, L2	25	CD2, CD7, CD10, CD34	Favorable

SOURCE: adapted from references 2 and 5. CALLA, common ALL antigen.

Table 13-6. Commonly Used Chemotherapy Regimens for Remission Induction in ALL

Regimen	Drugs	Dose and Schedule
VAD[a]	**V**incristine	0.4 mg/day × 4 days CIVI, days 1–4
	Doxorubicin (**A**driamycin)	12 mg/m^2 per day × 4 days CIVI, days 1–4
	Dexamethasone	40 mg/day PO/IV, days 1–4, 9–12, 17–20
Linker[b]	Vincristine	2 mg IV push q week × 4 weeks
	Daunorubicin	50 mg/m^2 per day IV × 3 days, days 1–3
	Asparaginase	6000 IU/m^2 per day × 12 days, days 17–28
	Prednisone	60 mg/m^2 per day PO days 1–28

CIVI, continuous intravenous infusion; PO, by mouth; IV, intravenously; q, every; IU, international units.
[a]Data from reference 20.
[b]Data from reference 21.

irritation with intrathecal chemotherapy administration. High-dose, systemic administration of methotrexate and cytarabine achieve therapeutic levels in the CNS and are an effective substitute for intrathecal administration of these agents for CNS prophylaxis and for treatment of CNS disease in patients with ALL. The simultaneous administration of high-dose, systemic cytarabine and intrathecal cytarabine should be avoided to decrease the risk of irreversible cerebellar toxicity. Treatment of documented CNS ALL usually involves intensive intraventricular administration (e.g., through an Ommaya reservoir) of methotrexate or cytarabine.

The value of postremission consolidation therapy for ALL is well documented. Various treatment strategies have been employed,[19] but the best combination of drugs for consolidation therapy of adult ALL has not been established. Most protocols use alternating cycles of numerous agents, including vincristine, high-dose methotrexate, doxorubicin or daunorubicin, etoposide (VP-16) or teniposide (VM-26), high-dose cytarabine, asparaginase, and prednisone or dexamethasone.[19]

In contrast to AML, long-term, low-dose maintenance therapy is effective in prolonging remission in patients with ALL. Maintenance therapy for ALL typically consists of low-dose oral methotrexate (e.g., 20 mg/m^2 weekly) and 6-mercaptopurine (e.g., 75 mg/m^2 per day; dose is divided three times daily and rounded to the nearest 25 mg). Maintenance therapy for ALL is continued for 2–3 years after complete remission has been achieved.

Complete remission rates following induction treatment for adult ALL are 70–80%.[19] The median duration of complete remission averages 19–27 months, with a 20–30% chance for long-term disease-free survival (continuous complete remission >5 years).[19] Response to further chemotherapy following relapse of ALL is usually poor. For patients with an eligible donor, BMT may improve survival in ALL. Whether BMT should play a role in postremission therapy for ALL or be reserved for refractory and relapsed patients has not been determined. (See further discussion of BMT in chapter 14.)

Treatment-Related Toxicities and Complications

Toxicities following treatment for ALL are similar to those following treatment for AML. Patients with ALL are at greater risk for complications from tumor lysis syndrome because WBC counts are frequently higher at the time of diagnosis in ALL. Moderate to severe nausea and vomiting, diarrhea, mucositis, and alopecia may occur with ALL treatment regimens. Myelosuppression, characterized by anemia, thrombocytopenia, and neutropenia, is also common. The degree of bone marrow suppression caused by the drugs used in treatment of ALL (e.g., vincristine, prednisone or dexamethasone, and asparaginase) is less than that caused by AML chemotherapy. Thus, much of the postremission therapy (consolidation and maintenance) can be administered in the outpatient setting. However, protocols using high-dose systemic steroids and cyclophosphamide may pose an increased risk of atypical, non-neutropenic infections with fungal and viral pathogens.

Prognosis

Many factors influence an ALL patient's chance for long-term survival. Age is a prognostic factor. In contrast to AML, in which adult patients have a better chance for cure than children, pediatric ALL patients are more likely to respond to chemotherapy and have a better chance of long-term survival than adult patients.[19] Presence of the Philadelphia chromosome is a poor prognostic factor, and most patients with this abnormality will eventually relapse.[19] FAB morphological classification may also be associated with prognosis (as discussed in *Diagnosis and Classification*, above). Evidence of major organ dysfunction before treatment for ALL is associated with a poor prognosis. As with AML, the longer it takes to achieve a complete remission, the less the chance of cure. Chemotherapy-refractory ALL is associated with a very dim prognosis.

The Role of Colony-Stimulating Factors in Acute Leukemias

Bone marrow suppression following chemotherapy for acute leukemias, particularly AML, is severe and prolonged, sometimes 3 weeks or more. Myelosuppression typically produces neutropenia, thrombocytopenia, and anemia. Patients may require blood product support for many weeks following treatment. The use of colony-stimulating factors (CSFs) to stimulate bone marrow recovery in patients with acute leukemia has been an issue of considerable controversy. Some myeloid leukemic cells express receptors for granulocyte CSF (G-CSF) and granulocyte-macrophage CSF (GM-CSF), and there is concern that the use of CSFs following treatment for AML could stimulate leukemic cell growth. However, there is also evidence that the use of CSFs following chemotherapy for acute leukemias, especially ALL, is safe and may shorten the duration of neutropenia. Recently, several studies have reported the use of CSFs in elderly patients following treatment for AML and ALL.[22-25] These studies were conducted to determine the effect of G-CSF [22,23] or GM-CSF [24,25] on duration of neutropenia and overall morbidity and mortality following induction treatment for AML or ALL in elderly patients. The results of these studies are mixed. None of the studies indicated that the use of CSFs had a detrimental effect by stimulating leukemic cell growth. Two studies showed a beneficial effect (decreased duration of neutropenia),[23,24] and two studies described no advantage to the addition of CSFs. [23,24]

The original American Society of Clinical Oncology (ASCO) guidelines for the use of CSFs in cancer patients suggested that their use in patients with acute leukemias should be limited to patients being treated in the setting of a clinical trial.[26] However, the 1996 modifications to the ASCO guidelines support the administration of CSFs in the postinduction chemotherapy period for patients over 55 years of age, which is an FDA-approved use of GM-CSF.[27]

CHRONIC LEUKEMIAS

Chronic Myelogenous Leukemia

Clinical Presentation

Chronic myelogenous leukemia (CML) accounts for approximately 15% of all leukemias diagnosed in the United States, with approximately 4300 cases diagnosed each year.[28] CML can occur at any age but is most common in middle-aged adults, with a median age at onset of 53 years (Table 13-1).[29] It is characterized by accumulation of differentiated leukemic cells. Normal myeloid cells are gradually replaced with abnormal cells that are insensitive to normal regulatory controls of cell growth.

The hallmark feature of CML is the presence of the Philadelphia chromosome in leukemic cells. The Philadelphia chromosome was first identified in Philadelphia; it represents a translocation of genetic material between chromosomes 9 and 22 [t(9,22)] and is present in >90% of patients with CML.

CML typically occurs in three phases: chronic phase, accelerated phase, and blast crisis. The chronic phase, sometimes called the "benign phase," is the indolent stage of CML. Patients may be totally asymptomatic during the early chronic phase of CML. The chronic phase usually lasts for 3.5–5 years following the diagnosis of CML.[29] The accelerated phase of CML is a transitional phase, in which symptoms begin to worsen as leukemic cells accumulate more rapidly, eventually progressing to blast crisis. Blast crisis represents a transformation to acute leukemia.

Signs and symptoms of CML are nonspecific but may include fever, weight loss, fatigue, and general malaise. Anemia and thrombocytopenia usually occur, as normal blood cell precursors are crowded out of the bone marrow by high numbers of leukemic blast cells. As a result, symptoms of pallor, bleeding, easy bruising, and shortness of breath or exercise intolerance may develop. Because the leukemic cells in CML are mature and functional, infections are not a common presenting sign. This contrasts with AML, in which the leukemic cells are poorly differentiated and ineffective. Enlargement of the spleen, caused by accumulation of WBCs, is present in about 50% of patients at the time of diagnosis.[29] Splenomegaly can lead to complaints of left upper quadrant pain and early satiety with eating.

Laboratory findings in CML often include a high WBC count, sometimes well over 100,000 cells/mm^3. However, because the leukemic cells in CML tend to be smaller and more mature than the leukemic cells present in acute leukemias, leukostasis related to high WBC counts is uncommon in the chronic phase. As CML progresses to the more aggressive accelerated and blast crisis phases, the leukemic cells take on the characteristics of acute leukemic cells, and complications from leukostasis can occur. Uric acid and serum LDH levels may be elevated as a result of high cell turnover and rapid proliferation.

Diagnosis and Classification

In chronic phase CML, the peripheral blood smear typically shows WBCs in all stages of maturation, from blast cells to mature granulocytes, that look morphologically normal.[29] The diagnosis of CML is confirmed with a bone marrow biopsy, which typically reveals a hypercellular bone marrow (a bone marrow packed with cells) and an elevated myeloid-to-erythroid ratio.[29] A normal myeloid-to-erythroid ratio is approximately 2:1; in CML the ratio is 10–30:1.[29] In chronic phase CML, promyelocytes and blast cells account for <10% of all cells in the bone marrow.[30]

Treatment

Treatment of CML varies, depending on the phase of disease and whether or not the patient is a BMT candidate.

Chronic Phase

There are three major goals in treating chronic phase CML:

1. delay onset of blast crisis,
2. provide palliation and control signs and symptoms, and
3. eradicate the Philadelphia chromosome.

Hydroxyurea and busulfan are the two agents that have historically been used to delay the onset of blast crisis and provide symptomatic relief to patients in chronic phase CML. Both agents lower WBC counts, reducing symptoms of anemia, thrombocytopenia, splenomegaly, and malaise. The use of busulfan has fallen out of favor because of irreversible liver toxicity and pulmonary fibrosis associated with chronic use. Busulfan should be avoided in any patient who is a BMT candidate, because its use prior to BMT predisposes patients to more post-transplant treatment-related complications. Hydroxyurea is at least as effective as busulfan and offers a more favorable toxicity profile.[29,30] Hydroxyurea is administered intermittently in doses of 20–30 mg/kg per day orally until WBC counts decrease. Hydroxyurea provides a rapid onset of disease control, but some patients require daily maintenance therapy to sustain remission.[28] Because of its better toxicity profile, hydroxyurea is the drug of choice for acute symptom control in CML patients who are BMT candidates.

In the past decade, interferon alfa (INF-α) has become the standard of practice in the treatment of chronic phase CML because it can decrease the number of Philadelphia chromosome–positive cells in CML patients. Suppression of the Philadelphia chromosome correlates with improved survival.[31] There appears to be a relationship between the dose of the drug and response: higher doses of INF-α are associated with higher response rates.[29,30] The most effective dose of INF-α in treatment of CML appears to be 5 million units/m^2 of body surface area administered daily as a subcutaneous injection.[29,30] Because of the side effects associated with INF-α therapy, it is generally recommended that patients start at a lower dose of 3 million units/m^2 per day and titrate up to the target dose of 5 million units/m^2 per day.[29,30] To achieve the maximum benefits from INF-α therapy, INF-α treatment must be continued throughout the chronic phase. INF-α2a is approved by the FDA for this indication.

Response to traditional treatment with hydroxyurea or busulfan in chronic phase CML is 70–80%,[32] with a median survival time of 3–5 years. This compares with a median survival of <2 years in untreated patients.[28] Treatment with INF-α in CML produces response rates similar to those seen with conventional therapy. However, duration of response and survival time are longer in INF-α–treated patients because of the reduction in the number of Philadelphia chromosome–positive cells. Kantarjian et al.[31] recently reported estimated median survival times of ≥7 years with INF-α. Most patients with CML will, however, eventually progress to blast crisis because of the persistence of the Philadelphia chromosome.

Accelerated Phase and Blast Crisis

As patients enter the accelerated phase of CML, their symptoms become more difficult to manage. Response to palliative drug therapy is markedly decreased in the accelerated phase. Hydroxyurea is usually administered in an attempt to control elevated WBC counts, but most patients progress rapidly, over a period of weeks or months, to blast crisis. CML blast crisis represents a transformation to acute leukemia and must be treated as such. Approximately half of patients exhibit acute leukemia with myeloid features, a quarter exhibit acute leukemia with lymphoid features, and the remaining patients exhibit undifferentiated acute leukemia.[29] Therapy for CML in blast crisis usually incorporates AML- or ALL-type chemotherapy regimens. Response to treatment of CML blast crisis is extremely poor and duration of response is short. Survival beyond 1 year after progression to blast crisis is rare.[29]

Treatment-Related Toxicities and Complications

For patients in chronic phase CML, treatment-related toxicities and complications are primarily associated with side effects of drug therapy, since the disease itself produces few symptoms in the absence of high WBC counts. Hydroxyurea is usually well tolerated. Mild nausea and vomiting, bone marrow suppression, and skin rash are some of the toxicities associated with hydroxyurea. Busulfan causes mild to moderate nausea and vomiting, hyperpigmentation of the skin, and bone marrow suppression with short-term use. Chronic use can lead to pulmonary fibrosis and hepatotoxicity.

Most patients treated with INF-α experience an acute flu-like syndrome with symptoms of fevers, headache, chills, and muscle aches. Chronic side effects include anorexia, fatigue, and mild leukopenia and thrombocytopenia. (See further discussion of specific chemotherapy-related toxicities in chapters 7 and 8.)

Patients receiving chemotherapy for CML in the accelerated phase or in blast crisis experience treatment-related toxicities and complications similar to those of patients being treated for acute leukemias. Tumor lysis syndrome can occur in patients with high WBC counts. Severe and prolonged bone marrow suppression is common, and patients are at risk for secondary complications, such as neutropenic infections and bleeding.

Prognosis

The estimated 5-year survival rate for patients with CML is approximately 50–60% (Table 13-1).[32] Survival is expected to increase as INF-α therapy becomes the standard of care.

Allogeneic BMT offers the best chance for long-term survival in CML, although outcomes depend on the stage of disease at the time of transplantation. The greatest benefit is seen in patients who undergo BMT in the chronic phase; patients have a 40–70% chance of long-term disease-free survival.[30] In the accelerated phase, the 5-year survival rates decrease to 15–30%.[30] Survival rates for patients who receive BMT during the blast crisis phase are 10–20%.[30] Because BMT provides the best chance for long-term survival in CML, eligible patients with suitable bone marrow donors should be offered BMT as a treatment option early in the course of their disease. (See chapter 14 for further discussion of BMT in treating CML.)

Chronic Lymphocytic Leukemia

Clinical Presentation

Approximately 7400 new cases of chronic lymphocytic leukemia (CLL) are diagnosed each year in the United States, representing about 25% of new leukemia diagnoses. The median age at onset of CLL is 65 years, and the incidence of CLL increases with age. For people in the 35- to 59-year-old age group, the incidence of CLL is approximately 5 cases per 100,000 persons. In the 80- to 84-year-old age group, the incidence of CLL increases to 30 cases per 100,000 persons.[33]

CLL is approximately twice as common in men as in women.[33] In contrast to the other types of leukemias discussed, the etiology of CLL does not appear to be related to exposure to radiation or alkylating agents.[33] There does appear to be a hereditary component to the development of CLL.

CLL is characterized by massive accumulation of small, mature, dysfunctional lymphocytes. Like CML, CLL displays a more chronic, indolent course than that of the acute leukemias. Some patients with CLL can live for many years without treatment, depending on the extent of their disease at the time of diagnosis.

CLL is commonly diagnosed in asymptomatic patients on a routine physical examination. For other patients, CLL presents with symptoms such as fever, night sweats, fatigue, exercise intolerance, or weight loss. Infection may also be a presenting feature of CLL. Approximately 75% of patients develop infectious complications as a result of their disease. Neutropenia and decreased levels of circulating immunoglobulins may compromise the immune system of CLL patients. As a result, they are predisposed to bacterial and fungal infections.[28] Patients in later stages of CLL may exhibit gross lymphadenopathy, splenomegaly, and hepatomegaly caused by massive lymphocyte accumulation.

Laboratory findings in CLL are marked by dramatically elevated WBC counts, which frequently approach or exceed 100,000 cells/mm^3, with a predominance of lymphocytes (70–90%). This lymphocytosis is the hallmark feature of CLL.[33] Many patients exhibit evidence of bone marrow failure, with neutropenia, thrombocytopenia, and anemia.

Diagnosis and Classification

Diagnosis of CLL is determined by clinical findings, absolute lymphocyte count (ALC), and bone marrow biopsy. A persistently elevated ALC (>10,000/mm^3) with >30% lymphocytes in the bone marrow is diagnostic of CLL.[33] CLL is staged by the extent of organ and bone marrow involvement and resulting symptoms. The Rai Staging System is the system most commonly used to classify CLL in the United States (Table 13-7). A modification of the Rai Staging System groups patients into low-, intermediate-, and high-risk categories. The majority of patients are diagnosed in the early stages of CLL (Table 13-7). Staging of CLL is important because treatment decisions are based on clinical stage.

Treatment

Because CLL occurs most commonly in the elderly, the benefits of treating patients with chemotherapy must be weighed very carefully against the risks of treatment. Traditionally, chemotherapy has been shown to neither decrease progression nor improve survival in CLL patients.[28] Chemotherapy-related toxicities may worsen quality of life and even shorten survival. Thus, for patients who are not experiencing symptoms, no treatment is a viable therapeutic option. The primary goal in treating CLL is palliation of symptoms. Asymptomatic patients with lymphocytosis only (e.g., Rai stage 0) do not benefit from treatment.[34] In patients with anemia (hemoglobin <11 g/dl) and/or thrombocytopenia (platelets <100,000/mm^3), Rai stages III and IV, treatment should be initiated for symptom management. Patients with Rai stages I and II may also benefit from treatment, depending on the degree of lymphocytosis, lymphadenopathy, splenomegaly, and/or presence of symptoms.[33] Surgery and/or radiation therapy play a role in palliative local treatment of extensive splenomegaly or lymphadenopathy in CLL patients.

Chlorambucil is the mainstay of treatment in CLL because it is effective in reducing symptoms and is generally well tolerated. Chlorambucil is administered orally in pulse doses of 0.4–0.7 mg/kg (for a 70-kg patient, this means 14-24 2-mg tablets) every 2–4 weeks or in daily doses of 0.1–0.4 mg/kg until lymphocyte counts decrease, symptoms resolve, or

Table 13-7. Rai Staging System for CLL

Stage	Modified Rai	Frequency (%)	Lymphocytosis	Lymphadenopathy	Liver or Spleen Enlargement	Hemoglobin (g/dl)	Platelets (× 10^3/mm^3)	Median Survival (years)
0	low risk	30	+	−	−	≥11	≥100	14.5
I	intermediate	60	+	+	−	≥11	≥100	7.5
II	risk		+	±	+	≥11	≥100	
III	high risk	10	+	±	±	<11	≥100	2.5
IV			+	±	±	any	<100	

SOURCE: adapted from references 29, 33, and 34. +, present; −, not present; ±, may or may not be present.

bone marrow toxicity develops. When treatment is no longer producing a therapeutic effect, it should be discontinued to minimize toxicities.[33] Oral prednisone is often used in combination with chlorambucil but has no proven impact on response rates or patient survival.[33] Glucocorticoids help reduce symptoms in patients with severe lymphadenopathy and splenomegaly and may improve anemia and thrombocytopenia in some patients. Cyclophosphamide is sometimes used as an alternative to chlorambucil, but it does not offer any therapeutic gain in terms of efficacy or toxicity profile.[33] Conventional treatment of CLL provides patients with adequate relief of symptoms but is not curative (complete remission rates <10%) and has little impact on overall survival.[33]

Fludarabine is an antimetabolite drug with significant activity in CLL.[30,33] Fludarabine is administered intravenously in doses of 25 mg/m^2 per day for 5 days, repeated monthly for 4–6 months. Fludarabine is effective for initial treatment of CLL and in patients refractory to traditional treatment. In contrast to traditional therapy for CLL, fludarabine can induce complete remissions in up to 60% of patients, depending on the extent of their disease at the time of treatment.[30,33] The significance of this remission rate in CLL is not clear, however. Follow-up on initial studies with fludarabine in treatment of patients with CLL is incomplete, so the impact of fludarabine on survival has not been established. In addition, fludarabine has many toxicities that warrant caution, especially in the elderly. Of particular concern is fludarabine's propensity to cause immunosuppression with neutropenia and decreased numbers of functional T lymphocytes. The neutropenia seen with fludarabine is acute and self-limiting, but the lymphocytopenia may persist for several months following treatment and predisposes patients to atypical opportunistic infections, such as *Pneumocystis carinii* pneumonia (PCP). Although preliminary results with fludarabine in the treatment of CLL look promising, the benefits of treatment must be carefully weighed against the risks of toxicity.

Treatment-Related Toxicities and Complications

Treatment-related toxicities in CLL are primarily related to side effects of the chemotherapy. Treatment for CLL is typically administered in the outpatient setting. Common side effects with the alkylating agents chlorambucil and cyclophosphamide include bone marrow suppression and mild to moderate nausea and vomiting. With fludarabine, bone marrow suppression and immunosuppression, as discussed above, are common toxicities. (See further discussion of specific chemotherapy-related toxicities in chapters 7 and 8.)

Other complications associated with the pathophysiology of CLL include decreased production of immunoglobulins and cytopenias (e.g., anemia, thrombocytopenia, and neutropenia). Low immunoglobulin levels put CLL patients at increased risk for bacterial and atypical opportunistic infections. Administration of intravenous immune globulin every 3–4 weeks may decrease the incidence of infections but is very expensive and does not improve survival in CLL patients.[34]

Prognosis

The prognosis for patients with CLL is variable, depending on the patient's stage at the time of diagnosis (Table 13-7). Survival ranges from 2 years in patients with advanced disease to more than 20 years for patients with early asymptomatic disease.[33]

Because CLL is a malignancy that most commonly afflicts the elderly, few patients are BMT candidates. Thus, the role of BMT in treatment of CLL is not well established and is therefore limited.

LYMPHOMAS

Lymphomas are a group of malignancies of the lymphatic system. They are classified as hematological malignancies because the malignant cells arise from the bone marrow. However, lymphomas often behave like solid tumors in that they can be slow-growing and bulky; patients often present with visible or palpable masses that are enlarged lymph nodes. Lymphomas are divided into two main categories: Hodgkin's disease (HD) and non-Hodgkin's lymphoma (NHL). Lymphomas account for approximately 5% of all new cancers in the United States each year and approximately 5% of all cancer deaths.[1] Most of these new cancers are NHL. Approximately 55,400 patients were diagnosed with NHL in 1998, compared with only 7100 new cases of HD.[1] Lymphomas have a relatively low death rate because they are often responsive to treatment and are frequently curable. However, the incidence of lymphomas in the United States is climbing each year. Acquired immunodeficiency syndrome (AIDS)-related lymphomas are a major factor contributing to the increasing incidence of lymphomas.[35]

Clinical Presentation

HD and NHL are similar in their clinical presentation but are histologically very distinct diseases. Table 13-8 compares the clinical features and prognostic factors of HD and NHL. As with most types of cancer, the etiology of lymphomas is uncertain. There are many risk factors for the development of lymphoma, including exposure to radiation, environmental exposures (e.g., pesticides), occupational exposures (e.g., woodworkers), and viruses (Epstein-Barr virus and HIV).[36,37] There appears to be a hereditary predisposition to the development of lymphomas. Immunosuppression, whether congenital, acquired (e.g., through AIDS), or drug-induced (e.g., following organ transplantation), is also a risk factor.[36,37] In addition, NHLs may arise many years following treatment with alkylating drugs or other chemotherapy agents.[35]

HD and NHL occur most commonly in adults but can occur in almost any age group. HD exhibits a bimodal distri-

Table 13-8. Comparison of Hodgkin's Disease (HD) and Non-Hodgkin's Lymphoma

	Etiology/Risk Factors	Tissue Pathology	Classification	Presentation Signs and Symptoms	Negative Prognostic Factors
Hodgkin's disease	Viral: EBV Ionizing radiation Genetic Environmental/occupational exposure	**Reed-Sternberg cell:** characteristic malignant cell	Lymphocyte-predominant Nodular sclerosing Mixed cellularity Lymphocyte depleted	**Bimodal distribution:** peak incidence age 15–34 and >50 years **Lymphadenopathy:** painless, rubbery; often in the mediastinal and neck regions **B symptoms** (40%): fever, weight loss, night sweats Contiguous, regional spread Extranodal involvement uncommon	Advanced age Male Presence of B symptoms Lymphocyte-depleted histology Large mediastinal or abdominal involvement Subdiaphragmatic, lower abdominal, mesenteric, or pelvic lymph node involvement Extranodal extension Bone marrow or liver involvement
Non-Hodgkin's lymphoma	Viral: EBV (Burkitt's), HTLV, HIV Immunodeficiency: acquired (AIDS; postorgan transplant) and congenital Genetic Ionizing radiation Environmental	Monoclonal proliferation of malignant B or T lymphocytes	Low grade Intermediate grade High grade	**Median age:** at onset 56 years; can occur at any age **Lymphadenopathy:** painless, rubbery; cervical, supraclavicular regions **B symptoms** (20%): less common than with HD **Extranodal involvement:** bone marrow, GI tract, testes, brain	Advanced age Elevated LDH Large tumor burden ≥Stage II disease Lymphoblastic or Burkitt's lymphoma Presence of B symptoms Bone marrow or GI tract involvement Conversion from low to high grade

EBV, Epstein-Barr Virus; HTLV, human T-cell leukemia virus; HIV, human immunodeficiency virus; AIDS, acquired immunodeficiency virus; HD, Hodgkin's disease; B symptoms: fever, night sweats, weight loss; GI, gastrointestinal; LDH, lactate dehydrogenase.

bution, with peaks in incidence between the ages of 15 and 34 years and again over the age of 50.[37] NHLs are more common in middle-aged persons, with an average age of onset of 56 years.[35]

Most patients with lymphomas present with complaints of lymphadenopathy. In HD, enlarged lymph nodes are most common in the neck and in the mediastinum (visible on chest X-ray). In NHL, lymphadenopathy is also common in the neck area, primarily in the supraclavicular and cervical regions. Spread of HD is contiguous, so the disease is usually localized to regional lymph nodes. With the exception of the spleen, involvement outside the lymph nodes is rare.[38] HD seldom spreads to the bone marrow or liver. NHL spreads hematogenously and noncontiguously, so many nodal and extranodal sites may be involved. Gastrointestinal tract involvement is common. NHL also frequently spreads to the brain, bone marrow, and testes. So-called "B" symptoms, designated by the Ann Arbor Staging Classification for Lymphomas (Table 13-9) as the presence of fevers, weight loss, and night sweats, are present in approximately 40% of HD patients and approximately 20% of NHL patients at the time of diagnosis.[39] Many patients with lymphoma also complain of severe, relentless itching.

Laboratory findings in lymphoma patients commonly include an elevated LDH level due to high cell turnover rates. LDH levels may correlate with tumor burden, and higher LDH levels suggest more extensive disease.[35] If the bone marrow is involved, patients usually have evidence of bone marrow failure, including anemia, neutropenia, and thrombocytopenia. With very aggressive, high-grade lymphomas (e.g., Burkitt's or adult T-cell lymphomas), patients may present with signs of tumor lysis syndrome, including elevated uric acid, potassium, phosphate, and serum creatinine levels.

Diagnosis

The diagnostic workup for patients with presumed lymphoma is very extensive. A comprehensive physical examination and laboratory evaluation, including liver and kidney function, chemistries, and complete blood count, must be performed. The definitive diagnostic study is a tissue biopsy. Typically, an enlarged lymph node is removed and studied to confirm the diagnosis of HD or NHL. The characteristic pathological finding in HD is the Reed-Sternberg cell, a large multinucleated lymphocyte.[37] The Reed-Sternberg cell is considered to be the malignant culprit in HD. In NHL, tissue biopsy usually reveals a monoclonal (i.e., arising from a single mutant cell line) proliferation of B or T lymphocytes.

Lymphomas are staged according to the extent of disease and the presence of B symptoms. Radiographic studies are very important in staging lymphomas, as they help determine the extent of disease. Radiographic studies typically include a chest X-ray and a chest, abdominal, and/or pelvic computed tomography (CT or "CAT") scan. Some clinicians also

Table 13-9. Ann Arbor Staging Classification for Lymphomas

Stage	Characteristics
I	Involvement of a single lymph node region (I) or a single extralymphatic region or site (I_E)
II	Involvement of two or more lymph node regions on the same side of the diaphragm (II) or localized involvement of an extralymphatic organ or site (II_E)
III	Involvement of lymph node regions on both sides of the diaphragm (III), localized involvement of an extralymphatic site (III_E) or spleen (III_S), or both
IV	Diffuse or disseminated involvement of one or more extralymphatic organs with or without associated lymph node involvement
Any Stage	A: asymptomatic B: presence of B symptoms (fever, night sweats, weight loss)

SOURCE: adapted from reference 38.

include lymphangiography, a radiographic study that helps to visualize the lymphatic system.[36] Lymphangiograms are more sensitive than other radiographic studies, such as CT scans, and may detect disease that cannot be picked up by other studies. Bilateral bone marrow biopsies are usually done to look for bone marrow involvement.

The Ann Arbor Staging Classification is the most commonly used system to stage HD and NHL (Table 13-9). Ann Arbor stages I and II represent regional or limited spread and are generally considered localized disease. Ann Arbor stages III and IV represent widespread involvement and are considered advanced disease. Patients who present at any stage without constitutional symptoms of fever, night sweats, or weight loss are subclassified as "A" (e.g., stage III_A). Patients who present with constitutional (or "B") symptoms are subclassified as "B" (e.g., stage III_B).

Classification

Lymphomas are classified on the basis of tissue pathology. HD and NHLs are classified separately. The Rye classification system divides HD into four histological categories: lymphocyte predominant, nodular sclerosing, mixed cellularity, and lymphocyte depleted. The most common types of HD are nodular sclerosing and mixed cellularity.[38] There are many, ever-changing tissue classification systems for NHLs. The currently accepted *Working Formulation for Classification of Non-Hodgkin's Lymphomas* (the "Working Formulation") was

Table 13-10. Working Formulation for Classification of Non-Hodgkin's Lymphoma

Low Grade
- Small lymphocytic
- Follicular, small cleaved
- Follicular, mixed small cleaved and large cell

Intermediate Grade
- Follicular large cell
- Diffuse small cleaved cell
- Diffuse mixed, small cleaved and large cell
- Diffuse large
- Diffuse large cell

High Grade
- Immunoblastic, large cell
- Lymphoblastic
- Small, noncleaved cell

SOURCE: adapted from reference 40.

put together by an international group of pathologists in the early 1980s.[40] The Working Formulation classifies NHL according to morphological features of the affected lymph node tissue. Essentially, the Working Formulation divides NHLs into three main categories: low-, intermediate-, and high-grade lymphomas, with many subcategories (Table 13-10). In general, low-grade lymphomas are very slow-growing and usually incurable tumors, but patients can live for many years without treatment because of their indolent nature (much like CLL, which is often classified as a low-grade lymphoma). Intermediate- and high-grade lymphomas are typically more aggressive, rapidly growing tumors that can be rapidly fatal if not treated. However, they are usually responsive to chemotherapy and are more frequently curable with appropriate treatment than low-grade lymphomas. The significance of tissue classification of lymphomas relates mainly to prognosis. Certain histological subtypes are associated with a better or worse prognosis (Table 13-8). The REAL (Revised European American Lymphoma) Classification system has recently been developed and classifies lymphomas by T- or B-cell histology. The REAL classification system has not been as widely incorporated into clinical practice as the Working Formulation.

Treatment

Chemotherapy regimens for treatment of lymphomas are based on two basic principles. First, most lymphomas are dose-responsive tumors. Thus, it is important to maintain dose-intensity when treating lymphomas with chemotherapy. Second, lymphomas are typically heterogeneic tumors. Therefore, chemotherapy regimens for lymphomas incorporate multiple agents with different mechanisms of action and nonoverlapping toxicities.

Treatment plans for lymphomas frequently employ a multimodal approach that includes surgery, radiation, and chemotherapy. Treatment for patients with localized disease often includes surgery and/or radiation without chemotherapy, whereas patients with advanced disease usually require systemic treatment with chemotherapy. Chemotherapy for lymphomas is generally administered in repeated 2- to 4-week cycles for a minimum of six courses.

Table 13-8 describes many prognostic factors that are associated with a patient's chance for cure following treatment for lymphoma. In addition, initial response to chemotherapy is an indicator of outcome. Patients who fail to respond to initial chemotherapy have a limited chance for cure or long-term survival.

Hodgkin's Disease

There are numerous drugs that have established efficacy in HD, including mechlorethamine, vinca alkaloids, corticosteroids, procarbazine, chlorambucil, dacarbazine, doxorubicin, and bleomycin. Single-agent therapy for HD does not improve survival, but combinations of active drugs can produce cures in ≥60% of patients treated.[37] Table 13-11 displays a list of commonly used combination chemotherapy regimens that are effective in the treatment of HD. Response and long-term survival rates are similar regardless of the combination used, so selection of a chemotherapy regimen for HD is based largely on toxicity profile.[37] MOPP (*m*echlorethamine, vincristine [*O*ncovin], *p*rocarbazine, and *p*rednisone) was the first combination regimen to show significant activity against HD. However, some of the long-term toxicities (such as sterility and secondary malignancies) associated with this regimen are highly undesirable, especially in young and potentially curable patients. ABVD (doxorubicin [*A*driamycin], *b*leomycin, *v*inblastine, and *d*acarbazine) produces similar response rates with a lower risk of these long-term toxicities.[38] A

Table 13-11. Combination Chemotherapy Regimens in Treatment of Hodgkin's Disease

Drug Combination	
MOPP	Mechlorethamine Vincristine (Oncovin) Procarbazine Prednisone
ABVD	Doxorubicin (Adriamycin) Bleomycin Vinblastine Dacarbazine
MOPP/ABVD	(MOPP alternating monthly with ABVD)
MOPP/ABV hybrid	(no dacarbazine)

SOURCE: adapted from reference 37.

recent study conducted by the CALGB compared combination chemotherapy with a hybrid regimen (MOPP/ABV) and ABVD in advanced HD.[41] There was no significant difference in efficacy between the two regimens, but the study was closed prematurely because of concerns about excessive treatment-related deaths and secondary cancers associated with the MOPP/ABV arm.[41] Accumulating evidence supports ABVD as initial treatment for HD in patients who require systemic treatment.[38] Second-line or salvage combination chemotherapy regimens for HD incorporate drugs with different mechanisms of cytotoxicity, such as etoposide, methotrexate, cisplatin, cytarabine, cyclophosphamide, ifosfamide, or melphalan.

Non-Hodgkin's Lymphomas

Low-grade lymphomas are not commonly curable with chemotherapy. However, chemotherapy may offer some survival benefit and provide palliative relief for symptomatic patients. Recent data suggests that chemotherapy followed by maintenance therapy with INF-α improves disease-free survival in patients with low-grade lymphomas.[42]

Intermediate- and high-grade lymphomas are responsive to treatment, and patients with these malignancies are frequently curable with chemotherapy alone. As with HD, no single-agent therapy has had a significant impact on outcome in the management of NHL, but combinations of active drugs can produce long-term survival and cure. Response rates may depend on prognostic factors. For patients with good prognostic factors, combination chemotherapy can produce complete remission rates as high as 87%, with 73% long-term survival.[35] For patients with poor prognostic factors, indicating a higher risk of relapse, complete remission rates are closer to 40% and long-term survival is only 26%.[35]

Drugs active in the treatment of NHL include cyclophosphamide, doxorubicin, vinca alkaloids, corticosteroids, methotrexate, bleomycin, etoposide, and cytarabine. Table 13-12 lists common combination chemotherapy regimens active in the treatment of NHL. CHOP (*c*yclophosphamide, doxorubicin [*h*ydroxydaunorubicin], vincristine [*O*ncovin], and *p*rednisone) is the standard regimen at present for initial treatment of NHL. Studies comparing CHOP with more complicated regimens containing as many as eight drugs, such as ProMACE/CytaBOM, have shown no difference in response rates or survival and more toxicity than CHOP therapy.[35] More complicated regimens are generally reserved for second-line therapy.

Bone Marrow Transplantation

Because the cure rate is so high with conventional-dose chemotherapy and/or radiation, BMT in the treatment of HD is generally reserved for salvage therapy in relapsed or refractory patients. In treatment of NHL, the role of BMT is more controversial. Currently, the accepted use of BMT in the management of NHL is for the treatment of relapsed or refractory disease. The controversy concerns whether or not to incorporate BMT earlier in the course of treatment, especially for patients with poor prognostic factors, in whom the chance for relapse is high. Autologous BMT is an acceptable procedure for lymphoma patients without bone marrow involvement; otherwise, allogeneic BMT is preferred. (See chapter 14 for additional information on BMT.)

Table 13-12. Combination Chemotherapy in Non-Hodgkin's Lymphoma

CHOP	Cyclophosphamide Doxorubicin (Hydroxydaunorubicin) Vincristine (Oncovin) Prednisone
CHOP-Bleo	Chop + Bleomycin
ProMACE/CytaBOM	Prednisone Doxorubicin (Adriamycin) Cyclophosphamide Etoposide Cytarabine Bleomycin Vincristine (Oncovin) Methotrexate/Leucovorin
ESHAP	Etoposide Methylprednisolone (Solu-medrol) Cytarabine (High-dose Ara-C) Cisplatin (Platinol)
M-BACOD	Methotrexate Bleomycin Doxorubicin (Adriamycin) Cyclophosphamide Vincristine (Oncovin) Dexamethasone

Treatment-Related Toxicities and Complications

Acute chemotherapy-related toxicities, such as bone marrow suppression, mucositis, nausea, vomiting, and infection, are common with lymphoma therapy. In most patients, however, toxicities are not severe enough to require hospitalization for treatment. Late and long-term toxicities, such as anthracycline-induced cardiac toxicity, infertility, and secondary malignancies, are unfortunate risks following treatment for lymphomas.

SUMMARY

Hematological malignancies are much less common than solid tumors, but they are among the few types of malignancies that are potentially curable with drug therapy. Because some of these diseases are potentially curable, treatment is often aggressive and may be associated with significant toxicities and complications. During their course of treatment, patients with hematological malignancies will experience a wide array of therapy-related side effects, including nausea, vomiting, infection, and mucositis. By combining an understanding of the basic disease processes of hematological malignancies with knowledge of the medications used in treatment and supportive care of these patients, a pharmacist is able to become an integral member of the patient care team.

REFERENCES

1. Landis SH, Murray T, Bolden S, et al. Cancer statistics, 1998. *CA Cancer J Clin* 1998;48:6–29.
2. Skarin AT, editor. *Diagnostic Oncology*. London: Gower Medical; 1991. Chapter 11, Acute and chronic leukemias. p. 11.1–11.40.
3. Vogel VG, Fisher RE. Epidemiology and etiology of leukemia. *Curr Opin Oncol* 1993;5:26–34.
4. Sandler DP, Ross JA. Epidemiology of acute leukemia in children and adults. *Semin Oncol* 1997;24:3–16.
5. Scheinberg DA, Maslak P, Weiss M. Acute leukemias. In: DeVita VT, Hellman S, Rosenberg SA, editors. *Cancer: Principles and Practices of Oncology*. 5th ed. Philadelphia, PA: JB Lippincott; 1997. p. 2293–321.
6. Stone RM, Mayer RJ. Treatment of the newly diagnosed adult with de novo acute myelogenous leukemia. *Hematol Oncol Clin North Am* 1993;7:47–64.
7. Berman E, Heller G, Santorsa J, et al. Results of a randomized trial comparing idarubicin and cytarabine with daunorubicin and cytarabine in adult patients with newly diagnosed acute myelogenous leukemia. *Blood* 1991;77:1666–74.
8. Wiernik PH, Banks PC, Case DC, et al. Cytarabine plus idarubicin or daunorubicin as induction and consolidation therapy for previously untreated adults with acute myelogenous leukemia. *Blood* 1992;79:313–9.
9. Vogler WR, Velez-Garcia E, Omura G, et al. A phase III trial comparing daunorubicin or idarubicin combined with cytarabine arabinoside in acute myelogenous leukemia. *J Clin Oncol* 1992;10:1103–11.
10. Fenaux P, Le Delay MC, Castaigne S, et al. Effect of all-*trans*-retinoic acid in newly diagnosed acute promyelocytic leukemia: results of a multi-center randomized trial. *Blood* 1993;82(11):3241–9.
11. Degos L, Dombret H, Chomienne C, et al. All *trans*-retinoic acid as a differentiating agent in treatment of acute promyelocytic leukemia. *Blood* 1995;85:2643–53.
12. Fenaux P, Chomienne C, Degos L. Acute promyelocytic leukemia: biology and treatment. *Semin Oncol* 1997;24:92–102.
13. Mayer RJ, Davis RB, Schiffer CA, et al. Intensive postremission chemotherapy in adults with acute myelogenous leukemia. *N Engl J Med* 1994;331:896–903.
14. Bishop JF. The treatment of adult acute myeloid leukemia. *Semin Oncol* 1997;24:57–69.
15. Fenaux P, Chastang CL, Sanz M, et al. Effect of ATRA in newly diagnosed acute promyelocytic leukemia: validation of short-term effect in a large multi-center trial (APL 93 Trial) and assessment of long-term benefit (APL 91 Trial) [abstract 824]. *Blood* 1996;88(10 Suppl 1):209a.
16. Laport GF, Larson RA. Treatment of adult acute lymphoblastic leukemia. *Semin Oncol* 1997;24:70–82.
17. Copelan EA, McGuire EA. The biology and treatment of acute lymphoblastic leukemia. *Blood* 1995;85:1151–68.
18. Teresi ME, Crom WM. Childhood leukemias and lymphomas. In: DiPiro JT, Talbert RL, Hayes PE, et al., editors. *Pharmacotherapy: A Pathophysiologic Approach*. 2nd ed. East Norwalk, CT: Appleton & Lange; 1993. p. 2051–67.
19. Hoelzer DF. Therapy of the newly diagnosed adult with acute lymphoblastic leukemia. *Hematol Oncol Clin North Am* 1993;7:139–60.
20. Kantarjian HM, Walters RS, Keating MJ, et al. Results of vincristine, doxorubicin, and dexamethasone regimen in adults with standard- and high-risk acute lymphocytic leukemia. *J Clin Oncol* 1990;8:994–1004.
21. Linker CA, Levitt LJ, O'Donnell M, et al. Treatment of adult lymphoblastic leukemia with intensive cyclical chemotherapy: a follow-up report. *Blood* 1991;78:2814–22.
22. Ottman OG, Hoelzer D, Gracien E, et al. Concomitant granulocyte colony-stimulating factor and induction chemoradiotherapy in adult acute lymphoblastic leukemia: a randomized phase III trial. *Blood* 1995;86:444–50.
23. Dombret H, Chastang C, Fenaux P, et al. A controlled study of recombinant human granulocyte colony stimulating factor in elderly patients after treatment for acute myelogenous leukemia. *N Engl J Med* 1995;332:1678–83.
24. Stone RM, Berg DT, George SL, et al. Granulocyte-macrophage colony-stimulating factor after initial chemotherapy for elderly patients with primary acute myelogenous leukemia. *N Engl J Med* 1995;332:1671–77.
25. Rowe JM, Anderson JW, Mazza JJ, et al. A randomized placebo-controlled phase III study of granulocyte-macrophage colony-stimulating factor in adult patients (> 55–70 years of age) with acute myelogenous leukemia: a study of the Eastern Cooperative Oncology Group. *Blood* 1995;86:457–62.
26. American Society of Clinical Oncology. Recommendations for the use of hematopoietic colony-stimulating factors: evidence-based, clinical practice guidelines. *J Clin Oncol* 1994;12(11):2471–508.
27. American Society of Clinical Oncology. Update of recommendations for the use of hematopoietic colony-stimulating factors: evidence-based, clinical practice guidelines. *J Clin Oncol* 1996;14(6):1957–60.
28. Morrison VA. Chronic leukemias. *CA Cancer J Clin* 1994;44:353–77.
29. Cortes JE, Talpaz M, Kantarjian H. Chronic myelogenous leukemia: a review. *Am J Med* 1996;100:555–70.
30. Deisseroth AB, Kantarjian H, Andreef M, et al. Chronic leukemias. In: DeVita VT, Hellman S, Rosenberg SA, editors. *Cancer: Principles and Practices of Oncology*. 5th ed. Philadelphia, PA: JB Lippincott; 1997. p. 2321–43.
31. Kantarjian HM, Smith TL, O'Brien S, et al. Prolonged survival in chronic myelogenous leukemia after cytogenetic response to interferon-alpha therapy. *Ann Intern Med* 1995;122:254–61.
32. Kantarjian HM, Deisseroth AB, Kurzrock R, et al. Chronic myelogenous leukemia: a concise update. *Blood* 1993;82:691–703.
33. Faguet GB. Chronic lymphocytic leukemia: an updated review. *J Clin Oncol* 1994;12:1974–90.

34. Rozman C, Montserrat E. Chronic lymphocytic leukemia. *N Engl J Med* 1995;333(16):1052–7.
35. Shipp MA, Mauch P, Harris NL. Non-Hodgkin's lymphomas. In: DeVita VT, Hellman S, Rosenberg SA, editors. *Cancer: Principles and Practices of Oncology*. 5th ed. Philadelphia, PA: JB Lippincott; 1997. p. 2165–242.
36. Armitage JO. Treatment of non-Hodgkin's lymphoma. *N Engl J Med* 1993;328:1023–30.
37. Urba WJ, Longo DL. Hodgkin's disease. *N Engl J Med* 1992;326:678–87.
38. DeVita VT, Hellman S, Jaffe ES. Hodgkin's disease. In: DeVita VT, Hellman S, Rosenberg SA, editors. *Cancer: Principles and Practices of Oncology*. 5th ed. Philadelphia, PA: JB Lippincott; 1997. p. 1819–58.
39. Koeller J, Adams V. Malignant lymphomas. In: DiPiro JT, Talbert RL, Yee GC, et al., editors. *Pharmacotherapy: A Pathophysiologic Approach*. 3rd ed. East Norwalk, CT: Appleton & Lange; 1997. p. 2559–86.
40. The Non-Hodgkin's Lymphoma Pathologic Classification Project. National Cancer Institute–sponsored study of classifications of non-Hodgkin's lymphomas: summary and description of a working formulation for clinical usage. *Cancer* 1982;49:2112–35.
41. Duggan D, Petroni J, Johnson K, et al. MOPP/ABV versus ABVD for advanced Hodgkin's disease—a preliminary report of CALGB 8952 (with SWOG, ECOG, NCIC) [abstract 43]. *Proc ASCO* 1997;16:12a.
42. Unterhalt M, Hermann R, Koch P, et al. Long-term interferon-alpha maintenance prolongs remission duration in advanced low-grade lymphoma and is related to efficacy of initial cytoreductive chemotherapy [abstract 1801]. *Blood* 1996;88(10 Suppl 1):453a.

SELF-STUDY QUESTIONS

Questions 1–4: Match the following descriptions with the corresponding type of leukemia:

a. acute leukemia
b. chronic leukemia
c. myeloid leukemia
d. lymphoid leukemia

1. This type of leukemia is characterized by the presence of mature cells, gradual onset of symptoms, and natural history measured in years.
2. Cell lines affected include B and T lymphocytes.
3. Cell lines affected include neutrophils, megakaryocytes, and erythrocytes.
4. This type of leukemia is characterized by the presence of very immature cells, with a rapid onset of symptoms and progression over weeks to months.

Questions 5–9: Match the following clinical features with the corresponding type of leukemia (each answer may be used more than once):

a. acute myelogenous leukemia (AML)
b. acute lymphocytic leukemia (ALL)
c. chronic myelogenous leukemia (CML)
d. chronic lymphocytic leukemia (CLL)

5. high white blood cell (WBC) count; bone marrow biopsy reveals >30% leukemic blast cells, myeloperoxidase negative; terminal deoxynucleotidyl transferase (TdT) positive; central nervous system (CNS) is sanctuary site
6. median age at onset is 65 years; often diagnosed on a routine physical examination; associated with massive lymphadenopathy
7. associated with the presence of the Philadelphia chromosome; occurs in three phases; may progress to more aggressive leukemia
8. most common malignancy in childhood
9. WBC count may be high, low, or normal; bone marrow biopsy reveal >30% blast cells; myeloperoxidase positive; subtype may respond to treatment with vitamin A derivative

Questions 10–14: Match each of the following phases of treatment for acute leukemia with the corresponding definition:

a. induction
b. intensification
c. consolidation
d. maintenance
e. CNS prophylaxis

10. Low doses of chemotherapy are administered daily or weekly to sustain an established remission.
11. Chemotherapy, in standard doses, is administered after complete remission has been achieved, with the goal of destroying any residual leukemic cells.
12. Chemotherapy, in high doses, is administered after complete remission has been achieved, with the goal of destroying any residual leukemic cells.
13. Chemotherapy and/or radiotherapy is administered to prevent CNS leukemia.
14. Initial chemotherapy is administered to try to produce a complete remission.

15. The 7 + 3 regimen for treatment of AML may include cytarabine and:

a. ara-C
b. methotrexate
c. idarubicin
d. vincristine

16. For a 45-year-old patient in complete remission following 7 + 3 chemotherapy, which of the following chemotherapy regimens would be the most appropriate for

postremission therapy?

   a. high-dose cytarabine
   b. low-dose cytarabine
   c. daily methotrexate with weekly 6-mercaptopurine
   d. interferon alfa (IFN-α)

17. Which of the following chemotherapy regimens would be most appropriate for induction treatment for a patient with the M3 (acute promyelocytic leukemia [APL]) subtype of AML?

   a. 7 + 3 chemotherapy
   b. high-dose cytarabine
   c. all-*trans*-retinoic acid (ATRA)
   d. IFN-α

18. Select the true statement:

   a. Therapy for AML incorporates four phases of treatment: induction, consolidation, CNS prophylaxis, and maintenance therapy.
   b. Therapy for ALL incorporates four phases of treatment: induction, consolidation, CNS prophylaxis, and maintenance therapy.
   c. Therapy for AML incorporates only two phases of treatment: induction and maintenance therapy.
   d. Therapy for ALL incorporates only two phases of treatment: induction and maintenance therapy.

19. Induction therapy for ALL typically includes which of the following chemotherapy agents?

   a. cytarabine and idarubicin
   b. cytarabine and asparaginase
   c. idarubicin, asparaginase, dexamethasone, and prednisone
   d. doxorubicin, vincristine, asparaginase, and prednisone

20. Treatment with which of the following agents in CML has been shown to increase survival and decrease expression of the Philadelphia chromosome?

   a. IFN-α
   b. chlorambucil
   c. busulfan
   d. hydroxyurea

21. The use of IFN-α in treatment of CML is indicated for patients in which phase of the disease?

   a. chronic phase
   b. accelerated phase
   c. blast crisis
   d. any phase

22. Initiation of chemotherapy in CLL should be considered when:

   a. patients are in the asymptomatic phase of their disease.
   b. absolute lymphocyte counts are >10,000/mm³.
   c. patients begin to develop symptoms (e.g., anemia or thrombocytopenia).
   d. CLL is diagnosed, to prolong survival.

23. Which of the following agents has been shown to induce the highest complete remission rate in CLL patients?

   a. chlorambucil
   b. prednisone
   c. cyclophosphamide
   d. fludarabine

24. Which of the following is a complication of treatment with fludarabine?

   a. predisposition to development of opportunistic infections, such as *Pneumocystis carinii* pneumonia (PCP)
   b. predisposition to development of severe lung and liver toxicity
   c. flu-like syndrome (fevers, muscle aches, headache)
   d. predisposition to the development secondary cancers

25. Treatment-related toxicities and complications following chemotherapy are common in AML and ALL. Which of the following complications occurs more frequently with ALL?

   a. tumor lysis syndrome
   b. infectious and bleeding complications resulting from bone marrow suppression
   c. nausea and vomiting
   d. alopecia

26. Select the true statement:

   a. The ASCO guidelines on colony-stimulating factor (CSF) use state that CSFs should never be used in patients with acute leukemias.
   b. The ASCO guidelines on CSF use state that only granulocyte-macrophage CSF (GM-CSF) should be used in patients with acute leukemias.
   c. The ASCO guidelines on CSF use state CSFs should be included as standard treatment to decrease the severity and duration of neutropenia following chemotherapy for all patients with an acute leukemia.
   d. The ASCO guidelines on CSF use support the use of CSFs following induction chemotherapy for acute leukemia in elderly patients (>55 years of age).

Questions 27–30: Match the following clinical feature with the corresponding type of lymphoma (each answer may be used more than once):

   a. non-Hodgkin's lymphoma (NHL)
   b. Hodgkin's disease (HD)

27. bimodal distribution of incidence, with peaks in patients between the ages of 15 and 34 and >50 years

28. malignancy associated with human immunodeficiency virus (HIV) infection

29. classification by the Working Formulation into low, intermediate, and high grades

30. characterized by the presence of the Reed-Sternberg cell

31. Which of the following is considered a poor prognostic factor in patients with NHL?

    a. high-grade classification
    b. involvement below the diaphragm
    c. presence of lymphadenopathy
    d. presence of B symptoms

32. The CHOP regimen for treatment of NHL includes which of the following chemotherapy agents?

    a. cyclophosphamide, doxorubicin, vincristine, and prednisone
    b. cisplatin, doxorubicin, vincristine, and prednisone
    c. cisplatin, high-dose cytarabine, vincristine, and prednisone
    d. cyclophosphamide, hydroxyurea, cisplatin, and prednisone

33. Select the true statement:

    a. Chemotherapy has no role in the management of low-grade lymphomas.
    b. Low-grade lymphomas are curable with combination chemotherapy.
    c. Low-grade lymphomas are typically more sensitive to chemotherapy than high-grade lymphomas.
    d. High-grade lymphomas are typically more sensitive to chemotherapy than low-grade lymphomas.

34. Select the true statement:

    a. In the treatment of HD, MOPP chemotherapy has been proved to be more effective than ABVD chemotherapy.
    b. In the treatment of HD, ABVD chemotherapy has been proved to be more effective than MOPP chemotherapy.
    c. In the treatment of HD, MOPP chemotherapy has been proved approximately equal in efficacy to ABVD chemotherapy, but greater in toxicity.
    d. In the treatment of HD, ABVD chemotherapy has been proved approximately equal in efficacy to MOPP chemotherapy, but greater in toxicity.

35. Select the true statement:

    a. CHOP is less effective and less toxic than more complicated regimens, such as ProMACE/CytaBOM, in the treatment of NHL.
    b. CHOP is as effective as and less toxic than more complicated regimens, such as ProMACE/CytaBOM, in the treatment of NHL.
    c. CHOP is as effective and toxic as more complicated regimens, such as ProMACE/CytaBOM, in the treatment of NHL.
    d. CHOP is more effective and more toxic than more complicated regimens, such as ProMACE/CytaBOM, in the treatment of NHL.

36. Which of the following is/are late (long-term) complications following chemotherapy for HD with the MOPP chemotherapy regimen?

    a. infertility
    b. pulmonary fibrosis
    c. cardiomyopathy
    d. secondary malignancies
    e. a and d
    f. b and d
    g. all of the above

37. In the management of CML, patients have the best chance for long-term survival following bone marrow transplantation (BMT) when they receive the transplant in which phase of the disease?

    a. chronic phase
    b. accelerated phase
    c. blast crisis
    d. any phase

38. Because of the typical patient's age at the time of diagnosis, BMT is usually not a treatment option for patients with which type of leukemia?

    a. AML
    b. ALL
    c. CML
    d. CLL

39. Patients with CML who are candidates for BMT should not receive which of the following chemotherapy agents for treatment in the chronic phase of their disease?

    a. hydroxyurea
    b. busulfan
    c. IFN-α
    d. any of the above

40. At what point in the management of HD is BMT typically considered?

    a. BMT is considered as initial therapy to improve chances for long-term survival.
    b. BMT is considered as consolidation therapy, following induction, to improve chances for long-term survival.
    c. BMT is considered as salvage therapy for relapsed or refractory patients.
    d. BMT is not considered a treatment modality in the management of HD.

Chapter 14: Bone Marrow Transplantation

Laura E. Wiggins, Pharm.D., B.C.P.S.
Oncology Clinical Pharmacist
The Cancer Institute
Good Samaritan Medical Center
West Palm Beach, Florida

Bone Marrow Transplantation	252
Types of BMT	252
Peripheral Stem Cell Transplantation	253
Bone Marrow Harvest and Infusion	253
Applications of BMT	254
Hematological Malignancies	254
Solid Tumors	255
Pediatric Tumors	255
Complications	256
Hepatic Veno-occlusive Disease	256
Prevention of Hepatic VOD	256
Treatment of Hepatic VOD	256
Graft-Versus-Host Disease	256
Acute GVHD	256
GVHD Prophylaxis	257
Toxicity of GVHD Prophylaxis	258
Treatment of Acute GVHD	259
Chronic GVHD	259
Treatment of Chronic GVHD	260
Infectious and Related Complications	260
Interstitial Pneumonitis	261
Hematopoietic Growth Factors in BMT	262
Recent Advances in BMT	262
Summary	262
References	262
Self-Study Questions	266

Bone marrow transplantation (BMT) has increasingly been utilized in the treatment of patients with many types of cancer. Although initially developed as treatment for patients with acute leukemia, BMT with high-dose chemotherapy is rapidly becoming an integral part of the treatment of patients with a variety of diagnoses, including hematological malignancies (such as lymphoma or multiple myeloma) and solid tumors (such as breast cancer). The application of BMT in the treatment of cancer has grown, and clinical research in this field is rapidly expanding.

After completing this chapter, the reader should be able to:

1. Explain the rationale for the use of BMT to treat patients with cancer.
2. Compare the regimen-related complications of allogeneic BMT with those of autologous BMT.
3. Describe which patients may be at risk for developing graft-versus-host disease following BMT.
4. Assess the risks and benefits of current therapies used to prevent and treat graft-versus-host disease in BMT patients.
5. Outline the types, course, prevention, and management of common infectious complications that can occur in patients who have undergone BMT.
6. Compare peripheral stem cell transplantation with traditional autologous BMT in the following areas: source of cells, need for hospitalization, complications, time to recovery, and efficacy.

BONE MARROW TRANSPLANTATION

Bone marrow, a liquid substance found within bones, is the source of hematopoietic stem cells. Stem cells proliferate and differentiate, producing white blood cells, red blood cells, and platelets. Bone marrow transplantation (BMT) has been used to treat a variety of malignant and nonmalignant disorders.[1-3] Many oncological disorders are caused by a defect in the function of bone marrow or stem cells, including leukemias, lymphomas, and aplastic anemia. Another person's marrow can be infused to treat these diseases. For some kinds of cancer (e.g., solid tumors), BMT is used to improve the dose intensity of the chemotherapy.

Standard-dose chemotherapy has improved overall survival among patients with cancer; many times, however, a cure is not achieved. Studies of chemotherapy doses and tumor responses indicate that, for chemotherapy-sensitive tumors, as the chemotherapy dose increases, overall survival often improves; this is reflected in the dose-response curve. Unfortunately, bone marrow toxicity is frequently the dose-limiting toxicity observed with most chemotherapy agents. Increases in chemotherapy doses may produce permanent bone marrow suppression, resulting in an inadequate production of white blood cells or platelets that may put the patient at risk for life-threatening infections or bleeding. This major limitation to dose intensification can be overcome with intensive bone marrow support. BMT is one method of providing such support.

The BMT process consists of the administration of high doses of chemotherapy followed by the intravenous infusion of healthy, intact hematopoietic stem cells. These healthy stem cells serve to "rescue" the patient from irreversible bone marrow suppression. Thus, the phrase *bone marrow transplantation* is misleading; it may be more appropriate to think of BMT as intensive chemotherapy followed by bone marrow rescue. Bone marrow rescue therefore provides a means of intensifying doses of chemotherapy.

TYPES OF BMT

Because healthy bone marrow cells can come from several sources, BMTs are classified by the source of the cells (Table 14-1). The first BMTs were allogeneic BMTs, in which the bone marrow was harvested, or collected, from someone other than the patient. Allogeneic BMT is the most complicated type of transplantation, because the donor bone marrow must be immunologically compatible with the patient. Compatibility is assured by testing and matching the human leukocyte antigens (HLAs) on the patient and donor cells. HLAs are antigens present on white blood cells that are important in antigen recognition and immune stimulation. To minimize unwanted or adverse immunologic interactions and serious side effects, the HLA type of the patient and the donor must match. As will be discussed later in this chapter, many of the serious side effects associated with allogeneic BMT are immunologically based. In allogeneic BMT, bone marrow ideally comes from an HLA-identical sibling donor. An allogeneic BMT from an identical twin donor is referred to as a syngeneic BMT; in this situation, the donor is genetically iden-

Table 14-1. Types of Bone Marrow Transplantation

Type of Transplant	Stem Cell Donor
Autologous	Patient (either bone marrow or peripheral stem cells)
Allogeneic	Someone other than the patient, usually an HLA-matched sibling or unrelated donor (either bone marrow or peripheral stem cells)
Syngeneic	Identical twin

SOURCE: references 1 and 3. HLA, human leukocyte antigen.

tical to the patient and graft-versus-host complications do not occur. In the absence of a matched related donor, bone marrow from a partially matched related donors or an HLA-matched unrelated donor may be used.[1,4] Transplants from an HLA-matched unrelated donor are commonly referred to as "MUD" (matched unrelated donor) BMTs. Unrelated donors can be identified through the U.S. National Marrow Donor Program (NMDP), a network of donors, bone marrow collection, and transplantation centers throughout the United States and other countries. The NMDP cooperates with donor registries world-wide to expand the pool of potential donors.[5]

Unfortunately, a majority of patients never find a suitable bone marrow donor; therefore, in recent years, autologous bone marrow transplantation (ABMT) has become more widely used.[1,6] In this process, the patient's own bone marrow is harvested before chemotherapy is begun. It is then frozen and stored. After the patient receives high-dose chemotherapy and/or radiation therapy, the bone marrow is administered. ABMT has an advantage over allogeneic BMT: because patients receive their own bone marrow (or stem cells), there is no concern about the development of rejection or graft-versus-host disease. ABMT is most often used to treat patients with solid tumors, such as breast cancer; this approach, however, is also used for patients with hematological malignancies. ABMT may be used to treat conditions in which the bone marrow is affected by the disease; such involvement frequently occurs in leukemia and in some lymphomas. In these cases, the bone marrow may be treated, or purged, to remove diseased cells or any residual tumor from the bone marrow before freezing. By removing these cells from the bone marrow, the chance that the patient will relapse after BMT is decreased. Purging is most often used in treating patients with acute leukemia; effective purging methods are less well developed for many other kinds of cancer.

Peripheral Stem Cell Transplantation

Unfortunately, bone marrow collection is not possible for all patients. Patients with extensive bone marrow fibrosis or bone marrow involvement may not be suitable candidates for autologous bone marrow harvest. These patients have an option called *peripheral stem cell transplantation* (PSCT), also referred to as peripheral blood progenitor cell transplantation (PBPCT).[7–10] Under normal circumstances, very few stem cells circulate in the peripheral blood. Administration of chemotherapy or hematopoietic growth factors (such as granulocyte colony-stimulating factor or granulocyte-macrophage colony-stimulating factor) causes greater numbers of stem cells to be mobilized from the bone marrow into the peripheral blood. These stem cells are collected from the peripheral blood by leukapheresis, a procedure similar to dialysis. A catheter is placed, and blood is fed into a centrifuge-like device. The desired stem cells are separated and removed, and the remaining blood components are returned to the circulation. The collected cells are then frozen and stored like autologous bone marrow. When the patient undergoes PSCT, the cells are thawed and infused into the patient in place of bone marrow. These cells are capable of reestablishing hematopoiesis, and the quality of bone marrow recovery observed following PSCT is equivalent to that seen with ABMT.[11–13] In addition, the time to engraftment (the process in which the transplanted stem cells begin producing new blood cells in the bone marrow) following PSCT is significantly decreased when compared with ABMT.[14,15]

Peripheral stem cells have a number of other advantages over bone marrow. Collection of these cells is much less invasive than a bone marrow harvest, and it can be performed in an outpatient setting. PSCT allows high-dose chemotherapy and bone marrow rescue to be performed on patients who would otherwise not be able to undergo BMT. Because of the shorter time to engraftment, the duration of neutropenia, the need for intravenous antibiotic therapy, and the length of inpatient hospital stay are all decreased.[16] In many institutions, PSCT has become an outpatient procedure.[17] In addition, current data indicate that PSCT is a more cost-effective approach than traditional ABMT in the treatment of certain cancers.[16]

BONE MARROW HARVEST AND INFUSION

For allogeneic BMT, the bone marrow harvest is performed in the operating room, while the donor is under general anesthesia.[4] The bone marrow is collected in multiple aspirations, most commonly from the posterior iliac crest; large-bore needles are repeatedly inserted, and the liquid bone marrow is aspirated. During the procedure, blood cell counts are performed on the harvested bone marrow to ensure that an adequate number of cells has been collected. The final volume of bone marrow collected is usually <1L. While in the operating room, the bone marrow is filtered to remove any unwanted particles, such as pieces of tissue or bone fragments. After the bone marrow cells are transferred to an empty bag, they can be taken to the lab for further processing (such as purging or freezing) or transferred directly to the patient for intravenous administration. The donor usually experiences pain from the harvest site that requires analgesics for a few days.

For ABMT, the bone marrow harvest is performed on the patient before high-dose chemotherapy begins.[6] The harvest technique is the same one used for allogeneic BMT. The collected bone marrow is filtered, frozen, and stored until the patient is ready for BMT. To preserve the stem cells (either bone marrow or peripheral stem cells) during the freezing process, dimethyl sulfoxide (DMSO) is often added.[11,13] Bone marrow is cryopreserved at very low temperatures; under these conditions the cells can retain viability for several years.[11,13] At the time of bone marrow infusion, the frozen bone marrow is thawed (usually at the patient's bedside) and then administered intravenously.

In both allogeneic BMT and ABMT, the transplanted cells are infused into circulating blood, where complex intrinsic homing mechanisms allow the stem cells to move from the peripheral circulation into the bone medullary space.[18] Once in the medullary space, the cells proliferate and divide, reestablishing hematopoiesis. The recovery of hematopoiesis is referred to as *engraftment*; when a patient has engrafted, the patient's bone marrow is producing cells. For most patients, it takes 2–4 weeks after transplantation for engraftment to occur, although this can vary. In some patients, engraftment never takes place. A number of factors influence the time to engraftment, such as the number of stem cells transplanted, the type of transplant, manipulation of the bone marrow, and the type of chemotherapy regimen.

APPLICATIONS OF BMT

High-dose chemotherapy with BMT has been used to treat a variety of malignant (Table 14-2) and nonmalignant diseases.[1-3] Although this chapter focuses on the use of BMT in the treatment of cancer, BMT has the potential to treat or cure patients with a number of other nonmalignant disorders, including aplastic anemia, immunodeficiency diseases, lysosomal storage disorders (such as Gaucher's disease),[19] sickle cell anemia, and thalassemias.

Hematological Malignancies

BMT has been widely used in the treatment of many hematological cancers, including leukemias, lymphomas, and myeloma. Allogeneic BMT and ABMT have become widely accepted forms of therapy for acute myelogenous leukemia (AML) and acute lymphocytic leukemia (ALL).[1,20-23] Long-term (i.e., ≥5 years) survival rates in patients with AML undergoing BMT may be as high as 50–60%.[24-29] Patients who undergo BMT in first complete remission (CR) or first early relapse generally tend to have better survival rates than those who undergo BMT in second CR or later. Generally, long-term disease-free survival (DFS) is greater among allogeneic BMT patients than among ABMT patients.[24-29]

ALL, the most common form of childhood leukemia, is highly responsive to treatment with standard chemotherapy. Although ALL in adults generally carries a poorer prognosis, BMT is usually reserved for patients who relapse after initial treatment or whose disease is refractory to conventional therapy. In adult ALL patients, long-term survival rates without BMT average ≤10%; BMT may produce up to 30–40% long-term survival. Response rates tend to be higher for allogeneic BMT than for ABMT. Both approaches produce responses in >50% of patients, but ABMT is associated with a higher rate of relapse.[30-32] Although more data support the superiority of allogeneic BMT over ABMT in treating ALL, both methods are currently used.[22,23]

Table 14-2. Applications of Bone Marrow Transplantation (BMT) in the Treatment of Cancer

Disease	Type of BMT	Potentially Curative in Advanced Disease?	Accepted Therapy
Acute leukemias	Allogeneic (most)	Yes	Yes
	Autologous	?	?
Chronic myelogenous leukemia	Allogeneic	Yes	Yes
	Autologous	?	No
Chronic lymphocytic leukemia	Allogeneic (most)	?	No
Multiple myeloma	Uncertain but mostly autologous	?	No
Non-Hodgkin's lymphoma			
• Aggressive	Autologous (most)	Yes	Yes
• Indolent	Autologous (most)	?	Yes
Hodgkin's disease	Autologous	Yes	Yes
Breast cancer	Autologous	?	Yes
Testicular cancer	Autologous	Yes	Yes
Neuroblastoma	Uncertain	Probably	Yes

SOURCE: adapted with permission from reference 1.

Similarly, BMT has become a common form of therapy in the treatment of patients with chronic myelogenous leukemia (CML).[1,33] CML remains relatively indolent for a period of time; during this chronic phase (which lasts an average of 3–5 years), interferon and/or hydroxyurea therapy controls signs of the disease (see chapter 13). CML eventually reaches an accelerated stage and then progresses to a blast crisis that resembles acute leukemia. Once this blast crisis occurs, the disease progresses rapidly and the chance of long-term survival is very poor. Allogeneic BMT is the only therapeutic modality for CML that consistently results in cure or prolonged (i.e., ≥5 years) DFS. Patients who undergo allogeneic BMT within 1 year of their diagnosis (while their disease is in the chronic phase) may have long-term survival rates as high as 75–80%. Patients with more advanced disease (either accelerated disease or blast crisis) who undergo BMT have a survival rate of <30%.

Both allogeneic BMT and ABMT have been reported to produce long-term DFS in patients with intermediate or aggressive non-Hodgkin's lymphoma (NHL) as well as in patients with recurrent or aggressive Hodgkin's disease (HD).[34-37] As a general rule, results are better when patients undergo BMT early in the course of their disease, before the tumor has a chance to develop significant resistance to chemotherapy. Overall, 2- to 3-year DFS has been reported as high as 60–80% in some groups of patients. Allogeneic BMT has generally been used only for those patients with bone marrow involvement, who are unable to have an autologous bone marrow harvest. With the development of PSCT, however, these patients now have a safer effective alternative. Consequently, the use of allogeneic BMT in the treatment of lymphomas has become much less frequent.

The use of BMT to treat other hematological cancers, such as chronic lymphocytic leukemia (CLL) or multiple myeloma, is less well defined, although studies indicate that BMT may play a role in the treatment of patients with these diseases.[38,39]

Solid Tumors

In contrast to BMT's well-described utility in the treatment of hematological malignancies, the role of BMT in the treatment of solid tumors is less clearly defined. Any disease that demonstrates dose-responsiveness to chemotherapy (i.e., with increasing doses of chemotherapy, a greater antitumor response is seen) has the potential to be treated with BMT. As a result, many transplantation centers are currently conducting studies to further assess this approach. The use of ABMT and PSCT in the management of breast cancer is now well established.[40,41] Breast cancer displays a dose-response relationship, encouraging the application of high-dose chemotherapy to this patient population in an effort to improve outcome and survival rates.

BMT has been used to treat patients with metastatic breast cancer, as well as patients with locally advanced disease. Historically, patients with metastatic disease have a very poor prognosis, with a median survival of approximately 2 years; these patients are considered incurable with standard chemotherapy. Use of ABMT or PSCT in these patients produces improved response rates as high as 60–70%.[42-44] Bezwoda et al.[45] reported a randomized evaluation comparing high-dose chemotherapy plus stem cell/bone marrow support with standard chemotherapy; response rates were significantly higher with high-dose chemotherapy, as was duration of survival (90 weeks in the high-dose arm vs. 45 weeks in the standard arm). This study has generated a great deal of criticism, because the duration of survival in the standard arm was significantly shorter than that seen in other studies of standard chemotherapy. It is too soon to determine whether survival of patients with metastatic breast cancer is improved following high-dose chemotherapy.

The relapse rate of patients with locally advanced breast cancer increases with increased lymph node involvement. Patients with stage II or III breast cancer who have extensive lymph node involvement (≥10 positive nodes) also have a poor prognosis with standard chemotherapy, and most will progress within 5 years.[41] ABMT or PSCT in this patient population has resulted in relapse-free survival rates at 2 years as high as 85–90%.[41,46,47] This data appears promising, although whether these results will translate into durable responses and improved DFS remains to be seen. Randomized trials are under way to determine whether high-dose chemotherapy can improve long-term survival. Although initial results suggest that patients with chemotherapy-sensitive breast cancer may benefit from ABMT, this modality remains controversial and should be considered experimental until studies that definitively describe the efficacy of BMT in treating this disease are complete.[41]

In testicular cancer, ABMT has produced durable responses in patients with relapsed or refractory disease. These responses have led some researchers to explore the application of ABMT earlier in the course of the disease. ABMT has also been used to treat patients with other solid tumors, such as ovarian cancer, other gynecological malignancies, and soft-tissue sarcomas. Early results in these patient populations appear positive, leading to a number of clinical trials to further define the usefulness of BMT in treating such patients.

Pediatric Tumors

BMT has been widely used in the pediatric patient population. As with adults, leukemias and some lymphomas are treated with BMT. BMT is also employed in the treatment of neuroblastoma, which can be difficult to treat with standard chemotherapy doses.[48] In trials utilizing BMT to treat advanced neuroblastoma, 2-year DFS rates as high as 40% have been reported. Results achieved with ABMT appear to equal those seen with allogeneic BMT. These data are preliminary, and further studies need to be completed. For a summary of the more common applications of BMT, see Table 14-2.

COMPLICATIONS

A significant number of complications occur among BMT patients. Many of these are related to the very high doses of chemotherapy used. Because severe bone marrow suppression is expected (and will be treated with stem cell infusion), chemotherapy doses are often pushed to their nonhematological toxicities. As a result, patients commonly experience serious side effects, which may be life threatening. Many of these adverse effects are well-described toxicities of the chemotherapy agents. For example, neurotoxicity, mucosal damage, or cyclophosphamide- or ifosfamide-induced hemorrhagic cystitis are common toxicities that are seen in patients undergoing BMT. A few toxicities, however, are unique to BMT.

Hepatic Veno-occlusive Disease

Hepatic veno-occlusive disease (VOD) is a serious clinical syndrome. BMT greatly increases a patient's risk of developing this syndrome. Hepatic VOD most commonly occurs 10–20 days following BMT. Clinical manifestations of hepatic VOD consist of a triad of findings: elevated bilirubin and jaundice, ascites and weight gain, and an enlarged liver and right upper quadrant tenderness.[50-54] Hepatic VOD occurs in up to 20% of patients undergoing BMT, although some centers report incidences of ≥50%. Mortality rates range from 25–50% to 95%, with higher mortality rates among patients with more severe disease. Although patients with hepatic VOD can develop hepatic failure and subsequent encephalopathy, not all mortality is due to liver failure. Many patients go on to develop multiorgan failure (e.g., renal and cardiopulmonary failure). Risk factors for the development of hepatic VOD include increased age, elevation in transaminases before BMT, liver metastases, and exposure to certain antineoplastic agents (e.g., busulfan, methotrexate, and cyclophosphamide).[50,55-57]

Hepatic VOD is believed to be caused by chemotherapy-induced damage to the endothelial lining of the hepatic venules and to centrilobular hepatocytes. Endothelial injury triggers activation of the coagulation cascade, which results in platelet aggregation and thrombus formation in the small blood vessels of the liver, leading ultimately to occlusion of small blood vessels.[57,58] Hepatocyte involvement and injury can lead to necrosis. In addition, a number of cytokines have been associated with hepatic VOD, including tumor necrosis factor alpha (TNF-α) and interleukin 1β (IL-1β). Levels of these cytokines appear to be elevated in patients just prior to the clinical onset of hepatic VOD and other complications following BMT.[54] The exact relationship between these cytokines and hepatic VOD is not clear, because these cytokines may be elevated in response to many insults, including chemotherapy, radiation, and infection. Because of the high degree of morbidity associated with hepatic VOD, there have been extensive efforts to prevent and treat it.

Prevention of Hepatic VOD

Most efforts to prevent hepatic VOD focus on interruption of the coagulation cascade. Heparin was used initially, and several trials administering continuous low-dose heparin (100–150 units/kg per day) have produced conflicting results. Although the safety of low-dose heparin has been demonstrated, the efficacy of this approach is still undetermined.[59,60] Prostaglandins that have antithrombotic and vasodilatory effects, such as prostaglandin E_1 (PGE_1 or alprostadil), have also been used to prevent hepatic VOD,[61] as has pentoxifylline, an agent that inhibits TNF-α activity.[62-64] These approaches, however, have not been supported by prospective, randomized studies and are still considered investigational.[65,66]

Treatment of Hepatic VOD

Management of hepatic VOD has conventionally consisted of providing supportive care until the liver injury healed or the patient died of multiorgan failure. Recently, other approaches have been tried. As discussed above, agents that can alter or reverse the coagulation cascade, such as heparin or prostaglandins, have been used with varying degrees of success. One of the more promising approaches is the use of recombinant tissue plasminogen activator (alteplase or rt-PA). In a number of case reports and a small trial in which alteplase was administered with low-dose heparin infusions, initial results were promising and bleeding complications were minimal.[67-70] Perhaps the most aggressive approach in the management of severe, life-threatening hepatic VOD has been the use of liver transplantation. Such an approach is highly controversial and at this time is not recommended for routine use.[71]

Graft-Versus-Host Disease

First described in animals in the 1950s, "secondary disease" was a wasting syndrome seen in animals who received allogeneic spleen cells in an effort to reverse the toxicity of irradiation. When it was recognized that the clinical findings of this disease were due to the activity of immunocompetent donor cells against the immunocompromised recipient, this syndrome was termed "graft-versus-host disease" (GVHD). GVHD is one of the most serious complications of allogeneic BMT. The pathophysiology of GVHD is very complex; the basic mechanism involves the immunocompetent T cells in the donor bone marrow recognizing the host (patient) as foreign, triggering an immune response similar to that seen in organ rejection in solid organ transplantation.[72] GVHD is classified as acute or chronic, depending on the time of presentation and clinical findings.

Acute GVHD

Acute GVHD generally occurs in the first 100 days following allogeneic BMT, although some patients may present after day 100 with symptoms consistent with acute GVHD.[72] Acute

Table 14-3. Clinical Staging of GVHD According to Organ Involvement

Stage	Skin	Liver	GI Tract
+	Maculopapular rash over <25% of body	Bilirubin 2–3 mg/dl	500–1000 ml/day of diarrhea
++	Maculopapular rash over 25–50% of body	Bilirubin 3–6 mg/dl	1000–1500 ml/day of diarrhea
+++	Generalized erythroderma	Bilirubin 6–15 mg/dl	>1500 ml/day of diarrhea
++++	Generalized erythroderma with bullae formation and desquamation	Bilirubin >15 mg/dl	Severe abdominal pain +/– ileus

SOURCE: reference 2. GVHD, graft-versus-host disease; GI, gastrointestinal.

GVHD involves primarily three organ systems: skin, liver, and gastrointestinal (GI) tract. The initial manifestation of acute GVHD is often a maculopapular rash. This rash, which usually appears in the first 3 weeks after allogeneic BMT and coincides with evidence of engraftment (elevation in the white blood cell count), frequently looks and feels like a sunburn and may be itchy or painful. Initially, the rash typically appears on the palms of the hands or the soles of the feet, but the face and the trunk can also be involved. As the rash intensifies, it can become more confluent; in the most severe cases, bullous lesions and desquamation may be seen.

The other organ systems most frequently involved are the liver and GI tract. Liver GVHD initially manifests as an increase in liver function tests, particularly of bilirubin (direct or conjugated). Cholestatic jaundice occurs frequently, although fulminant liver failure is uncommon. Although a clinical diagnosis of liver GVHD can be made based on elevated bilirubin in the presence of skin and/or GI tract involvement, definitive diagnosis of liver GVHD can only be made with a liver biopsy. This procedure is associated with significant risks, most notably bleeding. GVHD of the GI tract manifests initially as diarrhea in the form of loose, watery stools. As the disease progresses, patients may have very large stool volumes, bloody stools, abdominal pain, nausea, and vomiting, and may even develop ileus. Patients with GVHD involving the intestine will usually have GVHD of other organ systems also.

Acute GVHD is staged according to a clinical grading scale. Staging of each organ system is based on the severity of organ involvement, and then an overall clinical grade is assigned (Tables 14-3 and 14-4).[2,72] Grade I GVHD indicates very mild disease, and grade IV disease is considered life threatening.

GVHD Prophylaxis

Most clinical trials addressing GVHD have focused on prevention. Because the pathophysiology of GVHD involves T-cell activation and differentiation, much of the current therapy is directed at inhibiting the proliferation and function of T cells.[72,73] Agents initially used to treat GVHD included methotrexate, cyclophosphamide, and corticosteroids. Although these agents were effective in decreasing the incidence of GVHD, they did not improve overall survival. Cyclosporine (cyclosporin A or CsA), a T cell–specific immunomodulatory agent, was introduced in the late 1970s. Although initial results demonstrated cyclosporine's efficacy in preventing GVHD, subsequent studies failed to demonstrate a survival benefit of cyclosporine over methotrexate.[74] These initial negative outcomes led to studies investigating the use of cyclosporine in combination with other agents, such as corticosteroids and methotrexate. A number of studies have demonstrated that the combination of cyclosporine and a corticosteroid (such as methylprednisolone or prednisone) is superior to either cyclosporine alone, methotrexate plus corticosteroids, or cyclophosphamide plus corticosteroids.[75,76] Similarly, the combination of cyclosporine plus methotrexate has been shown to be superior to single-agent therapy in preventing the development of serious GVHD.[77–80] More recently, there is evidence that the addition of a third agent leads to improvement over double-agent therapy. In one study, methotrexate plus cyclosporine plus prednisone was more effective in preventing grade II–IV acute GVHD than cyclosporine plus prednisone.[81]

Table 14-4. Clinical Grading of GVHD Severity

Grade	Stage
I	+ to ++ skin involvement no GI tract, no liver involvement no decrease in clinical performance
II	+ to +++ skin involvement + GI tract or + liver or both involved mild decrease in clinical performance
III	++ to +++ skin involvement ++ to +++ GI tract or ++ to ++++ liver or both involved mild decrease in clinical performance
IV	like grade III ++ to ++++ organ involvement extreme decrease in clinical performance

SOURCE: reference 2.

Table 14-5. Examples of GVHD Prophylaxis Regimens

Drug	Dose and Schedule	Comments
Cyclosporine	3–7.5 mg/kg per day IV as CI or divided doses	divided doses = q12hr
Methotrexate	15 mg/m² IV day 1, 10 mg/m² days 3, 6, and 11	short-course methotrexate; associated with mucositis, hepatic VOD
Cyclosporine	3–5 mg/kg per day IV as above	CI or q12hr
Methylprednisolone	0.5–1 mg/kg per day in divided doses	corticosteroids may start day 7, then increase day 14
Antithymocyte globulin	7–10 mg/kg IV QOD × 6 doses	+ methotrexate
	15 mg/kg IV QOD × 7 days	+ methotrexate + prednisone

SOURCE: references 77–79, 84, and 85. IV, intravenous; CI, continuous infusion; VOD, veno-occlusive disease; QOD, every other day.

Tacrolimus, also known as FK 506, is a newer immunosuppressive agent that has been studied in GVHD. Although tacrolimus is structurally different from cyclosporine, it is similar in that it also inhibits interleukin 2 activation of T cells. In early studies, tacrolimus appears to be at least as effective as cyclosporine in preventing GVHD.[82,83] More studies are in progress to better define the role of this new immunosuppressant in BMT.

Antithymocyte globulin (ATG) is a polyclonal immunoglobulin that binds to T cells, allowing them to be removed from the circulation by the reticuloendothelial system. Antithymocyte globulin has been used in combination with methotrexate to prevent GVHD, but it has not been shown to be any more effective than methotrexate alone.[84] The combination of antithymocyte globulin, prednisone, and methotrexate has resulted in a lower incidence of acute GVHD when compared with methotrexate alone.[85] See Table 14-5[77–79,84,85] for examples of GVHD prophylaxis regimens.

Because T cells are major mediators of GVHD, T-cell depletion of donor bone marrow prior to BMT has been used to decrease the incidence of GVHD. Several studies using T-cell depletion have produced significant decreases in the incidence and severity of GVHD. Drawbacks to T-cell depletion include increased rates of graft failure and increased relapse rates. These are serious concerns, so this technique remains controversial.[86,87]

Toxicity of GVHD Prophylaxis

The agents used to prevent GVHD are associated with a number of side effects (Table 14-6). Patients receiving cyclosporine commonly experience renal insufficiency, hypertension, tremors, hypokalemia, hypomagnesemia, and hirsutism. More serious effects include liver toxicity and severe neurological toxicity, including headaches, cortical blindness, and seizures. Methotrexate use can result in delayed engraftment and severe mucositis, as well as in increased incidence of hepatic VOD in the week following administration of a dose. Corticosteroids, especially when used for long periods, produce numerous side effects. These include cushingoid effects,

Table 14-6. Side Effects Associated with GVHD Prophylaxis

Agent	Side Effect
Cyclosporine	renal toxicity hepatic toxicity CNS symptoms: tremors, headaches, cortical blindness, seizures electrolyte abnormalities: hypokalemia, hypomagnesemia hirsutism hypertension
Methotrexate	delayed engraftment mucositis increased hepatic VOD in the week following dose
Corticosteroids	cushingoid effects myopathies osteoporosis hyperglycemia hypertension avascular necrosis of the hip
Antithymocyte globulin	fevers chills myalgias nausea/vomiting serum sickness

SOURCE: references 72–88. CNS, central nervous system.

myopathies, osteoporosis, hyperglycemia, hypertension, and an increased risk of ulcer disease. Corticosteroid use in GVHD prophylaxis may be associated with a higher incidence of infections.[88] Long-term use of corticosteroids also increases the risk of aseptic necrosis of the femoral head, necessitating hip replacement surgery. Antithymocyte globulin administration causes fever, chills, myalgias, nausea, vomiting, and serum sickness. Because antithymocyte globulin is of equine origin, some patients may have an allergic or hypersensitivity reaction. A skin test of ATG is usually performed before the first dose is administered.

Treatment of Acute GVHD

Management of established GVHD is extremely difficult; the greatest chance of success lies in its prevention. Many therapeutic strategies use the same agents used in prophylaxis. Often, no therapy is started for very mild grade I GVHD, because it frequently resolves on its own.

An antileukemic or antitumor effect has also been observed in patients experiencing GVHD. Groups of patients who do not experience any GVHD tend to have higher relapse rates than groups that develop GVHD. This antileukemic effect is referred to as the graft-versus-leukemia (GVL) effect, and it appears to reflect immunologic activity of donor bone marrow cells against tumor.[89] As a result, mild GVHD may be desirable, particularly in patients with leukemia, as the immunologic interactions that occur in GVHD may ultimately result in improved overall survival. More severe (grade II–IV) or worsening GVHD requires prompt intervention.

Corticosteroids are considered first-line therapy in the treatment of acute GVHD.[90] Corticosteroids are usually administered in high doses (e.g., 2–2.5 mg/kg per day of methylprednisolone), with a subsequent taper. For patients who fail to respond to corticosteroids, overall survival is very poor.[91] Agents used to treat these patients include antithymocyte globulin or very high doses of corticosteroids or cyclosporine. Newer investigational approaches include the use of monoclonal antibodies or immunologically active agents that target other cytokines active in GVHD. Muromonab-CD3 (Orthoclone OKT3), a pan-T-cell antibody, has been studied in cases of corticosteroid-resistant GVHD. Although modest responses were seen, they were generally transient, and administration of the antibody was associated with TNF-α release and significant toxicity.[92–94] Other approaches currently under investigation include monoclonal antibodies and cytokine antagonists that target other cytokines involved in GVHD, such as interleukin 1 or interleukin 2, and their receptors.[95] In addition, a number of novel immunosuppressive agents are currently under investigation for use in both the prevention and management of acute GVHD.[96]

Chronic GVHD

Chronic GVHD is a late complication in patients undergoing allogeneic BMT. By definition, chronic GVHD occurs after day 100 following BMT. Many patients will develop features of chronic GVHD before this time.[97] Like acute GVHD, chronic GVHD is caused by immunologic recognition of host (patient) cells by donor cells. Chronic GVHD occurs in up to 60% of patients receiving allogeneic BMT.[98] The risk of developing chronic GVHD is increased in patients with prior acute GVHD, increased HLA mismatch between patient and donor, and increased age.[99] Chronic GVHD can develop in different ways. The most severe disease is seen in patients whose acute GVHD evolves into chronic GVHD (progressive GVHD). Less severe disease is likely when chronic GVHD occurs after a period in which acute GVHD has not been active (quiescent disease after acute GVHD) or when chronic GVHD occurs without any evidence of prior acute GVHD (de novo GVHD).[97]

Chronic GVHD is a systemic disease, and many organ systems are involved. It shares clinical features with many autoimmune or collagen vascular disorders. The most common sites of organ involvement include the skin, liver, mouth, and eyes, although virtually every organ system may be involved. Skin involvement usually manifests as changes in pigmentation, erythematous patches, scaly skin, and red or purple papules. Fibrosis of the dermal and subcutaneous layers of the skin can lead to thickening and hardening of the skin. Hair loss in affected areas of the skin is quite common. Severe skin involvement can lead to the formation of joint contractures and skin ulcers. In the mouth, both the mucosa and the salivary glands may be affected. Patients may develop white striae on mucosal areas and ulcerations in the mouth. Because of the salivary gland involvement, patients may experience decreased saliva production and dry mouth. Consequently, many patients experience mouth pain and have difficulty eating.

Liver involvement manifests as a cholestatic, obstructive disease. Elevations in serum bilirubin and other liver function tests may be seen, but fulminant liver failure is rare. Many patients have eye involvement, with decreased tear production leading to dry, gritty eyes (Sjögren's syndrome). Conjunctival ulceration may also occur. Less frequently, chronic GVHD affects the esophagus and GI tract, causing difficulty swallowing, diarrhea, and abdominal pain.

Pulmonary involvement of chronic GVHD has increasingly been recognized.[100] This involvement is termed *bronchiolitis fibrosa obliterans*, and it usually involves small airways. The risk of developing this particular syndrome may be increased with certain prophylactic methotrexate regimens and with low levels of serum immunoglobulin G.[101,102] The clinical course of bronchiolitis obliterans varies from slowly progressing mild disease to fatal necrotizing involvement of the small airways. Although patients may present with an obstructive disease, bronchodilators are usually not effective. Immunosuppression (e.g., with corticosteroids) may be helpful.[103] For more examples of organ involvement with chronic GVHD, see Table 14-7.[104,105]

Staging of chronic GVHD is based on the extent of organ involvement. Patients with limited-stage disease have only skin or liver involvement; these patients are likely to do

Table 14-7. Organ Involvement in Chronic GVHD

Organ	Early	Late
Skin	erythematous maculopapular or lichen planus–like rash, photosensitivity	scleroderma-like reaction with joint contractures, alopecia, nail dystrophy, hypohydrosis
Mouth	mucositis, lichenoid changes, dryness	ulcers, mucosal atrophy, caries
Eyes	decreased tear production, gritty sensation, conjunctivitis, uveitis	keratoconjunctivitis, corneal ulceration and scarring
Liver	hepatomegaly, ↑ alkaline phosphatase, ↑ transaminases, ↑ bilirubin	persistent ↑ alkaline phosphatase, hepatomegaly
Lungs	subclinical or clinical bronchitis with obstructive pattern	cough, marked dyspnea, severe obstructive pattern, respiratory failure
GI tract	difficulty swallowing, esophagitis, diarrhea	difficulty swallowing, changes in motility, web formation with stenosis, malabsorption
Musculoskeletal system	arthralgia, arthritis, pleural effusion, pericardial effusion, polymyositis	
Immune system	functional asplenia, polyclonal hypogammaglobulinemia, immunoglobulin subclass deficiencies, poor specific cellular and antibody responses, autoantibodies, multiple or recurrent infections	
Blood	thrombocytopenia, eosinophilia	

SOURCE references 104 and 105. ↑, increase.

well with minimal therapy. Patients with extensive-stage disease have multiple organ involvement and will usually require therapy; these patients are less likely to do well.

Treatment of Chronic GVHD

To date there are no recognized effective prophylactic measures for chronic GVHD. The best prevention of chronic GVHD is to minimize acute GVHD. Agents used to treat chronic GVHD are similar to those used in acute disease and include cyclosporine, corticosteroids, antithymocyte globulin, and tacrolimus.[97,104–106] As a rule, more benefit is obtained with early initiation of therapy. As in acute GVHD, chronic GVHD has also been associated with a GVL effect, in which patients who experience mild acute and chronic GVHD appear less likely to relapse with their malignant disease.

Corticosteroids are considered first-line therapy. In one trial, prednisone at 1 mg/kg was administered every other day with either cyclophosphamide, procarbazine, or azathioprine. Patients receiving prednisone and azathioprine responded after about 1 year of therapy.[107] These authors then conducted a study comparing prednisone with prednisone plus azathioprine; they found that overall survival in the prednisone group was better than in the group receiving combination therapy. The decreased survival seen with combination therapy was largely due to an increase in fatal infections in patients receiving additional immunosuppression.[108] Patients who have failed initial primary therapy with corticosteroids have been treated with cyclosporine (often alternating with prednisone), azathioprine, or thalidomide. In addition, psoralens combined with ultraviolet A radiation (PUVA) therapy has been used for some patients with mostly skin involvement and minimal visceral organ involvement.[109]

Thalidomide has been investigated in the treatment of chronic GVHD.[110,111] Despite the severe birth defects associated with this drug, thalidomide remains available in certain countries. It is known that thalidomide is immunologically active, and as a result, it has continued to be used in the treatment of a variety of autoimmune and immunologically mediated diseases. Because of its immunologic activity, it has been studied in the treatment of corticosteroid-refractory GVHD. In one trial, patients with high-risk chronic GVHD had an actuarial survival rate of 48%, compared with a projected actuarial survival rate of 20%. Patients receiving salvage therapy for refractory disease had a 78% actuarial survival rate.[110] Side effects of thalidomide include sedation, constipation, and neuropathies. Although the mechanism of action of thalidomide is not clearly understood, it appears to inhibit TNF-α production and may alter T-cell function.

Infectious and Related Complications

Along with GVHD, infections are among the most serious complications that occur after BMT. Advances in the prevention and management of infections in these patients are largely responsible for the increasing success of BMT.[112] The infections that are most commonly seen tend to occur in three time periods.

During the early period, usually the first 30 days after BMT, the major infections are related to the destruction of host defenses by chemotherapy and radiation and to the profound neutropenia that these patients experience. The types of infections in this period of time tend to be bacterial, including both gram-negative and gram-positive organisms, and fungal. These infections are similar to those seen in neutropenic patients after chemotherapy. Viral infections at this time are usually caused by reactivation of latent herpesviruses. As a result, prophylactic antiviral and antibacterial therapy are frequently used in the BMT setting (see chapter 15).

In the middle period, generally from day 30 to day 100 after BMT, neutropenia is of less concern, and the risk of bacterial infection decreases. This period is characterized by viral infections with cytomegalovirus, fungal infections with *Aspergillus* spp., and protozoal infections with *Pneumocystis carinii*. The risk of developing these infections is directly related to the active immunosuppression used to prevent and treat GVHD in allogeneic BMT patients and the resultant decrease in both cellular and humoral immune function. Although ABMT patients also have decreased immune function following the procedure, the degree of immunosuppression is much less than that following allogeneic BMT, because immunosuppressive therapy for the prevention or treatment of GVHD is not required. As a result, serious infections in these patients are much less frequent and less severe than in the allogeneic BMT population.

After day 100, or in the late period, the risk of serious infection decreases significantly. Patients gradually recover immune function over many months. Bacterial infections still occur, but they tend to be less severe; the most common pathogens tend to be encapsulated organisms, such as *Streptococcus pneumoniae* (pneumococcus) or *Haemophilus influenzae*. Viral infections also become less frequent in this period, although some patients may develop herpes simplex virus infections (Table 14-8).[96] Patients who do not develop chronic GVHD and are able to be tapered off immunosuppressive therapy usually recover normal immune function within 1–2 years. Patients who develop chronic GVHD require prolonged immunosuppression and remain at risk for infection for a long time. For a more complete discussion of the types of infections and their prevention and management, refer to Chapter 15, Infectious Complications.

Interstitial Pneumonitis

Interstitial pneumonitis, another serious complication, accounts for up to 40% of allogeneic BMT-related deaths.[113] Patients with interstitial pneumonitis develop fever, shortness of breath, dry cough, and hypoxemia, and diffuse interstitial infiltrates are visible on their chest X-rays. The etiology of interstitial pneumonitis appears to be multifactorial. The most common causes of interstitial pneumonitis are infectious, with the most common infecting organisms being viral (cytomegalovirus), fungal (*Aspergillus* spp.), and protozoal (*Pneumocystis carinii*). Frequently, however, interstitial pneumonitis can also be caused by damage to the lungs resulting from chemotherapy and/or radiation therapy. Pulmonary damage has been seen with a number of chemotherapy agents used in BMT, including cyclophosphamide, busulfan, and carmustine (BCNU).[114,115] Similarly, the incidence of interstitial pneumonitis is increased in patients receiving radiation to the chest, particularly total body irradiation. Patients undergoing allogeneic BMT are at greater risk than those undergoing ABMT. Among allogeneic BMT patients, other risk factors include age >20 years, CML as an underlying disease, prior splenectomy, and the presence of GVHD.[116,117]

Interstitial pneumonitis is associated with a high degree of morbidity and mortality, particularly following allogeneic BMT. Management of these patients is largely supportive, and many patients will experience progressive pulmonary failure, often evolving into an acute respiratory distress syndrome (ARDS), necessitating intubation and mechanical ventilation. Historically, BMT patients who require mechanical

Table 14-8. Common Infections Following BMT

Time Period	Infection Type	Risk Factors
days 0–30	bacterial: gram negative, gram positive fungal: *Candida* spp. viral: HSV	neutropenia, indwelling catheters
days 30–100	bacterial: as above, frequency usually less fungal: *Aspergillus* spp. viral: CMV other: *Pneumocystis carinii*	immunosuppression, presence of GVHD
after day 100	bacterial: encapsulated organisms viral: VZV	presence of GVHD

SOURCE: reference 96. Day 0 is defined as the day of bone marrow infusion. HSV, herpes simplex virus; CMV, cytomegalovirus; VZV, varicella-zoster virus.

ventilation have had an extremely poor overall survival.[118]

One type of pulmonary toxicity that occurs soon after BMT is diffuse alveolar hemorrhage. The clinical manifestations are similar to those described above; patients develop a fever, cough, dyspnea, and hypoxia. Diagnosis of diffuse alveolar hemorrhage is made by the recovery of increasingly bloody fluid from bronchovesicular lavage. This syndrome has an extremely high mortality rate and appears to be increased in patients with age >40 years old and in patients with severe mucositis, high fevers, or renal insufficiency.[119] Historically, the development of diffuse alveolar hemorrhage has almost always been fatal; more recently, it appears that high-dose corticosteroids may reverse this disorder. In one small study, patients who developed diffuse alveolar hemorrhage were treated with high-dose methylprednisolone, 1 g/day, with subsequent taper. All patients responded to therapy, with no increase in infectious complications.[120]

Hematopoietic Growth Factors in BMT

The development and subsequent clinical use of hematopoietic growth factors have had a tremendous impact in the field of BMT.[121-123] The major benefit has come from the positive effect of growth factors on bone marrow recovery after BMT. Both granulocyte colony-stimulating factor (G-CSF) and granulocyte-macrophage colony-stimulating factor (GM-CSF) have been administered after BMT.[123-126] Administration of these CSFs after BMT results in a significantly shorter duration of neutropenia and a reduction in the infectious complications associated with prolonged neutropenia. The CSFs were initially used in patients with nonmyeloid malignancies (e.g., solid tumors or lymphoid disease, such as lymphoma or Hodgkin's disease). They have been used successfully following allogeneic BMT and ABMT in patients with myeloid malignancies. Initial concerns that use of G-CSF or GM-CSF might stimulate leukemic activity after BMT appear to be unfounded, and it is becoming more common for these growth factors to be used to treat AML patients, without a resultant increase in leukemia.[127]

Another growing application of growth factors in BMT is their use in PSCT. Both G-CSF and GM-CSF are routinely used to mobilize circulating stem cells, as described in *Peripheral Stem Cell Transplantation*, above. Growth factors are also used to enhance the rate of engraftment and shorten the duration of neutropenia following PSCT.

RECENT ADVANCES IN BMT

One of the most exciting advances in BMT is the use of peripheral stem cells or peripheral blood progenitor cells as an alternative source of hematopoietic cells for bone marrow reconstitution. Patients undergoing PSCT have a much more rapid engraftment than patients undergoing ABMT, which translates into fewer days of neutropenia and fewer infectious complications. Unfortunately, there are some drawbacks to autologous PSCT. Patients who have had extensive prior chemotherapy often have very poor stem cell collections, and it can take as many as 10–12 leukapheresis sessions to obtain an adequate number of cells. It is sometimes necessary to harvest bone marrow if a patient's stem cell collection is extremely inadequate. In addition, there is some concern about potential tumor contamination of collections, although the risk appears to be low. Allogeneic PSCT has been employed as an alternative to allogeneic bone marrow harvest. PSCT is gaining acceptance and becoming an increasingly utilized technique.

Because of the many improvements in BMT, including the use of peripheral stem cells and hematopoietic growth factors, the application of BMT in the outpatient setting is now possible.[17] Outpatient BMT has most often consisted of autologous PSCT. Patients are usually admitted for high-dose chemotherapy and then discharged as outpatients after its completion, with very close (i.e., daily) follow-up by the BMT service.[17]

SUMMARY

High-dose chemotherapy with stem cell support is a widely growing area of oncology practice. New advances in the support of these patients, such as the use of peripheral stem cells and hematopoietic growth factors, have significantly reduced the toxicity and morbidity associated with traditional bone marrow transplantation. As a result, this approach is becoming available for an ever-increasing number of patients.

REFERENCES

1. Armitage JO. Bone marrow transplantation. *N Engl J Med* 1994;330:827–38.
2. Thomas ED, Storb R, Clift RA, et al. Bone-marrow transplantation. *N Engl J Med* 1975;292:832–43, 895–902.
3. Smith BR. Stem cell transplantation. In: DeVita VT, Hellman S, Rosenberg SA, editors. *Cancer: Principles and Practice of Oncology*. 5th ed. Philadelphia, PA: Lippincott-Raven; 1997. p. 2621–39.
4. Chao NJ, Blume KG. Reconstitution of hematopoiesis following allogeneic bone marrow transplantation. In: Armitage JO, Antman KH, editors. *High Dose Cancer Therapy: Pharmacology, Hematopoiesis, Stem Cells*. Baltimore, MD: Williams & Wilkins; 1992. p. 151–61.
5. Anasetti C, Howe C, Petersdorf EW, et al. Marrow transplants from HLA matched unrelated donors: an NMDP update and the Seattle experience. *Bone Marrow Transplant* 1994;13:693–5.
6. Keating A. Autologous bone marrow transplantation. In: Armitage JO, Antman KH, editors. *High Dose Cancer Therapy: Pharmacology, Hematopoiesis, Stem Cells*. Baltimore, MD: Williams & Wilkins; 1992. p. 162–81.
7. Juttner CA, To LB. Autologous peripheral blood stem cell transplantation: potential advantages, practical considerations, and initial clinical results. In: Atkinson K, editor. *Clinical Bone*

Marrow Transplantation. New York: Cambridge Univ Pr; 1994. p. 142–52.
8. Mangan KF. Peripheral blood stem cell transplantation: from laboratory to clinical practice. *Semin Oncol* 1995;22:202–9.
9. Vose JM, Armitage JO, Kessinger A. High-dose chemotherapy and autologous transplant with peripheral-blood stem cells. *Oncology* 1993;7:23–9.
10. Gray TF III, Shea TC. Current status of peripheral blood progenitor cell transplantation. *Semin Oncol* 1994;21(5 *Suppl* 12):93–101.
11. Kessinger A. Reestablishing hematopoiesis after dose-intensive therapy with peripheral stem cells. In: Armitage JO, Antman KH, editors. *High Dose Cancer Therapy: Pharmacology, Hematopoiesis, Stem Cells*. Baltimore, MD: Williams & Wilkins; 1992. p. 182–94.
12. Stadtmauer EA, Schneider C, Silberstein LE. Peripheral blood progenitor cell generation and harvesting. *Semin Oncol* 1995;22:291–300.
13. Lee J-H, Klein HG. Collection and use of circulating hematopoietic progenitor cells. *Hematol Oncol Clin North Am* 1995;9:1–22.
14. To LB, Roberts M, Haylock DN, et al. Comparison of haematological recovery times and supportive care requirements of autologous recovery phase peripheral blood stem cell transplants, autologous bone marrow transplants and allogeneic bone marrow transplants. *Bone Marrow Transplant* 1992;9:277–84.
15. Sheridan WP, Begley CG, Juttner CA, et al. Effect of peripheral-blood progenitor cells mobilised by filgrastim (G-CSF) on platelet recovery after high-dose chemotherapy. *Lancet* 1992;339:640–4.
16. Smith TJ, Hillner BE, Schmitz N, et al. Economic analysis of a randomized clinical trial to compare filgrastim-mobilized peripheral-blood progenitor cell transplantation and autologous bone marrow transplantation in patients with Hodgkin's and non-Hodgkin's lymphoma. *J Clin Oncol* 1997;15:5–10.
17. Peter WP, Ross M, Vredenburgh JJ, et al. The use of intensive clinic support to permit outpatient autologous bone marrow transplantation for breast cancer. *Semin Oncol* 1994;21(4 *Suppl* 7):25–31.
18. Tavassoli M, Hardy CL. Molecular basis for homing of intravenously transplanted stem cells to the marrow. *Blood* 1990;76:1059–70.
19. Hoogerbrugge PM, Brouwer OF, Bordigoni P, et al. Allogeneic bone marrow transplantation for lysosomal storage disorders. *Lancet* 1995;345:1398–402.
20. Burnette AK. Autologous bone marrow transplantation for acute nonlymphocytic leukemia. In: Atkinson K, editor. *Clinical Bone Marrow Transplantation*. New York: Cambridge Univ Pr; 1994. p. 111–6.
21. Gorin NC. High-dose therapy for acute myelocytic leukemia. In: Armitage JO, Antman KH, editors. *High Dose Cancer Therapy: Pharmacology, Hematopoiesis, Stem Cells*. Baltimore, MD: Williams & Wilkins; 1992. p. 569–606.
22. Weisdorf DJ. Autologous bone marrow transplantation for acute lymphoblastic leukemia. In: Atkinson K, editor. *Clinical Bone Marrow Transplantation*. New York: Cambridge Univ Pr; 1994. p. 112–23.
23. Billet AL. High-dose therapy in acute lymphoblastic leukemia. In: Armitage JO, Antman KH, editors. *High Dose Cancer Therapy: Pharmacology, Hematopoiesis, Stem Cells*. Baltimore, MD: Williams & Wilkins; 1992. p. 607–18.
24. Thomas ED, Buckner CD, Clift RA, et al. Marrow transplantation for acute nonlymphoblastic leukemia in first remission. *N Engl J Med* 1979;301:597–9.
25. Champlin R, Gale RP. Bone marrow transplantation for acute leukemia: recent advances and comparison with alternative therapies. *Semin Hematol* 1987;24:55–67.
26. Santos GW, Tutschka PJ, Brookmeyer R, et al. Marrow transplantation for acute non-lymphocytic leukemia after treatment with busulfan and cyclophosphamide. *N Engl J Med* 1983;309:347–53.
27. Hurd D. Allogeneic and autologous bone marrow transplantation for acute non-lymphocytic leukemia. *Semin Oncol* 1987;14:407–15.
28. Ball ED, Vredenburgh JJ, Mills LE, et al. Autologous bone marrow transplantation for acute myeloid leukemia following in vitro treatment with neuraminidase and monoclonal antibodies. *Bone Marrow Transplant* 1990;6:277–80.
29. Yeager A, Kaizer H, Santos GW, et al. Autologous bone marrow transplantation in patients with acute nonlymphocytic leukemia using ex-vivo marrow treatment with 4-hydroperoxycyclophosphamide. *N Engl J Med* 1986;315:141–7.
30. Chao NJ, Forman SJ. Allogeneic bone marrow transplantation for acute lymphoblastic leukemia. In: Forman SJ, Blume KG, Thomas ED, editors. *Bone Marrow Transplantation*. Cambridge, MA: Blackwell Scientific; 1994. p. 618–28.
31. Kersey JH, Weisdorf D, Nesbit ME, et al. Comparison of autologous and allogeneic bone marrow transplantation for treatment of high risk refractory acute lymphoblastic leukemia. *N Engl J Med* 1987;317:461–7.
32. Ritz J, Ramsay NKC, Kersey JH. Autologous bone marrow transplantation for acute lymphoblastic leukemia. In: Forman SJ, Blume KG, Thomas ED, editors. *Bone Marrow Transplantation*. Cambridge, MA: Blackwell Scientific; 1994. p. 731–42.
33. Gale RP, Butturini A. Intensive therapy of chronic myelogenous leukemia. In: Armitage JO, Antman KH, editors. *High Dose Cancer Therapy: Pharmacology, Hematopoiesis, Stem Cells*. Baltimore, MD: Williams & Wilkins; 1992. p. 619–25.
34. Bierman PJ, Armitage JO. Autologous bone marrow transplantation for non-Hodgkin's lymphoma. In: Atkinson K, editor. *Clinical Bone Marrow Transplantation*. New York: Cambridge Univ Pr; 1994. p. 99–104.
35. Goldstone AH, McMillan AK, Chopra R. High-dose therapy for the treatment of non-Hodgkin's lymphoma. In: Armitage JO, Antman KH, editors. *High Dose Cancer Therapy: Pharmacology, Hematopoiesis, Stem Cells*. Baltimore, MD: Williams & Wilkins; 1992. p. 662–76.
36. Mills W, Goldstone A. Autologous bone marrow transplantation for Hodgkin's disease. In: Atkinson K, editor. *Clinical Bone Marrow Transplantation*. New York: Cambridge Univ Pr; 1994. p. 105–10.
37. Vose JM, Phillips GL, Armitage JO. Autologous bone marrow transplantation for Hodgkin's disease. In: Armitage JO, Antman KH, editors. *High Dose Cancer Therapy: Pharmacology, Hematopoiesis, Stem Cells*. Baltimore, MD: Williams & Wilkins; 1992. p. 651–61.
38. Barlogie B, Jagannath S. Autologous bone marrow transplantation for multiple myeloma. In: Forman SJ, Blume KG, Thomas ED, editors. *Bone Marrow Transplantation*. Cambridge,

MA: Blackwell Scientific; 1994. p. 754–66.
39. Gahrton G. Allogeneic and syngeneic bone marrow transplantation for multiple myeloma. In: Forman SJ, Blume KG, Thomas ED, editors. *Bone Marrow Transplantation*. Cambridge, MA: Blackwell Scientific; 1994. p. 640–6.
40. Antman KH. Dose-intensive therapy in breast cancer. In: Armitage JO, Antman KH, editors. *High Dose Cancer Therapy: Pharmacology, Hematopoiesis, Stem Cells*. Baltimore, MD: Williams & Wilkins; 1992. p. 701–18.
41. Crilley P, Goldstein LJ. Peripheral blood stem cell transplantation in breast cancer. *Semin Oncol* 1995;22:238–49.
42. Peters WP. Autologous bone marrow transplantation for breast cancer. *Curr Opin Oncol* 1992;4:279–82.
43. Antman K, Ayash L, Elias A, et al. A phase II study of high-dose cyclophosphamide, thiotepa, and carboplatin with autologous marrow support in women with measurable advanced breast cancer responding to standard dose therapy. *J Clin Oncol* 1992;10:102–10.
44. Kennedy MJ, Beveridge RA, Rowley SD, et al. High-dose chemotherapy with reinfusion of purged autologous bone marrow following dose intensive induction as initial therapy for metastatic breast cancer. *J Natl Cancer Inst* 1991;83:920–6.
45. Bezwoda WR, Seymour L, Dansey RD. High-dose chemotherapy with hematopoietic rescue as primary treatment for metastatic breast cancer: a randomized trial. *J Clin Oncol* 1995;13:2483–9.
46. Peters WP, Ross M, Vredenburgh JJ, et al. High-dose chemotherapy and autologous bone marrow support as consolidation after standard-dose adjuvant therapy for high-risk primary breast cancer. *J Clin Oncol* 1993;11:1132–43.
47. Gianni AM, Siena S, Bregni M, et al. Growth-factor supported high-dose sequential (HDS) adjuvant chemotherapy in breast cancer ≥10 positive nodes [abstract]. *Proc Am Soc Clin Oncol* 1992;11:68.
48. Graham-Pole JR. Myeloablative treatment supported by marrow infusions for children with neuroblastoma. In: Armitage JO, Antman KH, editors. *High Dose Cancer Therapy: Pharmacology, Hematopoiesis, Stem Cells*. Baltimore, MD: Williams & Wilkins; 1992. p. 735–49.
49. Storb R. HLA-identical bone marrow transplantation for severe aplastic anemia. In: Atkinson K, editor. *Clinical Bone Marrow Transplantation*. New York: Cambridge Univ Pr; 1994. p. 230–7.
50. McDonald GB, Sharma P, Matthews DE, et al. Venocclusive disease of the liver after bone marrow transplantation: diagnosis, incidence, and predisposing factors. *Hepatology* 1984;4:116–22.
51. Jones RJ, Lee KSK, Beschorner WE, et al. Venocclusive disease of the liver following bone marrow transplantation. *Transplantation* 1987;44:778–83.
52. Shulman HM, Hinterberger W. Hepatic veno-occlusive disease—liver toxicity syndrome after bone marrow transplantation. *Bone Marrow Transplant* 1992;10:197–214.
53. McDonald GB, Hinds MS, Fisher LD, et al. Veno-occlusive disease of the liver and multi-organ failure after bone marrow transplantation: a cohort study of 355 patients. *Ann Intern Med* 1993;118:255–67.
54. Bearman SI. The syndrome of hepatic veno-occlusive disease after marrow transplantation. *Blood* 1995;85:3005–20.
55. Grochow LB, Jones RJ, Brundrett RB, et al. Pharmacokinetics of busulfan: correlation with veno-occlusive disease in patients undergoing bone marrow transplantation. *Cancer Chemother Pharmacol* 1989;25:55–61.
56. Essell JH, Thompson JM, Harman GS, et al. Marked increase in veno-occlusive disease of the liver associated with methotrexate use for graft-versus-host disease prophylaxis in patients receiving busulfan/cyclophosphamide. *Blood* 1992;79:2784–8.
57. Shulman HM, McDonald GB, Matthews D, et al. An analysis of hepatic venocclusive disease and centrilobular hepatic degeneration following bone marrow transplantation. *Gastroenterology* 1980;79:1178–91.
58. Shulman HM, Gown AM, Nugent DJ. Hepatic veno-occlusive disease after bone marrow transplantation: immunohistochemical identification of the material within occluded central venules. *Am J Pathol* 1987;127:549–58.
59. Bearman SI, Hinds MS, Wolford JL, et al. A pilot study of continuous infusion heparin for the prevention of hepatic veno-occlusive disease after bone marrow transplantation. *Bone Marrow Transplant* 1990;5:407–11.
60. Attal M, Huguet F, Rubie H, et al. Prevention of hepatic veno-occlusive disease after bone marrow transplantation by continuous infusion heparin: a prospective, randomized trial. *Blood* 1992;79:2834–40.
61. Gluckman E, Jolivet I, Scrobohaci ML, et al. Use of prostaglandin E_1 for prevention of liver veno-occlusive disease in leukaemic patients treated by allogeneic bone marrow transplantation. *Br J Hematol* 1990;74:277–81.
62. Holler E, Kolb HJ, Möller A, et al. Increased serum levels of tumor necrosis factor α precede major complications of bone marrow transplantation. *Blood* 1990;75:1011–6.
63. Bianco JA, Nemunaitis J, Almgren J, et al. Pentoxifylline (PTX) diminishes regimen related toxicity (RRT) in patients undergoing bone marrow transplantation. *Proc Am Soc Clin Oncol* 1990;9:528a.
64. Bianco JA, Appelbaum FR, Nemunaitis J, et al. Phase I–II trial of pentoxifylline for the prevention to transplant-related toxicities following bone marrow transplantation. *Blood* 1991;78:1205–11.
65. Attal M, Huguet F, Rubie H, et al. Prevention of regimen-related toxicities after bone marrow transplantation by pentoxifylline: a prospective, randomized trial. *Blood* 1993;82:732–6.
66. Clift RA, Bianco JA, Appelbaum FR, et al. A randomized controlled trial of pentoxifylline for the prevention of regimen-related toxicities in patients undergoing allogeneic bone marrow transplantation. *Blood* 1993;82:2025–30.
67. Baglin TP, Harper P, Marcus RE. Veno-occlusive disease of the liver complicating ABMT successfully treated with recombinant tissue plasminogen activator (rt-PA) [case report]. *Bone Marrow Transplant* 1990;5:439–41.
68. LaPorte JP, Lesage S, Tilleul P, et al. Alteplase for hepatic veno-occlusive disease after bone-marrow transplantation [letter]. *Lancet* 1992;339:1057.
69. Rosti G, Bandini G, Belardinelli A, et al. Alteplase for hepatic veno-occlusive disease after bone-marrow transplantation [letter]. *Lancet* 1992;339:1481–2.
70. Bearman SI, Shuhart MC, Hinds MS, et al. Recombinant

human tissue plasminogen activator for the treatment of established severe venocclusive disease of the liver after bone marrow transplantation. *Blood* 1992;80:2458–62.
71. Rapaport AP, Doyle HR, Starzl T, et al. Orthotopic liver transplantation for life-threatening veno-occlusive disease of the liver after allogeneic bone marrow transplantation [case report]. *Bone Marrow Transplant* 1991;8:421–4.
72. Ferrara JLM, Deeg HJ. Graft-versus-host disease. *N Engl J Med* 1991;324:667–74.
73. Schwinghammer TL, Bloom EJ. Pharmacologic prophylaxis of acute graft-versus-host disease after allogeneic bone marrow transplantation. *Clin Pharm* 1993;12:736–61.
74. Storb R, Deeg HJ, Thomas ED, et al. Marrow transplantation for chronic myelocytic leukemia: a controlled trial of cyclosporine versus methotrexate for prophylaxis of graft-versus-host disease. *Blood* 1985;66:698–702.
75. Santos GW, Tutschka PJ, Brookmeyer R, et al. Cyclosporine plus methylprednisolone versus cyclophosphamide plus methylprednisolone as prophylaxis for acute graft-versus-host disease: a randomized double-blind study in patients undergoing allogeneic marrow transplantation. *Clin Transplant* 1987;1:21–8.
76. Forman SJ, Blume KG, Krance RA, et al. A prospective randomized study of acute graft-versus-host disease in 107 patients with leukemia: methotrexate/prednisone vs. cyclosporine A/prednisone. *Transplant Proc* 1987;19:2605–7.
77. Storb R, Deeg HJ, Whitehead J, et al. Methotrexate and cyclosporine versus cyclosporine alone for prophylaxis of acute graft-versus-host disease after marrow transplantation for acute leukemia. *N Engl J Med* 1986;314:729–35.
78. Mrsic M, Labar B, Bogdanic V, et al. Combination of cyclosporin and methotrexate for prophylaxis of acute graft-versus-host disease after allogeneic bone marrow transplantation for leukemia. *Bone Marrow Transplant* 1990;6:137–41.
79. Gondo H, Harada M, Taniguchi S, et al. Cyclosporine combined with methylprednisolone or methotrexate in prophylaxis of moderate to severe acute graft-versus-host disease. *Bone Marrow Transplant* 1993;12:437–41.
80. Shepherd JD, Shore TB, Reece DE, et al. Cyclosporine and methylprednisolone for prophylaxis of acute graft-versus-host disease. *Bone Marrow Transplant* 1988;3:553–8.
81. Chao NJ, Schmidt GM, Niland JC, et al. Cyclosporine, methotrexate, and prednisone compared to cyclosporine and prednisone for prophylaxis of acute graft-versus-host disease. *N Engl J Med* 1993;329:1225–30.
82. Masaoka T, Shibata H, Kakishita E, et al. Phase II study of FK 506 for allogeneic bone marrow transplantation. *Transplant Proc* 1991;23:3228–31.
83. Nash RA, Etzioni R, Storb R, et al. Tacrolimus (FK506) alone or in combination with methotrexate or methylprednisolone for the prevention of acute graft-versus-host disease after marrow transplantation from HLA-matched siblings: a single-center study. *Blood* 1995;85:3746–53.
84. Weiden PL, Doney K, Storb R, et al. Antihuman thymocyte globulin for prophylaxis of graft-versus-host disease: a randomized trial in patients with leukemia treated with HLA-identical sibling marrow grafts. *Transplantation* 1979;27:227–30.
85. Ramsay NK, Kersey JH, Robison LL, et al. A randomized study of the prevention of acute graft-versus-host disease. *N Engl J Med* 1982;306:392–7.
86. Schattenberg A, DeWitte T, Preijers F, et al. Allogeneic bone marrow transplantation for leukemia with marrow grafts depleted of lymphocytes by counterflow centrifugation. *Blood* 1990;75:1356–63.
87. Amici C, Carlo-Stella C, Donnenberg AD, et al. Counterflow centrifugal elutriation: present and future. *Bone Marrow Transplant* 1993;12:105–8.
88. Sayer HG, Longton G, Bowden R, et al. Increased risk of infection in marrow transplant patients receiving methylprednisolone for graft-versus-host disease prevention. *Blood* 1994;84:1328–32.
89. Sullivan KM, Storb R, Buckner CD, et al. Graft-versus-host disease as adoptive immunotherapy in patients with advanced hematologic neoplasms. *N Engl J Med* 1989;320:828.
90. Vogelsang GB, Morris LE. Prevention and management of graft-versus-host disease: practical recommendations. *Drugs* 1993;45:668–76.
91. Martin PJ, Schoch G, Fisher L, et al. A retrospective analysis of therapy for acute graft-versus-host disease: initial treatment. *Blood* 1990;76:1464–72.
92. Gratama JW, Jansen J, Lipovich RA, et al. Treatment of acute graft-versus-host disease with monoclonal antibody OKT3: clinical results and effect on circulating T lymphocytes. *Transplantation* 1984;38:469–74.
93. Gluckman E, Devergie A, Varin F, et al. Treatment of steroid resistant severe acute graft-vs.-host disease with a monoclonal pan T OKT3 antibody. *Exp Hematol* 1984;12:66.
94. Gleixner B, Kolb HJ, Holler E, et al. Treatment of GVHD with OKT3: clinical outcome and side-effects associated with release of TNFα. *Bone Marrow Transplant* 1991;8:93–8.
95. Byers VS, Henslee JP, Kernan NA, et al. Use of an anti-pan T-lymphocyte ricin A chain immunotoxin in steroid-resistant graft-versus-host disease. *Blood* 1990;75:1426–32.
96. Herve P, Tiberghien P, Racadot E, et al. Prevention and treatment of acute GvHD—new modalities. *Bone Marrow Transplant* 1990;11(*Suppl* 1):103–6.
97. Atkinson K. Chronic graft-versus-host disease. *Bone Marrow Transplant* 1990;5:69–82.
98. Sullivan KM, Agura E, Anasetti C, et al. Chronic graft-versus-host disease and other late complications of bone marrow transplantation. *Semin Hematol* 1991;28:250–9.
99. Wingard JR, Piantadosi S, Vogelsang GB, et al. Predictors of death from chronic graft-versus-host disease after bone marrow transplantation. *Blood* 1989;74:1428–35.
100. Schwarer AP, Hughes JMB, Trotman-Dickenson B, et al. A chronic pulmonary syndrome associated with graft-versus-host disease after allogeneic marrow transplantation. *Transplantation* 1992;54:1002–8.
101. Sullivan KM, Shulman HM. Chronic graft-versus-host disease, obliterative bronchiolitis, and graft-versus-leukemia effect: case histories. *Transplant Proc* 1989;21(3 *Suppl* 1):51–62.
102. Holland HK, Wingard JR, Beschorner WE, et al. Bronchiolitis obliterans in bone marrow transplantation and its relationship to chronic graft-versus-host disease and low serum IgG. *Blood* 1988;72:621–7.
103. Deeg HJ. Delayed complications and long-term effects after bone marrow transplantation. *Hematol Oncol Clin North Am* 1990;4:641–57.
104. Sullivan KM. Graft-versus-host disease. In: Forman SJ, Blume KG, Thomas ED, editors. Bone marrow transplantation. Cambridge, MA: Blackwell Scientific; 1994. p. 339–62.

105. Sullivan KM, Deeg HJ, Sanders JE, et al. Late complications after marrow transplantation. *Semin Hematol* 1984;21:53–63.
106. Tzakis AG, Abu-Elmagd K, Fung JJ, et al. FK 506 rescue in chronic graft-versus-host disease after bone marrow transplantation. *Transplant Proc* 1991;23:3225.
107. Sullivan KM, Shulman HM, Storb R, et al. Chronic graft-versus-host disease in 52 patients: adverse natural course and successful treatment with combined immunosuppression. *Blood* 1981;57:267–76.
108. Sullivan KM, Witherspoon RP, Storb R, et al. Prednisone and azathioprine compared with prednisone and placebo for treatment of chronic graft-versus-host disease: prognostic influence of prolonged thrombocytopenia after allogeneic marrow transplantation. *Blood* 1988;72:546–54.
109. Atkinson K, Weller P, Rayman W, et al. PUVA therapy for drug-resistant graft-versus-host disease. *Bone Marrow Transplant* 1986;1:227–36.
110. Vogelsang GB, Farmer E, Hess AD, et al. Thalidomide for the treatment of chronic graft-versus-host disease. *N Engl J Med* 1992;326:1055–8.
111. Heney D, Norfolk DR, Wheeldon J, et al. Thalidomide treatment for chronic graft-versus-host disease. *Br J Hematol* 1991;78:23–7.
112. Wingard JR. Advances in the management of infectious complications after bone marrow transplantation. *Bone Marrow Transplant* 1990;6:371–83.
113. Weiner RS, Bortin MM, Gale RP, et al. Interstitial pneumonitis after bone marrow transplantation: assessment of risk factors. *Ann Intern Med* 1986;104:168–75.
114. Seiden MV, Elias A, Ayash L, et al. Pulmonary toxicity associated with high dose chemotherapy in the treatment of solid tumors with autologous marrow transplant: an analysis of four chemotherapy regimens. *Bone Marrow Transplant* 1992;10:57–63.
115. Morgan M, Dodds A, Atkinson K, et al. The toxicity of busulphan and cyclophosphamide as the preparative regimen for bone marrow transplantation. *Br J Hematol* 1991;77:529.
116. Cordonnier C, Bernaudin JF, Bierling P, et al. Pulmonary complications occurring after allogeneic bone marrow transplantation: a study of 130 consecutive transplanted patients. *Cancer* 1986;58:1047–54.
117. Grañena A, Carreras E, Rozman C, et al. Interstitial pneumonitis after BMT: 15 years experience in a single institution. *Bone Marrow Transplant* 1993;11:453–8.
118. Afessa B, Tefferi A, Hoagland HC, et al. Outcome of recipients of bone marrow transplants who require intensive-care unit support. *Mayo Clin Proc* 1992;67:117–22.
119. Robbins RA, Linder J, Stahl MG, et al. Diffuse alveolar hemorrhage in autologous bone marrow transplant recipients. *Am J Med* 1989;87:511–8.
120. Chao NJ, Duncan SR, Long GD. Corticosteroid therapy for diffuse alveolar hemorrhage in autologous marrow transplant recipients. *Ann Intern Med* 1991;114:145–6.
121. Grigg A, Sheridan WP. The role of hemopoietic growth factors in autologous bone marrow and peripheral blood stem cell transplantation. In: Atkinson K, editor. *Clinical Bone Marrow Transplantation*. New York: Cambridge Univ Pr; 1994. p. 153–63.
122. Lieschke GJ, Burgess AW. Granulocyte colony-stimulating factor and granulocyte-macrophage colony-stimulating factor (part 2). *N Engl J Med* 1992;327:99–106.
123. Sheridan WP, Morstyn G, Wolf M, et al. Granulocyte colony-stimulating factor and neutrophil recovery after high-dose chemotherapy and autologous bone marrow transplantation. *Lancet* 1989;891–4.
124. Nemunaitis J, Rabinowe SN, Singer JW, et al. Recombinant granulocyte-macrophage colony-stimulating factor after autologous bone marrow transplantation for lymphoid malignancies. *N Engl J Med* 1991;324:1773–8.
125. Gorin NC, Coiffier B, Hayat M, et al. Recombinant human granulocyte-macrophage colony-stimulating factor after high-dose chemotherapy and autologous bone marrow transplantation with unpurged and purged marrow in non-Hodgkin's lymphoma: a double-blind placebo-controlled trial. *Blood* 1992;80:1149–57.
126. Taylor KM, Jagannath S, Spitzer G, et al. Recombinant human granulocyte colony-stimulating factor hastens granulocyte recovery after high-dose chemotherapy and autologous bone marrow transplantation in Hodgkin's disease. *J Clin Oncol* 1989;7:1791–9.
127. Gupta P, Tiley C, Powles R, et al. No increase in relapse in patients with myeloid leukemias receiving rhGM-CSF after allogeneic bone marrow transplantation. *Bone Marrow Transplant* 1992;9:491–3.

SELF-STUDY QUESTIONS

1. Bone marrow transplantation (BMT) is being used more frequently in an attempt to increase dose intensity of chemotherapy agents.

    a. true
    b. false

2. BMT is a proven therapeutic modality in all of the following *except*:

    a. acute myelogenous leukemia.
    b. metastatic breast cancer.
    c. chronic myelogenous leukemia.
    d. non-Hodgkin's lymphoma.

3. Patients with leukemia can only receive a bone marrow transplant if the marrow comes from a separate donor.

    a. true
    b. false

4. What is the difference between allogeneic BMT and autologous BMT?

5. Why are patients undergoing BMT more likely to experience therapy-related toxicity than patients receiving standard doses of chemotherapy?

6. Which of the following are clinical features of hepatic veno-occlusive disease?

   a. hepatomegaly
   b. jaundice
   c. weight gain
   d. all of the above

7. All of the following BMT-related complications are potentially life threatening *except:*

   a. hepatic veno-occlusive disease
   b. interstitial pneumonitis
   c. graft-versus-host disease
   d. nausea and vomiting

8. Recent evidence supports the treatment of hepatic veno-occlusive disease with:

   a. prostaglandin
   b. alteplase
   c. pentoxifylline
   d. tacrolimus

9. Graft-versus-host disease (GVHD) following allogeneic BMT is initiated by the activation of which of the following?

   a. B cells
   b. T cells
   c. neutrophils
   d. natural killer cells

10. Acute GVHD is most likely to occur after which kind of bone marrow transplantation?

    a. allogeneic transplantation
    b. autologous transplantation
    c. peripheral stem cell transplantation
    d. syngeneic transplantation

11. GVHD involves all of the following organ systems *except:*

    a. liver
    b. skin
    c. kidneys
    d. gastrointestinal tract

12. Patients who have clinical grade IV GVHD have a very poor survival rate.

    a. true
    b. false

13. What is the rationale for the use of cyclosporine in the prevention of GVHD?

14. Which of the following is considered the treatment of choice for patients who have acute GVHD?

    a. muromonab-CD3 (OKT3)
    b. corticosteroids
    c. immunotoxin
    d. tacrolimus (FK 506)

15. List three common side effects associated with cyclosporine therapy.

16. All of the following are effective in the prevention of acute GVHD *except:*

    a. cyclosporine + corticosteroids.
    b. cyclosporine + methotrexate.
    c. thalidomide.
    d. cyclosporine + corticosteroids + methotrexate.

17. *Pneumocystis carinii* infections are a common complication in patients who have received an autologous bone marrow transplant.

    a. true
    b. false

18. Patients who have received an allogeneic bone marrow transplant are at risk for which of the following infections?

    a. cytomegalovirus
    b. *Pneumocystis carinii*
    c. *Aspergillus* spp.
    d. all of the above

19. Infections seen early in the post-BMT period are primarily related to neutropenia caused by chemotherapy and/or radiation.

    a. true
    b. false

20. Why do patients with chronic GVHD have a greater risk of developing infection than patients without GVHD?

Chapter 15: Infectious Complications

James A. Trovato, Pharm.D.
Pharmacy School Assistant Professor
Department of Pharmacy Practice and Science
University of Maryland
Assistant Professor of Oncology
Greenebaum Cancer Center
University of Maryland Medicine
Baltimore, Maryland

Rebecca S. Finley, Pharm.D., M.S.
Chair and Associate Professor
Department of Pharmacy Practice and
  Pharmacy Administration
Philadelphia College of Pharmacy
Philadelphia, Pennsylvania

Predisposing Factors 270
Common Sites of Infection and Predominant Pathogens 271
Managing the Febrile Granulocytopenic Patient 272
    Antibiotic Selection 272
    Antimicrobial Resistance 274
    Factors That Influence Response to Antimicrobials 274
    Duration of Therapy 275
    Outpatient Management 275
Fungal Infections 276
Viral Infections 278
    Herpes Simplex Virus 278
    Varicella-Zoster Virus 278
    Cytomegalovirus 278
    Epstein-Barr Virus 279
Preventing Infection 279
    Reducing Patient Exposure to Nosocomial Organisms 279
    Suppressing Organisms 280
    Avoiding Invasive Procedures 281
    Bolstering Host Defense Mechanisms 281
Summary 282
References 282
Self-Study Questions 286

Infectious complications are a major cause of morbidity and mortality in patients with cancer. The malignant disease, its therapy, or both alter the body's normal defense mechanisms, increasing the patient's risk of serious infections (Table 15-1). In recent years, major advances have been made in managing many malignancies with aggressive chemotherapy. However, these aggressive regimens are frequently associated with an even greater incidence of infectious sequelae. Early diagnosis, effective management, and successful prevention of infectious complications in patients with cancer depend on understanding the factors that place these patients at increased risk.

This chapter first discusses the predisposing factors and common sites of infection for the patient with cancer. Strategies and guidelines for controlling bacterial, fungal, and viral infections are then discussed; methods for preventing infections close the chapter.

After completing this chapter, the reader should be able to:

1. Describe factors that predispose a patient with cancer to infectious complications.
2. Discuss considerations that influence antibiotic selection for infectious complications.
3. Discuss factors that affect antibiotic effectiveness for infectious complications.
4. Describe therapy for cancer patients with fungal and viral infections.
5. Discuss methods for preventing various infections in the patient with cancer.

PREDISPOSING FACTORS

Several well-recognized factors predispose patients with cancer to serious infections. Granulocytopenia is considered the most significant. Granulocytes (or neutrophils) are the white blood cells that provide the body's major cellular defense against bacterial and fungal infections. Patients with cancer may experience granulocytopenia secondary to invasion of the bone marrow (which produces the granulocytes) by the malignancy or after cytotoxic chemotherapy. Radiation therapy may also suppress the bone marrow, resulting in a decline of the granulocyte count.

The risk of serious infections is inversely related to the absolute neutrophil count (ANC) in the systemic circulation. As shown in Figure 15-1, the risk of infection does not rise appreciably until the ANC drops below 500 cells per cubic millimeter of blood, and the most severe infections (especially bacteremias) occur at levels below 100 cells/mm³.[1] The risk of serious infections is directly related to the duration of granulocytopenia; most infections occur after prolonged granulocytopenia.[2] For example, most patients who undergo initial treatment for acute myelogenous leukemia experience at least one infection during the 2–4 weeks in which they are granu-

Table 15-1. Defects in Host Defense Mechanisms in Patients with Cancer

Defect	Causes
Granulocytopenia	Acute leukemia; chemotherapy
Abnormal cell-mediated immunity	Hodgkin's disease; corticosteroids; chemotherapy
Abnormal immunoglobulins	Multiple myeloma; chronic lymphocytic leukemia; corticosteroids
Disruption of skin or mucosal surfaces	Invasive procedures (biopsies or venipuncture); erosion due to tumor or decubitus ulcers

locytopenic. In contrast, a much lower percentage of patients with solid tumors become infected after chemotherapy, because their ANCs generally remain very low for only a few days. The treatment regimens for many solid tumors, such as small cell lung carcinoma, advanced breast cancer, and aggressive lymphomas, are beginning to include aggressive high-dose cancer chemotherapy, and, as a result, a greater number of these patients experience serious infections. Today, colony-stimulating factors are frequently administered following these

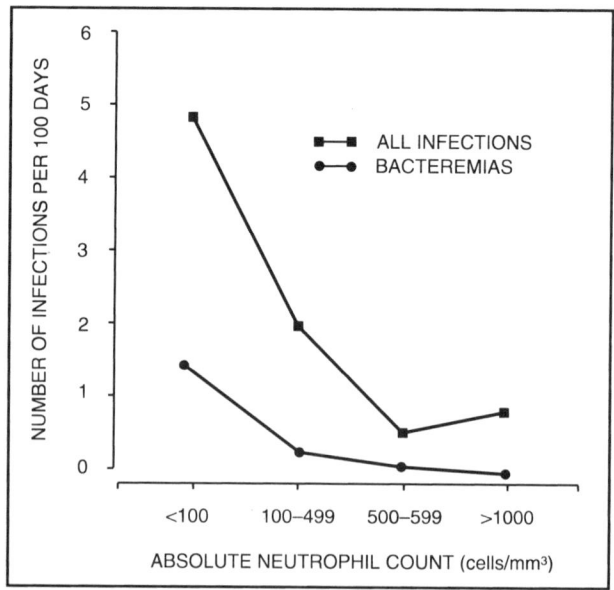

Figure 15-1. Relationship between risk of infection and absolute neutrophil count

SOURCE: reprinted with permission from Schimpff SC. Infections in the compromised host: an overview. In: Mandell GL, Douglas RJ Jr., Bennett JE, editors. *Principles and Practice of Infectious Diseases*, 3rd ed. New York: Churchill Livingstone; 1990. p. 2259.

regimens to decrease the period of granulocytopenia and reduce the risk of infection.

The malignant disease and its therapy are responsible for other factors that increase the risk of infection. The skin and mucosal linings normally provide the body's primary host defense against invasion by microorganisms. Radiation therapy and many cancer chemotherapy agents damage the mucosa that lines the gastrointestinal (GI) and respiratory tracts, creating a portal of entry for pathogenic organisms. Likewise, the skin may be damaged by radiation therapy, invasive procedures (e.g., venipunctures or bone marrow aspirations), decubitus ulcers, and tumor erosion. Over the past two decades, widespread use of right atrial catheters (e.g., Hickman or Broviac catheters) has become associated with an increased risk of gram-positive infections in particular.[3,4] Tumors may also cause obstruction of the bronchi, biliary tract, and ureters, thus increasing the possibility of postobstructive infection.

COMMON SITES OF INFECTION AND PREDOMINANT PATHOGENS

The most common sites of infection in granulocytopenic cancer patients are

- the alimentary tract (periodontium, pharynx, esophagus, and perirectal area),
- the respiratory tract (lungs and sinuses), and
- the skin.

Unfortunately, the usual inflammatory signs of infection (redness, pain, and swelling) are often absent because of the lack of functioning granulocytes, and the only evidence of infection may be fever.

The pathogens most often responsible for infections in this setting are the endogenous microbial flora that frequently colonize at or near the site of infection (Table 15-2). Many of these organisms are nosocomial, and they include enteric gram-negative bacilli (*Pseudomonas aeruginosa*, *Klebsiella pneumoniae*, and *Escherichia coli*), which colonize the mouth, pharynx, and stool of cancer patients soon after hospitalization.[5] This colonization is presumably due to chemotherapy-induced alterations in the epithelial adherence of these organisms.[6] The hospital environment, including the air, water, food, medical equipment, and procedures, as well as staff-to-patient and patient-to-patient contact, contributes to microbial colonization.[7] Although these gram-negative bacilli still cause the majority of bacteremias in granulocytopenic patients, the frequency of such infections appears to be decreasing.[3] In contrast, the frequency of gram-positive infections appears to be rising.

The gram-positive cocci *Staphylococcus aureus* and *S. epidermidis* are also common pathogens in patients with cancer. *S. epidermidis* is reportedly a major pathogen in patients with intravenous (IV) catheters.[4] A common gram-positive anaerobic bacillus that colonizes the GI tract of cancer patients is *Clostridium difficile*. *C. difficile* colonization is promoted by alterations in the normal GI flora caused by prolonged use of broad-spectrum antibiotics. An outbreak of *C. difficile* in an isolated oncology unit is a major risk factor for colonization, because the organism is easily transmitted from patient to patient via health care providers. Wearing gowns and gloves and washing hands frequently are critical in preventing transmission when caring for patients with *C. difficile*.

Table 15-2. Predominant Pathogens Associated with Infections in Cancer Patients

Host Defect	Bacteria	Fungi	Viruses	Other Pathogens
Granulocytopenia	*Escherichia coli*, *Pseudomonas aeruginosa*, *Klebsiella* sp., *Staphylococcus aureus*, *S. epidermidis*, *Enterococcus* sp.	*Candida* sp., *Aspergillus* sp., *Mucor* sp.		
Abnormal cell-mediated immunity	*Mycobacterium* sp., *Salmonella* sp., *Legionella* sp., *Listeria* sp., *Nocardia* sp.	*Cryptococcus* sp., *Candida* sp., *Histoplasma* sp., *Coccidioides* sp.	Cytomegalovirus, Varicella-zoster virus, Epstein-Barr virus, Herpes simplex virus types 1 and 2	*Pneumocystis carinii*, *Toxoplasma gondii*
Anatomical abnormalities	*Staphylococcus* sp., *Streptococcus* sp.	*Candida* sp., *Torulopsis* sp.		
Abnormal immunoglobulins	*Pneumococcus* sp., *Hemophilus influenzae*, *Meningococcus* sp.			*Pneumocystis carinii*, *Giardia lamblia*

Yeasts (*Candida* sp.) and filamentous fungi (*Aspergillus* sp.) are rarely responsible for initial infections but may account for serious subsequent infections, especially in patients who experience prolonged periods of granulocytopenia and extended courses of broad-spectrum antibiotics. Opportunistic fungal infections are also common in patients with abnormal cell-mediated immunity. It is important to remember that management of these patients may be complicated by multiple concurrent infections.

Parasitic and viral infections are also common in patients with cancer. *Pneumocystis carinii* is a major pulmonary pathogen in patients receiving corticosteroids and in patients with acquired immunodeficiency syndrome (AIDS). Herpes simplex, varicella-zoster, and cytomegalovirus are viral pathogens of great concern to immunosuppressed patients, especially allogeneic bone marrow transplant patients and those with lymphoid malignancies who may have associated abnormalities of cell-mediated immunity.

MANAGING THE FEBRILE GRANULOCYTOPENIC PATIENT

The majority of fevers that occur in cancer patients, especially those who are granulocytopenic, are of infectious origin, even though fevers may be caused by drugs, blood transfusions, or the underlying malignancy.[7] Ultimately, about 60% of these febrile episodes are defined as infectious episodes; a specific pathogen is identified in approximately 40% of the cases.[3]

A very careful history, physical examination, chest X-ray, and blood and urine cultures must be obtained to try to document the infection site and pathogen. The practice of initiating antimicrobial therapy before obtaining documentation of infection, such as culture results, is referred to as empiric antibiotic therapy and has dramatically reduced morbidity and mortality in febrile granulocytopenic patients.

Antibiotic Selection

Selection of an appropriate empiric antimicrobial regimen must take into account the incidence and susceptibility patterns of pathogenic organisms at a particular institution. Historically, combinations of broad-spectrum antimicrobial agents have been considered superior to single-agent regimens. The availability of agents with high bactericidal activity (e.g., imipenem or ceftazidime) has allowed single-agent therapy to become acceptable in some settings.[8] More recently, newer broad-spectrum antimicrobial agents, such as cefepime[9–11] and meropenem,[12,13] have been considered for single-agent therapy in febrile granulocytopenic patients.

Bacteremias account for approximately 20% of all febrile episodes in granulocytopenic cancer patients.[3] These infections are generally very severe, and death frequently occurs within 24 hours if the infection is not appropriately treated. Most granulocytopenic patients with gram-negative bacteremias did not survive before empiric broad-spectrum antimicrobial therapy was routinely used. For example, in 1969, 20 of 25 patients (80%) with *Pseudomonas aeruginosa* bacteremias at the Baltimore Cancer Research Center died of their infections despite single-agent therapy with gentamicin or polymyxin. After combination empiric therapy with carbenicillin and gentamicin was started, 25 of 43 patients (58%) with microbiologically documented infections improved, including 8 of 13 patients (62%) with *P. aeruginosa* bacteremias.[14]

Since that time, most empiric antibiotic regimens have employed an antipseudomonal penicillin or third-generation cephalosporin with an aminoglycoside agent or the combination of two extended-spectrum β-lactam antibiotics, as shown in Table 15-3.[15–57] Other regimens include the combination of a fluoroquinolone plus a penicillin or an aminoglycoside plus a β-lactamase–resistant penicillin.

Because of the increasing frequency of gram-positive infections,[58] some institutions have advocated the addition of an empiric antistaphylococcal agent to the initial regimen. Others, however, recommend that adding such an agent is necessary only when staphylococcal resistance to the original regimen is demonstrated or when the patient does not respond promptly to the original regimen.[59] A penicillinase-resistant penicillin is appropriate therapy for most strains of *S. aureus*. However, many strains of *S. epidermidis* are now resistant to β-lactam antibiotics and aminoglycosides, leaving vancomycin as the drug of choice.

Most published studies report response rates from empiric antibiotic regimens ranging from 60 to 80%.[15–24,35–40,42,45,46,48,55] The major differences among regimens have been the cost and the pattern of toxicities associated with the various combinations. Many studies have incorporated third-generation cephalosporins or extended-spectrum penicillins or both into empiric antibiotic regimens. More recent studies have incorporated the use of high-dose ciprofloxacin in combination with an aminoglycoside or an extended-spectrum penicillin. An alternative agent for patients allergic or intolerant to β-lactam antibiotics, such as imipenem or ceftazidime, may use aztreonam for initial empiric synergistic gram-negative coverage. Routine use of such agents is tempting, given their broad spectrum of activity (particularly against gram-negative bacteria), their minimal toxicity, and their high bactericidal activity. However, many of these agents are significantly more costly, and their use should be restricted to cases in which the microbial susceptibility patterns indicate they are needed.

The double β-lactam combinations, such as the ceftazidime-plus-piperacillin regimen,[27] are very costly. These combinations are, however, devoid of the nephrotoxicity and ototoxicity associated with aminoglycoside use. These regimens should be reserved for patients who are at high risk for developing aminoglycoside toxicity (e.g., prior renal insufficiency, prior ototoxicity, or concomitant therapy with other nephrotoxic or ototoxic drugs). Single daily dosing of aminoglycosides has been considered as a means of reducing nephrotoxicity. A few clinical trials comparing the standard three-times-a-day aminoglycoside dosing to single daily dosing have

Table 15-3. Examples of Antibiotic Regimens Used as Empiric Therapy for Fever in Granulocytopenic Patients

Regimen	Reference
Penicillin plus aminoglycoside	
Carbenicillin + gentamicin	15–17
Carbenicillin + amikacin	15, 18
Ticarcillin + gentamicin	19
Ticarcillin + tobramycin	20–22
Ticarcillin + amikacin	19, 23, 24
Piperacillin + amikacin	18, 23
Mezlocillin + tobramycin	22
Azlocillin + amikacin	24
Piperacillin + netilmicin	25
Piperacillin + gentamicin	26, 27
Azlocillin + gentamicin	28
Azlocillin + netilmicin	29
β-lactamase inhibitor penicillin plus aminoglycoside	
Piperacillin/tazobactam + gentamicin	30
Piperacillin/tazobactam + amikacin	31–33
Ticarcillin/clavulanate + amikacin	34
Cephalosporin plus aminoglycoside	
Cephalothin + gentamicin	16
Cefotaxime + amikacin	24
Cefoperazone + amikacin	35
Ceftazidime + tobramycin	36, 37
Moxalactam + amikacin	38–40
Ceftazidime + amikacin	31, 32, 41
Double β-lactam combinations	
Carbenicillin + cephalothin	16
Moxalactam + piperacillin	39, 40
Moxalactam + ticarcillin	21, 42
Ceftazidime + piperacillin	36
Fluroquinolone plus aminoglycoside	
Ciprofloxacin + netilmicin	25
Fluroquinolone plus penicillin	
Ciprofloxacin + azlocillin	28, 41
Ciprofloxacin + benzylpenicillin	43
Ciprofloxacin + piperacillin	44
Monotherapy	
Imipenem	45–47
Ceftazidime	47–52
Cefepime	9–11
Meropenem	12, 13
Ciprofloxacin	29, 51–54
Other Combinations	
Trimethoprim–sulfamethoxazole + carbenicillin	17
Trimethoprim–sulfamethoxazole + ticarcillin	55
Trimethoprim–sulfamethoxazole + amikacin	49
Aztreonam + vancomycin + amikacin	42
Aztreonam + vancomycin	27, 56
Ciprofloxacin + teicoplanin	26
Imipenem + vancomycin	56
Ticarcillin/clavulanate + vancomycin	57
Ticarcillin/clavulanate + ceftazidime + vancomycin	57

documented similar clinical efficacy and no greater incidence of nephrotoxicity in granulocytopenic patients.[60-62] As in prior regimens, a broad-spectrum β-lactam antibiotic should be used in combination with single-daily-dose aminoglycoside therapy.

The exceptional antibacterial properties of the newer agents raise the question of whether they could be used as single-agent therapy. Pickard et al.[20] compared moxalactam with ticarcillin plus tobramycin. Pizzo et al.[48] compared ceftazidime with gentamicin, carbenicillin, and cephalothin. Both studies reported that single-agent therapy was equivalent to the combination. Newer comparative trials continue to support single-agent therapy with ceftazidime.[49,50] Imipenem has also been used as single-agent therapy.[45] The most recent randomized comparison of ceftazidime versus imipenem as monotherapy for febrile granulocytopenic patients concluded that both agents are equally efficacious.[47] Modifications, such as the addition of vancomycin or aminoglycosides, were similar between the two agents. The frequency of additional anaerobic coverage was greater with ceftazidime. Imipenem was associated with greater side effects (e.g., nausea and vomiting) and *C. difficile*–associated diarrhea. Factors to consider when choosing between imipenem and ceftazidime include cost, dosing frequency, side effects, and patient drug allergies. More recently ciprofloxacin, cefepime, and meropenem have been studied as single-agent therapy.[9-13,29,51-54] Patients must be carefully monitored if monotherapy is used. Therapy should be modified immediately if evidence of clinical deterioration or resistant organisms emerges.

Antimicrobial Resistance

Unfortunately, the widespread use of vancomycin has resulted in the development of vancomycin-resistant enterococci (VRE). *Enterococcus faecalis* and *E. faecium* are the predominant VRE species among granulocytopenic patients. This resistance is due to the enterococci's ability to produce a modified cell-wall precursor to which vancomycin has a low binding affinity. This low binding affinity allows the pathogen to continue cell wall production uninterrupted. A report by Montecalvo and colleagues[63] identified 29 cases of vancomycin-resistant *E. faecium* in 413 adult oncology patients over a 1-year period. Seven neutropenic patients (1.7%) developed VRE bacteremia and 22 of 167 patients evaluated (13%) were noninfected stool carriers. Five of the 7 bacteremia patients received high-dose ampicillin with an aminoglycoside, which resulted in survival for only 1 patient. One of the remaining bacteremia patients died, and the other showed signs of clinical improvement. Duration of antibiotic therapy and prolonged neutropenia due to leukemia were the most significant risk factors associated with VRE bacteremia. Prolonged use of multiple antibiotics and intestinal epithelial damage from chemotherapy were also suggested to be risk factors.

A recent study of vancomycin-resistant *E. faecium* on an oncology unit[64] concluded that the use of antibiotics, such as metronidazole and imipenem, with activity against anaerobic pathogens and GI colonization with VRE were the two greatest risk factors for the development of VRE bacteremia. These investigators discussed the possibility that VRE infection occurred by transmission from another patient via a health care provider and changes in the patient's GI flora, caused by broad-spectrum antibiotics, that allowed the enterococci to thrive. Factors that contribute to the spread of VRE in hospitalized granulocytopenic patients include duration of hospital stay, prolonged use of broad-spectrum antibiotics, previous vancomycin use, duration and severity of immunosuppression, GI colonization by VRE, and transmission due to poor prevention or infection control.

Although a variety of antibiotics, such as teicoplanin (not commercially available in the U.S.), chloramphenicol, novobiocin, and rifampin have potential activity against VRE, there are limited clinical data to support their efficacy. Measures to prevent transmission, such as wearing gowns and gloves and washing hands frequently, are the best intervention against VRE.[65] Guidelines for the use of vancomycin at your institution to minimize VRE should include reserving vancomycin for only methicillin-resistant *S. aureus* and *S. epidermidis* infections; adjusting treatment as soon as possible, based on culture and sensitivities; avoiding empiric use of single positive blood cultures; and using oral vancomycin only for *C. difficile* infections that have not responded to two courses of metronidazole.[65] Empiric vancomycin therapy remains controversial, and its use should be based on institution-specific guidelines.

Over the past decade, enteric gram-negative bacilli, such as *Pseudomonas* and *Enterobacter* sp., have acquired the ability to produce β-lactamases capable of destroying extended-spectrum cephalosporins, including ceftazidime, ceftriaxone, and even aztreonam. One study reported the outbreak of ceftazidime-resistant *Klebsiella pneumoniae* and *E. coli* in 13 pediatric oncology patients receiving ceftazidime monotherapy for febrile granulocytopenia.[66] Colonization and infection with β-lactamase–producing pathogens in the blood, urine, or respiratory tract of febrile granulocytopenic patients have led to prolonged hospitalization. Patients may show clinical signs and symptoms of sepsis, urinary tract infection, or pneumonia. Other patients may only present with persistent fever. The identification of β-lactamase–producing pathogens in positive cultures should be considered, especially if the patient is not responding to broad-spectrum β-lactam therapy. Antimicrobial therapy for resistant organisms should be guided by culture and susceptibility results.

Factors That Influence Response to Antimicrobials

The goal of empiric antibiotic therapy is the prevention of premature death and other morbidity. Favorable responses to empiric antibiotic therapy include the resolution of fever and other clinical signs and symptoms of infection and the eradication of the pathogen (for documented infections) without a change in antibiotic therapy. The response of infectious episodes to antimicrobial interventions is influenced by a number of factors. The most crucial factor, however, is prompt initiation of antimicrobial therapy when fever or other evidence of infection becomes apparent. The mortality rate rises if antimicrobial therapy is not begun immediately or if therapy is inadequate. Therefore, broad-spectrum antimicrobial therapy must be initiated immediately when fever occurs during granulocytopenia.

Favorable response is also strongly influenced by regeneration of bone marrow and the return of functioning granulocytes to the circulation. In an analysis of 75 gram-negative bacteremias, DeJongh et al.[67] reported an 85% (29 of 34) response rate when the granulocyte count recovered, but only a 29% (12 of 41) response rate in patients whose granulocyte count remained severely depressed (i.e., <100/mm^3).

Historically, gram-negative bacteremias have also demonstrated a more favorable response when the infecting organism is susceptible to both antibiotics included in the combination. In 1980, Love et al.[68] reported that 28 of 33 patients (85%) improved when the pathogen was susceptible to both antibiotics used, 18 of 27 (67%) improved when the pathogen was susceptible to only one antibiotic, and only 2 of 7 (29%) improved when the pathogen was resistant to both antibiotics. As mentioned previously, the availability of antibacterial agents with enhanced activity against many gram-negative pathogens has dramatically improved the response rates to single-drug therapy.

The clinical outcome of gram-negative bacteremias in granulocytopenic patients has also improved when synergistic combinations (rather than nonsynergistic or antagonistic ones) are used. Two studies reported by Klastersky et al.[69,70] reported a combined overall response rate of 80% (80 of 100) in patients receiving synergistic combinations but only a 50% (52 of 105) response rate in those receiving nonsynergistic regimens. Likewise, Lau et al.[15] reported a mortality rate of 18% (4 of 22) in patients given synergistic combinations, compared with 44% (4 of 9) in patients receiving combinations that were additive but not synergistic.

Duration of Therapy

Deciding when to alter or discontinue antimicrobial therapy is often difficult in the management of granulocytopenic patients. After bacterial infection is documented, therapy should be adjusted if the pathogen is resistant to one or more agents in the regimen or if less expensive or less toxic regimens are suitable. If the pathogen is sensitive to low concentrations of the antimicrobial agent or agents, consideration may be given to narrowing the antimicrobial regimen.

Such an alteration may lessen the risk of antimicrobial resistance and superinfection in addition to decreasing cost and potential toxicity. However, this alteration places granulocytopenic patients at greater risk for developing a second bacterial infection. Regardless of whether the regimen is narrowed, all granulocytopenic patients must be monitored carefully for fever and other signs of new infectious complications, and therapy should be adjusted or reinstituted whenever indicated.

Therapy should be continued until the site of infection has healed and the fever has subsided. Antibiotics may be discontinued after a 10- to 14-day course for bacteremias or another serious infection in patients whose granulocyte counts recover. A 7- to 10-day course of therapy is usually sufficient for less severe infections.[71]

Deciding when to stop therapy in patients who remain granulocytopenic is more controversial. Joshi and Schimpff[71] recommend that therapy be continued for 4–5 days after the fever and all other signs of infection have resolved. On the other hand, Pizzo and colleagues[8,72] recommend that antimicrobials be continued until the granulocyte count recovers. Several potential risks and benefits of stopping therapy must be evaluated carefully in patients who remain febrile and granulocytopenic without a demonstrable source of infection (i.e., fever of unknown origin). Pizzo et al.[73] reported that 9 of 16 such patients developed infection or shock or both after therapy was discontinued, and Joshi et al.[74] also reported that the reinstitution of antibiotics is necessary in approximately 50% of such patients. Evidence like this certainly favors continuing antibiotics in persistently febrile granulocytopenic patients. However, complications associated with long-term antimicrobial therapy (e.g., development of resistant organisms, antibiotic toxicity, or fungal superinfections) may weigh toward stopping therapy. If antibiotics are discontinued, the patient should undergo frequent evaluations to detect subtle evidence of infection.

Outpatient Management

Traditionally, the management of febrile granulocytopenic patients has involved the administration of broad-spectrum IV antibiotics in the hospital for the duration of the granulocytopenia. More recently, the outpatient setting has been explored as an alternative for patients who have a low risk of developing serious complications during their period of febrile granulocytopenia. The outpatient setting is attractive because of the problems associated with hospital treatment: extra costs, exposure to hospital pathogens, and possibly a negative impact on the patient's overall quality of life. The first step in managing the febrile granulocytopenic outpatient is to identify which patients fit into the low-risk category.

Buchanan and colleagues[75] identified several factors that define a low-risk patient. These include an ANC >100, cancer in remission, ≥10 days following chemotherapy, and absence of underlying organ disease, mucositis, and diarrhea. Other important patient characteristics that allow for outpatient management of febrile granulocytopenia include patient willingness and compliance, 24-hour family or caregiver support, living <30 miles from an acute care facility, and appropriate medical insurance.

The next step is to decide whether the outpatient should be treated with IV or oral antibiotics. Febrile granulocytopenic patients who are started on IV antibiotics in the hospital may be candidates for home IV antibiotic therapy when the patient is deemed clinically stable. It has been shown that low-risk patients discharged early from the hospital can be successfully treated with IV antibiotics at home.[76] Advances in infusion devices, skilled nursing care, and educated family members have made home IV antibiotic therapy a convenient and viable option.

More recently, there has been a desire to use oral antibiotics to manage the febrile granulocytopenic patient in the inpatient as well as the outpatient setting. The most common oral agents used in these settings are the fluoroquinolones. They can be used as monotherapy, are well tolerated, and provide excellent gram-negative and adequate gram-positive coverage. Several clinical trials in low-risk febrile granulocytopenic patients have demonstrated the safety and efficacy of the oral fluoroquinolones either alone or in combination with other oral agents such as clindamycin, amoxicillin/clavulanate, and rifampin.[77–82] The definition of a low-risk patient is usually more strict when considering oral antibiotics for the outpatient management of febrile granulocytopenic patients. For example, patients at the Greenebaum Cancer Center are eligible for outpatient management only if they have a controlled solid tumor, an expected duration of granulocytopenia of ≤7 days, no sites of infection on physical exam, no comorbid diseases, a caregiver living with them within 25 miles of the cancer center, and a telephone and are able to read a thermometer. Patients meeting these criteria are started on oral ofloxacin 400 mg twice daily and are observed for 2 hours before being sent home. Patients who do not develop complications are followed daily for the first 2 days and then every other day in the outpatient clinic.

FUNGAL INFECTIONS

Fungal infections have long been recognized as serious complications in patients with cancer. However, these opportunistic infections have gained importance over the past decade as patient morbidity and mortality associated with them have risen.[83] Various reasons have been proposed for this increase in serious fungal infections. It is generally assumed that prolonged granulocytopenia increases the likelihood of a serious or fatal fungal infection. The average duration of granulocytopenia has lengthened as chemotherapy regimens have become more aggressive. Chemotherapy may also cause more severe host defense abnormalities, resulting in more opportunistic fungal infections. Over the years, advances in antibiotic therapy have enabled more patients to survive serious bacterial infections, increasing the potential for subsequent fungal complications. Also, cancer patients generally survive longer now and are more likely to develop a fungal infection at some point during their illness.

Candida and *Aspergillus* spp. account for >90% of all fungal infections in patients with cancer.[71] *Mucor, Torulopsis,* and *Cryptococcus* spp. are also responsible for infections in these patients.[71] Histoplasmosis and coccidioidomycosis are occasionally seen outside endemic areas among cancer patients.[71] Particular fungi cause infections in patients with specific types of host defense abnormalities. *Candida, Aspergillus,* and *Mucor* spp. are the most common fungal pathogens identified in granulocytopenic patients, whereas *Cryptococcus* and *Candida* spp. are common in cancer patients with cellular immunity defects (Table 15-2).[7] *Candida* and *Torulopsis* spp. are the most common fungi in patients with disruptions of the integument of the skin or mucosal barriers.

Candidiasis usually begins as a superficial infection of the GI mucosa (especially the distal esophagus), but it often spreads via the bloodstream to cause invasive disease of one or more visceral organs (kidneys, lungs, spleen, or liver) in the presence of granulocytopenia. Disseminated candidiasis may be associated with multiple small skin nodules and painful myalgias. Disseminated candidiasis is often difficult to diagnosis despite its frequent multiorgan involvement. Positive blood cultures are seen in <50% of patients found during autopsy to have disseminated disease.[71]

Aspergillosis is most commonly seen in patients with leukemia or lymphoma and in patients receiving allogeneic bone marrow transplants, although it may also be seen in patients with solid tumors. The infection is usually confined to the lungs, the GI tract, and the central nervous system, but other organs may be involved. *Aspergillus* sp. have a tendency to invade and obstruct blood vessels in the lung, resulting in hemorrhagic pulmonary infarctions characterized by wedge-shaped pulmonary infiltrates and pleuritic chest pain. These organisms may also cause a necrotizing bronchopneumonia and cavitation of the lungs.[71] Diagnosing aspergillosis is even more difficult than diagnosing candidiasis; a biopsy of the infected tissue is necessary for a definitive diagnosis.

Mucormycosis occurs less commonly than either candidiasis or aspergillosis and most frequently occurs in patients with leukemias or lymphomas during periods of granulocytopenia.[84] The lungs are the most common site of *Mucor* sp. infection, resulting in pulmonary infarction and cavitation.[71] Dissemination to the brain, liver, kidneys, and spleen may also occur.[71] Rhino-orbital disease, associated with diabetes mellitus, may also occur in patients with malignancies. Diagnosis of mucormycosis is established by demonstrating the characteristic nonseptate hyphae on tissue biopsy.[71]

The most common clinical syndrome associated with cryptococcal infection in cancer patients is chronic or subacute meningitis, which may progress rapidly and result in severe neurological abnormalities if therapy is not instituted promptly. Cryptococcal disease in cancer patients may also include brain lesions, diffuse bilateral pneumonias, and dissemination to other visceral organs. Cryptococcal disease is most easily diagnosed by testing serum or cerebrospinal fluid to demonstrate the presence of cryptococcal antigens.

Amphotericin B, administered intravenously, is the drug of choice for treating invasive candidiasis, aspergillosis, mucormycosis, and cryptococcosis.[71] A favorable clinical outcome in each of these diseases depends on initiating therapy early in the course of the disease. Therapy should be initiated promptly whenever microbiological or histological evidence of invasive disease is demonstrated.

However, these infections are life threatening in patients with cancer and are frequently difficult to diagnose definitively. Therefore, it may be appropriate sometimes to initiate empiric therapy with amphotericin B, particularly in patients who have been granulocytopenic for a long time or received prolonged courses of broad-spectrum antibacterial therapy. Indications for empiric amphotericin B therapy include the following:

- persistent fever despite 4–7 days on broad-spectrum antibacterial therapy (especially when there is extensive mucosal damage or evidence of fungal colonization);
- symptoms suggestive of esophageal candidiasis;
- development of a new pulmonary infiltration while receiving broad-spectrum antibiotics; and
- development of a skin rash characteristic of candidiasis, with or without muscle pain and tenderness.

The optimal dose and duration of amphotericin B therapy are not clearly defined. Fortunately, resistance to this agent is rarely clinically significant. Total cumulative doses of 500–750 mg (e.g., 0.5 mg/kg per day for 14–20 days) for disseminated candidiasis and 1.5 grams (e.g., 1 mg/kg per day for 21 days) for aspergillosis have been suggested.[71] Clinical parameters, such as the resolution of fever and other evidence of infection, may be helpful indicators in deciding how long to continue therapy. Various schedules for escalating amphotericin B doses have been recommended and are outlined in Table 15-4.[85]

Chills and fever, which often accompany the infusion of amphotericin B, may be prevented or diminished by premedicating the patient with acetaminophen, antihistamines, or corticosteroids.[86] Also, IV meperidine has been reported to shorten the duration of chills when they occur.[87]

The desire for less toxicity and greater clinical efficacy has prompted the development of various lipid amphotericin

Table 15-4. Suggested Amphotericin B Regimens for Immunocompromised Cancer Patients

Regimen	Reference
Give 0.3 mg/kg over 2 hr on day 1, then 0.6 mg/kg over 2 hr daily	71
Give 1-mg test dose, followed by the remaining dose of 0.5 mg/kg within 8 hr on day 1, then 0.5 mg/kg daily	73
Give 1-mg test dose over 2–4 hr, then escalating doses at 6-hr intervals so that a total of 0.6–1.0 mg/kg is given over the first 24 hr, then 0.6–1.0 mg/kg over 4–6 hr daily	85

SOURCE: reference 85.

B formulations. These lipid formulations allow for equally efficacious doses of amphotericin with less nephrotoxicity. The three lipid formulations in clinical use are amphotericin B lipid complex (ABLC; Abelcet), amphotericin B colloidal dispersion (ABCD; Amphocil), and liposomal amphotericin B (AmBisome); all except AmBisome are commercially available. Clinical studies have been conducted evaluating AmBisome,[88–91] Abelcet,[92,93] and Amphocil[94] for the prophylaxis and treatment of invasive fungal infections in febrile granulocytopenic patients. Although all three lipid formulations have demonstrated efficacy comparable with conventional amphotericin, a greater therapeutic effect has not been shown. The major factor limiting the use of lipid formulations is their high cost. At most institutions, these products are restricted to the treatment of aspergillosis in patients refractory or intolerant to conventional amphotericin and for the treatment of fungal infections in patients with rapidly deteriorating renal function. Lipid amphotericin products are also used in allogeneic bone marrow transplant patients receiving multiple nephrotoxins (e.g., cyclosporine, tacrolimus, or aminoglycosides).

Although flucytosine (Ancobon) is effective against many *Candida* and *Cryptococcus* spp., these organisms may develop resistance to it, making it inappropriate as single-agent therapy.[71] Combined, amphotericin B and flucytosine have demonstrated synergistic activity against a variety of fungi in animal and in vitro studies.[95] This combination has shown superiority to amphotericin alone in treatment of cryptococcal meningitis.[95] Rifampin and amphotericin B have also shown synergistic effects against a variety of fungi.[96] The clinical effectiveness of these combinations has not been evaluated in controlled clinical trials.

Fluconazole (Diflucan) is a synthetic bistriazole antifungal agent with demonstrated effectiveness in treating candidiasis and cryptococcal meningitis. It has undergone extensive clinical evaluations for the treatment of oropharyngeal and esophageal candidiasis in both patients with cancer and those with AIDS. When oral fluconazole was compared to ketoconazole in cancer patients with oropharyngeal candidiasis, response rates were similar, but patients receiving ketoconazole appeared to relapse sooner.[97] As stated earlier, IV amphotericin B is the drug of choice for treating invasive candidiasis and cryptococcosis; therefore, fluconazole therapy for these fungal infections should be reserved for patients intolerant to amphotericin B.

Fluconazole is available in both oral and IV formulations and achieves good penetration in all body fluids, including cerebrospinal fluid.[98,99] Its half-life is approximately 30 hours, so only a single daily dose is required. Because it is eliminated almost completely by the kidneys, the dose must be adjusted in patients with renal dysfunction.[100] Fluconazole is well tolerated; the most common side effects are mild nausea, headache, diarrhea, skin rash, and abdominal pain. Several significant drug interactions between fluconazole and other drugs commonly used in cancer patients (e.g., phenytoin, cimetidine, oral contraceptives, rifampin, and warfarin) have been reported. Patients receiving such concomitant therapy require careful observation.[101]

Itraconazole (Sporanox) is a synthetic triazole antifungal agent indicated for the treatment of blastomycosis, histoplasmosis, and aspergillosis in both immunocompromised and immunocompetent patients. Overall, the use of itraconazole in cancer patients is limited. A small number of trials have studied its use in the treatment of invasive aspergillosis in patients with leukemia.[102–104] Although a favorable response was seen in these clinical trials, there was great variability among patients regarding site of infection, degree of granulocytopenia, and methods used to measure response, making it difficult to interpret itraconazole's efficacy. Itraconazole should be reserved as second-line therapy for patients infected with susceptible organisms who experience toxicity to amphotericin B therapy. Itraconazole, available only in an oral formulation, is known to have erratic absorption, so it may be wise to monitor itraconazole plasma concentrations to ensure adequate absorption and optimal efficacy of the drug. Clinical trials in granulocytopenic patients have suggested maintaining itraconazole plasma concentrations at >250 µg/L.[105,106] The usual dose of itraconazole is 200 mg twice daily, taken with food to enhance absorption. The most common adverse effects of itraconazole are nausea, vomiting, edema, skin rash, and headache.

Clinical experience using the systemic imidiazole derivatives, miconazole and ketoconazole, in managing invasive fungal infections in patients with cancer is very limited. The use of these agents has been superseded by the newer agents. The only exception is in treating *Petriellidium boydii* infections, for which miconazole is the agent of choice.

VIRAL INFECTIONS

The most common and troublesome pathogens in cancer patients with cellular immunity defects are the herpesviruses. The herpesviruses are a group of DNA viruses that include herpes simplex virus types 1 and 2, Epstein-Barr virus, varicella-zoster virus, and cytomegalovirus. These viruses share certain characteristics, including the ability to produce clinically apparent disease or become clinically latent. The clinical disease usually involves severe and prolonged skin infection, often characterized by extensive localized spread. These infections may, however, disseminate to other organs, sometimes resulting in death. In general, primary infections with herpesviruses cause more disease than reactivation of a latent virus, and the severity of the symptoms and extent of the disease correlate with the degree of immunosuppression.

Herpes Simplex Virus

Reactivation of herpes simplex virus (HSV) is common in cancer patients and normal individuals. However, these infections are often more prolonged and more severe in immunosuppressed patients. HSV reactivation is usually characterized by large, painful skin and mucous membrane lesions that eventually ulcerate. These lesions may provide a portal of entry for bacteria and fungi that may cause either systemic or local superinfections. Patients with esophageal damage after radiation, chemotherapy, or intubation may be prone to herpetic esophagitis. The lungs (and, less commonly, other organs) may become involved also.

Cutaneous HSV lesions may be cosmetically distressing and quite painful to the patient; oral and esophageal lesions may interfere with eating. HSV also contributes to the mucositis that occurs with some chemotherapy regimens. Perirectal and genital lesions may alter bowel and bladder habits. It may be necessary to delay the next course of chemotherapy when lesions are very severe.

Acyclovir is effective (250 mg/m^2 IV every 8 hours) for mucocutaneous HSV[107,108] and is probably effective for disseminated disease. However, HSV dissemination is rare, and conducting a controlled trial with so few patients is difficult. Bone marrow transplant patients are commonly given IV acyclovir as prophylaxis if they are HSV seropositive. Oral acyclovir may be useful for mucocutaneous disease.[109]

Varicella-Zoster Virus

Varicella-zoster virus can reactivate and cause herpes zoster (HZ or shingles) in any individual who has had varicella (chickenpox). The risk of reactivation is much higher in patients with cancer—especially those with Hodgkin's disease and non-Hodgkin's lymphomas—and may be related to the extent and type of cancer, the type of chemotherapy, or prior radiation therapy.

HZ lesions in patients with cancer are generally more extensive, deeper, and more necrotizing than in normal hosts. Cutaneous dissemination distant from the primary lesions occurs in 15–50% of patients; about 10% of them develop other, possibly life-threatening organ involvement. Neurological complications, postherpetic neuralgias, and bacterial superinfections may also develop.

Although HZ is generally a self-limited disease, IV acyclovir (500 mg/m^2 every 8 hours for 7 days) appears to be effective in reducing progression and complications of acute HZ.[110] Famciclovir (Famvir), a prodrug of penciclovir, and valacyclovir (Valtrex), the L-valyl prodrug of acyclovir, are indicated for the treatment of HZ in immunocompetent adults. There are currently no published data on the efficacy of valacyclovir for the prevention or treatment of HZ or herpes simplex in the febrile granulocytopenic patient. A small pilot study by Tucker and colleagues[111] showed famciclovir to be very effective in the treatment of herpes labialis in immunocompromised cancer patients.

Cytomegalovirus

Cytomegalovirus (CMV) infections can arise from reactivation of an endogenous virus or after an infusion of CMV-infected blood products. Many patients with CMV are asymptomatic. However, CMV may produce severe interstitial pneumonitis, retinitis, and liver disease in the immunocompromised patient. In fact, interstitial pneumonia due to CMV is a frequent and often fatal complication after allogeneic bone marrow transplantation. CMV may also cause a gastroenteritis with severe diarrhea and GI bleeding in immunocompromised patients. In addition, CMV infection may enhance the patient's susceptibility to bacterial and fungal infections.

Ganciclovir has demonstrated clinical benefit in patients with symptomatic CMV infections.[112,113] Early clinical studies suggest that ganciclovir is more effective for treating viremia, hepatitis, retinitis, and colitis than for treating pneumonia. Improved response and survival have been reported when ganciclovir is combined with high-dose IV immune globulin containing CMV antibodies.[114] Prophylactic high-dose IV immune globulin has also decreased the incidence and severity of CMV pneumonia after bone marrow transplantation.[115]

Clinical trials are evaluating the prophylactic use of valacyclovir for the suppression of CMV infection in bone marrow transplant patients. Oral valacyclovir, when compared with oral acyclovir, has the advantage of better absorption. According to data from Glaxo Wellcome, oral valacyclovir doses of 1–2 g four times a day has bioequivalence equal to acyclovir 5–10 mg/kg IV every 8 hours.

Epstein-Barr Virus

Epstein-Barr virus causes infectious mononucleosis, and reactivation may occur in patients receiving treatment for cancer. Symptoms are generally mild. It has also been implicated in the pathogenesis of Burkitt's lymphoma and nasopharyngeal carcinoma.

PREVENTING INFECTION

Because of the considerable morbidity associated with infections in patients with cancer, a great deal of emphasis must be placed on preventing infection, particularly in patients who are rendered granulocytopenic for >10 days. The factors that predispose these high-risk patients to serious infections lead logically to the techniques that are most commonly employed in infection prevention:

- reducing patient exposure to nosocomial organisms;
- suppressing organisms that colonize at or near common sites of infection (especially the GI tract);
- avoiding invasive procedures; and
- bolstering host defense mechanisms.

Preventing infection is critically important in the overall management of patients with cancer; it should be considered the responsibility of all who care for these patients to understand and reinforce these principles.

Reducing Patient Exposure to Nosocomial Organisms

Hospitalized patients may become colonized with microbial organisms through a number of sources. Sources of potential contamination include contact with staff, visitors, or other patients, and contaminated medical instruments, blood products, or parenteral medications.

Some very simple procedures may be used to decrease patients' exposure to new and potentially pathogenic organisms. All personnel and patients should be carefully trained in a program of personal hygiene that includes careful and frequent hand washing with a germicidal soap. An effective approach is to teach patients to refuse contact with people who have not washed their hands. Patients should also be instructed to bathe and shampoo daily with germicidal soap. Simple housekeeping procedures, such as daily disinfection of floors, sinks, and horizontal surfaces in patient rooms, may also help reduce patients' exposure to microorganisms.

Food is a common source of pathogenic organisms; a diet of low microbial content (i.e., a cooked-food diet) may help the patient reduce this acquisition. Uncooked fruits and vegetables are frequently contaminated with *Pseudomonas aeruginosa*, *Klebsiella pneumoniae*, and *Escherichia coli*, whereas meats, vegetables, and desserts prepared by cooking are generally acceptable. The water supply may also be contaminated with microorganisms in some institutions. Therefore, water supplies should be evaluated periodically. Removing a faucet aerator often reduces bacterial contamination.

In the past, simple reverse or protective isolation techniques that included placing the patient in a private room and requiring all staff and visitors to wear masks, gowns, and gloves when entering the room were advocated in caring for profoundly granulocytopenic patients. However, these practices appear to offer no significant benefit in preventing infection by new organisms and reducing the incidence of subsequent infections.

Total protected environments have been developed to prevent the acquisition of exogenous organisms while the patient's endogenous flora are eradicated. A total protected environment consists of a laminar airflow room with high-efficiency particulate air (HEPA) filters along one wall. Air entering the room is pumped through the filters at uniform velocity, producing a laminar airflow similar to that in laminar airflow cabinets used in sterile product preparation areas. The room is rendered virtually sterile when surfaces are disinfected, and all objects entering the room are sterilized, including medical equipment and personal objects. Total protected environments are recommended for patients who are at high risk of aspergillosis,[116,117] such as allogeneic bone marrow transplant patients. Uncomplicated autologous bone marrow transplant patients can be safely treated in simple isolated rooms with strict hand washing as the only protective measure.[117] Immunocompromised patients being treated in an environment undergoing construction or where there is a known outbreak of aspergillosis should also be confined to a total protected environment.

Suppressing Organisms

Many organisms responsible for serious infections in granulocytopenic cancer patients are presumed to enter the body through the GI tract. These are the organisms that constitute the normal flora of the GI tract. However, in many cases they may be more resistant, hospital-acquired strains. Therefore, antimicrobial regimens have been developed to reduce the endogenous flora and, it is hoped, prevent infection.

The antimicrobial prophylaxis strategy used to decrease the incidence of infections in granulocytopenic patients is called selective suppression or selective decontamination (Table 15-5).[82,118-121] In the 1960s, van der Waaij and colleagues[122] recognized that normal anaerobic flora in the GI tract tend to prevent colonization by other organisms. They called this mechanism colonization resistance. In animals with normal flora, they found a resistance to colonization when large inoculums of organisms were given orally. However, colonization in germ-free animals (in which both aerobic and anaerobic flora had been eradicated) could be established with a relatively small inoculum of organisms. Animals in which only the aerobic flora were suppressed (the anaerobic flora were preserved) could resist colonization even when large inoculums of aerobic flora were given orally.

The concept of colonization resistance has been applied to infection prevention strategies in granulocytopenic patients. It might be possible to selectively decontaminate the patient of the organisms most likely to cause infection rather than the historical attempt to suppress all of the GI tract flora with broad-spectrum antibiotic regimens. Keep in mind that most bacterial infections in the granulocytopenic patient are caused by aerobic flora. An antibiotic should be selected that suppresses only these organisms. Oral antibiotics that fulfill these criteria include trimethoprim–sulfamethoxazole (Bactrim or Septra), nalidixic acid (NegGram), ciprofloxacin (Cipro), norfloxacin (Noroxin), ofloxacin (Floxin), and rifampin (Rifadin) (Table 15-5). These agents are effective against a wide spectrum of enterobacters, and ofloxacin, norfloxacin, and ciprofloxacin have the added advantage of having activity against *Pseudomonas aeruginosa*.

Trimethoprim–sulfamethoxazole (TMP–SMZ) has currently been replaced by the fluoroquinolones as the most widely used antibiotic in this setting. Overall, it appears that TMP-SMZ may offer some benefit in reducing the incidence of fever and infections in granulocytopenic patients, although reports of efficacy have been conflicting. However, disadvantages associated with TMP-SMZ have included development of resistance, prolongation of granulocytopenia, and skin rashes. Nalidixic acid has also been used to achieve selective decontamination. However, in a randomized trial, it was less effective than TMP-SMZ and was also associated with the emergence of resistant organisms.[118] More recently, norfloxacin

Table 15-5. Prophylactic Oral Antibiotic Regimens Used in Granulocytopenic Cancer Patients

Selective Decontamination	Reference
Trimethoprim–sulfamethoxazole 160 mg/800 mg q8hr	118
Naladixic acid 2 g q6hr	118
Norfloxacin 400 mg q12hr	119
Ciprofloxacin 500 mg q12hr	120
Ofloxacin 400 mg q12hr	121
Rifampin 300 mg q12hr	82

and ofloxacin have been evaluated in granulocytopenic patients. The results of several trials have indicated that both ofloxacin and norfloxacin treatment were well tolerated and effective in preventing serious infections by gram-negative bacilli.[119,121]

Selective suppression using TMP–SMZ or one of the fluoroquinolones should be reserved for patients expected to be profoundly granulocytopenic for >10 days (remember that the incidence of serious infections increases as the duration of granulocytopenia increases). Patients receiving this type of prophylaxis should have cultures taken regularly to monitor for the emergence of resistant organisms.

Antifungal prophylaxis with topical agents, such as nystatin suspension, clotrimazole troches (Mycelex), and oral solutions of amphotericin B, are not the most effective means of preventing fungal infections. Although topical antifungal agents decrease the fungal burden in the GI tract, nystatin and oral solutions of amphotericin B have limited efficacy in this regard. On the other hand, clotrimazole troches are effective in decreasing oropharyngeal candidiasis. All of these topical antifungal agents have failed to show a benefit in preventing candidemia. Another drawback is poor patient compliance due to the taste of these agents.

A second and more effective means of preventing fungal infections is the use of fluconazole. Fluconazole, which can achieve high concentrations in both the GI tract and blood, is better tolerated and more effective than topical agents and oral solutions of amphotericin B in preventing oropharyngeal candidiasis in granulocytopenic patients.[123,124] Prevention of candidemia with fluconazole has been best demonstrated in the bone marrow transplant population. Fluconazole 400 mg daily has been shown to decrease superficial and hematological candidiasis and mortality in this population.[125,126] Both fluconazole 400 mg IV daily and low-dose amphotericin B 0.5 mg/kg IV three times weekly are equally effective in preventing candidiasis in adult leukemia and bone marrow transplant patients.[127,128] Patients receiving fluconazole experienced fewer adverse effects than did those receiving low-dose amphotericin. Lower doses of fluconazole (50–200 mg/day) have also proved effective in preventing oropharyngeal candidiasis in granulocytopenic patients. Comparative trials of oral nystatin, amphotericin, and clotrimazole in leukemia and bone marrow transplant patients have shown efficacy similar to or better than lower oral doses of fluconazole.[129–132]

Avoiding Invasive Procedures

Any disruption of the normal protective barrier created by the skin or mucous membranes (e.g., venipuncture sites, mucositis, or decubitus ulcers) is a potential portal of entry for pathogenic organisms that may cause serious local infections or bacteremias. Therefore, invasive and traumatic procedures should be avoided whenever possible. Peripheral IV catheters should be avoided. Small-gauge butterfly needles, changed at least every 48 hours, should be used to administer IV medications and blood products. Permanent access devices, such as the Hickman and Broviac catheters or mediports, are acceptable alternatives when they are inserted under proper, sterile conditions and are properly cared for. All IV tubing, bottles, and dressings should be changed daily. Urinary catheters should be avoided in granulocytopenic patients unless they are necessary for managing obstruction or if the patient is severely ill (e.g., in septic shock).

Firm pressure should be applied to reduce the chance of blood extravasation and subsequent infection after venipuncture, fingersticks, and bone marrow aspirations. Patients should also be advised to use only electric razors to reduce the chance of skin cuts and irritation.

Bolstering Host Defense Mechanisms

The most important approach is, of course, to reverse the patient's underlying condition so that granulocytopenia and immunosuppression will be avoided or will resolve as quickly as possible. Hematopoietic growth factors or colony-stimulating factors (CSFs), such as granulocyte CSF (G-CSF) and granulocyte-macrophage CSF (GM-CSF), have decreased the period of neutropenia following aggressive chemotherapy.[133] Experience with these factors has resulted in a significant decline in the incidence and severity of infections in patients receiving chemotherapy.[133] To date, clinical trials supporting the use of CSFs in febrile granulocytopenic patients do not show a clear-cut benefit in all patients. However, the use of CSFs may be appropriate in febrile granulocytopenic patients with existing complications, such as sepsis or pneumonia. It has been recommended that the use of CSFs in granulocytopenic patients who are already febrile be reserved for those patients with a persistent (>7–10 days) ANC of <100, severe gram-negative or streptococcal bacteremia, or subsequent infection. Adult acute leukemia and allogeneic bone marrow transplant patients tend to be the populations at highest risk for these complications and may benefit the most from CSFs. A recent study looked at the use of G-CSF in febrile granulocytopenic patients with cancer.[134] Greatest efficacy was seen in patients with documented infections and an ANC of <100. Despite the decrease in the number of days of granulocytopenia, the duration of antibiotic use and length of hospital stay were not reduced.

The most common situations in which CSFs may be used include:

- when the expected incidence of febrile granulocytopenia from chemotherapy is high,
- when trying to avoid chemotherapy dose reduction in patients with prior documented febrile granulocytopenia who have experienced infectious complications with prior chemotherapy, and
- when high-dose chemotherapy is followed by bone marrow or peripheral blood cell support.[135]

The usual adult dose of G-CSF (filgrastim) is 5 µg/kg per day and 250 µg/m² per day for GM-CSF (sargramostim). Both agents can be given subcutaneously or intravenously. It is general practice to start growth factors at least 24 hours after the completion of chemotherapy and continue until the ANC reaches 10,000/mm³.[135,136] It has been proposed that immunomodulators such as Bacillus Calmette-Guérin vaccine and lithium may accelerate granulocyte recovery, but these strategies have not proved helpful.

Overall, prophylactic granulocyte transfusions have not been beneficial in preventing infection either, although the approach seems logical. Unfortunately, no amount of granulocytes collected for transfusion by means of current technology can approach the number of granulocytes produced by normal bone marrow. Furthermore, granulocytes are probably not as functionally effective after collection and transfusion as they are in their native host. Prophylactic granulocyte transfusions have reduced the incidence of bacteremias in some controlled trials,[137–139] but they have also been associated with severe transfusion-related reactions, CMV infections, and increased incidence of pneumonias in some patients.[137,140]

Immunocompromised patients, especially bone marrow transplant, leukemia, and lymphoma patients, have an increased risk of influenza, streptococcal pneumonia, and *Haemophilus influenzae* type b (HIB) diseases. The efficacy of active immunization with influenza, pneumococcal, and HIB vaccines is very controversial, because these patients may be unable to mount a sufficient antibody response.[141] Despite the controversy, it is recommended that immunocompromised patients receive yearly immunization with influenza vaccine. Immunization with 23-valent pneumococcal vaccine and HIB conjugate vaccine is recommended 1–2 weeks before chemotherapy or >3 months after chemotherapy.[142] Bone marrow transplant patients should receive these same vaccines at 12 and 24 months following transplant.[143] There are no existing data on the efficacy of influenza vaccine in bone marrow transplant patients.

SUMMARY

Infections among patients with cancer are both frequent and serious. Granulocytopenia is considered the most significant factor in the development of life-threatening infections, but other risk factors include damage to the skin and mucosal linings. Susceptibility to infections may result from the spread of the malignancy or from chemotherapy or radiation therapy.

The mortality rate is high among granulocytopenic patients who experience infections. Single-agent therapy is generally preferred over combination antimicrobial therapy; quick initiation of therapy is the single most important factor for patient survival. Other factors influencing favorable outcomes are bone marrow regeneration, using more than one drug that is effective against the infecting organism, and choosing synergistic drugs. Some newer single-agent therapies appear to be as effective as combination therapy. Disagreement continues to exist about how long therapy should continue.

Fungal infections are becoming increasingly frequent and fatal for patients with cancer; *Candida* and *Aspergillus* spp. account for >90% of cases. Because these fungi are difficult to diagnose, empiric therapy may be appropriate for individuals who have been granulocytopenic for a long time.

Patients with cancer may also experience infection from one of the herpesviruses, which may be clinically apparent or latent. These types of infections, which are most common among patients with cellular immunity defects, include herpes simplex viruses types 1 and 2, Epstein-Barr virus, varicella-zoster virus, and cytomegalovirus. Some herpesviruses result in extremely painful lesions, which can provide a portal of entry for bacteria and fungi.

The first line of defense against infection among cancer patients is prevention. Germicidal soaps, shampoos, and cleansers reduce the number of nosocomial organisms that come into contact with the cancer patient. Partial or total decontamination of the gastrointestinal tract in a total protected environment may also decrease incidence of infection. Whenever possible, avoid any disruption of the skin and mucous membranes that would permit entry of pathogenic organisms. Finally, colony-stimulating factors reduce the length of neutropenia after chemotherapy.

REFERENCES

1. Schimpff SC. Infections in the compromised host: an overview. In: Mandell GL, Douglas RJ Jr., Bennett JE, editors. *Principles and Practice of Infectious Diseases*. 3rd ed. New York: Churchill Livingstone; 1990. p. 2258–65.
2. Bodey GP, Buckley M, Sathe YS, et al. Qualitative relationships between circulating leukocytes and infection in patients with acute leukemia. *Ann Intern Med* 1966;64:328–40.
3. Klastersky J. Concept of empiric therapy with antibiotic combinations: indications and limits. *Am J Med* 1986;80(Suppl 5C):2–12.
4. Wade JC, Schimpff SC, Newman KA, et al. Staphylococcus epidermidis: an increasing cause of infection in patients with granulocytopenia. *Ann Intern Med* 1982;97:507–8.
5. Schimpff SC, Young VM, Greene WH, et al. Origin of infection in acute nonlymphocytic leukemia. *Ann Intern Med* 1972;77:707–14.
6. Beachey EH. Bacterial adherence: adhesin-receptor interactions mediating the attachment of bacteria to mucosal surfaces. *J Infect Dis* 1981;143:325–45.
7. Freifeld AG, Walsh TJ, Pizzo PA. Infections in the cancer patient. In: DeVita VT, Hellman S, Rosenberg SA, editors. *Cancer: Principles and Practice of Oncology*. 5th ed. Philadelphia, PA: JB Lippincott; 1997. p. 2659–704.
8. Rubin M, Hathorn JW, Pizzo PA. Controversies in the management of febrile neutropenic cancer patients. *Cancer Invest* 1988;6:167–84.
9. Del Favero A, Bucaneve G, Menichetti F. Empiric monotherapy in neutropenia: a realistic goal? *Scand J Infect Dis* 1995(Suppl 96):34–7.
10. Eggimann P, Glauser M, Aoun M, et al. Cefepime monotherapy for the empirical treatment of fever in granulocytopenic cancer patients. *J Antimicrob Chemother* 1993;32(Suppl B):151–63.
11. Ramphal R, Gucalp R, Rotstein C, et al. Clinical experience with single agent and combination regimens in the management of infection in the febrile neutropenic patients. *Am J Med* 1996;100(Suppl 6A):83s–89s.
12. Cometta A, Calandra T, Gaya H, et al. Monotherapy with meropenem versus combination therapy with ceftazidime plus amikacin as empiric therapy for fever in granulocytopenic patients with cancer. *Antimicrob Agents Chemother* 1996;40:1108–15.
13. [Anonymous]. Equivalent efficacies of meropenem and ceftazidime as empirical monotherapy of febrile neutropenic patients. The meropenem study group of Leuven, London and Nijmegen. *J Antimicrob Chemother* 1995;36:185–200.
14. Schimpff SC. Therapy of infection in patients with granulocytopenia. *Med Clin North Am* 1977;61:1101–18.
15. Lau WK, Young LS, Black RE, et al. Comparative efficacy and toxicity of amikacin/carbenicillin versus gentamicin/carbenicillin in leukopenic patients: a randomized trial. *Am J Med* 1977;62:959–66.
16. European Organization for Research and Treatment of Cancer [EORTC]. Three antibiotic regimens in the treatment of infection in febrile granulocytopenic patients with cancer. *J Infect Dis* 1978;137:14–29.
17. Stuart RK, Braine HG, Lietman PS, et al. Carbenicillin-trimethoprim/sulfamethoxazole versus carbenicillin-gentamicin as empiric therapy of infection in granulocytopenic patients: a prospective, randomized, double-blind study. *Am J Med* 1980;68:876–85.
18. Winston DJ, Ho WG, Young LS, et al. Piperacillin plus amikacin therapy versus carbenicillin plus amikacin therapy in febrile, granulocytopenic patients. *Arch Intern Med* 1982;142:1663–7.
19. Love LJ, Schimpff SC, Hahn DM, et al. Randomized trial of empiric antibiotic therapy with ticarcillin in combination with gentamicin, amikacin, or netilmicin in febrile patients with granulocytopenia and cancer. *Am J Med* 1979;66:603–10.
20. Pickard W, Durack D, Gallis H. A randomized trial of moxalactam versus tobramycin plus ticarcillin in 50 febrile neutropenic patients [abstract]. Proceedings of the 22nd Interscience Conference on Antimicrobial Agents and Chemotherapy. Miami Beach, FL; 1982.

21. Feld R, Louie TJ, Mandell L, et al. A multicenter comparative trial of tobramycin and ticarcillin vs moxalactam and ticarcillin in febrile neutropenic patients. *Arch Intern Med* 1985;145:1083–8.
22. Lawson RD, Gentry LO, Bodey GP, et al. A randomized study of tobramycin plus ticarcillin, tobramycin plus cephalothin and ticarcillin, or tobramycin plus mezlocillin in the treatment of infection in neutropenic patients with malignancies. *Am J Med Sci* 1984;287:16–23.
23. Wade JC, Schimpff SC, Newman KA, et al. Piperacillin or ticarcillin plus amikacin: a double-blind prospective comparison of empiric antibiotic therapy for febrile granulocytopenic cancer patients. *Am J Med* 1981;71:983–90.
24. Klastersky J, Glauser MP, Schimpff SC, et al. Prospective randomized comparison of three antibiotic regimens for empirical therapy of suspected bacteremic infection in febrile granulocytopenic patients. *Antimicrob Agents Chemother* 1986;29:263–70.
25. Chan CC, Oppenheim BA, Anderson H, et al. Randomized trial comparing ciprofloxacin plus netilmicin versus piperacillin plus netilmicin for empiric treatment of fever of neutropenic patients. *Antimicrob Agents Chemother* 1989;33:87–91.
26. Kelsey SM, Weinhardt B, Collins PW, et al. Teicoplanin plus ciprofloxacin versus gentamicin plus piperacillin in the treatment of febrile neutropenic patients. *Eur J Clin Microbiol Infect Dis* 1992;11:509–14.
27. Kelsey SM, Shaw E, Newland AC. Aztreonam plus vancomycin versus gentamicin plus piperacillin as empirical therapy for the treatment of fever in neutropenic patients: a randomised controlled study. *J Chemother* 1992;4:107–13.
28. Philpott-Howard JN, Barker KF, Wade JJ, et al. Randomized multicentre study of ciprofloxacin and azlocillin versus gentamicin and azlocillin in the treatment of febrile neutropenic patients. *J Antimicrob Chemother* 1990;26(Suppl F):89–99.
29. Johnson PR, Liu Yin JA, Tooth JA. A randomized trial of high-dose ciprofloxacin versus azlocillin and netilmicin in the empirical therapy of febrile neutropenic patients. *J Antimicrob Chemother* 1992;30:203–14.
30. Kelsey SM, Weinhardt B, Pocock CE, et al. Piperacillin/tazobactam plus gentamicin as empirical therapy for febrile neutropenic patients with hematological malignancy. *J Chemother* 1992;4:281–5.
31. Marie JP, Vekhoff A, Cony-Makhoul P, et al. A randomized trial of piperacillin-tazobactam plus amikacin versus ceftazidime plus amikacin in 222 febrile neutropenic patients [abstract]. Proceedings of the 33rd Interscience Conference on Antimicrobial Agents and Chemotherapy, 1993.
32. Gaya H. Piperacillin/tazobactam plus amikacin versus ceftazidime plus amikacin as empirical therapy for fever in patients with granulocytopenia: a prospective, randomized, multicenter study (efficacy, safety, and tolerance) [abstract]. Proceedings of the 33rd Interscience Conference on Antimicrobial Agents and Chemotherapy, 1993.
33. Micozzi A, Nucci M, Venditti M, et al. Piperacillin/tazobactam/amikacin versus piperacillin/amikacin/teicoplanin in the empirical treatment of neutropenic patients. *Eur J Clin Microbiol Infect Dis* 1993;12:1–8.
34. Shenep JL, Hughes WT, Roberson PK, et al. Vancomycin, ticarcillin, and amikacin compared with ticarcillin-clavulanate and amikacin in the empirical treatment of febrile, neutropenic children with cancer. *N Engl J Med* 1988;319:1053–8.
35. Klastersky J. New antibacterial agents: the role of new penicillins and cephalosporins in the management of infection in granulocytopenic patients. *Clin Haematol* 1984;587–8.
36. Joshi J, Ruxer R, Newman K, et al. Ceftazidime plus piperacillin vs. ceftazidime with/without tobramycin for empiric therapy in febrile, granulocytopenic cancer patients [abstract]. Proceedings of the 23rd Interscience Conference on Antimicrobial Agents and Chemotherapy. Miami, FL; 1983.
37. Fainstein V, Bodey GP, Elting L, et al. A randomized study of ceftazidime compared to ceftazidime and tobramycin for the treatment of infections in cancer patients. *J Antimicrob Chemother* 1983;12(Suppl A):101–10.
38. DeJongh CA, Wade JC, Schimpff SC, et al. Empiric antibiotic therapy for suspected infection in granulocytopenic cancer patients: a comparison between the combination of moxalactam plus amikacin and ticarcillin plus amikacin. *Am J Med* 1982;73:89–96.
39. Winston DJ, Barnes RC, Ho WG, et al. Moxalactam plus piperacillin versus moxalactam plus amikacin in febrile, granulocytopenic patients. *Am J Med* 1984;77:442–50.
40. DeJongh CA, Joshi JH, Thompson BW, et al. A double beta lactam combination versus an aminoglycoside-containing regimen as empiric antibiotic therapy for febrile granulocytopenic cancer patients. *Am J Med* 1986;80(Suppl 5C):96–111.
41. Flaherty JP, Waitley D, Edlin B, et al. Multicenter randomized trial of ciprofloxacin plus azlocillin versus ceftazidime plus amikacin for empiric treatment of febrile neutropenic patients. *Am J Med* 1989;87(Suppl 5A):278S–82S.
42. Jones P, Rolston K, Fainstein V, et al. Aztreonam plus vancomycin (plus amikacin) vs. moxalactam plus ticarcillin for the empiric treatment of febrile episodes in neutropenic cancer patients. *Rev Infect Dis* 1985;7(Suppl 4):S741–6.
43. Kelsey SM, Wood ME, Shaw E, et al. Intravenous ciprofloxacin as empirical treatment of febrile neutropenic patients. *Am J Med* 1989;87(Suppl 5A):274S–7S.
44. Samuelsson J, Nilsson PG, Wahlin A, et al. A pilot study of piperacillin and ciprofloxacin as initial therapy for fever in severely neutropenic leukemia patients. *Scand J Infect Dis* 1992;24:467–75.
45. Wade JC, Bustamante C, Devlin A, et al. Imipenem vs. amikacin plus piperacillin, empiric therapy for febrile, neutropenic patients: a double blind trial [abstract]. Proceedings of the 27th Interscience Conference on Antimicrobial Agents and Chemotherapy. Los Angeles, CA; 1987.
46. Bodey GP, Alvarez ME, Jones PG, et al. Imipenem-cilastatin as initial therapy for febrile cancer patients. *Antimicrob Agents Chemother* 1986;30:211–4.
47. Freifeld AG, Walsh T, Marshall D, et al. Monotherapy for fever and neutropenia in cancer patients: a randomized comparison of ceftazidime versus imipenem. *J Clin Oncol* 1995;13:165–76.
48. Pizzo PA, Hathorn JW, Hiemenz J, et al. A randomized trial comparing ceftazidime alone with combination antibiotic therapy in cancer patients with fever and neutropenia. *N Engl J Med* 1986;315:552–8.
49. Engervall P, Gunther G, Ljungman P, et al. Trimethoprim-sulfamethoxazole plus amikacin versus ceftazidime monotherapy as empirical treatment in patients with neutropenia and fever. *Scand J Infect Dis* 1996;28:297–303.

50. Sanders JW, Powe NR, Moore RD. Ceftazidime monotherapy for empiric treatment of febrile neutropenic patients: a metaanalysis. *J Infect Dis* 1991;164:907–16.
51. Lim SH, Smith MP, Goldstone AH, et al. A randomized prospective study of ceftazidime and ciprofloxacin with or without teicoplanin as an empiric antibiotic regimen for febrile neutropenic patients. *Brit J Haematol* 1990;76(Suppl 2):41–4.
52. Bayston KF, Want S, Cohen J. A prospective, randomized comparison of ceftazidime and ciprofloxacin as initial empiric therapy in neutropenic patients with fever. *Am J Med* 1989;87(Suppl 5A):269S–73S.
53. Meunier F, Zinner SH, Gaya H, et al. Prospective randomized evaluation of ciprofloxacin versus piperacillin plus amikacin for empiric antibiotic therapy of febrile granulocytopenic cancer patients with lymphomas and solid tumors. *Antimicrob Agents Chemother* 1991;35:873–8.
54. Johnson PR, Yin JA, Tooth JA. High dose intravenous ciprofloxacin in febrile neutropenic patients. *J Antimicrob Chemother* 1990;26(Suppl F):101–7.
55. Keating MJ, Lawson R, Grose W, et al. Combination therapy with ticarcillin and sulfamethoxazole-trimethoprim for infections in patients with cancer. *Arch Intern Med* 1981;141:926–30.
56. Raad II, Whimbey EE, Rolston KV, et al. A comparison of aztreonam plus vancomycin and imipenem plus vancomycin as initial therapy for febrile neutropenic cancer patients. *Cancer* 1996;77:1386–94.
57. Bodey GP, Fainstein V, Elting LS, et al. Beta-lactam regimens for the febrile neutropenic patient. *Cancer* 1990;65:9–16.
58. Karp JE, Dick JD, Angelopulos C, et al. Empiric use of vancomycin during prolonged treatment-induced granulocytopenia: randomized, double-blind, place-controlled clinical trial in patients with acute leukemia. *Am J Med* 1986;81:237–42.
59. Rubin M, Hathorn JW, Marshall D, et al. Gram-positive infections and the use of vancomycin in 550 episodes of fever and neutropenia. *Ann Intern Med* 1988;108:30–5.
60. Hansen M, Achen F, Carstensen C, et al. Once versus thrice daily dosing of netilmicin in febrile immunocompromised patients: a randomized, controlled study of efficacy and safety. *J Drug Dev* 1988;1(Suppl 3):119–24.
61. Rozdzinski E, Kern WV, Reichle T, et al. Once-daily versus twice-daily dosing of netilmicin in combination with beta-lactam antibiotics as empirical therapy for febrile neutropenic patients. *J Antimicrob Chemother* 1993;31:585–98.
62. International Antimicrobial Therapy Cooperative Group of the European Organization for Research and Treatment of Cancer [EORTC]. Efficacy and toxicity of single daily doses of amikacin and ceftriaxone versus multiple daily doses of amikacin and ceftazidime for infection in patients with cancer and granulocytopenia. *Ann Intern Med* 1993;119:584–93.
63. Montecalvo MA, Horowitz H, Gedris C, et al. Outbreak of vancomycin-, ampicillin-, and aminoglycoside-resistant enterococcus faecium bacteremia in an adult oncology unit. *Antimicrob Agents Chemother* 1994;38:1363–7.
64. Edmond MB, Ober JF, Weinbaum DL, et al. Vancomycin-resistant enterococcus faecium bacteremia: risk factors for infection. *Clin Infect Dis* 1995;20:1126–33.
65. [Anonymous]. Recommendations for preventing the spread of vancomycin resistance: recommendations of the Hospital Infection Control Practices Advisory Committee [HICPAC]. *MMWR* 1995;44(RR-12):1–13.
66. Naumovski L, Quinn JP, Miyashiro D, et al. Outbreak of ceftazidime resistance due to a novel extended-spectrum beta-lactamase in isolates from cancer patients. *Antimicrob Agents Chemother* 1992;36:1991–6.
67. DeJongh CA, Newman KA, Moody MR, et al. Antibiotic synergism and response in gram-negative bacteremias among granulocytopenia cancer patients [abstract]. Proceedings of the 22nd Interscience Conference on Antimicrobial Agents and Chemotherapy. Miami Beach, FL; 1982.
68. Love LJ, Schimpff SC, Schiffer CA, et al. Improved prognosis for granulocytopenic patients with gram-negative bacteremia. *Am J Med* 1980;68:643–8.
69. Klastersky J, Cappel R, Daneau D. Clinical significance of in vitro synergism between antibiotics in gram-negative infections. *Antimicrob Agents Chemother* 1972;2:470–5.
70. Klastersky J, Meunier-Carpentier F, Prevost JM. Significance of antimicrobial synergism for the outcome of gram-negative sepsis. *Am J Med Sci* 1977;273:157–67.
71. Joshi JH, Schimpff SC. Therapy of infection in granulocytopenic patients with cancer. *Clin Oncol* 1983;2:611–34.
72. Pizzo P, Thaler M, Hiemenz J, et al. Duration of empiric antibiotic therapy in granulocytopenic patients with cancer. *Am J Med* 1979;67:194–200.
73. Pizzo PA, Robichaud KJ, Gill FA, et al. Empiric antibiotic and antifungal therapy for cancer patients with prolonged fever and granulocytopenia. *Am J Med* 1982;72:101–11.
74. Joshi JH, Schimpff SC, Tenney JH, et al. Can antibacterial therapy be discontinued in persistently febrile granulocytopenic cancer patients? *Am J Med* 1984;76:450–7.
75. Buchanan GR. Approach to treatment of the febrile cancer patient with low-risk neutropenia. *Hemat Oncol Clin North Am* 1993;7:919–35.
76. Talcott JA, Whalen A, Clark J, et al. Home antibiotic therapy for low-risk cancer patients with fever and neutropenia: a pilot study of 30 patients based on a validated prediction rule. *J Clin Oncol* 1994;12:107–14.
77. Rolston K, Rubenstein E, Frisbee-Hume S, et al. Outpatient treatment of febrile episodes in low-risk neutropenic cancer patients [abstract]. *Proc Am Soc Clin Oncol* 1993;12:436.
78. Malik IA, Khan WA, Karim M, et al. Feasibility of outpatient management of fever in cancer patients with low-risk neutropenia: results of a prospective randomized trial. *Am J Med* 1995;98:224–31.
79. Rubenstein EB, Rolston K, Benjamin RS, et al. Outpatient treatment of febrile episodes in low-risk neutropenic patients with cancer. *Cancer* 1993;71:3640–6.
80. Malik IA, Khan WA, Aziz Z, et al. Self-administered antibiotic therapy for chemotherapy-induced, low-risk febrile neutropenia in patients with nonhematologic neoplasms. *Clin Infect Dis* 1994;19:522–7.
81. Gilbert C, Meisenberg B, Vredenburgh J, et al. Sequential prophylactic oral and empiric once-daily parenteral antibiotics for neutropenia and fever after high-dose chemotherapy and autologous bone marrow support. *J Clin Oncol* 1994;12:1005–11.
82. Bow EJ, Mandell LA, Louie TJ, et al. Quinolone-based antibacterial chemoprophylaxis in neutropenic patients: effect of aug-

mented gram-positive activity on infectious morbidity. *Ann Intern Med* 1996;125:183–90.
83. Meunier-Carpentier F, Kiehn TE, Armstrong D. Fungemia in the immunocompromised host: changing patterns, antigenemia, high mortality. *Am J Med* 1981;71:363–70.
84. Meyer RD, Rosen P, Armstrong D. Phycomycosis complicating leukemia and lymphoma. *Ann Intern Med* 1972;77:871–9.
85. Hawkins C, Armstrong D. Fungal infections in the immunocompromised host. *Clin Haematol* 1984;559–630.
86. Maddux MS, Barriere SL. A review of complications of amphotericin B therapy: recommendations for prevention and management. *Drug Intell Clin Pharm* 1980;14:177–81.
87. Burks LC, Aisner J, Fortner CL, et al. Meperidine for the treatment of shaking chills and fever. *Arch Intern Med* 1980;140:483–4.
88. Andstrom EE, Ringden O, Remberger M, et al. Safety and efficacy of liposomal amphotericin B in allogeneic bone marrow transplant recipients. *Mycoses* 1996;39:185–93.
89. Goldstone AH, O'Driscoll A. Early AmBisome in febrile neutropenia in patients with haematological disorders. *Bone Marrow Transplant* 1994;14(*Suppl* 5):S15–7.
90. Mills W, Chopra R, Linch DC, et al. Liposomal amphotericin B in the treatment of fungal infections in neutropenic patients: a single-centre experience of 133 episodes in 116 patients. *Br J Haematol* 1994;86:754–60.
91. Tollemar J, Ringden O, Andersson S, et al. Randomized double-blind study of liposomal amphotericin B (AmBisome) prophylaxis of invasive fungal infections in bone marrow transplant recipients. *Bone Marrow Transplant* 1993;12:577–82.
92. Hospenthal DR, Byrd JC, Weiss RB. Successful treatment of invasive aspergillosis complicating prolonged treatment-related neutropenia in acute myelogenous leukemia with amphotericin B lipid complex. *Med Pediatr Oncol* 1995;25:119–22.
93. Oravcova E, Mistrilk M, Sakalova A, et al. Amphotericin B lipid complex to treat invasive fungal infections in cancer patients: report of efficacy and safety in 20 patients. *Chemother* 1995;41:473–6.
94. Bowden RA, Cays M, Gooley T, et al. Phase I study of amphotericin B colloidal dispersion for the treatment of invasive fungal infections after marrow transplant. *J Infect Dis* 1996;173:1208–15.
95. Bennett JE, Dismukes WE, Duma RJ, et al. A collaborative study comparing amphotericin B alone or combined with flucytosine in the treatment of cryptococcal meningitis. *N Engl J Med* 1979;301:126–31.
96. Meunier-Carpentier F. Combination of antifungal agents for systemic mycotic diseases. In: Klastersky J, Staquet M, editors. *Combination Antibiotic Therapy in the Compromised Host*. EORTC Monograph Series. New York: Raven; 1982. p. 167–221.
97. Meunier F. Fluconazole treatment of fungal infections in the immunocompromised host. *Semin Oncol* 1990;17(*Suppl* 6):19–23.
98. Humphrey MJ, Jevons S, Tarbit MH. Pharmacokinetic evaluation of UK-49,858, a metabolically stable triazole antifungal drug, in animals and humans. *Antimicrob Agents Chemother* 1985;28:815–8.
99. Foulds G, Brennan DR, Wajszczuk C. Fluconazole penetration into cerebrospinal fluid in humans. *J Clin Pharmacol* 1988;28:363–6.
100. Lazar JD, Hilligoss DM. The clinical pharmacology of fluconazole. *Semin Oncol* 1990;17(*Suppl* 6):14–8.
101. Lazar JD, Wilner KD. Drug interactions with fluconazole. *Rev Infect Dis* 1990;12(*Suppl* 3):S327–33.
102. DeBeule K, De Doncker P, Cauwenbergh G, et al. The treatment of aspergillosis and aspergilloma with itraconazole: clinical results of an open international study (1982–1987). *Mycoses* 1988;31:476–85.
103. Dupont B. Itraconazole therapy in aspergillosis: study in 49 patients. *J Am Acad Dermatol* 1990;23:607–14.
104. Kreisel W, Kochling G, Von Schilling C, et al. Therapy of invasive aspergillosis with itraconazole: improvement of therapeutic efficacy by early diagnosis. *Mycoses* 1991;34:385–94.
105. Persat F, Marzullo C, Guyotat D, et al. Plasma itraconazole concentrations in neutropenic patients after repeated high-dose treatment. *Eur J Cancer* 1992;28A:838–41.
106. Boogaerts MA, Verhoef GE, Zachee P, et al. Antifungal prophylaxis with itraconazole in prolonged neutropenia: correlation with plasma levels. *Mycoses* 1989;32:103–8.
107. Wade JC, Newton B, McLaren C, et al. Intravenous acyclovir to treat mucocutaneous herpes simplex virus infection after marrow transplantation: a double-blind trial. *Ann Intern Med* 1982;96:265–9.
108. Meyers JD, Wade JC, Mitchell CD, et al. Multicenter collaborative trial of intravenous acyclovir for the treatment of mucocutaneous herpes simplex virus infection in the immunocompromised host. *Am J Med* 1982;73:229–35.
109. Shepp DH, Newton BA, Dandliker PS, et al. Oral acyclovir therapy of mucocutaneous herpes simplex virus infection in immunocompromised patients. *Ann Intern Med* 1985;102:783–5.
110. Balfour HH Jr, Bean B, Laskin OL, et al. Acyclovir halts progression of herpes zoster in immunocompromised patients. *N Engl J Med* 1983;308:1448–53.
111. Tucker R, Perry MC, Young CL. A pilot study to evaluate famciclovir treatment of herpes labialis in immunocompromised cancer patients. Proceedings of the 33rd Annual Meeting of the American Society of Clinical Oncology 1997;16:83a.
112. Winston DJ, Ho WG, Bartoni K, et al. Gancyclovir therapy for cytomegalovirus infections in recipients of bone marrow transplants and other immunosuppressed patients. *Rev Infect Dis* 1988;10(*Suppl* 3):S547–53.
113. Crumpacker C, Marlowe S, Zhang JL, et al. Treatment of cytomegalovirus pneumonia. *Rev Infect Dis* 1988;10(*Suppl* 3):S538–46.
114. Bratanow NC, Ash RC, Turner PA, et al. Successful treatment of serious cytomegalovirus disease with (1,3-dihydroxy-2-propoxymethyl) guanine (ganciclovir, DHPG) and intravenous immunoglobulin in bone marrow transplant patients. [abstract]. *Exp Hematol* 1987;15:541.
115. Winston DJ, Ho WG, Lin CH, et al. Intravenous immune globulin for prevention of cytomegalovirus infection and interstitial pneumonia after bone marrow transplantation. *Ann Intern Med* 1987;106:12–8.
116. Fenelon LE. Protective isolation: who needs it? *J Hosp Infect* 1995;30(*Suppl*):218–22.
117. Rowe JM, Lazarus HM. In response: are protected environments necessary for recipients of bone marrow transplants? *Ann Intern Med* 1994;121:76.

118. Wade JC, DeJongh CA, Newman KA, et al. Selective antimicrobial modulation as prophylaxis against infection during granulocytopenia. Trimethoprim-sulfamethoxazole vs. nalidixic acid. *J Infect Dis* 1983;147:624–34.
119. Karp JE, Merz WG, Hendrickson C, et al. Oral norfloxacin for prevention of gram-negative bacterial infections in patients with acute leukemia and granulocytopenia. *Ann Intern Med* 1987;106:1–7.
120. Dekker AW, Rozenberg-Arska M, Verheof J. Infection prophylaxis in acute leukemia: a comparison of ciprofloxacin with trimethoprim–sulfamethoxazole and colistin. *Ann Intern Med* 1987;106:7–12.
121. Bow EJ, Mandell LA, Louie TJ, et al. Quinolone-based antibacterial chemoprophylaxis in neutropenic patients: effect of augmented gram-positive activity on infectious morbidity. National Cancer Institute of Canada Clinical Trials Group. *Ann Intern Med* 1996;125:183–90.
122. Van der Waaij D. Colonization resistance of the digestive tract of mice during systemic antibiotic treatment. *J Hyg (Camb)* 1972;70:605–10.
123. Samonis G, Rolston K, Karl C, et al. Prophylaxis of oropharyngeal candidiasis with fluconazole. *Rev Infect Dis* 1990;12(*Suppl* 3):S369–73.
124. Winston DJ, Chandrasekar PH, Lazarus HM, et al. Fluconazole prophylaxis of fungal infections in patients with acute leukemia: results of a randomized, placebo-controlled, double-blind, multicentre trial. *Ann Intern Med* 1995;118:495–503.
125. Goodman JL, Winston DJ, Greenfield RA, et al. A controlled trial of fluconazole to prevent fungal infections in patients undergoing bone marrow transplantation. *N Engl J Med* 1992;326:845–51.
126. Slavin M, Bowden R, Osborne B, et al. Fluconazole prophylaxis in marrow transplant recipients: a randomized placebo-controlled, double-blind study [abstract]. Proceedings of the 32nd Interscience Conference on Antimicrobial Agents and Chemotherapy, 1992.
127. Bodey GP, Anaissie EJ, Elting LS, et al. Antifungal prophylaxis during remission induction therapy for acute leukemia: fluconazole versus intravenous amphotericin B. *Cancer* 1994;73:2099–106.
128. Wolff S, Fay J, Stevens D, et al. Fluconazole (Fluc) versus low dose amphotericin B (Ampho) for the prevention of fungal infections in patients (pts) undergoing marrow transplantation (BMT): a study of the North American Bone Marrow Transplant Group (NAMTG) [abstract]. *Blood* 1993;82(*Suppl* 1):[abstract no. 1686].
129. Rozenberg-Arska M, Dekker AW, Branger J, Verhoef J. A randomized study to compare oral fluconazole to amphotericin B in the prevention of fungal infections in patients with acute leukaemia. *J Antimicrob Chemother* 1991;27:369–76.
130. Menichetti F, Del Favero A, Martino P, et al. Preventing fungal infection in neutropenic patients with acute leukemia: fluconazole compared with oral amphotericin B. The GIMEMA Infection Program. *Ann Intern Med* 1994;120:913–8.
131. Philpott-Howard JN, Wade JJ, Mufti GJ, et al. Randomized comparison of oral fluconazole versus oral polyenes for the prevention of fungal infection in patients at risk of neutropenia. Multicentre Study Group. *J Antimicrob Chemother* 1993;31:973–84.
132. Ellis ME, Clink H, Ernst P, et al. Controlled study of fluconazole in the prevention of fungal infections in neutropenic patients with haematological malignancies and bone marrow transplant recipients. *Eur J Clin Microbiol Infect Dis* 1994;13:3–11.
133. Laver J, Moore MAS. Clinical use of recombinant human hematopoietic growth factors. *J Natl Cancer Inst* 1989;81:1370–82.
134. Maher DW, Lieschke GJ, Green M, et al. Filgrastim in patients with chemotherapy-induced febrile neutropenia: a double-blind, placebo-controlled trial. *Ann Intern Med* 1994;121:492–501.
135. Ozer H, Miller LL, Anderson PN, et al. American Society of Clinical Oncology recommendations for the use of hematopoietic colony-stimulating factors: evidence-based, clinical practice guidelines. *J Clin Oncol* 1994;12:2471–508.
136. American Society of Clinical Oncology. Update of recommendations for the use of hematopoietic colony-stimulating factors: evidence-based clinical practice guidelines. *J Clin Oncol* 1996;14:1957–60.
137. Strauss RG, Connett JE, Gale RP, et al. A controlled trial of prophylactic granulocyte transfusions during initial induction chemotherapy for acute myelogenous leukemia. *N Engl J Med* 1981;305:597–603.
138. Clift RA, Sanders JE, Thomas ED, et al. Granulocyte transfusions for the prevention of infection in patients receiving bone-marrow transplants. *N Engl J Med* 1978;298:1052–7.
139. Gomez-Villagran JL, Torres-Gomez A, Gomez-Garcia P, et al. A controlled trial of prophylactic granulocyte transfusions during induction chemotherapy for acute nonlymphoblastic leukemia. *Cancer* 1984;54:734–8.
140. Hersman J, Meyers JD, Thomas ED, et al. The effect of granulocyte transfusions upon the incidence of cytomegalovirus infection after allogeneic marrow transplantation. *Ann Intern Med* 1982;96:149–52.
141. Freifeld AG, Walsh TJ, Pizzo PA. Infections in the cancer patient. In: DeVita VT, Hellman S, Rosenberg SA, editors. *Cancer: Principles and Practice of Oncology*. 5th ed. Philadelphia, PA: JB Lippincott; 1997. p. 2659–704.
142. Advisory Committee on Immunization Practices [ACIP] of the Centers for Disease Control. Recommendations of the ACIP: use of vaccines and immune globulins for persons with altered immunocompetence. *MMWR* 1993;42 (No. RR-4): 1–12.
143. Ambrosino DM, Molrine DC. Critical appraisal of immunization strategies for prevention of infection in the compromised host. *Hematol Oncol Clin North Am* 1993;7:1027–50.

SELF-STUDY QUESTIONS

1. Risk of infection becomes significant after the granulocyte count drops below _____ /mm^3, and the most severe infections occur below _____ /mm^3.

2. In what way does radiation damage create a portal of entry for pathogenic organisms?

3. Most empiric antibiotic regimens combine _____ or _____ with an aminoglycoside in treating infectious complications in cancer patients.

4. Disagreement exists among authorities about whether to add an antistaphylococcal agent to initial antibiotic regimens.

   a. true.
   b. false.

5. What is the single most important factor influencing the effectiveness of antibiotics for infectious complications in granulocytopenic patients?

6. What is the drug of choice for treating invasive candidiasis, aspergillosis, mucormycosis, and cryptococcosis?

7. Why would you begin antimicrobial therapy in the absence of a definitive diagnosis of a fungal infection?

8. Varicella-zoster virus and herpes simplex virus respond favorably to which common drug?

9. Ganciclovir combined with _____ may improve response and survival of patients with cytomegalovirus infections.

10. What should patients be instructed to do to reduce exposure to nosocomial organisms?

Chapter 16 | Pain Management

David S. Johnson, Major USAF, B.S., Pharm.D., B.C.P.S.
Chairman, Department of Pharmacy
3rd Medical Group/SGSAP
24-800 Hospital Drive
Elmendorf Air Force Base, Alaska

Trust: The Patient-Practitioner Relationship	290
Overview of Cancer Pain	291
Prevalence	291
Causes and Contributing Factors	291
Acute Versus Chronic Pain	292
Management of Cancer Pain	292
Patient Assessment	293
Baseline Assessment	294
Pain History	294
McGill Pain Questionnaire	294
Psychosocial Assessment	294
Physical Evaluation	295
Reassessment	295
Patient Education and Goal Setting	295
Designing an Effective Treatment Plan	295
As-Needed Versus Around-the-Clock Dosing	296
Primary Regimen	297
Nonopioid Analgesics	297
Opioid Analgesics	298
Breakthrough Pain Analgesic Regimen	301
Tolerance, Addiction, and Physical Dependence	301
Tolerance	301
Addiction	302
Physical Dependence	302
Adverse Effects	302
Alternative Methods of Drug Delivery	303
Transdermal Administration of Fentanyl	303
Sublingual Administration of Opioids	303
Rectal Administration of Opioids	303
Spinal Administration of Opioids	303
Continuous Intravenous or Subcutaneous Administration of Opioids	303
Adjuvant Drugs	304
Antidepressants	304
Anticonvulsants	304

David S. Johnson is serving on active duty in the U.S. Air Force.
The contributions made by Nicky Dozier, Pharm.D., to this chapter are gratefully acknowledged.

Corticosteroids 304
Bone Pain Adjuvants 304
Nerve Blocks 305
AHCPR Guidelines for the Management of Cancer Pain 305
Summary 305
References 306
Self-Study Questions 307

Pain in patients with cancer is a complex and recurring process. For many of these patients, persistent pain becomes the most incapacitating aspect of their disease. However, in >90% of patients, pain control can be accomplished by relatively simple means throughout the course of the disease.[1-3] Pain is a subjective experience and is often difficult to define, describe, and interpret. The past few decades have presented an abundance of new information regarding the pathophysiology of pain and modalities for its treatment. A persistent lack of understanding, societal pressures, and popular misconceptions, however, continue to undermine the effective treatment of cancer pain. These barriers to effective cancer pain management are endemic to the medical system and include shortcomings of health care providers, patients, and the health care system.[1,4] Drug therapy remains the cornerstone of effective pain management, and the application of the principles outlined in this chapter will assist in preparing a regimen that will provide adequate pain relief to patients with cancer.

After completing this chapter, the reader should be able to:

1. Identify the barriers and fears that impede effective cancer pain management and discuss the importance of a trustful patient-practitioner relationship.
2. Discuss the causes, contributing factors, and multi-dimensional aspects of pain associated with various types and stages of cancer.
3. Discuss strategies for obtaining a detailed pain history and an ongoing pain assessment plan.
4. Discuss appropriate therapies for pain associated with cancer, cancer treatment, and concomitant medical conditions.
5. Using patient-specific information, select an individualized analgesic regimen for the management of cancer pain.
6. Discuss alternate methods for delivering analgesia for patients unable to tolerate oral analgesics.
7. Discuss the role of adjuvant drugs in cancer pain management.

This chapter examines the evaluation and management of cancer pain. Topics covered include patient assessment, pharmacologic treatment, administration and side effects of treatment, adjuvant treatments, and a discussion of alternative drug delivery methods.

TRUST: THE PATIENT-PRACTITIONER RELATIONSHIP

The importance of a trusting patient-practitioner relationship and proper patient education to the success of a pain control regimen cannot be overemphasized. Diminished quality of life, suffering, and loss of self-control are major fears facing most cancer patients. Ongoing, unrelenting pain becomes the greatest factor perpetuating these fears. Establishment of a trusting relationship with the provider and reassurance to the patient and family that most pain can be relieved safely and effectively are key to the patient's comfort and quality of life.

Several coexistent sources and types of pain may compound the emotional and cognitive responses to pain (symptoms of depression, helplessness, anxiety, and hostility). Successful management requires the understanding and support of the patient, practitioner, family, and friends and may require the integration of various nonpharmacologic interventions (such as psychological and psychiatric support, biofeedback, physical therapy, and neurosurgical procedures) with pharmacologic measures. With appropriate treatment, pain should not interfere with a patient's level of function, even as the disease progresses.

For the clinician, the only direct source of information on the subjective pain experience is the patient. Consequently, successful assessment and control of pain depend on a positive relationship between caregiver and patient. The clinician must recognize a patient's common fears that may impede effective pain reporting and assessment. Failure of the practitioner to deliver effective analgesia has been shown to be multifactorial (Table 16-1).[3]

An inability to openly communicate with health care providers and a lack of confidence in the provider's ability to treat pain are a constant source of fear and anxiety for patients and their families. Such fear intensifies the perception of pain and may adversely influence the patient's willingness to cooperate or find relief with therapy (Table 16-1).

There are also confounding problems within the health care system that contribute to the undertreatment of cancer pain.[1,6] Health care workers may be reluctant to prescribe, stock, or dispense opioids because they fear regulatory questioning (or even professional license suspension or revocation) in cases in which large quantities of opioids are provided to an individual, even though the medical needs for such drugs can be

Table 16-1. Barriers to Cancer Pain Management

Problems related to health care professionals
- Inadequate knowledge of pain management
- Lack of understanding of the pharmacology of analgesics
- Overestimating the analgesic efficacy of the drug
- Poor assessment of pain
- Concern about regulation of controlled substances
- Fear of patient addiction
- Concern about side effects of analgesics (i.e., respiratory depression)
- Concern about patients becoming tolerant to analgesics

Problems related to patients
- Reluctance to report pain
  - Concern about distracting physicians from treating the underlying disease
  - Fear that pain means disease is worsening
  - Concern about not being a "good" patient
- Reluctance to take pain medications
  - Fear of addiction or of being thought of as an addict
  - Worries about unmanageable side effects
  - Concern about becoming tolerant to pain medications

Problems related to the health care system
- Low priority to cancer pain treatment
- Inadequate reimbursement
- The most appropriate treatment may not be reimbursed or may be too costly for patients and family
- Restrictive regulation of controlled substances
- Problems of availability of treatment or access to it

SOURCE: adapted from reference 1.

justified.[1] In addition, reimbursement, or lack of it, influences the manner in which pain is treated, where it is treated, and the supportive care that is available (Table 16-1).[1]

In the patient-practitioner relationship, negative consequences are much easier to avoid than correct. A constructive relationship with the patient begins with willingness to listen to the patient's subjective report of the pain experience. Open communication and understanding become invaluable in the monitoring and titration of the therapeutic regimen. Ongoing discussion among providers, patients, and families must be maintained for continual reassessment of pain control and reestablishment of pain management goals.

The deceptive use of placebos and the misinterpretation of the placebo response to discredit the patient is not acceptable, because it ultimately leads to lack of confidence in the analgesic regimen and mistrust of the prescriber.[1,7] Potential mechanisms of placebo analgesia include behavioral and psychological influences and the induction of the endogenous opioids (β-endorphins and enkephalins). Placebos are effective in a few patients for a short period of time only and should not be used in the management of cancer pain.[1,7]

OVERVIEW OF CANCER PAIN

Pain management is largely an empiric practice, predominantly because of the complex and subjective nature of the pain experience. However, the approach has become increasingly specific as our understanding of the neurobiological mechanisms involved in the initiation and transmission of pain impulses has grown. Pain, by definition, is an unpleasant sensory and emotional experience associated with actual or potential tissue damage, or described in terms of such damage.[7] Pain is a symptom of an underlying disorder, not a diagnosis in itself. The treatment of cancer pain is often difficult and frustrating because there is no universal formula for success. It is important to understand the various mechanisms and stimuli that may be involved in producing cancer pain. Cancer pain management requires a treatment regimen easily understood by the patient and the immediate caregivers that has sufficient flexibility to adapt to changing needs. The practitioner must formulate a planned and individualized approach to the pain, applying the physiological and pharmacologic principles of analgesia to the subjective pain experience and needs described by the patient.

Prevalence

The frequency and severity of pain experienced by cancer patients vary considerably among patients with different stages and types of disease. It is evident that pain occurs with increasing frequency and severity as the disease progresses and that refractory pain is avoidable with all types of cancer. Moderate to severe pain is estimated to occur among 15% of patients with limited malignant disease, 30–50% of patients with intermediate-stage disease, and 60–90% of patients with more advanced disease.[1,5,8-11]

Causes and Contributing Factors

The cause of pain is not always clear, but the factors identified as contributing to the pain process in cancer patients include:

- direct tumor infiltration of a tissue, especially nervous tissue;
- tissue damage due to treatment (e.g., radiation therapy, chemotherapy, or phlebitis); and
- factors that are unrelated to the cancer itself (i.e., other concurrent medical conditions).

Specific examples of etiologic factors are outlined in Table 16-2. It is estimated that 75% of the pain experienced by cancer patients is directly attributable to the cancer, about 20% is the result of therapy, and <5% of the pain problems are completely unrelated to the cancer.[12]

Epidemiologic studies have underscored the significant variation in the likelihood of pain according to the type of

Table 16-2. Etiologies of Pain in Cancer Patients

Cancer-related factors
- Pressure due to direct tumor invasion of organs and tissues
- Vascular engorgement due to blockage of blood egression from a tissue
- Arterial ischemia
- Tissue damage due to necrosis, ulceration, or inflammation
- Bone pain
- Neurologic pain due to infiltration, inflammation, or stimulation of nerves
- Obstruction of an internal organ

Treatment-related factors
- Postsurgical pain
- Sequelae to chemotherapy, such as peripheral neuropathy, postherpetic neuralgia, aseptic necrosis of bone, or mucositis
- Postradiation pain due to burns, fibrosis of a nerve, myelopathy, or radiation enteritis

Factors unrelated to cancer
- Diabetic neuropathy
- Degenerative joint disease
- Migraine headache
- Decubitus ulcers
- Peptic ulcer disease

malignancy. Prevalence of pain varied widely, from significant pain among 85% of patients with primary bone tumors, 50% of breast cancer patients, and 45% of lung cancer patients. In contrast, about 20% of patients with lymphoma and 5% of patients with leukemia have pain requiring potent analgesics.[9]

Recognizing causative or contributing factors may have significant implications for the choice of analgesic therapy and consideration of adjunctive measures. For example, pain associated with tumor infiltration of bone generally responds to palliative radiation to the involved area and to nonsteroidal anti-inflammatory drugs (NSAIDs). On the other hand, pain caused by infiltration of other tissues, especially if the pain is associated with inflammation, may be more responsive to the anti-inflammatory effects of corticosteroids.

Identifying causative factors is often helpful in formulating the regimen. However, it is equally important to note that the occurrence of pain often precedes radiological or other clinical evidence of disease progression. Lacking clinical findings, therefore, pharmacists should not underestimate the patient's report of pain. Any such report deserves the serious attention of all health care providers.

Acute Versus Chronic Pain

Many cancer patients experience more than one distinct type of pain, often simultaneously. Cancer pain may be acute, intermittent, or chronic. Unlike most chronic nonmalignant pain, chronic cancer pain usually progresses over time. The psychological and sociological aspects of the underlying malignancy and the extent they impact the patient's sense of well-being and quality of life may have a significant influence on the perception of chronic cancer pain.

The experience of acute pain generally serves as a warning that some aspect of one's health requires immediate attention. The patient with acute pain can normally give a clear description of its location, severity, and timing. Acute pain has subjective and objective physical signs. Acute pain causes the patient to relate unpleasant sensory and emotional experiences, such as anxiety and fear, and behavioral responses, such as grimacing, moaning or screaming, guarding (covering or protecting), and splinting (favoring unnaturally). Acute pain is generally characterized by autonomic nervous system hyperactivity (i.e., tachycardia, hypertension, tachypnea, muscle tension, diaphoresis, mydriasis, pallor, nausea, or vomiting).

Chronic pain differs from acute pain in that it no longer serves a protective or warning function. The patient's descriptions of location, severity, and timing of pain are often vague. The autonomic nervous system adapts to chronic pain, and the objective signs associated with acute pain are often absent. For these reasons, the expression of pain as a chronic ailment is often poorly understood and mismanaged. The treatment of chronic pain is more difficult and may require a multidisciplinary and multimodal approach.

The frequently chronic nature of cancer pain presents two dimensions to the pain syndrome: first, the pain experience itself, and second, the patient's emotional or cognitive reaction to the pain. The emotional and physiological components aggravate each other, creating a destructive cycle that intensifies suffering. As a result, the pain becomes an all-consuming experience for the patient, one that is very difficult to treat if the interplay of emotional and physical variables is not recognized and addressed. As pain becomes chronic it becomes increasingly burdensome to the patient. Effective pain control with minimal analgesic side effects generally improves the patient's emotional well-being and quality of life.

Breaking this chronic pain cycle requires careful attention to both the emotional and the physiological dimensions. The specific cause of pain should be treated, if possible. Patients with malignancies responsive to treatment might benefit from further treatment with chemotherapy, surgery, or radiation therapy to reduce pain caused by large tumor masses. At the same time, emotional support for the patient is extremely important.

MANAGEMENT OF CANCER PAIN

Most cancer pain can be effectively and safely managed on an outpatient basis, in many cases throughout the last few days of life. The fact remains, however, that in this country and others throughout the world, cancer pain remains inadequately treated because of inherent shortcomings in the delivery of needed care.[3] Some surveys have indicated that >40–50% of cancer patients receive inadequate pain management. In addition, patients seen at medical centers that treat predominantly minorities were three times more likely to have received inadequate pain management.[3] These numbers clearly demonstrate that undertreatment of cancer pain is a major health care issue facing practitioners today. Ineffective pain management results in unnecessary suffering by patients and families and can effectively nullify a patient's opportunity to lead a meaningful and productive life even when the cancer is stable or in remission. Cancer pain is most often multidimensional, and its intensity is not always proportional to the type or extent of tissue damage. The different components of cancer pain that influence a patient's interpretation and must be taken into consideration when planning therapy include:

- physiological components (i.e., nociceptive is the process of pain transmission);
- sensory components (i.e., a patient's nociception, such as pain location, intensity, and quality);
- affective components (i.e., mood and anxiety response);
- cognitive components (i.e., how the pain affects a patient's thought processes and self-image; and
- behavioral components (i.e., pain behaviors, such as analgesic intake or activity level).[13]

Patient Assessment

The critical first step in formulating a pain control regimen is the assessment phase (Figure 16-1). In this step, the nature and scope of the problem must be defined. Time spent assessing the nature of the report of pain before starting or adjusting therapy may abate unnecessary suffering caused by under- or overmedicating. Proper treatment relies on an accurate assessment of pain. The United States Agency for Health Care Policy and Research (AHCPR) *Clinical Practice Guideline on the Management of Cancer Pain* summarizes the approach to pain assessment and management with the mnemonic *ABCDE*:

A Ask about pain regularly.
    Assess pain systematically.
B Believe the patient and family in their report of pain and what relieves it.
C Choose pain control options appropriate for the patient, family, and setting.
D Deliver interventions in a timely, logical, and coordinated fashion.
E Empower patients and their families.
    Enable patients to control their course to the greatest extent possible.[1]

The key to attaining an accurate initial appraisal is to assemble a detailed pain history and then factor in the findings from the physical examination, diagnostic studies, and the psycho-

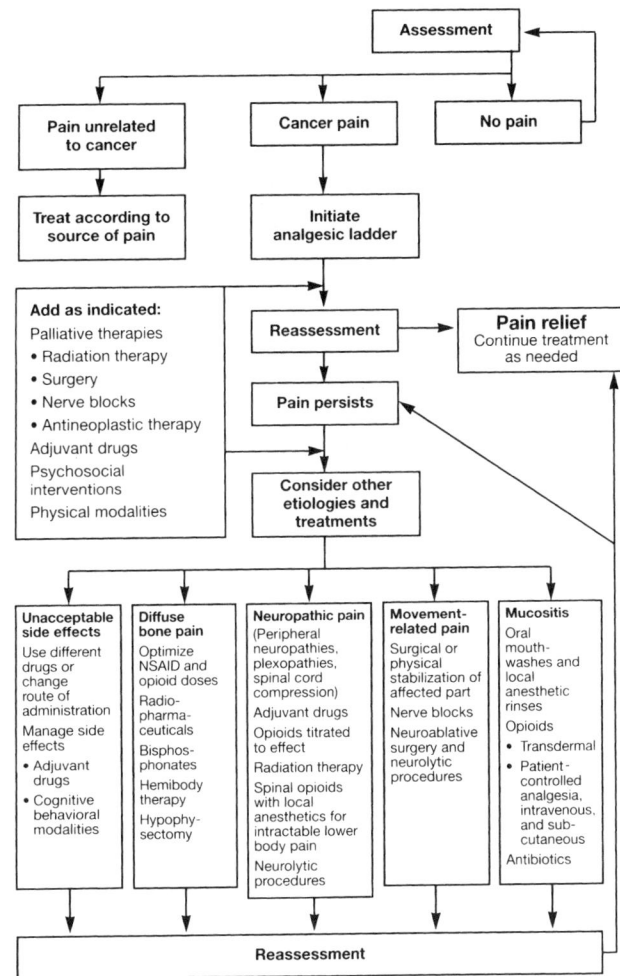

Figure 16-1. Continuing pain management in patients with cancer. NSAID, nonsteroidal anti-inflammatory drug.

SOURCE: Jacox AK, Carr DB, Payne R, et al. Management of cancer pain. Clinical practice guideline no. 9. Rockville, MD: Agency for Health Care Policy and Research; 1994. [AHCPR publication no. 94-0592].

social assessment. The patient's self-report should be the primary source of the assessment. Pain assessment is an ongoing process, with particular attention to changes in pain patterns and the onset of new pain. Steps similar to the initial assessment should follow each new report of pain. Persistent pain suggests the need to consider other causes and alternative, perhaps more invasive, treatments.

Special attention in assessment of pain must be emphasized in recognizing the unique needs and circumstances presented in treating children, the elderly, the cognitively impaired, and other special patient categories. Behavioral observation should be the primary assessment method for preverbal and nonverbal children and should be used as an adjunct to assessment for verbal children and cognitively impaired adults. The elderly are more vulnerable to drug accumulation because of age-related changes in pharmacokinetics of analgesic medications; aggressive pain assessment and management are as necessary for them as for younger age groups.[1]

Baseline Assessment

The initial assessment of a cancer patient in pain is important because it is a baseline for evaluating the effectiveness of any subsequent interventions. Because pain is such a complex phenomenon, several parameters should be identified and quantified as thoroughly as possible in the initial assessment. The initial evaluation should include:

- a systematic and thorough pain history, including assessment of the pain and intensity;
- an assessment of any pertinent psychosocial factors that may be involved;
- a review of findings from the physical and clinical examination; and
- a review of previously used methods for pain control.

Pain History

The pain history should be specific and systematic so that the baseline information needed to assess therapeutic efficacy is collected. A careful tracing of the progression of the pain over time and of any sites where the pain seems localized may provide clues to possible causes. The information obtained should focus on identifying the causes of the pain and developing a pain management plan. Failure to accurately assess pain can often lead to its undertreatment. Several pain characteristics are addressed by specific questions:[1]

- What are the onset and temporal pattern of the pain?
- What is the site of the pain?
- What are the quality and intensity of the pain?
- Are there any exacerbating or relieving factors?
- Are there any associated signs and symptoms?
- What has been the response to previous and current analgesic regimens?
- What are the effects on physical and social function?

The answers to these questions may suggest possible pain mechanisms involved and indicate the circumstances in which more aggressive therapy is needed. The initial assessment should elicit information about changes in activities of daily living, including work and recreational activities, sleep patterns, mobility, appetite, sexual function, and mood. If these phenomena are known in advance, they can be addressed specifically in the pain control regimen. An assessment of pain intensity must include an evaluation of not only the present pain intensity but also pain at its least and worst. Subsequent assessments with each new report of pain and/or increased pain or lack of response can then be accomplished by simpler means of appraisal.

Many validated pain assessment tools have been used for quantifying pain intensity. Most clinicians quantify the

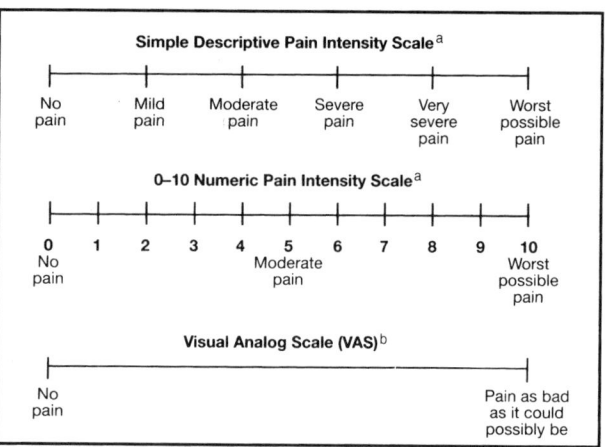

Figure 16-2. Pain intensity scales
SOURCE: Jacox AK, Carr DB, Payne R, et al. Management of cancer pain. Clinical practice guideline no. 9. Rockville, MD: Agency for Health Care Policy and Research; 1994. [AHCPR publication no. 94-0592]
[a]If used as a graphic rating scale, a 10-cm baseline is recommended.
[b]A 10-cm baseline is recommended for VAS scales.

pain indirectly, rating the patient's own report according to a scale or categorical ranking (Figure 16-2). The Visual Analog Scale (VAS)[14] and the McGill Pain Questionnaire[15,16] are two examples of clinical techniques for patient pain reporting. To use the VAS, the clinician asks the patient to indicate the intensity of the pain experience by striking a mark along a horizontal scale on which one extreme is no pain and the other is the worst pain imaginable. The VAS is quick and easy to use, although its reliability may sometimes be questioned.[12] It is especially useful when administered following major modification of the regimen. Patients can keep a log of their pain intensity scores and report them during follow-up visits or by telephone.

McGill Pain Questionnaire

The McGill Pain Questionnaire is a multidimensional tool for clinical assessment of pain that has the patient select from 20 sets of word descriptors representing the sensory, emotional, and cognitive aspects of the pain experience. This instrument is more comprehensive for evaluating pain both quantitatively and qualitatively. However, it is more difficult and time consuming to administer and score than the VAS, and its applicability is limited by its vocabulary and language constraints.

Psychosocial Assessment

The psychosocial assessment should emphasize the effect of pain on patients and their families, as well as patients' preferences among pain management methods. Other important components of the psychosocial assessment include the patient's acceptance and understanding of the cancer diagnosis, significant past experiences with pain, coping mechanisms for stress or pain, the economic impact of the pain and its treatment, and the patient's concerns about using controlled substances.¹ Anxiety and depression, common among patients facing devastating illness, can enhance pain perception and may necessitate a psychological or psychiatric consult. The patient's emotional reaction to pain can exacerbate suffering. Many cultural, linguistic, or other psychosocial factors may impair adequate pain assessment. Cultural and social pressures may also influence a patient's willingness to report pain. Judging pain by just observing the patient's behavior may lead to an underestimation of its severity.[17] Thus, in developing a pain treatment plan, clinicians need to be aware of the unique needs and circumstances of patients from various ethnic and cultural backgrounds.

Physical Evaluation

Physical findings and appropriate diagnostic evaluations should be reviewed to assist in identifying the primary source of pain and for evidence of advancing disease or alternative sources of pain. The physical examination should focus on each site of pain, include a pertinent neurological evaluation, and evaluate common sites of pain referral.[1] It is important to remember, however, that the absence of clinical findings does not rule out the presence of metastatic disease or other clinically undetectable problems. Even when no apparent cause is found, the clinician should proceed with the analgesic regimen and maintain a diligent effort to identify treatable factors.

Reassessment

With baseline pain evaluation completed, an initial treatment plan may be formulated. An ongoing reassessment plan is then needed to track the therapeutic efficacy of the regimen, the incidence of adverse effects, the patient's satisfaction with pain management, and its impact on the patient's quality of life. Reassessment detects any changes or progression in the pain process itself. Continual reassessment of the patient's response to therapy provides the best method to provide adequate pain control through dosage and therapy adjustments. Reassessment is also important because malignant diseases are rarely stable processes. A patient's log of daily pain experiences is one particularly helpful tool for evaluating the regimen and retitrating when necessary. In this record, the patient is asked to note the intensity, location, and frequency of the pain experience, as well as pain medication requirements: how often the medication is required, what degree and duration of analgesia are achieved, and what problems are being experienced with the medications.

Specific information permits a more structured approach to tailoring the regimen. To simply record a patient's responses to the question "how is your pain?" invites misunderstanding and impedes quantification.

The particular tool used for pain evaluation is clinically less important than assuring that an effective assessment and documentation tool is used. Evaluating therapy or changes in the pain process is difficult without a system for estimating or quantifying the pain experience. For most clinical situations, the simpler methods are probably more efficient and useful and should be done at regular intervals and systematically after starting the treatment plan, with each new report of pain and at a suitable interval after each pharmacologic or nonpharmacologic intervention.

Patient Education and Goal Setting

Patient education entails providing patients and families with accurate and understandable information about pain, pain assessment, the use of drugs, and other methods of pain relief. Common misconceptions, such as those concerning addiction and tolerance, should be addressed before rather than after problems are encountered. Patients generally need reassurance that their pain will be effectively managed and that the ultimate objective is to suppress pain continuously while allowing the patient an acceptable level of activity.

Designing an Effective Treatment Plan

Patient-specific therapy should begin promptly if pain from the cancer, the effects of cancer treatment, or concomitant medical conditions are identified in the initial assessment. It is important that patients and their families be involved in the discussion of treatment options, expectations, and anticipated effects. Painful disorders that benefit from specific therapy probably account for <50% of the major problems of patients with cancer, but they may exacerbate the pain process in a greater number of patients. Among the treatable causes of pain are bedsores, musculoskeletal disorders, headaches, peptic ulcer disease, and constipation (Table 16-2).

Drug therapy is the key component of cancer pain management because of its efficacy, rapid onset of action, and relatively low cost and risk. Successful planning of a pain control regimen requires individualizing the regimen to the patient. Pain control regimens are usually individualized by dividing the regimen into several parts: the primary pain control regimen, measures for managing breakthrough pain, and adjunctive agents for specific pain syndromes.

The primary pain control regimen is directed at suppressing pain during normal activity. The simplest, least invasive therapy should be attempted first. Additional agents or doses are essential for breakthrough pain (pain that increases at the end of a dosing interval as a result of insufficient analgesic use and occurs with or without a precipitating event) or incidental pain (pain that occurs as a result of action of the patient, such as movement, swallowing, urination, defecation, or cough).[18] It is important that these supplemental doses are adequate to allow the patient flexibility and confidence to participate in activities beyond the basic activities of daily living (e.g., doctor office visits or social functions) while the primary regimen is held constant.

Adjuvant drugs are useful as analgesics for specific painful states and can be initiated any time they are appropriate.

Table 16-3. Adjuvant Analgesic Drugs for Cancer Pain

Drug	Approximate Adult Daily Dose Range	Route of Administration	Type of Pain
Corticosteroids			
Dexamethasone	16–96 mg	PO, IV	Pain associated with brain metastases and epidural spinal cord compression
Prednisone	40–100 mg	PO	
Anticonvulsants			
Carbamazepine	200–1600 mg	PO	Neuropathic pain
Phenytoin	300–500 mg	PO	
Antidepressants			
Amitriptyline	25–150 mg	PO	Neuropathic pain
Doxepin	25–150 mg	PO	
Imipramine	20–100 mg	PO	
Trazodone	75–225 mg	PO	
Neuroleptics			
Methotrimeprazine	40–80 mg	IM	Neuropathic pain
Antihistamines			
Hydroxyzine	300–450 mg	IM	Adjuvant to opioids in postoperative and other types of pain; relief of complicating symptoms, including anxiety, insomnia, and nausea
Local Anesthestics/ Antiarrythmics			
Lidocaine	5 mg/kg	IV/SC	Neuropathic pain
Mexiletine	450–600 mg	PO	
Tocainide	20 mg/kg	PO	
Psychostimulants			
Dextroamphetamine	5–10 mg	PO	Improve opioid analgesia, decrease sedation
Methylphenidate	10–15 mg	PO	

SOURCE: Jacox AK, Carr DB, Payne R, et al. Management of cancer pain. Clinical practice guideline no. 9. Rockville, MD: Agency for Health Care Policy and Research; 1994. [AHCPR publication no. 94-0592]. PO, orally; IV, intravenous; IM, intramuscularly; SC, subcutaneously.

Their mechanisms of action are often still unclear; thus, their use is often empiric. Included in this group are phenothiazines, antidepressants, antiarrhythmics, butyrophenones, antihistamines, anticonvulsants, and other agents that, although not usually considered analgesics, have clinical data to support their use in restricted pain syndromes (Table 16-3).

As-Needed Versus Around-the-Clock Dosing

When pain is prevented from recurring by a continuous therapeutic level of an analgesic, the fear and memory of pain recede in the patient's mind. Pro re nata (PRN) dosing is effective in many clinical settings, including acute mild to moderate pain or for breakthrough pain during regular around-the-clock (ATC) analgesia. However, if pain is persistent during most of the day or frequently recurs, such as with severe acute pain or chronic malignant pain, ATC analgesia is most appropriate.[1,19,20] Using the PRN approach, the patient receives drugs only after he or she is in pain, receiving only intermittent relief. Persistent pain can quickly lead to "clock watching," stoicism, or fear of addiction. As the pain intensifies during this interval, the patient may need a larger dose to obtain relief and is thus subject to the side effects of larger doses, such as somnolence and nausea. In addition, the peak effect may not be realized for an hour or more following an oral dose, prolonging the pain experience. PRN dosing alone results in higher daily dosage requirements and leads to a cycle of undermedication and pain alternating with periods of overmedication and analgesic toxicity.

ATC analgesia will decrease anxiety, fear, and sensitivity to pain and may ultimately result in the patient using less analgesia for pain control. It is important to remember that cancer pain is typically always present and that administering analgesics on a scheduled ATC basis results in consistent relief with fewer variations in patient comfort and sedation.

The fixed-dose approach has practical value because it prevents the usual medical and nursing delays that occur when a patient on a PRN schedule requests medication. Similarly, for the patient who self-medicates at home, it may facilitate compliance. ATC dosing should always be accompanied by an order for rescue dosing for breakthrough pain on a PRN basis. The use of ATC with rescue dosing provides a method for reliable and sensible stepwise dose escalation and is appropriate to all routes of opioid administration.[1,19,20] The fixed-dose approach is potentially dangerous in an opioid-naive patient, particularly when drugs with long half lives are used, such as methadone and levorphanol. When these opioids are used, dose escalations must be slow and cautious to avoid dose-related side effects.

Primary Regimen

Selection of the primary analgesic for the pain control regimen is still largely an empiric decision. The World Health Organization (WHO) has endorsed a three-step analgesic ladder approach to the treatment of cancer pain (Figure 16-3). This method is a simple, well-validated, and effective method for assuring the rational titration of therapy for cancer pain. Several clinical and pharmacologic variables deserve consideration in making a rational choice: the relative severity of the pain, the responsiveness of the pain to previous therapy, and the suspected cause or causes of the pain process.

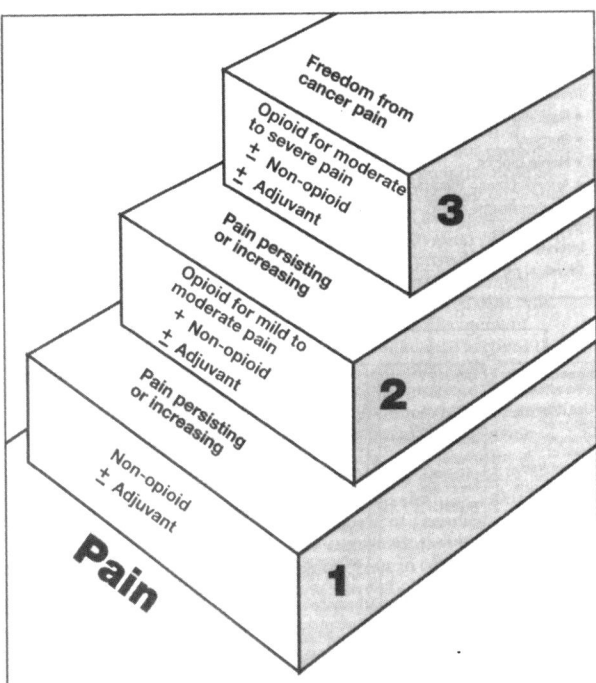

Figure 16-3. The World Health Organization three-step analgesic ladder

Source: reprinted with permission from World Health Organization [WHO]. Cancer pain relief and palliative care. Report of a WHO expert committee [WHO technical report series, no. 804]. Geneva, Switzerland: WHO; 1990.

Nonopioid Analgesics

Nonopioid analgesics, such as NSAIDs (including aspirin) or acetaminophen, are usually sufficient for mild to moderate pain (WHO Ladder, Step 1). NSAIDs act by inhibiting the synthesis of prostaglandins, inflammatory mediators known to sensitize peripheral nociceptors. Prostaglandin inhibition by NSAIDs occurs as a result of the inactivation of cyclooxygenase, an enzyme that catalyzes the formation of prostaglandin precursors (endoperoxides) from arachidonic acid. In addition, the effects of NSAIDs on the mechanism of action in the central nervous system (CNS) are thought to contribute to analgesia, but not by activation of opiate receptors.[1]

Pain response to individual NSAIDs varies considerably. It may be necessary to switch agents several times to achieve an acceptable response. Each agent should be allowed an adequate trial period (several days) on a fixed, continuous basis, using maximum doses, before switching to another drug. Table 16-4 lists the most commonly used NSAIDs and the recommended doses.

Acetaminophen is included with the NSAIDs because it has similar analgesic potency. The NSAIDs are superior to acetaminophen in their anti-inflammatory effects; however, acetaminophen lacks their associated renal, gastrointestinal, and hematopoietic toxicities. Chronic dosing of acetaminophen >4 g/day is a concern when using fixed combination products, because of the risk of hepatotoxicity with acetaminophen.

The anti-inflammatory and antipyretic properties, as well as the lack of potential for tolerance and physical dependence, are desirable qualities of the nonopioid analgesics. They are also useful in potentiating the effects of opioid analgesics for treatment of moderate to severe pain. The dose of nonopioid analgesics is limited by a maximum effective dose for pain relief, above which little or no additional analgesic effect is gained but the risk of adverse effects increases significantly. They also carry the risk of side effects with long-term use, including gastrointestinal ulceration, fluid retention, hypertension, CNS effects, platelet-inhibiting actions, and renal toxicity. Side effects can occur at any time, and patients, especially patients who are elderly or those with hepatic or renal insufficiency, should be monitored carefully. To reduce the risk of toxicity, it is reasonable to start at the minimally acceptable dose and titrate upward as needed (Table 16-4).

NSAIDs may be classified by chemical structure (e.g., acetic acids or propionic acids) and have different elimination half-lives, which determine their recommended dosing frequency. Most NSAIDs are organic acids and are highly bound to plasma proteins, properties that facilitate drug penetration into inflamed tissues. Patients receiving concomitant therapy with other highly protein-bound drugs (e.g., phenytoin, oral anticoagulants, sulfonamides, sulfonylureas, methotrexate, and cyclosporine) should be monitored closely for toxicity due to drug interactions.

The nonacetylated salicylate salts, such as salsalate and choline salicyclate and magnesium salicylate combinations,

Table 16-4. Nonsteroidal Anti-inflammatory Drugs (NSAIDs)

NSAID	Dose (mg)	Maximum Dose per Day (mg)
Acetaminophen[a]	650–1000 q4–6hr	4000
Salicylates		
Aspirin	650–1000 q4–6hr	4000
Salsalate[b]	1000–1500 q8–12hr	4000
Choline/magnesium trisalicylate[b] combinations	1000–1500 TID	4500
Choline salicylate liquid[b]	870 q3–4hr	5220
Diflunisal	500 q8–12hr	1500
Diclofenac	50–75 q8–12hr	200
Etodolac	200–400 q6–12hr	1200
Flurbiprofen	50–100 q6–12hr	300
Ibuprofen	200–800 q6–8hr	3200
Indomethacin	25–50 q8hr 75 q24hr (SR)	200
Ketoprofen	50–75 q6–8hr 200 q24hr (SR)	300
Ketorolac[c]	15–30 q6hr (IM/IV) 10 q4–6hr (PO)	120 40
Nabumetone	1000–2000 QD–BID	2000
Naproxen	200–500 q8–12hr	1250
Oxaprozin	600–1200 QD–BID	1800
Piroxicam	20 QD	20
Sulindac	150–200 BID	400
Tolmetin	400–600 BID–TID	1800

SR, sustained release.
[a]No anti-inflammatory activity.
[b]Fewer platelet effects than aspirin.
[c]For short-term use only.

have minimal effects on platelet aggregation and have fewer gastrointestinal side effects.[1] These attributes make these NSAIDs relatively safe to use in treating thrombocytopenic patients or patients with clotting impairment. These effects have only been studied in small numbers of patients, however, and have not been determined to be clinically definitive. Some newer NSAIDs (e.g., nabumetone and oxaprozin) are reputed to have fewer gastrointestinal and hematological effects, but these drugs lack a large body of evidence of enhanced safety in high-risk populations.

Ketorolac is the only NSAID available for parenteral analgesia. Because of its potent anti-prostaglandin effects and higher incidence of adverse effects, it is only indicated for short-term relief of pain (<5 days). Numerous reports of renal, gastrointestinal, and hematopoietic effects have been associated with its use. As a result, its use in chronic cancer pain is limited to isolated uses, such as perioperative analgesia or special acute pain episodes for which other routes are not viable.

NSAIDs have a distinct role in treating pain associated with bone metastases.[21] The benefit of NSAIDs in this setting is probably because of inhibition of prostaglandin synthesis. Bone metastases increase prostaglandin E_2 (PGE_2) production, which in turn causes an increase in osteolysis. The lytic process in bone further increases PGE_2 production. The accumulation of PGE_2 sensitizes free nerve endings, lowering the peripheral pain threshold.[22,23] Administering NSAIDs on a fixed, continuous basis, rather than PRN, is preferable for pain associated with metastatic bone disease.

Tramadol, a centrally acting analgesic that binds to μ-opioid receptors and inhibits the reuptake of norepinephrine and serotonin, is approved for the treatment of moderate to moderately severe pain. Its analgesic efficacy is reported to be equivalent to 60 mg of codeine or 30 mg of codeine plus acetaminophen in patients with procedural or cancer pain.[24] The side effect profile of tramadol includes nausea, dizziness, constipation, sedation, headache, and dose-limiting seizures. Although this drug was originally touted to have limited abuse potential, reports of physical dependence are now appearing. Its role in the treatment of cancer pain has yet to be clearly defined, but it may be best suited to those patients intolerant of NSAIDs for mild to moderate pain that cannot be relieved by acetaminophen.[24]

Opioid Analgesics

Opioids produce analgesia by binding to specific receptors inside and outside the CNS. An opioid is indicated when unsatisfactory relief is achieved after an appropriate trial at maximum doses of nonopioid agents or as initial therapy for patients with moderate to severe pain. Delays in switching to the more aggressive therapy serve no constructive purpose. In general, primary pain control is achieved by using a single opioid agonist with or without a concomitant NSAID in patients with moderate to severe pain (Figure 16-3).

The opioid analgesics are classified as agonists, partial agonists, or mixed agonist/antagonists according to their interaction with opioid receptors. The agonist opioids bind competitively to opioid receptors in the CNS and trigger intracellular changes that mediate analgesia. Agonist opioids are the most useful agents for cancer pain management. The partial agonist buprenorphine has only a limited role in treating cancer pain because of its ceiling effect. The mixed agonist/antagonists (pentazocine, dezocine, nalbuphine, and butorphanol) also bind to opioid receptors in the CNS, but binding does not elicit the full spectrum of responses seen with agonists. These agents have three disadvantages: they (1) produce psychotomimetic effects at higher doses, (2) are limited by a ceiling in efficacy, and (3) produce withdrawal syndromes in opioid-dependent patients. These problems seriously restrict the use of the mixed agonist/antagonists, making the opioid agonists the agents most frequently used for the management of cancer pain.

Products that combine a nonopioid, such as aspirin or acetaminophen, with an opioid take advantage of different mechanisms of action and different side effect profiles. The addition of nonopioids may permit lower doses of opioids to be used. The ceiling dose and toxicity of the nonopioid component limit the amount of opioids that can be delivered using these formulations, however.

Morphine is the standard by which the potency and effect of all other opioids are compared. Morphine, a potent opioid, is a good agent for initial therapy because it is available in various strengths and dosage forms, making it easy to titrate doses to pain management. The optimal dosage form and route of administration are generally the ones that allow the patient as much self-reliance as possible while providing an acceptable onset and duration of analgesia.

Related opioids have qualitatively similar actions that differ primarily in terms of potency and duration of effect. Drug availability, cost, and previous success or failure with particular agents may be important long-term considerations, especially for patients who will continue therapy as outpatients. Individual patient susceptibility to side effects is variable and may be agent specific. A change from one opioid to another may decrease side effects and improve analgesia. Several characteristics relevant to selecting an opioid are tabulated for comparison in Table 16-5.

Codeine and propoxyphene are considered to be weak opioids. They are effective for mild to moderate pain but have limited utility in more severe cancer-related pain because of the diminishing effect of dose increases above the suggested range. Above suggested dose levels, each incremental increase in dose provides a smaller incremental increase in pain relief but a full incremental increase in side effects.[1,19] Hydrocodone and oxycodone have also been classified as weak opioids, but only because they are usually prescribed in fixed combination products that limit their dose ranges. Oxycodone is also available as a single-entity product, which allows dosage titration and avoids the limitations (i.e., ceiling dose effect and toxicity) of the fixed combinations. A sustained-release formulation of oxycodone is now available and may be a viable alternative to sustained-release morphine.[24]

Meperidine is not a good choice for opioid analgesia in chronic cancer pain. Meperidine has a very short duration of action, is painful on injection, and has poor bioavailability when given orally. Meperidine causes a toxic metabolite, normeperidine, to accumulate in the CNS, especially in patients with renal dysfunction. This metabolite causes CNS hyperirritability, which manifests as myoclonus and may predispose the patient to seizures.[25] Consequently, meperidine is not a good choice for chronic cancer pain management.

The route of administration may influence therapeutic effectiveness and affect ease of administration, cost, and compliance. The oral route of opioid administration is generally preferred because it allows self-medication and relatively prolonged analgesia. Administration by subcutaneous (SC), intramuscular (IM), rectal (PR), or transdermal routes eliminates the need for a functioning gastrointestinal tract, but absorption may not be predictable. The IM route is not recommended, because of the discomfort and risk of hematomas caused by the injection. The intravenous (IV) route is the most efficient route of administration for immediate and predictable drug effect; however, it is invasive, must be closely supervised, has a shorter duration of action, has the potential for increased side effects, and is generally more expensive. Epidural and intrathecal routes of analgesic administration have been used effectively to treat postoperative and chronic pain. Epidural, intrathecal, and intravenous administration can be accomplished in an outpatient setting, but these routes require catheter placement and comprehensive patient or caregiver instruction and support.

The severity of the immediate problem must be considered first when selecting the dose of an opioid. If the pain is incapacitating, dosing should be started aggressively to rapidly control the pain. The patient should be closely monitored (e.g., for excessive sedation or respiratory rate) for the first few hours. When the patient is stabilized, the maintenance dose can be titrated down to the lowest effective dose. The severity of pain is also important in selecting the route of opioid administration. Patients with severe pain should generally be stabilized with intravenous opioids (e.g., morphine infusion) and then converted to an oral regimen (e.g., sustained-release morphine or oxycodone plus rescue doses), if possible. Rapid control of pain provides the patient with emotional comfort as well. For less severe pain, it may be possible to start with a lower dose (e.g., oxycodone/acetaminophen or hydrocodone/acetaminophen, or sustained-release morphine or oxycodone) and titrate up to the desired degree of pain control. The dose should generally be titrated up only after steady-state serum levels have been achieved. Peaks in the degree of analgesia do not correlate with peak serum levels. Duration of analgesia does not necessarily follow the serum-concentration-versus-time curve. Evaluating a regimen at steady state provides a gross indication of the clinical effect achieved when total drug accumulation is at its maximum. The short-acting agents (i.e., morphine and hydromorphone) have a short elimination half-life, so steady state is achieved within 24 hours. At that point, the patient's own report of pain relief may be used as a guide for titrating the dose as indicated.

Longer dosing intervals are usually desirable (e.g., 8–12 hours), if possible, because they allow the patient more freedom and easier compliance with the regimen. In addition, animal models have indicated that longer dosing intervals may be less likely to elicit the rapid development of analgesic tolerance than frequent dosing; however, this has not been well

Table 16-5. Comparison of Opioid Analgesics

Opioid	Equianalgesic Dose (mg)[a]	Route	Usual Oral Starting Dose[b]	Usual Parenteral Starting Dose[b]	Duration (hr)
Codeine Phosphate	130	IM	60 mg q3–4hr	60 mg q2hr	3–4
Codeine Sulfate	200	PO		(IM/SC)	
Hydrocodone	30	PO	10 mg q3–4hr	N/A	3–4
Hydromorphone	1.5 7.5	IV, IM, SC PO, PR	6 mg q3–4hr	1.5 mg q3–4hr	3–4
Morphine Sulfate	10 30	IV, IM, SC PO, PR, SL SR tab	30 mg q3–4hr 90–120 mg q8–24hr	10 mg q3–4hr	3–4
Oxycodone	30	PO, SR tab	10 mg q3–4hr 10–20 mg q8–12hr	N/A	3–4
Oxymorphone	1–1.5 10	IV, IM, SC PR	N/A	1 mg q3–4hr	3–4
Meperidine HCl[c]	75–100 300	IV, IM, SC PO	N/R	100 mg q3hr	2–4
Fentanyl transdermal	100 µg	TRANS	[d]	N/A	72
Methadone HCl	10 15–20	IV, IM, SC PO	20 mg q6–8hr	10 mg q6–8hr	6–8
Propoxyphene[c]	250[e]	PO		N/A	4–5
Levorphanol Tartrate	2 4	IV, IM, SC PO	4 mg q6–8hr	2 mg q6–8hr	4–6

SOURCE: adapted from reference 1. N/A, not applicable. PR, rectal; SL, sublingual; SR tab, sustained-release tablet; N/R, not recommended; TRANS, transdermal.
[a] Equianalgesic doses are not necessarily starting doses, especially with transdermal fentanyl.
[b] Usual starting doses for moderate to severe pain.
[c] Not considered an appropriate choice for managing chronic cancer pain.
[d] Transdermal fentanyl dosage is not calculated as equianalgesic to a single morphine dose. See the package insert for dosing calculations. Doses >25 µg/hr should not be used in opioid-naive patients.
[e] Exceeds received dose.

established in humans. The dosing interval should be scheduled rather than PRN and should reflect consideration of the duration of analgesia for the agent being used (Table 16-5). The use of a PRN dosing interval for the primary pain control regimen is irrational in chronic pain syndromes because it forces the patient to re-experience the pain before receiving the analgesic. In addition, it fails to achieve the desired continuous, uniform pain suppression. A reasonable scheduled dosing interval should be selected and modified in response to the patient's report of duration of analgesia. Although tolerance to opioids in pain treatment is a controversial issue, it is generally not considered a significant issue in cancer pain treatment. Dosage increases, which are necessary, are usually a result of disease progression or other mitigating circumstances rather than the development of tolerance.

Sustained-release morphine products may be dosed every 8–24 hours. In addition, there are sustained-release formulations of oxycodone available for dosing in intervals of 8 or 12 hours. Products with extended dosing intervals are preferred because of their simplicity and the potential to allow the patient to rest without interruption. Sustained-release formulation tablets should never be crushed, split, or chewed; altering the release vehicle may cause a rapid release of the drug into the systemic circulation. Appropriate supplemental doses with short-acting dosage forms (e.g., immediate-release morphine tablets or liquid or hydromorphone tablets) must be made available to manage breakthrough pain as it occurs.

Sustained-release products may display variations in bioequivalence between brand name products. Patients should be monitored when they are converted from one product to another, and therapy should be re-titrated as necessary.

Changes in the drug regimen should be made judiciously when treating patients with impaired renal and hepatic function or when using opioids with long half-lives. Accumulation of drugs with prolonged half-lives or of active drug metabolites may result in toxicity (e.g., respiratory sedation that may not be evident for several days following initiation). Opioids with a short half-life usually reach steady state within 24 hours in patients without profound organ dysfunction and can therefore be titrated rapidly according to pain needs. Methadone and levorphanol have relatively long half-lives (12–16 hours for levorphanol; 24–36 hours for methadone). Careful titration of these products is important because serum levels take 2–3 days for levorphanol and 4–7 days for methadone to reach a steady state and establish the full clinical impact. Patients with renal impairment may accumulate the active metabolites of propoxyphene (norpropoxyphene), meperidine (normeperidine), and morphine (morphine-6-glucuronide).[1,20,26] Meperidine, pentazocine, and propoxyphene have a decreased systemic clearance in cirrhotic patients, but morphine and methadone disposition are not significantly altered in cirrhotic patients.[26]

Breakthrough Pain Analgesic Regimen

The regimen for breakthrough pain is intended to address the patient's need for additional analgesic support during periods of stress or exacerbation of pain. This secondary regimen provides a dosing supplement (or "rescue dose") to the primary analgesic. This method is preferred to modifying an already adequate primary regimen and overcompensating for transient difficult periods. When selecting an agent for the secondary regimen, one should look for a short-acting agent that has a rapid onset and is easy to administer. Immediate-release morphine and hydromorphone are frequently used. The size of the rescue dose depends on the clinical situation. Some general guidelines include dosing with the equivalent of 5–15% of the total normal daily dose or approximately one third of the 12-hour requirement when using sustained-release morphine.[19, 20]

It may be helpful when initiating the secondary regimen (rescue dosing) to have the patient use a pain log to outline when and under what conditions the primary regimen is inadequate. This breakthrough regimen may be added for periods of exacerbation once the primary regimen provides continuous pain suppression under normal levels of activity. The PRN dosing frequency should be restricted so that the secondary regimen does not add significant toxicity to the primary regimen. Oral rescue dosing can be taken up to every 1–2 hours, and parenteral rescue doses can be taken up to every 15–30 minutes. The number of PRN doses should be recorded by the patient in the log so that the progression of the pain can be tracked and the primary regimen adjusted as required. As the requirement for PRN doses increases, or if PRN doses are required consistently each day, a portion of the PRN requirement should be incorporated into the primary regimen as a dose increase. This procedure is analogous to the treatment of diabetes mellitus, in which the requirements of supplemental insulin are added to the primary regimen. A dramatic change in rescue dosing warrants close reevaluation of the primary regimen and an aggressive workup for disease progression.[20]

TOLERANCE, ADDICTION, AND PHYSICAL DEPENDENCE

Tolerance

Tolerance describes the need for increasing analgesic doses to provide the same effect with repeated administration. Often patients report a shortened duration of analgesic effect or progressively less relief after continued administration of an opioid analgesic.[1] These may be signs of analgesic tolerance. Many clinicians believe that clinically significant analgesic tolerance does not usually develop in patients with chronic cancer pain and that decreased effectiveness usually indicates disease progression.[13,19] It is often difficult, however, to make this distinction, and in treating cancer pain, it need not be a major clinical problem. If signs of tolerance develop, the analgesic dose must be increased to re-establish pain control. Tolerance develops at different rates for the various opioid effects. Tolerance to respiratory depression, nausea, and sedation develops rapidly, in contrast to the slow development of tolerance, if any develops at all, to the constipating effect of opioids.[20,24,26]

Because cross-tolerance between different opioids is not complete, switching a patient from one opioid analgesic to an equianalgesic dose of another opioid may result in improved pain control.[27] When changing opioids, the successive regimen usually starts at 50–75% of the equianalgesic dose required on the previous regimen. The dose is then titrated up or down as clinically indicated by the degree of pain control achieved or the appearance of toxicities. The patient should be closely observed for effect, the doses promptly adjusted, and rescue doses made available for breakthrough pain.[27]

Table 16-5 lists the generally accepted equianalgesic doses of parenteral and oral opioid analgesics. However, there is considerable controversy regarding the accuracy of these suggested conversion ratios. There is also variability among individual patients in sensitivity to effects and toxicity. For example, a patient may report severe nausea to one opioid but tolerate an equal analgesic dose of another very well. If nausea and vomiting do not subside following pharmacologic management with antiemetics (e.g., prochlorperazine, haloperidol, or metoclopramide), another opioid regimen should be considered.[1,19,23] In addition, bioavailability may vary widely, especially with morphine and hydromorphone.

Addiction

Addiction, or psychological dependence, is defined as a pattern of compulsive drug use characterized by a continued craving for an opioid and the need to use the opioid for effects other than pain relief. The incidence of addiction is rare in the treatment of acute pain or chronic cancer pain. Drug-seeking behavior (i.e., pseudoaddiction) in patients with severe pain is generally an indication of inadequate analgesic doses or relates to a pre-existing substance abuse disorder. The fear of addiction among cancer patients is unfounded. Unfortunately, societal pressures have heightened the concerns of prescribers and patients, resulting in the undertreatment of many patients with advanced malignancies.

Physical Dependence

Physical dependence is often confused with addiction and tolerance. Physical dependence implies that an abstinence or withdrawal syndrome will occur upon abrupt discontinuation of the opioid or following administration of an opioid antagonist. Signs and symptoms of the withdrawal syndrome include yawning, lacrimation, frequent sneezing, anxiety, agitation, tremors, insomnia, fever, diaphoresis, diarrhea, abdominal cramps, nausea, and vomiting. These symptoms may be described as a flu-like syndrome. It may begin as early as 6–12 hours following the last dose (with short-acting opioids) and peak at 24–72 hours after discontinuation. If patients with cancer require abrupt discontinuation or drastic dose reductions, the opioid abstinence syndrome can be prevented by tapering the opioid on a schedule that provides half the prior daily dose for each of the first 2 days and then reduces the daily dose by 25% every 2 days until the total dose (in morphine equivalents) is 30 mg/day.[1]

ADVERSE EFFECTS

Certain opioid side effects warrant prophylactic therapy because of their common occurrence. Common adverse effects of opioids include constipation, nausea, vomiting, and sedation. Others include confusion, urinary retention, pruritus, dysphoria, euphoria, myoclonus, sleep disturbances, sexual dysfunction, and respiratory depression.[1] Opioid allergies are commonly reported, but true hypersensitivity is rare.

Constipation is one of the most common adverse effects of opioids and requires aggressive management and prophylaxis. Tolerance to this effect of opioids develops very slowly, if at all. Mild constipation may be managed by increasing dietary fiber; however, stimulant laxatives (e.g., senna concentrate, bisacodyl, or hyperosmotic agents, such as lactulose or sorbitol) are usually required with regular dosing of opioids. Stool softeners (e.g., docusate) are of limited usefulness and should not be considered a cornerstone of constipation management. Bulk laxatives should not be used, because they may increase the risk of impaction. Bowel function should be monitored very closely, and laxative therapy should be advanced aggressively as the condition dictates.

Nausea is less predictable and should be treated as it occurs. Because there may be direct medullary stimulation of the chemoreceptor trigger zone, as well as vestibular components to nausea, different antiemetics (e.g., prochlorperazine, haloperidol, or metoclopramide) may be chosen as single agents or in a combination regimen. Opioid-induced nausea is more frequently noted at the initiation of therapy and with dosage increases, and tolerance may develop. Barring these situations, other causes should also be explored (e.g., physiological changes or other medications). Some studies have shown that nausea and vomiting may be worse in ambulatory patients, suggesting that these drugs also alter vestibular sensitivity. Therefore, short-term bed rest may be helpful.[26] In addition, opioid-associated nausea is often caused by constipation. The prokinetic effects of metoclopramide may be helpful in alleviating constipation and its associated nausea. Antiemetics are usually not needed for extended periods, because most patients develop tolerance to this side effect.[1,19,24]

Sedation or confusion may occur in the first 1–2 days following initiation of opioid therapy, or after a significant dosage increase. It may suggest that the opioid dose is excessive, but the effect is usually only transient (2–3 days) if the dose is appropriate. A CNS stimulant may be useful with therapy initiation or change (e.g., starting with caffeinated beverages). Ongoing opioid-induced sedation is usually best treated by reducing the opioid in each dose and increasing the dosing frequency. The desired outcome is continuous pain suppression without sedation significant enough to interfere with the patient's desired level of function. Some patients may require the addition of a CNS stimulant, such as dextroamphetamine or methylphenidate, to increase attentiveness.[19,20,24] Some states prohibit the use of CNS stimulants to increase attentiveness.

Respiratory depression is a concern, particularly among patients that are opioid naive, elderly, or severely debilitated, or who receive excessive (i.e., ≥50%) dosage increases. Patients should be observed closely, but this effect is relatively uncommon among patients in intense pain. Pain is a physiological antagonist to this side effect. If reversal of respiratory depression becomes necessary, naloxone should be carefully titrated to the patient's respiratory rate to avoid withdrawal symptoms or re-emergence of severe pain. Among cancer patients whose opioid doses are carefully titrated, respiratory depression is rare. A dilute solution of naloxone (0.4 mg of naloxone diluted to 10 ml) should be given cautiously (1 ml every 1–2 minutes) to patients receiving opioids on a long-term basis. A severe withdrawal syndrome and return of pain often accompany a full return to alertness. Because naloxone has a short half-life, patients receiving long-acting opioids may require repeated doses of naloxone or an infusion to prevent recurrence of respiratory depression.[1,19,20]

Although commonly reported, true hypersensitivity to opioids is relatively rare. Most often the reported effect is attributable to an extension of the pharmacologic effects of these drugs (i.e., gastrointestinal intolerance, excess sedation, or pruritus) or caused by a nondrug entity in the formulation (e.g., dye or preservative). If a patient has a true allergy to an opioid (bronchoconstriction or anaphylaxis), the risk of cross-resistance can be decreased significantly if a drug is chosen from a different opioid chemical class. Methadone, a diphenylheptane, or fentanyl, a phenylpiperidine, would be a better choice than a morphine congener (phenanthrenes) if a severe allergy to codeine or morphine is reported. Cross-hypersensitivity cannot be completely ruled out, so patients should be closely monitored when using an alternative opioid.[1]

Other adverse effects associated less frequently with opioid use include myoclonus, sexual dysfunction, seizures, delirium, hallucinations, and sleep disturbances. Pruritus and urinary retention occur most frequently with spinal administration of opioids. Opioid-induced myoclonic jerks can be treated with benzodiazepines (e.g., clonazepam 0.25–0.5 mg PO TID) or by switching to a different opioid.[24]

ALTERNATIVE METHODS OF DRUG DELIVERY

A variety of methods for delivering analgesia to patients who cannot tolerate or who fail to respond to oral administration are available. Among these are transdermal administration of fentanyl, sublingual administration of opioids, rectal administration, spinal infusions, and continuous subcutaneous or intravenous infusion of opioids.

Transdermal Administration of Fentanyl

Transdermal fentanyl delivers 25, 50, 75, or 100 µg/hr of drug through a patch applied to the torso for a 72-hour period. This system is an efficacious alternative to oral therapy, but it also has several drawbacks that limit its application in treating cancer pain. With the initial application to the skin, onset of analgesia occurs gradually, with significant pain relief delayed 12–15 hours. The half-life of the system is about 21 hours, so it takes >72 hours to reach steady state, making rapid dose titration difficult. Fentanyl absorption continues for 24 hours once the patch is removed. Although more costly than many comparable oral therapies (e.g., immediate-release morphine sulfate), the patch is less expensive than parenteral therapy. This dosage form is best suited to patients with stable chronic pain who cannot tolerate oral opioids. Nausea, mental clouding, and skin irritation are the most frequent adverse effects of transdermal fentanyl. Other considerations include an increase in absorption by up to 30% in patients with a fever of 102°F and a tendency to become less adherent with oily skin or perspiration. Fentanyl patches should never be cut to titrate a dosage. Cutting the patch alters the barrier membrane, allowing active drug to be in direct contact with the skin, which could result in a large, bolus-type dose.[1]

Sublingual Administration of Opioids

For patients unable to swallow oral dosage forms, soluble tablets or oral concentrate of morphine may be given sublingually.[19,24] Administration by this route is limited by the low concentrations of available formulations and the need for frequent dosing (e.g., every 3–4 hours). Fentanyl citrate can be given buccally for episodic, breakthrough pain.[24]

Rectal Administration of Opioids

Rectal opioid administration results in absorption similar to that of oral opioids. Hydromorphone, oxymorphone, and morphine are commercially available in suppository form. This route is limited by a relatively slow onset of action, pain on insertion, contraindication in patients with diarrhea, and a dosage ceiling created by limited available dosage sizes. In addition, repeated manipulation of the rectal mucosa may introduce an avenue for infection or bleeding in neutropenic or thrombocytopenic patients. Rectal administration of sustained-release morphine tablets has been reported but is not an FDA-approved route of administration. This route may result in erratic absorption and is probably best reserved for patients with no suitable alternative.[19,28,29]

Spinal Administration of Opioids

Dose-dependent analgesia by spinal administration of opioids to patients with pain refractory to more conventional routes of administration has been demonstrated.[30-33] The main indication for long-term administration of intraspinal opioids is intractable pain in the lower part of the body, particularly when pain is bilateral or midline. Morphine is the most commonly used intraspinal drug. Hydromorphone, fentanyl, or sufentanil have also been used to treat cancer pain and may be useful alternatives when a patient experiences side effects from morphine.[32-37] Local anesthetics may be added to spinal opioids and may produce additive analgesia. All drugs given intraspinally should be free of preservatives because preservatives can cause neurotoxicity. Drawbacks to intraspinal administration of opioids include respiratory depression (which may be delayed up to 24 hours after administration), analgesic tolerance, nausea, vomiting, urinary retention, potential for infection at the catheter site, the need for close monitoring when therapy begins and when doses are increased, and pruritus.[38-41] Spinal opiate administration can provide effective analgesia in carefully selected patients, but it requires the care of experienced practitioners and is expensive to initiate and maintain.

Continuous Intravenous or Subcutaneous Administration of Opioids

Intravenous or subcutaneous infusions of opioids provide acceptable mechanisms for pain control in patients who cannot take medications orally. Continuous intravenous infusion provides the most consistent level of analgesia. Subcutaneous administration provides serum concentration levels comparable with those of intravenous doses. When incorporated into a patient-controlled analgesia (PCA) regimen, it provides the patient with a sense of control of their analgesic regimen and allows patients to accommodate transient changes in analgesic requirements.[42,43] High-potency agents, such as morphine and hydromorphone, are preferable for this type of therapy because effective doses can be administered in small volumes. Disadvantages of this modality include the need for experienced clinician support, irritation and induration at the infusion site, expensive pumps and supplies, and a limit to the volume that can be administered (i.e., 2–4 ml/hr for subcutaneous route).

Intravenous or subcutaneous infusion of opioids may benefit[1]:

- patients with persistent nausea and vomiting;
- patients with severe dysphagia or swallowing disorders;
- patients with delirium, confusion, stupor, or other mental status changes that contraindicate oral administration because of concerns about pulmonary aspiration in an unprotected airway;
- patients on high doses of oral medications that require numerous tablets;
- patients who experience undesirable side effects from each dose of a PRN medication; or
- patients who require rapid incremental doses of analgesia.

If continuous intravenous infusion must be used on a long-term basis, a permanent or long-term central catheter is desirable because of the risk of infection and infiltration at peripheral sites.

ADJUVANT DRUGS

Adjuvant drugs are those that (1) enhance the effects of opioid or nonopioid analgesics, (2) have independent analgesic activity in certain situations, or (3) treat concurrent symptoms that exacerbate pain (Table 16-3). Despite optimal prophylaxis and management of adverse effects, some patients do not achieve a satisfactory balance between pain relief and side effects. Adjuvant agents may be considered for their potential to add concurrent relief from pain with an acceptable side effect profile. Adjuvant agents are only useful in treating certain pain syndromes (e.g., neuropathic, bone, or visceral pain). These agents also may be helpful in relieving the anxiety, depression, and nausea that frequently accompany pain.

Adjuvant drugs are not without adverse effects. Therefore, practical guidelines for their use include:

- fully evaluating the most effective, least toxic therapy first;
- streamlining the existing regimen before adding adjuvants;
- administering adjuvants with caution to elderly patients because they may be more sensitive to the adverse effects.

Antidepressants

Tricyclic antidepressant agents (TCAs) potentiate opioid analgesia, presumably by potentiation of serotonergic mechanisms and by direct analgesic effects. In addition, they improve analgesia by their effects on mood and their sedative-hypnotic properties. They are useful in the treatment of chronic neuropathic and neuralgic pain, migraine and tension headaches, and other chronic pain syndromes.[44,45] In managing cancer pain, TCAs are indicated for neuropathic pain, psychiatric depression, and insomnia. Amitriptyline has commonly been used; however, among the TCAs it is often one of the most poorly tolerated, usually because of its potent anticholinergic and sedative effects. Nortriptyline and desipramine are alternative agents that may be better tolerated by cancer patients. The adjunctive analgesic effects of TCAs may be realized at lower doses than typically required for the antidepressant effect (e.g., amitriptyline 25–150 mg/day) in most adjunctive roles. Pain reduction usually begins within 1–2 weeks and peaks at 4–6 weeks with antidepressant agents.[1,19,20]

Anticonvulsants

The anticonvulsants have been useful in treating neuropathic pain, especially when the pain is lancinating or burning.[1,46,47] Phenytoin, carbamazepine, valproate, and clonazepam suppress abnormal neuronal firing activity in nociceptive pathways after nerve injury. In cancer pain, carbamazepine has been used to manage the acute shock-like neuralgic pain in the cranial and cervical nerve regions caused by tumor involvement or surgical-, chemotherapy-, or radiation-induced nerve injury. Carbamazepine should be used cautiously in cancer patients because it is known to cause leukopenia and thrombocytopenia.[1] The doses of the anticonvulsants in pain syndromes are similar to those used for seizure control. Care must be taken to avoid sudden withdrawal because this may induce seizures.

Corticosteroids

Corticosteroids are probably the most common adjuvant agents used in alleviating suffering in advanced malignancy. These agents improve mood and appetite, relieve pain caused by bone involvement, reduce spinal cord and intracranial pressure, have antiemetic activity, and reduce inflammation in nerve or soft tissue involvement. The high incidence of adverse effects remains a major drawback to this class of drugs.

Bone Pain Adjuvants

Osteoclast-induced bone resorption by the tumor is the likely cause of bone pain and may result in osteoporosis, hypercalcemia, microfractures, or pathological fractures. The bisphosphonates (etidronate and pamidronate), calcitonin, and the radiopharmaceutical strontium-89 are potentially useful adjuvants in treating severe bone pain, a frequent complication of bone metastases. Response to these agents may be variable and additional studies are warranted to determine criteria that may predict a response to these agents.[1] Table 16-3 contains a more complete list of adjuvant drugs used to treat cancer pain.

Nerve Blocks

Administering local anesthetics directly at the source or along the nociceptive pathways is the basis for nerve-blocking strategies. Nerve blocks help break the pain cycle and provide temporary relief until other, longer-term measures can be implemented. Nerve blocks are specialized procedures that should be undertaken only by experienced physicians. Some commonly used nerve-blocking agents, with their doses and duration of action, are listed in Table 16-6. Epinephrine can be used to retard the spread of anesthetics and facilitate localization of the anesthetic effect. Care should be taken to avoid accidental intravenous administration.

AHCPR GUIDELINES FOR THE MANAGEMENT OF CANCER PAIN

AHCPR has published clinical practice guidelines for the management of cancer pain. This collaborative effort was accomplished by an interdisciplinary panel of experts in an attempt to correct the problem of inadequate cancer pain treatment. These guidelines were devised for practitioners and patients, and single copies are available, currently at no cost.[1] Topics covered in this comprehensive guide include initial assessment, pharmacologic treatment, administration of medications, side effects of medications, adjuvant medications, cognitive-behavioral interventions, and discussion of other, more invasive palliative techniques. These guidelines call for a collaborative, interdisciplinary approach to the care of patients with cancer pain; an individualized pain-control plan developed and agreed upon by patients, their families, and practitioners; ongoing assessment and reassessment of the patient's pain; the use of both drug and nondrug therapies to prevent or control pain; and explicit institutional policies on the management of cancer pain, with clear lines of responsibility for pain management and for monitoring its effectiveness.

SUMMARY

The pain experience of cancer patients is a complex, multifactorial process. The vast majority of cancer pain can be well controlled with simple, readily available therapies. Overcoming the barriers that impede effective therapy, understanding the characteristics of cancer pain, and improving the use of analgesic agents for cancer pain management are important clinical challenges.

Table 16-6. Nerve-Blocking Agents

Agent	Concentration (%) Spinal Block Infiltration	Maximum Dose (mg/kg)	Speed of Onset	Duration of Action
Procaine	1.5–0.2 / 0.05	12	Moderate	Short
12-Chloroprocaine	1.0–0.2 / 0.5	15	Fast	Very short
Lidocaine	0.5–1.0 / 0.25	6	Fast	Moderate
Mepivacaine	0.5–1.0 / 0.25	6	Moderate	Moderate
Prilocaine	0.5–1.0 / 0.25	6	Moderate	Moderate
Tetracaine	0.1–0.2 / 0.05	2	Very slow	Long
Bupivacaine	0.25–0.5 / 0.05	2	Fast	Long
Etidocaine	0.5–1.0 / 0.1	2	Very fast	Long

REFERENCES

1. Jacox AK, Carr DB, Payne R, et al. Management of cancer pain. Clinical practice guideline no. 9. Rockville, MD: Agency for Health Care Policy and Research; 1994 [AHCPR publication no. 94-0592].
2. Jacox AK, Carr DB, Payne R. New clinical-practice guidelines for the management of pain in patients with cancer. *N Engl J Med* 1994;330:651–5.
3. Cleeland CS, Gonin R, Hatfield AK, et al. Pain and its treatment in outpatients with metastatic cancer. *N Engl J Med* 1994;330:592–6.
4. Ad Hoc Committee on Cancer Pain of the American Society of Clinical Oncology. Cancer pain assessment and treatment curriculum guidelines. *J Clin Oncol* 1992;10:1976–82.
5. Foley KM. Pain syndromes in patients with cancer. In: Bonica JJ, Ventafridda V, Fink RB, et al., editors. *Advances in Pain Research and Therapy*. Vol. 2. New York: Raven Pr; 1979. p. 59–75.
6. Joranson DE. Are health-care reimbursement policies a barrier to acute and cancer pain management? *J Pain Symptom Manage* 1994;9:244–53
7. International Association for the Study of Pain, Subcommittee on Taxonomy. Part II. Pain terms: a current list with definitions and notes on usage. *Pain* 1979;6:249–52 [updated 1982, 1986].
8. Foley KM. The treatment of cancer pain. *N Engl J Med* 1985;313:84–95.
9. Daut FL, Cleeland CS. The prevalence and severity of pain in cancer. *Cancer* 1982;50:1913–8.
10. Kanner RM, Foley KM. Patterns of narcotic use in a cancer pain clinic. *Ann NY Acad Sci* 1981;362:161–72.
11. Cleeland CS. The impact of pain on patients with cancer. *Cancer* 1984;54:2635–41.
12. Bonica JJ. Cancer pain. In: Bonica JJ, ed. *Pain*. New York: Raven Pr; 1980. p. 335–62.
13. Ashburn MA, Lipman AG. Management of pain in the cancer patient. *Anesth Analg* 1993;76:402–16.
14. Carlsson AM. Assessment of chronic pain. I. Aspects of the reliability of the Visual Analog Scale. *Pain* 1983;16:87–101.
15. Melzack R. The McGill Pain Questionnaire: major properties and scoring methods. *Pain* 1975;1:277–99.
16. Graham C, Bond SS, Gerlsousch MM, et al. Use of the McGill Pain Questionnaire in the assessment of cancer pain: replicability and consistency. *Pain* 1980;8:377–87.
17. Grossman SA, Sheidler VR, Swedeen K, et al. Correlation of patient and caregiver ratings of cancer pain. *J Pain Symptom Manage* 1991;6:53–7.
18. Portenoy RK, Hagen NA. Breakthrough pain: definition and management. *Oncology Supplement* 1989; 3:25–30.
19. Levy MH. Pharmacological management of cancer pain. *Semin Oncol* 1994;21:718–39.
20. Cherny NI, Portenoy RK. The management of cancer pain. *CA Cancer J Clin* 1994;44:262–303.
21. Ferreira SH. Prostaglandins, aspirin-like drugs, and analgesia. *Nature New Biol* 1972;240:200–3.
22. Galasko CSB. Mechanisms of bone destruction in the development of skeletal metastases. *Nature* 1976;263:507–10.
23. Watson CP, Evans RJ, Reed K, et al. Amitriptyline versus placebo in postherpetic neuralgia. *Neurology* 1982;32:671–3.
24. Levy MH. Pharmacologic treatment of cancer pain. *N Engl J Med* 1996;335:1124–32.
25. Kaiko RF, Foley KM, Grabinsky PY, et al. Central nervous system excitatory effects of meperidine in cancer patients. *Ann Neurol* 1983;13:180–5.
26. Inturrisi CE. Management of cancer pain. Pharmacology and principles of management. *Cancer* 1989;63:2308–20.
27. Houde RW. The use and misuse of narcotics in the treatment of chronic pain. *Adv Neurol* 1974;4:527–36.
28. Kaiko RF, Cronin C, Healy N, et al. Bioavailability of rectal and oral MS Contin [abstract] *Proc Am Soc Clin Oncol* 1989;8(Suppl):336.
29. Maloney CM, Kesner, RK, Klein G, et al. The rectal administration of MS Contin: clinical implications of use in end stage cancer. *Am J Hosp Care* 1989;6:34–5.
30. Wang JK, Nauss LE, Thomas JE. Pain relief by intrathecally applied morphine in man. *Anesthesiology* 1979;50:149–51.
31. Behar M, Olshwang D, Magora F, et al. Epidural morphine in the treatment of pain. *Lancet* 1979;1:527–9.
32. Cousins MJ, Mather LE. Intrathecal and epidural administration of opioids. *Anesthesiology* 1984;61:276–310.
33. Yaksh TL. Spinal opiate analgesia: characteristics and principles of action. *Pain* 1981;11:293–346.
34. Nurchi G. Use of intraventricular and intrathecal morphine in intractable pain associated with cancer. *Neurosurgery* 1984;15:801–3.
35. Payne R. Sole epidural and intrathecal narcotics and peptides in the management of cancer pain. *Med Clin North Am* 1987;71:313–27.
36. Tansen A, Sjostron S, Hartvid P, et al. CSF and plasma kinetics of morphine and meperidine after epidural administration [abstract]. *Anesthesiology* 1983;59:A196.
37. Glynn CJ, Mather LE, Cousins MJ, et al. Peridural meperidine in humans: analgesic response, pharmacokinetics, and transmission into CSF. *Anesthesiology* 1981;55:520–6.
38. Greenberg HA, Taren J, Ensminger WD, et al. Benefit from and tolerance to continuous intrathecal infusion of morphine for intractable cancer pain. *J Neurosurg* 1982;57:360–4.
39. Coombs DW, Saunders RL, Lachance D, et al. Intrathecal morphine tolerance: use of intrathecal clonidine, DADLE, and intraventricular morphine. *Anesthesiology* 1985;62:358–63.
40. Gustafsson LL, Schildt B, Jacobsen X. Adverse effects of extradural and intrathecal opiates: report of a nationwide survey in Sweden. *Br J Anaesth* 1982;54:479–85.
41. Bromage PR, Camporesi EM, Durant PAC, et al. Nonrespiratory side effects of epidural morphine. *Anesth Analg* 1982;51:490–5.
42. Mauskop A, Coyle N, Maggard J, et al. Continuous subcutaneous infusions of opiates in cancer patient with pain: safety and efficacy [abstract]. *Proc Am Soc Clin Oncol* 1985;4:39.
43. Drexel A, Dzien A, Spiegel RW, et al. Treatment of severe cancer pain by low-dose continuous subcutaneous morphine. *Pain* 1989;36:169–76.
44. Butler S. Present status of tricyclic antidepressants in chronic pain therapy. In: Benedetti C, Chapman CR, Moricca G, editors. *Advances in Pain Research and Therapy*. Vol. 7. New York: Raven Pr; 1984. p. 173–97.
45. Rosenblatt RM, Reich J, Dehringt D. Tricyclic antidepressants in the treatment of depression and chronic pain: analysis of the supporting evidence. *Anesth Analg* 1984;63:1025–32.

46. Crill WE. Carbamazepine. *Ann Intern Med* 1973;79:844–7.
47. Foley KM. Management of cancer pain. In: DeVita VT, Hellman S, Rosenberg SA, editors. *Cancer: Principles & Practice of Oncology*. 4th ed. Philadelphia, PA: JB Lippincott; 1993. p. 2417–48.

SELF-STUDY QUESTIONS

1. The percentage of cancer patients with advanced metastatic disease who suffer persistent moderate to severe pain is:

    a. 10–20%
    b. 20–40%
    c. 40–60%
    d. 60–90%
    e. 100%

2. The key person(s) in assessing and formulating an effective cancer pain analgesic regimen include:

    a. the physician.
    b. the patient.
    c. other medical disciplines (i.e., nurses and pharmacists).
    d. the patient's family or primary caregivers.
    e. all of the above

3. Most pain associated with cancer is:

    a. only fully managed in an inpatient setting.
    b. managed on an outpatient basis.
    c. best referred early to a hospice program.
    d. unmanageable regardless of the setting.
    e. none of the above.

4. When assessing a patient with pain, which of the following factors may cause a patient to hide or downplay their pain symptoms:

    a. concern that admission of pain means confirmation their disease is worse.
    b. fear of becoming "addicted."
    c. fear of disappointing their physician or being labeled a "complainer."
    d. side effects of the analgesic regimen are bothersome.
    e. all of the above.

5. The use of a nonopioid/opioid combination analgesic product in treating cancer pain:

    a. is usually safe even in very high doses.
    b. exposes the patient unnecessarily to the risk of side effects of two different drugs.
    c. results in additive analgesia and may reduce the side effects of higher doses of either single agent.
    d. eliminates the risk of addiction or physical dependence.

6. In assessing chronic cancer pain:

    a. always verify symptoms by measuring vital signs (indices of autonomic nervous system activity).
    b. the need for higher doses always signals disease progression.
    c. the patient's own report of pain generally is the most reliable assessment.
    d. try very small dosage increases to verify patient's report of inadequate analgesia.
    e. higher doses usually indicate psychological dependence (addiction).

7. What drug combinations are generally selected for primary pain control in patients with mild pain?

    a. opioid agonist/antagonist
    b. nonsteroidal anti-inflammatory drug (NSAID) or acetaminophen/opioid agonist
    c. corticosteroid/opioid agonist
    d. NSAID or acetaminophen/antidepressant
    e. corticosteroid/opioid antagonist

8. Longer dosing intervals are usually desired in a pain management regimen.

    a. true
    b. false

9. Short-acting opioids are better suited for the management of breakthrough pain.

    a. true
    b. false

10. Meperidine should not be used if continuous opioid use is anticipated because:

    a. it has a long duration of action.
    b. its toxic metabolite, normeperidine, may accumulate.
    c. it is "weaker" than other opioids.
    d. it is too expensive.
    e. its addiction potential is much higher.

11. Constipation is a common side effect associated with opioid administration, but:

    a. tolerance to this side effect occurs rapidly.
    b. it is usually always treatable with minor diet changes.
    c. it is a side effect of the malignancy rather than the drug, because opioids stimulate peristalsis.
    d. it merely indicates that the patient is not eating well.
    e. it is best prevented by dietary modifications and stimulant laxatives taken on a regular basis.

12. Sedation is frequently associated with opioid administration and:

    a. may occur initially, but tolerance to this effect develops rapidly.
    b. indicates an overdose, so the patient should be given an opioid antagonist.
    c. usually indicates that the patient is on other central nervous system depressants.
    d. probably indicates that the person is addicted.
    e. most often indicates that the patient is dosing more frequently than directed.

13. Which of the following statements is true?

    a. Chronic pain rarely affects the patient's psychological make-up.
    b. Acute pain has an identifiable cause that is likely unrelated to the patient's disease.
    c. Acute pain should elicit an assessment that may reveal a reversible noxious pain process.
    d. Chronic pain is probably caused by a readily reversible noxious process that remains undiscovered.
    e. Chronic and acute pain rarely occur in the same patient.

14. The following are barriers to proper cancer pain management, except:

    a. ignorance of the pharmacology of potent opioids by providers.
    b. fear of being labeled a "bad patient" if pain is reported.
    c. long-acting dosage forms.
    d. denial of symptoms to avoid facing possible disease progression.
    e. regulatory review of opioid prescriptions.

15. A mixed opioid agonist/antagonist is a good choice for cancer patients because they prevent addiction.

    a. true
    b. false

16. Opioid tolerance and physical dependence are expected with long-term opioid use and should not be confused with addiction.

    a. true
    b. false

17. The oral route of administration of analgesics:

    a. is not preferred, because of erratic absorption.
    b. is the most convenient and cost-effective route.
    c. should be given on an as-needed (PRN) basis except in cases of extremely severe pain.
    d. is subject to higher abuse potential.
    e. is rarely effective in advanced cancer.

18. The World Health Organization Ladder for titration of analgesic therapy:

    a. stresses early initiation of opioid therapy because opioid use is inevitable.
    b. suggests adding NSAIDs or acetaminophen when opioids are no longer effective.
    c. suggests avoiding combination products because more side effects will surely result.
    d. suggests around-the-clock dosing for persistent cancer-related pain.
    e. suggests using codeine and hydrocodone even for severe pain because they are less addictive than other opioids.

19. The following are adverse effects associated with NSAIDs use by cancer patients:

    a. fever production that mimics infection.
    b. gastric ulceration.
    c. renal dysfunction.
    d. bleeding.
    e. numerous potential drug interactions.

Chapter 17

Psychosocial and Palliative Care

Rowena N. Schwartz, Pharm.D.
Associate Professor of Pharmacy and Therapeutics
University of Pittsburgh School of Pharmacy
Coordinator, Pharmacy Programs
University of Pittsburgh Cancer Institute
Pittsburgh, Pennsylvania

Psycho-oncology	311
Depression	311
Management of Depression	312
Anxiety	313
Management of Anxiety	314
Confusion	314
Management of Confusion	315
Sleep Disorders	316
Management of Sleep Disorders	316
Dyspnea	316
Management of Dyspnea	317
Hospice Care	317
Socioeconomic Considerations	318
Summary	319
References	319
Self-Study Questions	320

Patients with cancer often experience multiple physical and nonphysical symptoms that affect their function and/or sense of well-being. The effect these symptoms have depends on personality, coping ability, social support, and medical factors, but these symptoms should be a primary consideration in the overall care of patients with cancer. The impact of the diagnosis of cancer may change during the course of the disease. Acute responses to cancer include shock, disbelief, fears about the future, sadness, anxiety, and feelings of hopelessness and/or helplessness, or a combination of these emotions. Responses to the diagnosis of cancer may change during the course of the disease and with time, but they may still affect a patient's ability to accept information and make decisions.

An important aspect of providing pharmaceutical care to a patient with cancer is understanding the impact treatment and treatment decisions have on the patient's quality of life. Many of the physical symptoms caused by cancer and cancer therapy affect quality of life, such as pain and nausea, and are addressed elsewhere in this book. This chapter discusses challenges involved in the palliative care of patients with cancer, focusing on the psychological issues that commonly face patients and health care practitioners during the course of the disease.

Palliative care has been described by the World Health Organization as

> *the active total care of patients whose disease is not responsive to curative treatment. Control of their pain, of other symptoms, and psychological, social and spiritual problems are paramount. The goal of palliative care is the achievement of the best quality of life for patients and their families. Many aspects of palliative care are applicable earlier in the course of the illness in conjunction with anticancer treatment.*[1]

The goals of palliative care are to alleviate suffering and to optimize the patient's quality of life until and through death. The intensity of suffering is determined by the number and severity of the factors that diminish quality of life. The physical and psychological symptoms that contribute to patient distress are numerous but can be complicated by distress caused by other concerns (Table 17-1).[2]

Palliative care includes the provision of care to patients with active, progressive, or advanced disease. Palliative care does not attempt to hasten or postpone death. Management of symptoms should be integrated into overall care to allow the patient to live as actively as possible until death and to help support the family and/or caregivers during the patient's illness and their own bereavement. Palliative care integrates the psychosocial and spiritual aspects of care; as providers of care, pharmacists should consider all these aspects when developing and implementing a pharmaceutical care plan.

Table 17-1. Factors Contributing to Patient Distress

Physical Symptoms
- pain
- lack of energy
- drowsiness
- xerostomia
- nausea
- feeling of fullness/bloating
- constipation/diarrhea
- itching
- dizziness
- problems with sexual interest/function
- difficulty swallowing

Psychological Symptoms
- anxiety
- depression
- sleep disturbances
- irritability
- impaired concentration
- nightmares
- delirium

Existential Concerns
- disrupted or distorted personal integrity
  - changes in body image
  - changes in body function
  - changes in intellectual function
  - increased dependency
- distress from retrospection
  - unfullfilled aspiration
  - deprecation of the value of previous achievements
  - remorse from unresolved guilt
- distress from future concerns
  - separation
  - hopelessness
  - futility
  - meaninglessness
  - concerns about death
- religious concerns
  - illness as a punishment
  - fear of divine retribution
  - fear of a void

SOURCE: reference 2.

After completing this chapter, the reader will be able to:
1. Discuss the concept of palliative care as it relates to the provision of care to the patient with cancer.
2. Describe the symptoms of depression in the patient with cancer and outline treatment options.
3. Discuss the types of anxiety seen in the patient with cancer and outline the treatment options.
4. Describe the pharmacotherapy issues in the management of confusion.

5. Discuss the assessment of sleep disturbances in the patient with cancer.
6. Outline the management of breathlessness in the patient with cancer.

PSYCHO-ONCOLOGY

The nonphysical problems associated with cancer are numerous. These issues can be attributed to the psychological distress caused by a progressive fatal illness; the disruption of personal, social, and work relationships produced by illness; and the demands imposed by cancer therapies. Nonphysical issues can be caused in part by the increasing reliance of a patient on family members and friends for care.[3] The stress of illness, including the stress of diagnosis and management of cancer, may precipitate reactive or situational distress, sadness, and grief. Two of the most common psychological disturbances of patients with cancer are depression and anxiety.[4] Although these responses to a diagnosis of cancer may be expected, recognition of pathological potential, complete assessment, and management of these disorders are often overlooked.

Depression

The reported frequency of depression among cancer patients ranges from 1.5 to 50%.[4-6] The prevalence of depression varies with the stage of disease, site of cancer, hospitalization, and the patient's physical performance status. Patients with compromised physical performance status are more likely to experience depression than those with a high level of functional performance.[7] Interpreting differences in the prevalence of depression by tumor site is difficult because published studies use a variety of diagnostic methods, definitions of depression, and disease status (i.e., stage of disease versus duration of disease). Patients with the highest risk of depression appear to be those with a history of an affective disorder, a history of alcoholism, pain that is not effectively managed, a concurrent illness, and/or who are taking medications that may produce symptoms of depression.[8] Cancer patients with a high level of disability and advanced illness also appear to have an increased incidence of depression.[7] Other risk factors that may predispose patients with cancer to the development of depression include social isolation, recent loss of family members or physical ability, tendency toward pessimism, and socioeconomic pressures.

Medications may also contribute to depression. Medications that are used to treat the cancer (e.g., interferons and corticosteroids), medications used to treat cancer-related or cancer therapy-related symptoms (e.g., opiates and benzodiazepines), and medications required to manage concurrent medical problems may cause or contribute to depression.

Research into the biological alterations associated with unipolar depression has identified biological markers that reflect the underlying pathophysiological processes of depression.[9] One of the best-characterized markers is hyperactivity of the hypothalamus-pituitary-adrenal (HPA) axis. The HPA axis hyperactivity appears to be induced through secretion of cytokines, such as the interleukins. This proposed biological alteration has not been well characterized in patients with cancer, but further study may aid in the standardization of methods to diagnose and manage patients.

Treatment of depression includes recognition, appropriate assessment, and work-up of all symptoms and possible etiologies. The difficulty in identifying depression in patients with cancer is that the reactive manifestations of grief that accompany an anticipated loss are similar to the symptoms of depression. Normal responses to a loss range from sadness to an adjustment disorder with a depressed mood to a major depression. Clinical evaluation is essential, but evaluation of cancer patients is complicated by the effects of the disease and its management. Symptoms of the cancer or cancer therapy may mimic the somatic or functional symptoms of depression. Fatigue, weight loss, anorexia, and insomnia may be caused by the cancer or cancer therapy or may be signs of depression. More useful indicators of depression in the patient with cancer are the severity of dysphoric mood; feelings of hopelessness, guilt, or worthlessness; and the presence of suicidal thoughts.[8] The difficulty of determining the extent of depression in the patient with cancer may make it difficult to determine an appropriate management strategy.

The clinical evaluation of any patient with depression includes an assessment of potential contributing factors, and the choice of factors may complicate the diagnosis. Identification of these factors is helpful when designing an appropriate plan of patient care. Metabolic, endocrine, and neurological disorders may contribute to depression. Brain metastases from the primary cancer, concurrent paraneoplastic syndromes, and metabolic complications (e.g., hypercalcemia) may present as depression and should be evaluated and managed prior to initiation of antidepressant therapy.

One of the symptoms most commonly associated with cancer and cancer therapy is fatigue,[10] which can contribute to depression. Fatigue, a subjective feeling that may be multifactorial in nature, can manifest in a patient's concentration, activity, appearance, and speech.[11] When evaluating depression in a patient with cancer, assessing the extent and impact of the patient's fatigue is essential. Management of fatigue can decrease some of the symptoms of depression[12]; treatment strategies should be guided by the etiology of fatigue, if it can be determined (e.g., administration of erythropoietin in a patient with anemia[13]). Review, evaluation, and management of medical conditions that may cause fatigue should be a routine part of the assessment in management of depression in the patient with cancer.

Medications should also be reviewed in the context of the patient's overall well-being. Medications that may contribute to depression or a decreased quality of life should be carefully evaluated and, if appropriate, adjusted to alleviate the symptoms. For example, corticosteroids cause mood changes, including depression, but they may be necessary for the optimal management of a cancer-related spinal cord compression. Discontinuation of corticosteroids may not be reasonable, but a reduction of the dose may be appropriate when all aspects of the patient's care are considered.

Management of Depression

The treatment of depression may include psychotherapy, pharmacotherapy, or a combination of both. Psychotherapy emphasizes the use of coping skills and behavioral techniques for the management of depression. Psychotherapeutic interventions have been shown to reduce the psychological distress and depression of cancer patients.[14] Cognitive-behavioral interventions, such as relaxation and distraction, have been shown to be effective in reducing symptoms in mild or moderate depression. Family and friends may benefit from taking part in therapy or individual counseling. Psychopharmacologic interventions are the mainstay in the treatment of cancer patients whose severe symptoms meet the criteria for major depressive episodes.[14]

The drug therapy of depression in patients with cancer mimics the pharmacotherapy of patients without other major illnesses. Historically, tricyclic antidepressant agents (TCAs) have been used as first-line therapy for depression in patients with cancer, based on numerous studies of physically healthy and ill patients. The side effects of TCAs can limit their use. Anticholinergic effects (e.g., dry mouth, constipation, blurred vision, urinary retention, dizziness, and tachycardia) can be problematic for patients on concurrent medications with additive effects. Dry mouth can be especially difficult for patients with certain cancers (e.g., head and neck cancers) or patients receiving radiation therapy. Sedation associated with some TCAs can be additive with medications used in the management of patients with cancer (e.g., opiates for pain management and phenothiazines for management of nausea and vomiting).

The proper dose of an antidepressant agent for a patient with cancer, as for all patients, is determined by individual response and effects. General recommendations for dosing of TCAs in ill patients suggests a low initial dose, given at bedtime, followed by increases every 1–3 days until a therapeutic benefit is seen. The maximum doses tolerated by ill patients may be lower than those tolerated by healthy patients.[15] These same recommendations are appropriate for ill patients with cancer, but they may be too conservative for cancer patients with no other medical problems. Studies of acutely depressed patients have demonstrated a correlation between antidepressant effect and the plasma concentrations of TCAs such as nortriptyline, desipramine, imipramine, and amitriptyline. Although the patient's clinical response should guide dosage adjustments, plasma level monitoring may be appropriate for patients with an inadequate response, serious or persistent adverse effects, or suspected noncompliance, or when pharmacokinetic drug interactions are suspected (Table 17-2).[16]

Selective serotonin reuptake inhibitors (SSRIs) are widely used in the management of depression, including the management of depression in patients with cancer, although few clinical studies support their use as first-line agents. One advantage of SSRIs is that they produce fewer anticholinergic and cardiovascular adverse effects than TCAs do. The side effects of SSRIs are also usually better tolerated than those of TCAs.

An initial concern with the use of fluoxetine was its apparent anorectic activity, but there appears to be less cause for concern with other agents of this class (e.g., fluvoxamine, paroxetine, and sertraline). Gastrointestinal side effects of SSRIs include nausea, vomiting, and diarrhea. These side effects can be a complicating factor in patients with disease- and/or treatment-related nausea and vomiting.

Headache, insomnia, a brief period of anxiety, and fatigue are also seen with SSRIs. Any of these symptoms should be evaluated and not simply attributed to the effects of the cancer or cancer therapy. Another potential concern are the drug-drug interactions that may occur between SSRIs and other drugs metabolized through the cytochrome P-450 system (e.g., warfarin). When SSRIs are initiated, concurrent medications should be evaluated for potential interactions.

Alprazolam decreases the depressive component of some anxiety disorders and has therefore been used in the management of mixed depressive-anxiety disorders.

The sympathomimetic stimulants are also used in the management of depression, but their use is somewhat controversial.[17] Stimulants have a rapid onset of action and improve attention, concentration, and overall performance on neuropsychological testing among the ill.[18] With prolonged use, tolerance develops and dose adjustments or alternative drug therapy are required, based on the patient's response.

Agents such as dextroamphetamine have been shown to improve mood and appetite in patients in the terminal phase of their illness. They have also been recommended for patients unable to tolerate TCAs and for patients with opiate-related daytime sedation. Methylphenidate has been evaluated in the treatment of depression in the physically ill elderly. Most clinical trials suggest a starting dose of 2.5–5 mg PO as a morning dose with a second dose at noon.[18-20] Doses can be slowly increased every 2–3 days to a maximum of 40 mg/day.

Side effects, such as nervousness, overstimulation, insomnia, increase in blood pressure, and tremor, may limit their use in patients with multiple medical problems. The availability of SSRIs may limit the necessity of using the sympathomimetic stimulants for depression.

Clinical trials of the newer antidepressant agents in patients with cancer are limited, but this scarcity of data should not exclude their use by patients that may benefit from their different side effect profile. Antidepressant therapy should be individualized on the basis of patient-specific factors. Consideration should be given to a patient's symptoms, as well as medical and psychological problems, when choosing an antidepressant agent. A single agent may be able to simplify drug

Table 17-2. Adult Dosages for Antidepressant Medications

Name	Suggested Therapeutic Plasma Concentration (ng/ml)	Initial Dosage (mg/day)	Dose Range (mg/day)
Tricyclics			
amitriptyline	120–250[a]	25–75	100–300
clomipramine		25	100–250
desipramine	125–300	25–75	100–300
doxepin	110–250[a]	25–75	100–300
imipramine	200–300[a]	25–75	100–300
nortriptyline	50–150	25–50	100–300
protriptyline	70–240	10–20	15–60
trimipramine		25–75	100–300
Dibenzoxazepine			
amoxapine	200–400[a]	50–150	100–400
Tetracyclic			
maprotiline	200–300[a]	25–75	100–225
Triazolopyridines			
nefazodone		200	300–600
trazadone		50–150	150–400
Aminoketone			
bupropion	50–100	200	300–450
Selective Serotonin Reuptake Inhibitors			
fluoxetine		10–20	10–80
fluvoxamine		50	50–300
paroxetine		20	20–50
sertraline		50	100–200
Serotonin/Norepinephrine Reuptake Inhibitor			
venlafaxine		75	75–375

SOURCE: references 4 and 16.
[a]Parent drug plus metabolite.

therapy while treating depression and another problem. For example, a patient with complaints of depression and anxiety may benefit from the triazolobenzodiazepine alprazolam. Patients with complaints of neuropathic pain and depression may receive relief from both symptoms with the initiation of a TCA. Patients with depression and problems with insomnia may benefit from a sedating TCA such as trazodone or amitriptyline. Medications should be optimized and, if possible, simplified when treating depression in patients with multiple medical problems.

The side effect profile of a specific antidepressant should be considered for each patient. The goal is to optimize benefit from the antidepressant while minimizing any unwanted side effects. A patient with chronically low blood pressure may have difficulty with the orthostatic hypotension seen with imipramine. After any agent is initiated, the side effect profile should be evaluated for the patient. Drug therapy should be modified if side effects are problematic, because palliative care focuses on the total care of the patient.

Anxiety

Anxiety, one of the most prevalent psychiatric complaints of the ill, is often unrecognized or not evaluated in the patient with cancer. Anxiety may be viewed by patients, families, and the health care team as a normal response to the fears and uncertainties associated with cancer, death, possible dependence, disability, and disruption of life and may therefore remain unaddressed. The frequency of anxiety in adult cancer patients has been reported to be as high as 44%; significant anxiety has been reported in 23%.[21,22] Anxiety in the patient with cancer may be a situational or reactive response to the stressors of cancer and its treatment. It may be caused by medical or physiological symptoms such as pain or insomnia, or it may be related to a pre-existing anxiety disorder (e.g., phobias, panic disorders, or chronic anxiety disorders) that is exacerbated by the medical illness. The patient experiencing anxiety may describe a feeling of tension, fear, dread, apprehension, distraction, and the inability to relax or may display subjective and/or physical symptoms.[23] Some of the more common physiological changes that may be present are listed in Table 17-3.[23] Physical or somatic manifestations of anxiety often overshadow psychological or cognitive symptoms in patients with advanced disease and may be the initial presenting symptom.[24] The high incidence of anxiety among patients with cancer requires a high level of scrutiny for this problem. Any complaints of anxiety should be evaluated and managed as early as possible.

Reactive anxiety is the most common anxiety disorder among cancer patients, occurring in as many as one third of these patients. The level of reactive anxiety seen in patients with cancer exceeds what is regarded as a normal and adaptive response to crisis brought on by illness.[25] Reactive anxiety is often seen in conjunction with depression. The symptoms of reactive depression are seen at crisis or transition points in the course of the disease: time of diagnosis, initiation of therapy, change in therapy, surgery, or in the terminal stages of the disease.

Another common type of anxiety among patients with cancer is anxiety caused by a direct effect of the cancer or cancer treatment. Anxiety may be caused by a change in metabolic state, addition or discontinuation of medications, or a direct effect of the cancer. Uncontrolled pain and the fear of pain caused by procedures are direct effects of cancer that could easily precipitate anxiety.

Table 17-3. Symptoms and Signs of Anxiety

Appearance
- flushed face
- tension
- restlessness
- smoking
- perspiration

Neurological
- poor concentration
- poor memory
- irritability
- dizziness
- fatigue
- insomnia
- nightmares
- headache

- panic attacks
- tremors

Cardiovascular
- palpitations
- sinus tachycardia

Respiratory
- dyspnea
- hyperventilation

Gastrointestinal
- anorexia
- diarrhea
- heartburn
- hyperphagia

SOURCE: reference 23.

Management of Anxiety

The management of anxiety related to cancer is directed at the elimination or correction of the precipitating problem. Unfortunately, the problem may not be easily treatable, and therapy may be required.

The management of reactive anxiety includes supportive psychotherapy, pharmacotherapy, and cognitive-behavioral interventions, or any combination of these. Supportive psychotherapy is intended to reduce perceived isolation and provide an outlet for the expression of fears and worries. Cognitive-behavioral interventions for anxiety include relaxation training, guided imagery, and hypnosis. These techniques involve the use of suggestion to induce physical and mental relaxation. Information and support can be provided to the patient, especially at the time of transition. Pharmacists are key providers of information and can confer support by providing information about drug therapy. Pharmacists, in cooperation with other members of the health care team, should outline the planned schedule of treatment, explain potential adverse reactions, and describe potential cancer or cancer-related symptoms to help coordinate care and minimize anxiety.

Medications, most commonly the benzodiazepines, may be used for a short course alone or with psychotherapy to manage reactive anxiety. To minimize the risk of accumulation, the shorter-acting benzodiazepines (lorazepam, alprazolam, and oxazepam) are recommended for patients with impaired elimination. Alprazolam has been shown to be effective in the management of reactive distress with or without a depressive component.[26] Pharmacotherapy is most useful during the period of acute distress and can be tapered when symptoms or situations resolve. Medications should not be abruptly discontinued, because this could precipitate anxiety symptoms.

Neuroleptics, such as haloperidol, are used in the treatment of anxiety when an organic etiology is suspected or when psychotic symptoms, such as delusions or hallucinations, are present.[23] The patient's family and/or caregivers should be counseled about potential side effects of these agents, such as extrapyramidal symptoms, because these side effects can be as frightening as delusions.

CONFUSION

One of the most upsetting problems for patients, family, friends, and caregivers is confusion. Confusion may, in effect, take the patient out of the decision-making process, and away from family and friends. Communication becomes difficult for patients with confusion, and clinicians may not be able to adequately assess symptoms. A challenge for the health care team is developing an appropriate pharmacotherapy plan without the patient's perception of symptoms.

Management of confusion requires evaluation and assessment of all possible contributing etiologies. The possible etiologies of confusion in the patient with cancer are numer-

Table 17-4. Etiology of Confusion in the Patient with Cancer

Medications
Hypoxia
Infection
Electrolyte disturbances (e.g., hypercalcemia)
Anemia
Psychosis
Depression
Alcohol or drug withdrawal
Paraneoplastic syndromes
Environment

SOURCE: reference 27.

ous and the cause is often multifactorial (Table 17-4).[27] Treatment should be directed at correcting the underlying cause of confusion if it can be identified.

Delirium has commonly been reported in patients with advanced-stage cancer, particularly in the last weeks of life. Prevalence may range from 25 to 85%.[28] Delirium is defined as an etiologically nonspecific, global, cerebral dysfunction manifested by concurrent disturbances of level of consciousness, attention, thinking, perception, memory, psychomotor behavior, emotions, and the sleep-wake cycle.[29] Delirium and dementia have some similar features, such as disorientation, but dementia generally appears in alert individuals and is accompanied by little or no clouding of consciousness. Delirium can be superimposed on an underlying dementia.

Delirium in the patient with cancer can be caused by numerous cancer and cancer treatment factors and is also often multifactorial. Delirium can be related to (1) a direct effect of the disease (e.g., brain metastasis or carcinomatous meningitis), (2) an indirect effect of the cancer (e.g., metabolic encephalopathy due to organ failure or paraneoplastic syndromes), (3) concurrent medical problems, (4) pharmacotherapy for cancer treatment (e.g., ifosfamide, interferon, or corticosteroids), (5) pharmacotherapy for disease-related symptom management (e.g., opioid analgesics or benzodiazepines), or (6) pharmacotherapy for treatment-related symptom management (e.g., phenothiazines for nausea and vomiting).

It is essential to reassess the appropriateness of the patient's overall pharmacotherapy at the onset or progression of confusion symptoms. The deterioration of a patient's status at the end of life may be signaled by new complaints of confusion, and chronic medications may need to be discontinued, or their doses reduced. Pharmacotherapy of confused patients may require adjustment, but all complaints of confusion should not arbitrarily be attributed to medication. For example, a patient on chronic opiates for pain should not have opiates withdrawn because of the onset of confusion. The dosage or the choice of opiate should be reviewed and evaluated, but a concurrent symptom of pain should be managed in the confused patient.

Other potential causes of confusion include the rapid escalation of a medication or the abrupt discontinuation of a chronic medication. An accurate medication history is essential to determining potential contributing factors of an abrupt change in mental status. Because the patient may not be able to provide an adequate history of drug use, family and caregivers are often relied on. Other potential sources of information include the patient's primary care physician, pharmacist, and home care team.

Management of Confusion

Unfortunately, the etiology of confusion in the terminal stages of cancer may not be apparent, and the cause may not be reversible. The assessment of confusion may be limited by the patient care setting (home or hospice) and the focus of care (palliative versus curative). Even when a patient evaluation is aggressive, the etiology may not be apparent. In one study, the etiology of cognitive failure was discovered in less than half of terminally ill patients.[30]

Supportive therapies, such as providing a quiet room with familiar objects and a visible clock and/or calendar, may help to reduce anxiety and disorientation.[29]

Pharmacologic management of the symptoms of confusion with neuroleptics has been shown to improve symptoms of abnormal sensorium and to improve cognition.[27] Haloperidol has been used to treat patients with abnormal behavior suggestive of hallucinations and altered cognition. If the patient is quiet and not distressed, sedating medications should be avoided.[31] Medications causing sedation may exacerbate the problem of misinterpreting information.

Delirium occurring in the last days of life is often referred to as terminal agitation or terminal restlessness in the palliative care literature. The use of sedation to manage delirium in the actively dying patient remains controversial.[29,32,33]

Fear is a very different issue from confusion, although the agitation seen in a severely frightened patient can appear to be confusion. Fear that does not respond to supportive techniques may be treated with benzodiazepines to blunt the frightening memory of distress and relieve severe agitation or insomnia.[27] Haloperidol should not be used to treat patients that are terrified but not confused.

Patients that are disruptive, confused, and perhaps paranoid may benefit from pharmacotherapy. Anxiolytics, such as lorazepam and midazolam, have been reported to be useful.[34]

Oral medications may present problems for some patients at the end of life, and alternate routes of administration of these medications that are appropriate for family or caregivers should be considered. Sedation may be appropriate, and the oral, rectal, and intramuscular administration of chlorpromazine has been described.[35]

SLEEP DISORDERS

Sleep disturbances occur and are reported as a range of different complaints in cancer patients. Problems with sleep can be witnessed by the health care team when patients are admitted to the hospital, but they are often present when the patient is at home and may go undetected. The International Classification of Sleep Disorders of the American Sleep Disorders Association classifies dyssomnias, parasomnias, and sleep disorders secondary to medical or psychiatric conditions. All of these types of sleep disorders may be seen in cancer patients.

Dyssomnias are a primary disorder that results in a disturbance to quantity, quality, or timing of nocturnal sleep. Excessive daytime sleep can be classified as a dyssomnia and is potentially disabling because it may compromise the patient's function and decrease the patient's ability to interact with others. Potential causes of excessive daytime sleepiness include disturbances of nighttime sleep, medications, metabolic disorders, and disruption of the sleep-wake cycle.

Insomnia, a dyssomnia, can be caused by depression, anxiety, pain, respiratory distress, nausea, vomiting, medications (e.g., corticosteroids or SSRIs), or substance abuse. Another common cause of dyssomnia is a sleep-wake schedule disorder caused by medication, procedures, or activities.

Parasomnias are events or conditions caused or exacerbated by sleep, such as nightmares or sleep terrors. Medications may precipitate nightmares and should be evaluated in the patient with cancer who describes this problem. A number of medications that a patient may require for management of cancer related issues or other health problems may cause vivid dreams (e.g., opioid analgesics and SSRIs). Patients should receive appropriate counseling about this possible side effect.

Management of Sleep Disorders

The management of sleep disorders includes a complete evaluation of the complaint. Patients should be asked to describe how they feel they sleep at night and whether they have symptoms of sleepiness during the day. A characterization of the complaint should be completed before developing a management plan. Evaluation should include documentation of the sleep-wake cycle and identification of possible precipitating factors.

Sleep hygiene is included in the nonpharmacologic management of sleep disorders.[36] Patients should be encouraged to maintain regular sleep-wake schedules. Patients should be encouraged to decrease unnecessary time in bed and to nap only when necessary, avoiding late afternoon and evening naps. If at all possible, patients should be encouraged to maintain some active daytime schedule that involves cognitive and physical stimulation. Every effort should be made to schedule activities to facilitate nighttime sleep and to avoid nighttime sleep interruptions. Scheduling of medications to allow an uninterrupted 6–8 hours of sleep, when possible, is optimal.

Review and modification of the patient's medication regimen is essential. Sedating medications should be administered at bedtime, when possible. Stimulants, including caffeine, should be avoided in the evening and at night. Pain management should be optimized to facilitate sleep uninterrupted by pain.

Sedative hypnotics are appropriate for patients whose symptoms cannot be managed with nonpharmacologic measures. As with any patient with a sleep disorder, appropriate therapy is tailored to the type and intensity of symptoms. A patient that has difficulty falling asleep may benefit from the initiation of a short-acting benzodiazepine. Patients that have problems with frequent nighttime waking may be more appropriately managed with a longer-acting agent.

Duration of therapy should be individualized on the basis of patient requirements. For example, a patient who complains of insomnia after the initiation of corticosteroids for the treatment of lymphoma may require pharmacotherapy for a relatively short time. After the corticosteroid is discontinued, the need for a sedative hypnotic should be reevaluated.

Care should be given to the effects of the medications used in the management of sleep and the evaluation of other patient problems. The sedating effects of sedative hypnotic agents may help a patient sleep through the night but may cause an unwanted hangover effect during the day. The dose of a medication should be carefully titrated to the desired effect, and the effects of disease or organ dysfunction on the pharmacodynamics of the medications should be considered for each patient.

DYSPNEA

One of the most distressing physical symptoms for patients and caregivers is breathlessness.[22] The sensation of breathlessness may occur in up to 70% of patients in the last 6 weeks of life.[37] Dyspnea, or "difficulty breathing," is an unpleasant sensation of difficult, labored breathing and, like pain, is subjective and includes the patient reaction to the sensation. Dyspnea and breathlessness are sometimes considered different sensations, but the terms are frequently used interchangeably. Breathlessness may contribute to fear, anxiety, and depression and may precipitate insomnia because of patient fears of not being able to control breathing while asleep.

The pathophysiology of dyspnea is not well defined and is likely complex. There are a number of possible causes of dyspnea in patients with cancer (Table 17-5).[27] Dyspnea may be a direct effect of the primary cancer or metastatic disease on the lung parenchyma. This direct effect is seen with nonsmall cell and small cell lung cancers, as well as breast, prostate and colorectal cancers. In addition, dyspnea may be caused by problems precipitated by the cancer, including pulmonary emboli, superior vena cava syndrome, anemia, congestive heart failure, and pleural or pericardial effusions. Radiation therapy or chemotherapy (e.g., bleomycin and alkylating agents) may contribute to the sensation of breathlessness. Other possible

Table 17-5. Potential Causes of Dyspnea in Advanced Cancer

Tumor progression
Endobronchial obstruction
Extrinsic bronchial compression
Pleural effusion
Lymphangitis carcinomatosa
Tracheoesophageal fistula
Pneumothorax
Postradiation pneumonitis
Infection
Airway obstruction
Pulmonary embolism
Heart failure
Ischemic heart disease
Arrhythmias
Pericardial effusions
Superior vena cava syndrome/obstruction
Ascites
Abdominal mass
Anemia

SOURCE: reference 27.

considerations include pre-existing cardiorespiratory disease, metabolic acidosis, and anxiety. Another, less obvious contributing factor to the patient's sensation of breathlessness is hyperventilation.

Dyspnea, like pain, is a sensation and is therefore affected by a patient's previous experiences and fears. Dyspnea is difficult to rate and to describe to caregivers. As with pain ratings, there appears to be disparity between physician and patient assessments of the severity of the symptom. Objective measurement of exertional activity required to evoke dyspnea in a patient has been used for assessment, but this method is not always feasible or appropriate for patients with advanced disease. There is controversy concerning subjective and objective measures of respiratory function. Therefore, the challenge is to listen to the patient's assessment and perception of the problem and modify therapy based on the patient's perceived benefit.

Management of Dyspnea

The fundamental approach to managing dyspnea is to identify and treat the cause. Treatment should be directed at the cause of the breathlessness, if it can be identified, and if the therapy can be tolerated by the patient. Dyspnea secondary to pleural effusion can frequently be alleviated by aspiration of the pleural effusions with or without concomitant pleurodesis. Surgery, chemotherapy, radiotherapy, or laser therapy may help relieve the dyspnea related to a malignancy affecting the lungs. The challenge lies in the treatment of breathlessness when interventions aimed at reversing the underlying disease process have failed.

Administration of oxygen is one of the interventions most commonly used to help alleviate the sensation of breathlessness. Oxygen is helpful if a patient is hypoxic on room air, but it is also used as a relatively nonspecific approach for some patients. Oxygen therapy has been demonstrated to improve both dyspnea and the general sense of well-being in patients with cancer-related breathlessness.[38]

Opiates, commonly morphine, have been used for relief of dyspnea in asthma, emphysema, pulmonary edema, and cancer.[39,40] Low-dose systemic opiates have an established place in the symptomatic management of breathlessness in patients with malignant disease,[41] but the mechanism of relief is not completely understood. The interaction of opiates and respiration is complex; opiates appear to improve lung function, decrease oxygen consumption, cause sedation, reduce anxiety, and cause respiratory depression.[42] In addition, the optimal dose, route, and schedule of opiates in dyspnea are not clearly defined. Dose ranges are patient specific, and initial doses should be low for opiate-naive patients. Oral opiates, including sustained release products, have been used. Nebulized opiates may offer an alternative method of delivery for some patients. At the end of life, intravenous or subcutaneous administration of opiates offer an alternative to other routes.

Psychological factors may also contribute to the perception of breathlessness. Historically, anxiolytics have been used to manage dyspnea, although the exact mechanism of action is not fully understood and controlled clinical trials are not available. It is believed that the primary benefit provided by these agents is due to their anxiolytic and sedative effects. Benzodiazepines (including oral diazepam, oral and sublingual lorazepam and, recently, parenteral midazolam) have been used to treat cancer-related breathlessness. Sedating antihistamines, such as promethazine and chlorpromazine, have also been used. Other medications that have been used to relieve dyspnea include theophylline, prostaglandins, nabilone, and respiratory stimulants. Clinical studies are not available, and all these agents require further evaluation.

HOSPICE CARE

One of the major changes in cancer care in the United States in the last 20 years has been the development of hospice services. Hospice is a term derived from the Latin word *hospes*, meaning host or receiver of guests. The movement toward the provision of care for support stems from the early hospice programs developed as Christian institutions to provide food and care for the sick. Cure was a goal, but with limited resources, care and spiritual comfort were emphasized. Hospices, as institutions for the care of the dying, opened first in Ireland and England, spreading eventually to the United States. Hospice care has grown to include hospice programs that function in the home, in acute care hospitals, or in independent institutions. The modern definition of hospice care focuses on the concept of care for terminally ill persons that concentrates on the management of physical and emotional symptoms of patients and their families.[43] Many hospice programs were originally designed for patients with cancer but now include other patient populations.

In the United States, the hospice movement has become a fully Medicare-funded service that provides a continuum of home and inpatient care for terminally ill patients and their families. The Tax Equity and Fiscal Responsibility Act of 1982 established the Medicare Hospice Benefit, defining patients who have a prognosis of 6 months or less to live as terminally ill.[44] A rationale for hospice reimbursement by Medicare and other insurance programs is that hospice care replaces hospital inpatient care and is theoretically less expensive. The care of patients is provided by an interdisciplinary team of health care professionals including, but not limited to, physicians, nurses, social workers, and pharmacists. Clergy and specially trained volunteers are also an essential part of the interdisciplinary team. Hospice care can be provided in a coordinated program of care across a variety of appropriate inpatient and outpatient settings. The primary setting for care is the patient's home, and hospice patients are encouraged to remain at home as long as possible.[45] Because care is primarily provided at home, a family member or caregiver is identified to actively participate in the care of the patient.

Hospice programs in the United States provide all medications, biological therapy, durable medical equipment, and health care services that are needed to manage the patient's symptoms.

A barrier to the provision of hospice or palliative care to patients with cancer is that the primary focus of such care is not cure. The basic premise of hospice care is the emphasis on palliation of symptoms for patients with terminal cancer, which is appropriate for many patients at some point in their disease. Despite this need, patients are still not referred to hospice programs routinely. In 1988, only 3% of Medicare recipients received the hospice benefit,[43] but a recent survey by the National Hospice Organization indicates that the number of patients and families served by hospices is growing. In 1994, >300,000 families were served by hospices, compared with 200,000 in 1990.[45] The majority of cancer patients in the United States are not presented with the option for hospice services or are referred late in the course of their disease.[46] It has only been in the last few years that the realization has grown within the oncology community that palliative care is an important focus of cancer care.[46,47]

Approximately half of all U.S. hospices are independent community programs, approximately a quarter are hospital-based programs, and the remainder are affiliated with home health agencies or nursing homes.[45] As the practice of palliative care expands through hospice care and other mechanisms, it expands the practice opportunities for pharmacists. Pharmacotherapy is essential in the management of most physical and emotional symptoms patients face during this time of their lives. The complexity of treating a patient who has numerous concurrent medical problems related to their cancer or cancer-related therapy, and who may also have changing functional abilities and social resources, requires continuous pharmacist intervention for modification and optimization of the treatment plan. Pharmacists have the opportunity to monitor efficacy and toxicity of therapy closely and to help tailor therapy appropriately when the physical and emotional status of the patient changes. Dosage formulations are a challenge when intravenous or oral routes are not available; pharmacists are the health care practitioners most capable of developing practical pharmacotherapeutic regimens that can be administered to the patient with the available resources. Hospice care strongly emphasizes a coordinated approach to care as a means of enhancing the combined skills and sensitivities of caregivers.

SOCIOECONOMIC CONSIDERATIONS

Cancer does not follow a predictable course, and it is difficult to determine what demands the disease and treatment will place on patients and their families. Patients with cancer and their caregivers are confronted with both obvious and hidden financial responsibilities. Financial problems occur for most families, regardless of economic status, because of insurance limitations, out-of-pocket health-related expenses, and the overall cost of care. Expenses that may not be obvious to the health care team include transportation, parking, child care, homemaker services, nonprescription medications, co-pays for insurance plans, and lost wages. If financial responsibilities are not met, the patient's treatment may be compromised, and the associated psychosocial needs and emotional stress may compromise quality of life.[48]

The impact of socioeconomic limitations on the provision of palliative care can be monumental. The cost of palliative medicine may not be as high as that of primary treatment, but the cost of other supportive services will decrease the financial resources available for the provision of palliative care. It has been shown that as a patient's functional status decreases with the advancement of disease, the cost of care to the family increases.[49] Patients without insurance may not have the resources for supportive care after a long and expensive treatment course. Gaps in insurance coverage or the total lifetime caps of some policies are restrictive for patients who do have insurance coverage.

The effects of these issues on the provision of palliative care to the patient with cancer must be included in the overall assessment of a patient and the plan.

SUMMARY

The care of a patient with cancer requires the management of all symptoms and problems encountered by the patient. The goal of palliative care is to provide the best quality of life possible throughout the course of the illness; palliative care should not be reserved for the terminal stages. Total care includes the management of medical, psychological, social, spiritual, and economic issues that face patients and their families. All treatment plans should address each of these aspects to provide optimal pharmacotherapy and optimal care.

REFERENCES

1. Cancer Pain Relief and Palliative Care. Technical Report Series 804 General. World Health Organization, 1990.
2. Cherney NI, Coyle N, Foley KM. Suffering in the advanced cancer patient: a definition and taxonomy. *J Palliat Care* 1994:10:57–70.
3. Walsh D. Palliative care: management of the patients with advanced cancer. *Semin Oncol* 1994;21(Suppl 7):100–6.
4. Breitbart E. Psycho-oncology: depression, anxiety, delirium. *Semin Oncol* 1994;21:754–69.
5. Maguire P. Barriers to psychological care of the dying. *Br Med J* 1985;291:1711–3.
6. Chochinov HM, Wilson KG, Enns M, et al. Prevalence of depression in the terminally ill: effects of diagnostic criteria and symptom threshold judgments. *Am J Psychiatry* 1994;151:537–40.
7. Bukberg J, Penman D, Holland JC. Depression in hospitalized cancer patients. *Psychosom Med* 1984;46:199–212.
8. Massie MJ. Depression. In: Holland JC, Rowland JH, editors. *Handbook of Psychooncology: Psychological Care of the Patient with Cancer*. New York: Oxford Univ Pr; 1990. p. 283–90.
9. McDaniel JS, Musselman DL, Porter MR, et al. Depression in patients with cancer: diagnosis, biology, and treatment. *Arch Gen Psychiatry* 1995;52:89–99.
10. Smets EMA, Garssen B, Schuster-Uitterhoeve ALJ, et al. Fatigue in cancer patients. *Br J Cancer* 1993;68:220–4.
11. Aistars J. Fatigue in the cancer patient: a conceptual approach to a clinical problem. *Oncol Nurs Forum* 1987;14:25–30.
12. Graydon JE, Bubela N, Irvine D, et al. Fatigue-reducing strategies used by patients receiving treatment for cancer. *Cancer Nurs* 1995;18:23–8.
13. Leitgeb C, Pecherstorfer M, Fritz E, et al. Quality of life in chronic anemia of cancer during treatment with recombinant human erythropoietin. *Cancer* 1994;73:2535–42.
14. Massie MJ, Holland JC. Depression and the cancer patient. *J Clin Psychiatry* 1990;51:12–7.
15. Massie M, Lesko LM. Psychopharmacological management. In: Holland JC, Rowland JH, editors. *Handbook of Psychooncology: Psychological Care of the Patient with Cancer*. New York: Oxford Univ Pr; 1990. p. 470–91.
16. Wells BG, Mandos LA, Hayes PA. *Depressive Disorders: Pharmacotherapy*. 3rd ed. Stamford, CT: Appleton & Lange; 1996. p. 1395–418.
17. Woods SW, Tesae GE, Murray GB, et al. Psychostimulant treatment of depressive disorders secondary to medical illness. *J Clin Psychiatry* 1986;47:12–5.
18. Wallace AE, Kofoed LL, West AN. Double-blind, placebo-controlled trial of methylphenidate in older, depressed medically ill patients. *Am J Psychiatry* 1995;152:929–1031.
19. Rosenberg PB, Ahmed I, Hurwitz S. Methylphenidate in depressed medically ill patients. *J Clin Psychiatry* 1991;52:263–7.
20. Emptage RE, Semla TP, Gonzales L. Depression in the medically ill elderly: a focus on methylphenidate. *Ann Pharmacother* 1996;30:151–7.
21. Schagg CC, Heinrich RL. Anxiety in medical situations: adult cancer patients. *J Clin Psychol* 1989;45:20–7.
22. Hockley PJ, Dunlop R, Davis RJ. Survey of distressing symptoms in dying patients and their families in hospital and the response to a symptom control team. *Br Med J* 1988;296:1715–7.
23. Massie MJ. Anxiety, panic, and phobias. In: Holland JC, Rowland JH, editors. *Handbook of Psychooncology: Psychological Care of the Patient with Cancer*. New York: Oxford Univ Pr; 1990. p. 300–9.
24. Holland JC. Anxiety and cancer: the patient and the family. *J Clin Psychiatry* 1989;50:20–5.
25. Derogatis LR, Morrow GR, Fetting J, et al. The prevalence of psychiatric disorders among cancer patients. *JAMA* 1983; 249:751–7.
26. Holland JC, Morrow GR, Schmale A, et al. A randomized clinical trial of alprazolam versus progressive muscle relaxation in cancer patients with anxiety and depressive symptoms. *J Clin Oncol* 1991;9:1004–11.
27. Fallon MT, Hanks GW. Control of common symptoms in advanced cancer. *Ann Acad Med Singapore* 1994;23:172–7.
28. Breitbart W, Bruera E, Chochinov H, et al. Neuropsychiatric syndromes and psychological symptoms in patients with advanced cancer. *J Pain Symptom Manage* 1995;10:131–41.
29. Jacobson PB, Breitbart W. Psychosocial aspects of palliative care. *Cancer Control* 1996;3:214–22.
30. Bruera E, Miller L, McCallian J. Cognitive failure in patients with terminal cancer: a prospective study. *J Pain Symptom Manage* 1992;7:192–5.
31. Stiefel F, Fainsinger R, Bruera M. Acute confusional states in patients with advanced cancer. *J Pain Symptom Manage* 1992;7:94–8.
32. Ventafridda V, Ripamanti C, De Conno F. Symptom prevalence and control during cancer patients' last day of life. *J Palliat Care* 1990;6:7–11.
33. Fainsinger R, Miller MJ, Bruera E. Symptom control during the last week of life on a palliative care unit. *J Palliat Care* 1991;7:5–11.
34. McNamara P, Minton M, Twycross RG. Use of midazolam in palliative care. *Palliat Med* 1991;5:244–9.
35. McIver B, Walsh D, Nelson K. The use of chlorpromazine for symptom control in dying cancer patients. *J Pain Symptom Manag* 1994;9:341–5.
36. Sateia MJ, Silberfarb PM. Sleep in palliative care. In: Doyle D, Hanks GWC, MacDonald N, editors. *Oxford Textbook of Palliative Medicine*. New York: Oxford Univ Pr; 1993. p. 472–86.
37. Reuben DB, Mor V. Dyspnea in terminally ill cancer patients. *Chest* 1986;89:234–6.
38. Bruera E, de Stoutz N, Velasco-Leiva A, et al. Effects of oxygen on dyspnea in hypoxemic terminal cancer patients. *Lancet* 1993;342:13–4.
39. Bruera E, MacEachern T, Ripamoniti C, et al. Subcutaneous morphine for dyspnea in cancer patients. *Ann Intern Med* 1993;119:906–7.

40. Cohen MH, Anderson AJ, Krasnow SH. Continuous intravenous infusion of morphine for severe dyspnea. *South Med J* 1991;84:229–34.
41. Ahmedzai S. Palliation of respiratory symptoms. In: Doyle D, Hanks GWC, MacDonald N, editors. *Oxford Textbook of Palliative Medicine.* New York: Oxford Univ Pr; 1993. p. 362–5.
42. Davis CL. The therapeutics of dyspnea. In: Hanks GW. *Cancer Surveys. Palliative Medicine: Problem Areas in Pain and Symptom Management.* New York: Cold Spring Harbor Laboratory Press; 1994. p. 85–98.
43. Hadlock DC. The hospice: intensive care of a different kind. *Semin Oncol* 1985:12:357–67.
44. Lubitz JD, Riley GF. Trends in medicare payments in the last year of life. *N Engl J Med* 1993;328:1092–6.
45. Showetter RS. Overview of hospice and palliative care in oncology. *Cancer Control* 1996;3:197–203.
46. Kinzbrunner BM. Hospice: what to do when anti-cancer therapy is no longer appropriate, effective, or desired. *Semin Oncol* 1994;21:792–8.
47. Davis CL, Hardy JR. Palliative care. *Br J Med* 1994;308:1359–62.
48. Berkman BJ, Sampson SE. Psychosocial effects of cancer economics on patients and their families. *Cancer* 1993;72:2846–9.
49. Mor V, Masterson S, Siegel K, et al. Cancer patients' home care needs and costs: a multisite longitudinal view. Brown University. Final Report (CA 46331). December 1990.

SELF-STUDY QUESTIONS

1. Palliative care is applicable in all stages of the disease in a patient with cancer.
   a. true
   b. false

2. List three symptoms that patients with cancer may experience during the course of their disease.

3. List three possible signs of depression that may be present in a patient with cancer because of the disease process and/or cancer therapy.

4. List useful indicators for depression in the patient with cancer.

5. Psychotherapy is always the first-line treatment for depression in the patient with cancer.
   a. true
   b. false

6. Tricyclic antidepressant agents are the preferred pharmacotherapy for the management of depression in all patients with cancer.
   a. true
   b. false

7. List three neurological signs or symptoms that may be seen in the patient with anxiety.

8. A patient's appearance may indicate anxiety.
   a. true
   b. false

9. Reactive anxiety is often seen at a crisis or transition point in the course of disease.
   a. true
   b. false

10. Uncontrolled pain may contribute to the feeling of anxiety in the patient with cancer.
    a. true
    b. false

11. Elimination of all opiates is appropriate for the patient that is confused and cannot report pain.
    a. true
    b. false

12. Sedation is the goal for all confused patients.
    a. true
    b. false

13. Name a medication that may be appropriate in the management of patients with hallucinations and confusion.

14. Describe the complaint of dyssomnia.

15. Excessive daytime sleepiness may compromise function in the patient with cancer.
    a. true
    b. false

16. List two potential causes of daytime sleepiness.

17. Sedative hypnotics should not be used in the management of insomnia in the patient with cancer.
    a. true
    b. false

18. Dyspnea is a subjective perception of a symptom.
    a. true
    b. false

19. List three potential causes of dyspnea in patients with advanced cancer.

20. Opiates should not be used in a patient with complaints of breathlessness.

    a. true
    b. false

21. List three medications that have been used in the management of dyspnea.

Chapter 18: Nutritional Support

Cynthia L. LaCivita, Pharm.D.
Clinical Coordinator, Department of Pharmacy
Shady Grove Adventist Hospital
Rockville, Maryland
Clinical Assistant Professor
University of Maryland School of Pharmacy
Baltimore, Maryland

Jeannine Schreiber, Pharm.D.
Clinical Coordinator
Department of Pharmacy
Fairview and Lutheran Hospitals
Cleveland Clinic Health System
Cleveland, Ohio

Malnutrition	324
Cancer Cachexia	324
Resting Energy Expenditure	324
Causes of Anorexia and Cachexia	324
Mechanical Problems	325
Malabsorption	325
Nausea and Vomiting	325
Taste Alterations, Xerostomia, and Mucositis	325
Psychological Effects	326
Hypothalamic Regulation of Eating Behavior	326
Humoral Factors	327
Normal Metabolism Versus Metabolism in Cancer Patients	327
Increased Activity of the Cori Cycle	327
Glucose Intolerance and Insulin Resistance	328
Increases in Gluconeogenesis	328
Alterations of Fat Storage and Lipid Utilization	328
Fluid and Electrolyte Imbalances	328
Patient Evaluation	329
Energy and Protein Needs	329
Management of Cancer Cachexia	330
Hormonal and Pharmacologic Interventions	331
Enteral Nutrition	331
Total Parenteral Nutrition	335
Prevention	336
Summary	337
References	337
Suggested Readings	340
Self-Study Questions	340

Malnutrition is often one of the most visible effects of advanced cancer. Many factors contribute to the development of anorexia (loss of appetite) and weight loss in patients with advanced cancer. Both the tumor and the treatment (chemotherapy, radiation, or surgery) can contribute to nutritional deficiencies. Pharmacists play an important role in helping distinguish drug-related causes of anorexia and nutritional deficits from other causes. They must also make appropriate therapeutic recommendations based on the causes of the nutritional problem and the patient's prognosis. Such therapeutic recommendations may include the use of drugs or nutritional support. Pharmacists are often responsible for monitoring the therapeutic and toxic effects of nutritional interventions. Therefore, it is essential that they understand the causes and range of nutritional problems that occur in cancer patients as well as the basis for specific therapeutic interventions. Nutritional support, a large specialty area of practice in itself, is beyond the scope of this chapter, which deals specifically with the nutritional complications of cancer patients. For general instruction in nutritional support, see the suggested readings at the end of the chapter, which cover nutritional support methods in more detail.

This chapter begins with a discussion of the many causes of anorexia and cancer cachexia, the syndrome of diminished appetite, fatigue, anemia, muscle wasting, organ atrophy, weight loss, and decreased performance status associated with cancer. The chapter continues with a description of the metabolic differences between starving individuals and cancer patients. The chapter then covers factors used to evaluate a cancer patient's nutritional status and guidelines for determining the patient's energy and protein needs. The following section describes the uses of hormonal and pharmacologic interventions, enteral nutrition, and total parenteral nutrition in managing cancer cachexia. Finally, prevention is described as part of total nutritional support.

After completing this chapter, the reader should be able to:

1. Distinguish the causes of weight loss in cancer patients that are related to the underlying malignancy from those that are related to the treatment.
2. Describe the differences in glucose, protein, and fat metabolism between patients with cancer and healthy individuals.
3. Discuss considerations in the nutritional evaluation of a cancer patient.
4. Describe factors that influence the determination of energy and protein needs of cancer patients.
5. Discuss the selection of pharmacologic interventions and parenteral or enteral nutritional support in managing cancer cachexia.
6. Discuss the role of diet in causing and preventing cancer.

MALNUTRITION

Malnutrition is common among cancer patients. Weight loss can be an early warning sign of a neoplasm, or it may manifest later in the course of the disease. The nutritional status of cancer patients influences disease treatment and prognosis. In many malignancies, a 5–10% weight loss before treatment is associated with a less favorable prognosis for duration of survival and response to therapy.[1] The deleterious effects of malnutrition include changes in body composition, depressed immunologic function, and decreases in both physical and mental performance.

Cancer Cachexia

Cancer cachexia is a syndrome of anorexia, fatigue, anemia, muscle wasting, organ atrophy, weight loss, and decreased performance status associated with cancer. Hypophagia and weight loss are the hallmarks of cancer cachexia. The signs and symptoms of cancer cachexia are estimated to occur in up to 50% of cancer patients at the time of diagnosis.[2] Tumor size, type, location, and rate of growth; type of treatment; other stresses; or any combination of these factors may contribute to cancer cachexia.

Resting Energy Expenditure

Resting energy expenditure (REE) tends to be higher in cancer patients with weight loss than in noncancer groups and cancer patients without weight loss if REE is calculated on the basis of total body weight.[3] This apparent difference disappears if the REE calculation is based on lean body mass, because lean body mass contributes more to energy expenditure than adipose tissue does.[3] To assume that all cancer patients have increased metabolic needs would be wrong, however; studies have shown that patients with malignancies demonstrate wide variation in REE.[4] The REE may be normal, hypermetabolic, or diminished. Lung cancer, Hodgkin's disease, and leukemia are examples of diseases that are reported to have energy expenditures that exceed predicted values.[5] The stage of disease, type of malignancy, and extent of weight loss at the time of estimating or measuring REE as well as the methods of determining REE may contribute to these apparent metabolic alterations.

Animal studies using experimental sarcomas have associated weight loss with tumor growth. Surgical removal of the tumor in these animals allowed them to return to their prior nutritional state, with weight gain and reversal of hypophagia.[6] In the clinical setting, ablating the tumor is the best therapy for reversing cancer cachexia.

CAUSES OF ANOREXIA AND CACHEXIA

Weight loss in cancer patients is a major prognostic indicator for survival and response to treatment.[7] Therefore, understanding and identifying causes of anorexia and cachexia in a specific patient are critically important, especially when selecting the most appropriate intervention and determining when the cause is not reversible (e.g., an advanced cancer not responding to therapy) or manageable.

Mechanical Problems

Anorexia, a common problem among patients with cancer, is defined as the loss of appetite. Patients may have mechanical or physical problems that contribute to inadequate enteral intake (Table 18-1). Depending on its location and size, a tumor may prevent chewing, swallowing, or passage of nutrients through the gastrointestinal (GI) tract. Surgical procedures can result in the loss of function for the involved organ. For example, radical head and neck surgery can leave a patient without access to the GI tract. Gastrectomy patients may complain of postprandial symptoms. When the stomach's function as a reservoir is lost, ingested contents are dumped directly into the small intestine, which usually does not tolerate bolus feedings or large fluid shifts. Patients who are intolerant may complain of nausea, bloating, early satiety, and abdominal cramping. Because their reservoir capacity has decreased, gastrectomy patients need to be counseled to eat smaller, more frequent meals to avoid discomfort and to prevent reduction of their enteral intake. Pharmacologic agents that promote GI motility may be added to patients' therapeutic regimens when GI stasis and early satiety are experienced.

Table 18-1. Mechanical and Physical Problems That Contribute to Inadequate Enteral Intake

- **Tumors likely to cause obstruction of the gastrointestinal tract**
  - Head and neck cancers
  - Gastric cancer
  - Colorectal cancer
  - Ovarian cancer
  - Non-Hodgkin's lymphoma
- **Chemotherapy**
  - Anorexia, nausea, and vomiting
  - Mucositis
    - Methotrexate
    - Doxorubicin
    - Fluorouracil
    - Bleomycin
    - Cytarabine
  - Diarrhea
  - Ileus
    - Vincristine
    - Vinblastine
- **Functional losses secondary to surgical resections**
  - Loss of ability to chew or swallow
  - Loss of access to gastrointestinal tract
  - Loss of stomach's ability to function as a reservoir
  - Decreased gastric motility
  - Decreased gastric acid production
  - Decreased absorptive capacity
- **Adverse effects associated with radiotherapy**
  - Anorexia, nausea, vomiting
  - Mucositis
  - Xerostomia, very dry mouth
  - Sore throat
  - Mouth blindness, taste alterations
  - Malabsorption
  - Diarrhea
  - Radiation enterocolitis
  - Enterocutaneous fistulas
  - Bowel obstruction
  - Perforation
  - Fibrosis

Malabsorption

Normal digestion and absorption of energy substrates, water, nutrients, and vitamins depend on an intact and functioning GI system (Figure 18-1).[7] Surgical removal or tissue damage from radiation or chemotherapy to the intestinal epithelium or other digestive organs often directly impairs the ability of the GI tract to absorb water and nutrients. Even with an intact GI tract and other digestive organs, GI mucosa and related tissues may be altered by radiation therapy or chemotherapy, leading to malabsorption. Weight loss and protein depletion may result from protein-losing enteropathies or draining fistulas. Biliary obstruction or exocrine dysfunction may cause a reduction in bile salts, resulting in impaired absorption of fats and fat-soluble vitamins.

Lactase deficiency may occur in patients who have received chemotherapy or abdominal radiation.[8] This deficiency may not lead to clinical signs and symptoms of lactose intolerance, so it is recommended that when resuming an oral diet these patients be started on a lactose-free diet and then advanced as tolerated.

Nausea and Vomiting

Some patients acquire food aversions during chemotherapy or radiation therapy because of severe nausea and vomiting (see chapter 9) or taste alterations. If those aversions are strong, foods that were eaten during that period may forever be avoided. A temporary decrease (2–4 days) in enteral intake is not a major concern, provided the patient's fluid requirements are met through parenteral routes. When nutritional status is compromised by protracted nausea, vomiting, or anorexia, supportive replacement needs to be implemented.

Taste Alterations, Xerostomia, and Mucositis

Taste abnormalities in cancer patients have been well documented. DeWys and Walters[9] studied 50 patients with a vari-

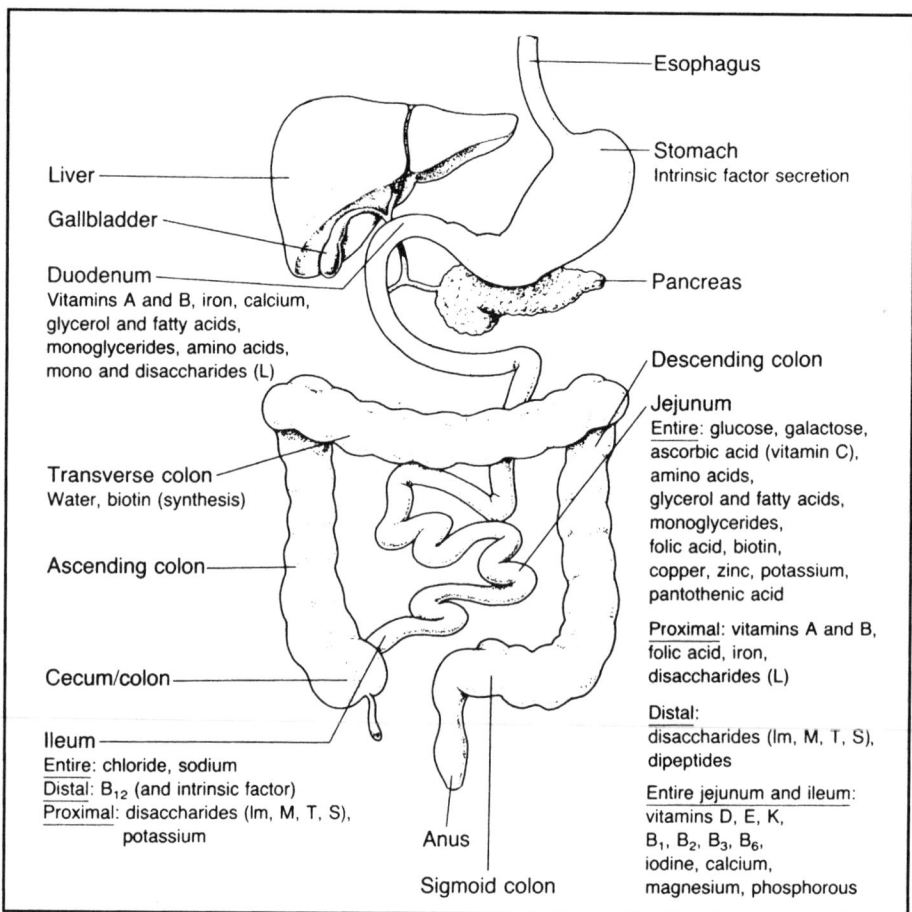

Figure 18-1. Normal function of the gastrointestinal system, with sites of nutrient absorption. L, lactose; Im, isomaltose; M, maltose; T, trehalose; S, sucrose.
SOURCE: reprinted with permission from reference 7.

ety of tumors for abnormalities of taste sensation. The patients' most common complaint was that foods lacked taste. A number of patients associated diminished ability to taste with reduced appetite. The ability of some patients to recognize sweetness may be decreased, whereas the ability to detect bitterness may be enhanced. There is a strong correlation between increased sensitivity to bitterness or urea and an aversion to meats. Taste alterations appear to correlate with total tumor burden[9] and often resolve if anticancer treatment is successful. It is unclear whether these taste abnormalities are caused by or precede nutritional deficiencies. Chemotherapy and numerous other medications can also result in taste alterations (e.g., cisplatin causes a metallic taste).

When radiation therapy includes portions of the GI tract, patients may experience a variety of adverse effects. Decreased salivation (xerostomia) severe enough to prevent normal chewing or swallowing of foods can occur. The microvilli of the taste buds may be damaged, resulting in "mouthblindness." Damage to the GI cells by radiation may also result in sore throat, mucositis, bowel obstruction, perforation, and fibrosis.

Chemotherapy and radiation therapy, although curative in intent, may result in severe mucosal damage. Mucositis can be extremely painful, diminishing patients' desire to continue oral intake (see chapter 9).

Psychological Effects

Depressed patients may have diminished appetites. Patients in severe or chronic pain are often anorectic. In these situations, the pleasurable sensations associated with eating are lost and interest in food can be significantly reduced.

Hypothalamic Regulation of Eating Behavior

Alterations in the hypothalamic satiety center were postulated as playing a role in the development of cancer cachexia. It was hypothesized that a dysfunctional hypothalamic satiety center would decrease the appetite; however, dysfunction of the hypothalamic satiety center did not prevent anorexia in animal models.[10,11]

Humoral Factors

Humoral factors probably play a significant role in the development of cancer cachexia.[2] In parabiotic models in which two animals shared a circulatory system but only one animal hosted a malignancy, both animals exhibited decreased food intake, weight loss, and similar blood abnormalities.[12] This data support the theory that tumor- or host-derived factors circulating through the circulatory system play a role in the development of cancer cachexia.

Tumor-derived factors have been identified from only a few specific cancers and probably play only a part in the development of cancer cachexia. Toxohormone-L, a lipid-mobilizing substance, was isolated by Masumo and colleagues.[13] Extracts of toxohormone-L caused a decrease in enteral intake when administered into the lateral ventricle of rats. Other researchers have identified another lipolytic factor that appears to cause weight loss in animal studies without obvious reductions in food intake.[14-16] Bombesin and serotonin, both of which are suspected to cause anorexia, are also produced by a few specific tumors.[17,18]

Cytokines are protein molecules produced by host macrophages and lymphocytes in response to noxious stimuli.[2,19] Cachectin—now thought to be the same factor as tumor necrosis factor (TNF)—has been found in the serum of patients with acute and chronic infections, chronic inflammatory processes, malignancies, and acquired immunodeficiency syndrome.[2] In vitro studies have shown that TNF is able to decrease the synthesis and activity of lipogenic enzymes and prevent accumulation of lipids in adipocytes.[20-24] It is proposed that in the disease states previously mentioned the adverse effects of TNF on peripheral protein lipase activity probably contribute to the extensive loss of body fat, even with adequate caloric intake. Although TNF may play a role in the progression of cachexia, detectable serum levels are not evident in all patients with anorexia or cachexia.[2]

Experimental data have produced some evidence that there are additional lipolytic factors that may contribute to cachexia.[19,25] Cytokines such as interleukin 1 (IL-1), interleukin 6 (IL-6), interferon β2, and interferon γ may be potential causes or mediators in the development of anorexia and cancer cachexia, although their exact contributions are currently unknown.[2]

It is certain that these circulating factors play a role in the development of cancer cachexia, but whether any of them plays a predominant role in producing cancer cachexia is unknown. It does not appear that the production of these humoral factors is exclusive to malignant states.

NORMAL METABOLISM VERSUS METABOLISM IN CANCER PATIENTS

During periods of inadequate enteral intake, the normal physiological response is to conserve energy. In the early days of starvation in normal, nonstressed individuals, the insulin level is greatly reduced, favoring gluconeogenesis (the formation of glucose from noncarbohydrate sources, such as glycogen and amino acids). Glycogen stores are only temporary energy reserves. When they are exhausted, glycogenolysis (the hydrolysis of glycogen to glucose) ceases, and protein (amino acid) catabolism can be used to produce glucose via gluconeogenesis and oxidative deamination. During acute starvation in normal individuals, up to 15% of muscle mass can be lost during the first 10 days.[26] This loss is attributed to rapid proteolysis and amino acid mobilization from muscle. As the body adapts, there is a decrease in urinary urea nitrogen (UUN) and ammonia production. As starvation becomes a chronic problem, fat is used as the predominant energy source, reducing protein catabolism. Adipose tissue is mobilized, producing free fatty acids that are used for oxidative purposes in body tissues and are the precursors for ketone body synthesis. Even the brain adapts to using ketone bodies as an energy source.[27] Total UUN losses can drop from 12 to 3 g/day with adaptation to starvation conditions.[26]

In summary, starvation in normal, nonstressed individuals results in decreased metabolism to conserve protein. The amount of glucose produced by the liver and utilized by peripheral tissues is greatly decreased as fat becomes the predominant energy source. These shifts in energy substrates reflect the normal individual's ability to adapt to starvation and minimize protein losses.

In contrast, cancer patients' ability to adapt to starvation conditions appears to be impaired (Table 18-2).[28] The host's inability to adapt to conditions of reduced caloric intake stems partly from the tumor's parasitic nature. Tumors exhibit autonomy with respect to growth and metabolic behavior, and their metabolic needs remain constant or increase regardless of the host's nutritional state. Controversy exists regarding the theory that feeding a cancer patient may stimulate tumor growth. Tumor-bearing animals administered parenteral nutrition have exhibited an increase in tumor and carcass mass.[29] In a review of more than 1000 oncology patients who received parenteral nutrition, no increase in the rate of tumor growth was apparent and nutritional support resulted in improved immune response and increased wound healing in some patient groups.[30] Because well-designed clinical studies in humans are lacking, it is inappropriate to withhold nutritional support for fear of stimulating tumor growth.

The metabolism of cancer patients is marked by certain abnormalities: (1) increased activity of the Cori cycle, (2) glucose intolerance and insulin resistance, (3) increases in gluconeogenesis, (4) alterations of fat storage and lipid utilization, and (5) fluid and electrolyte imbalances.

Increased Activity of the Cori Cycle

It appears that there is an increase in Cori cycle activity in cancer patients, particularly in patients who have lost weight.[31] The Cori cycle is an energy-consuming process that allows lactate, the end product of anaerobic glycolysis, to be recycled

Table 18-2. Comparison of Metabolic Parameters in Starved, Injured, and Cancer Patients

Parameter	Starvation	Injury	Cancer
Basal metabolic rate	↓	↑	↑
Alterations in carbohydrate metabolism and utilization			
Blood glucose	↓	↑	±
Blood lactate	±	↑	↑
Serum insulin	↓	↓	±
Plasma glucagon	↑	↑	±
Glucose tolerance	↓	↓	↓
Alterations in protein catabolism and synthesis			
Urinary nitrogen excretion	↓	↑	±
Whole body protein turnover	↓	↑	±
Whole body protein synthesis	↓	↑	±
Gluconeogenesis from alanine	↑	↑	↑

SOURCE: adapted from reference 28. ↑, increased; ↓, decreased; ±, may be increased or decreased.

back to glucose. Studies indicate that some animal and human tumors utilize glucose via anaerobic glycolysis.[32,33] Increased Cori cycle activity may contribute to alterations in carbohydrate metabolism, but it does not account for a significant portion of the daily energy expenditure of cancer patients who exhibit weight loss.[34]

Glucose Intolerance and Insulin Resistance

Abnormal insulin response to carbohydrates and peripheral insulin resistance have been well documented among cancer patients. In some instances, the cancer patient's response to glucose infusions is altered. The rate of clearing sugar from the body may be hampered, resulting in much slower clearance than normal individuals have.[34] Insulin levels have been noted to be lower in some cancer patients when they were subjected to a glucose bolus.[35] The lower insulin levels result from a decreased pancreatic response to carbohydrates.[36] Peripheral resistance to insulin also occurs in some cancer patients.[33] Peripheral insulin resistance and prolonged clearance of glucose are not unique to cancer patients; similar problems occur in patients who are in conditions of stress, such as surgery or trauma.

Increases in Gluconeogenesis

Gluconeogenesis from amino acids is an energy-wasting process. In the cachectic cancer population, the rate of gluconeogenesis from amino acids and the rate of protein degradation from muscle appear to be increased.[37–39]

When radiolabeled leucine was used as a tracer in cancer patients, both breakdown and turnover of protein synthesis appeared to be accelerated, with synthesis exceeding catabolic rates.[40] In weight loss, cancer patients lose a greater proportion of skeletal muscle mass than normal individuals do.[41]

Individual amino acids may play a specific role in tumor growth or inhibition. Arginine appears to enhance specific and nonspecific immune response while simultaneously displaying some inhibitory effects on tumor growth.[42,43] Glutamine is the primary amino acid consumed by both gut mucosa and rapidly dividing malignant cells.[28] Competition for this amino acid may occur between gut and malignant cells, with the malignant cells acting as a trap for glutamine. The competition for glutamine may have a detrimental effect on the integrity of the gut mucosa, predisposing the patient to bacterial translocation from the gut, which contributes to infectious complications.

Alterations of Fat Storage and Lipid Utilization

Lipid or fat storage and utilization appear to be altered as well. Some cancer patients apparently tend to preferentially use fat as an energy source, causing increased mobilization and decreased storage.[44] In normal individuals, glucose infusions suppress fatty acid oxidation. Glucose loading in cancer patients is ineffective in suppressing fatty acid oxidation.[45,46] It is possible that glucose is first converted to fat and then used as a fuel. These (and possibly other) disturbances lead to the ineffective utilization of energy sources.

Fluid and Electrolyte Imbalances

Cancer patients may have increased intracellular or extracellular water content. Fluid retention or shifts may occur secondary to low oncotic pressure (e.g., low serum protein), organ failure (renal or cardiac failure), or (in the critically ill patient) because of sepsis or capillary leak. Cancer-related medications can also cause fluid retention (e.g., corticosteroids, interleukin 2, and cyclophosphamide). Fluid retention may obscure or delay weight loss, decrease other objective measurements of nutritional status (e.g., percentage of ideal body weight and mid-upper-arm circumference), and contribute to fluctuations in serum proteins.

Electrolyte disturbances can result from paraneoplastic syndromes, organ dysfunction, tumor lysis syndrome, chemotherapy, anti-infectives, or other supportive therapy.

PATIENT EVALUATION

Nutritional assessments need not be complex. When patients are unable to quantitate exact weight changes, weight changes can be estimated from changes in clothing size or other approximations. Cancer patients should be evaluated for signs and symptoms of protein or protein-calorie malnutrition; the guidelines for that evaluation are the same guidelines used for the general population.

The nutritional assessment is a careful and thorough medical history that includes the patient's height, an estimate of ideal body weight (IBW), actual weight, weight trends over the past several months, weight before illness, measurements of triceps skin fold and mid-upper-arm circumference, serum albumin levels, nitrogen balance, prealbumin or transferrin levels, and record of current oral intake. Other parameters used for patient evaluation and monitoring include laboratory measures of retinol-binding protein (RBP), insulin-like growth factor, somatomedin-C, and fibronectin. Many of these parameters are good indicators of acute changes in protein status. Changes in these values may reflect recovery from stress as well as nutritional intervention.

The laboratory values that are widely used to monitor nutritional status may be affected by disease states, treatment, and nutritional intervention. Lymphocyte counts are often used as an indicator of nutritional status in noncancer patients. However, patients who have leukemia or have undergone aggressive chemotherapy have depressed white blood cell counts, so total lymphocyte counts may not reflect nutritional status accurately.

Albumin is commonly used as a nutritional marker for visceral protein status. The normal range for serum albumin is 3.5–5.0 mg/dl. A sudden drop in serum albumin usually results from a catabolic rate elevated by stress or sepsis rather than from inadequate protein intake. Hypoalbuminemia secondary to malnutrition has a tendency to occur over weeks to months. Severe liver disease could contribute to a decreased ability to synthesize albumin. Administering exogenous albumin may cause misinterpretation of serum albumin levels. If fluid is being retained or administered, serum albumin concentrations may be falsely decreased by the increased intravascular volume. When assessing serum albumin as a marker for protein repletion maintenance, it is important to remember that the half-life of albumin is 21 days. Prealbumin, with a half-life of 2–3 days, is a good indicator of acute changes in visceral protein status. The normal range for serum prealbumin is 16–40 mg/dl. A rising serum prealbumin level in the presence of renal dysfunction and dehydration can be misinterpreted as improved protein status.

Anthropometric measurements are important gross indicators of fat stores and muscle strength. These measurements may be distorted in edematous or dehydrated patients and may not reflect measurements of lean body tissue or fat stores accurately.

Cancer patients are frequently immunosuppressed and sometimes anergic, which may reflect their disease process rather than their current nutritional status. When the causes of weight loss can be identified, doing so is helpful. Patients may complain of persistent nausea and vomiting, diarrhea, alterations in taste, early satiety, difficulty swallowing, or organ dysfunction secondary to trauma or surgery. Excluding or identifying causes will allow the clinician to individualize the nutritional intervention.

A thorough patient interview and subsequent counseling provide invaluable insight into patient eating habits, aversions, and psychological issues that may hamper nutritional recovery. If previous efforts at nutritional counseling have been unsuccessful, the failure may be related to disease progression, patient noncompliance, or expense. Often what may appear to be noncompliance is mental or physical exhaustion caused by disease and its complications.

ENERGY AND PROTEIN NEEDS

Determining the caloric needs of cancer patients is usually left to the clinician. Despite abundant data, specific guidelines for calorie and protein requirements of cancer patients are not available because of wide patient-to-patient variation in energy expenditure and alterations in carbohydrate, protein, and fat metabolism and utilization.

The nutritional goal is to provide adequate calories and protein to rebuild or maintain peripheral and visceral protein stores and to minimize overall weight loss. Protein synthesis and ion pumping are the two processes responsible for establishing basal energy expenditure (BEE) (Table 18-3). Estimating energy expenditure for cancer patients is difficult because studies have revealed a wide range of variation in metabolic rates.[34] The Harris-Benedict equation is used to estimate BEE in kilocalories per day on the basis of the patient's sex, age, height, and total body weight (Table 18-3). BEE is then corrected for stress factors to estimate the patient's daily needs (Table 18-4).[47] This is an inexpensive method for estimating the patient's needs; however, the patient's needs may be overcalculated (e.g., for ventilated or obese patients) or undercalculated (e.g., for patients with cystic fibrosis). Clinical assessments and nutritional markers should be followed closely to ensure that nutritional needs are met.

Table 18-3. Harris-Benedict Equation for Estimating Basal Energy Expenditure (BEE) in Kilocalories

Men	BEE = 66 + (13.7 × weight in kilograms) + (5 × height in centimeters) − (6.8 × age in years)
Women	BEE = 655 + (9.6 × weight in kilograms) + (1.8 × height in centimeters) − (4.7 × age in years)

Table 18-4. Factors for Adjusting BEE for Activity and Injury

Activity and Injury	Adjustment Factor
Activity	
Confined to bed	1.20
Out of bed	1.30
Injury	
Minor operation	1.30
Skeletal trauma	1.35
Major sepsis	1.60
Severe thermal burn	2.10

SOURCE: adapted from reference 47. For example, for a patient confined to bed with skeletal trauma, multiply the BEE (Table 18-3) by 1.20, then multiply that result by 1.35.

Indirect calorimetry can be used to measure REE. Equipment is available to calculate oxygen consumption and carbon dioxide production from the patient's respirations and measure the individual's metabolic needs. The equipment needed is expensive and requires a trained operator, and it may not be available or practical in some institutions. Indirect calorimetry will assess the metabolic needs of the individual at one point in time. Fluctuations in oxygen consumption and carbon dioxide production will occur with changes in activity or disease state. If this method is used, measurements should be repeated periodically to reassess caloric needs.[47]

The normal, nonstressed individual can oxidize glucose at 2–4 mg/kg per minute.[48] Stressed patients with increased energy demands can oxidize glucose at a rate of up to 5 mg/kg per minute.[49]

In general, the presence of a tumor increases caloric needs. Caloric needs may also be increased by certain types of tumors. Energy expenditure is increased in lung cancer patients but not in GI and colon cancer patients when compared with controls.[50] In addition, Bozetti et al.[51] concluded that energy expenditure was greater in patients with more advanced cancer. Hypermetabolism is not present in all cancer patients. In a study conducted by Knox et al.,[4] REE was determined in 200 cancer patients. Results showed that 41% had normal, 25% increased, and 33% decreased REE.

The recommended daily allowance (RDA) for protein in healthy adults ranges from 0.5 to 1.0 g/kg per day. The quantity necessary to achieve positive nitrogen balance depends on the amount of nitrogen being lost. Protein requirements may be greater for the cancer patient, although specific ranges have not been determined. Studies support the belief that cancer patients have increased protein turnover.[40] It would be prudent to provide 1–2 g/kg of IBW per day of protein, depending on the patient's organ function and disease state. Protein intake should be adjusted, particularly when serum proteins reflect continued malnutrition or when the patient is in negative nitrogen balance. A 24-hour measurement of UUN provides an estimate of a patient's nitrogen losses for that day. The patient's urine is collected over a 24-hour period and analyzed for nitrogen content. That figure can then be used to calculate nitrogen balance. Nitrogen excreted renally and in the stool (4 g/day is routinely used as an estimate of nonrenal losses of nitrogen) are totaled and compared with the nitrogen (protein) consumed by or supplied to the patient in parenteral or enteral supplements.

$$\text{Nitrogen balance} = (\text{Nitrogen input} = \text{grams of protein}/6.25) - (\text{Nitrogen lost} = \text{UUN} + 4 \text{ g})$$

For extremely catabolic patients, a more realistic goal may be to achieve a less negative nitrogen balance than previously obtained, rather than a positive one. A UUN's reliability will be affected by protein losses from other organ systems (e.g., the GI tract or skin).

Essential fatty acids are required to maintain adequate platelet function; prostaglandin synthesis; wound healing; immunocompetence; and integrity of skin, hair, and nerve linings. To prevent fatty acid deficiency, approximately 1–2% of daily calories should be linoleic acid. The clinical signs of fatty acid deficiency generally occur 1–3 weeks after deprivation. Fats may be a useful source of calories, particularly in patients who have hyperglycemia, are fluid restricted, or may experience pulmonary complications when carbohydrates need to be limited.

Lipids and excessive calories may be especially harmful when feeding obese (>130% IBW) cancer patients. Glucose intolerance, fluid retention, and pulmonary compromise are complications often observed in these patients. Energy and essential fatty acid requirements can be met by a hypocaloric feeding. Hypocaloric feedings entail feeding the mildly to moderately stressed obese patient fewer calories than required, with adequate protein, and with or without lipids. Obese patients are able to mobilize their own endogenous adipose stores to meet energy needs.[52,53]

MANAGEMENT OF CANCER CACHEXIA

Because cancer patients are likely to experience nutritional deficits from either disease or treatment, they should be carefully monitored for changes in weight, oral intake, and serum proteins, as well as for GI complaints. Preventive measures are often necessary. When enteral intake is depressed for short periods, providing counseling to ensure adequate intake of fluids and calories may prevent hospital admission or shorten stays. If the initial methods are unsuccessful, it may be necessary to pursue other means of appetite stimulation or nutritional support. Enteral supplementation followed by pharmacologic stimulation of the patient's appetite are first- and second-line interventions. Enteral feeding tubes are considered when oral intake is unsuccessful in meeting nutritional needs and the GI tract is functioning. Parenteral nutrition should be reserved for patients for whom other interventions have failed or for those who have contraindications to other methods or therapies. Parenteral nutrition is not indicated as a method of hydration or for the terminally ill patient with resistant disease.

Feeding cancer patients by either the enteral or the parenteral route does not always reverse cancer cachexia, particularly when the cancer is progressive and/or the patient is stressed by infections, surgery, or antineoplastic therapy. Eradicating the tumor is the most effective therapy in alleviating the increased metabolic needs of the patient secondary to tumor presence. In many instances of advanced disease, this is not possible.

Hormonal and Pharmacologic Interventions

Insulin has been shown to reverse protein degradation and promote synthesis in both in vivo and in vitro studies.[24] Under normal circumstances, insulin activity inhibits or reduces lipolysis. Insulin can suppress lipolysis in tumor extracts containing TNF, supporting evidence that the effects of circulating substances may in part be modified. It has been proposed that the anabolic effects of insulin could benefit the cachectic cancer population. Clinical studies in humans of insulin as an anabolic hormone are lacking, so insulin cannot be recommended as a treatment for euglycemic patients.[54]

Weight gain and increased appetite have occurred in cancer patients who have received high-dose megestrol acetate. Stage IV breast cancer patients who received 480–1600 mg of megestrol acetate per day gained weight regardless of response to treatment, extent of disease, or pretreatment weight.[55] The weight gain was thought to reflect increased body mass, apparently due in part to an increase in adipose tissue, and not edema. It is proposed that the weight-enhancing effects are caused by presently undefined changes at the cellular level.[56] In double-blind, placebo-controlled, randomized trials, megestrol acetate has been shown to significantly improve appetite and food intake in patients with cancer cachexia associated with a variety of tumors.[57,58] Improvement in weight has also been reported, but it is uncertain what effect these outcomes have on the management of the underlying disease, quality of life, and overall survival. The effects of megestrol acetate are not immediate. A trial period of several weeks should occur before assessing the therapeutic effects. A once-daily dose of 800 mg is currently used to treat cachexia. Cost is another consideration; 800 mg daily for 3 weeks of therapy averages $250.

Cyproheptadine, an antihistamine with serotonin antagonist properties, was first noticed to cause weight gain in children being treated for asthma. Since then, a large, randomized, placebo-controlled study has been conducted in which cyproheptadine 8 mg TID produced mild appetite stimulation without significant weight gain.[59]

Hydrazine sulfate, a controversial agent, has been reported to stimulate enteral intake.[60,61] Hydrazine sulfate is thought to work by inhibiting phosphoenolpyruvate carboxykinase (GTP), which would inhibit gluconeogenesis. Conclusions regarding the efficacy of hydrazine sulfate are varied. It is not currently commercially available in the United States, so its use is limited to clinical studies.[62,63]

Other agents used in the management of cancer cachexia may be chosen according to specific patient complaints or clinical findings. Dexamethasone in doses of 0.75–1.5 mg QID may increase appetite without weight gain.[64] Selection of this agent may be good for patients in need of pain management, additional pain management, or anti-inflammatory action. Antidepressants may help cancer patients whose anorexia is secondary to depression. Patients who describe feelings of early satiety or dysmotility may be helped by a prokinetic agent.

Cancer patients who experienced both nausea and early satiety benefited from metoclopramide 10 mg before meals and at bedtime.[65] Delta-tetrahydrocannabinol (THC) may stimulate appetite and reduce nausea in some cancer patients. Studies have had varied results from increased appetite, minimal weight increase, and mood elevation.[66] Most notable with this agent is its effects on mental status, which some patients may find undesirable.

Enteral Nutrition

Nutritional support may be provided via enteral feedings when the GI tract is intact and functioning and there are no other contraindications (e.g., high risk for aspiration, bowel obstruction, ileus, or pancreatitis). In comparison with parenteral feedings, enteral feedings are simple, inexpensive, and generally well tolerated, and they have been as effective as total parenteral nutrition in suppressing gluconeogenesis.[67] In addition, enteral feedings are able to maintain the integrity of the gut, whereas total parenteral nutrition does not preserve the gut mucosa and can contribute to bacterial translocation.[68] Line sepsis is always a risk for these patients.

The enteral tube can be placed in the stomach, duodenum, or jejunum. Tubes are usually made of a soft, flexible polyurethane or silicone. Enteral feedings can be administered as continuous or intermittent infusions or as bolus feedings, depending on where the tube is placed in the GI tract and what the patient can tolerate. Nasogastric tubes are generally used for short-term support, although occasionally they have been used for several months. Esophagostomies, gastrostomies, or jejunostomies may be required for patients who require long-term nutritional support.

Enteral formulas range from blenderized foods to special formulations designed for patients with specific disease states (e.g., trauma or pulmonary disease). The products on the market today are formulated to meet the nutritional needs of virtually any patient who requires enteral feedings. Enteral formulations vary in caloric density, osmolarity, viscosity, and specific components. The protein content and source as well as the ratio of calories to protein content also vary among the available products (Table 18-5).[69]

Table 18-5. Nutritional Supplements for the Cancer Patient

Product (Manufacturer)	Carbohydrate Source	Protein (g/L)	Fat (g/L)	Carbohydrate (g/L)	Osmolarity (mOsm/kg H₂O)	Caloric Density (kcal/ml)	Comments
Cholesterol- and Gluten-Free							
Nutren 1 (Clintec)	maltodextrin, corn syrup solids	40	38	127	300	1	lactose- and gluten-free; for normal to mildly impaired digestive function; 24% of fat as MCT; vitamins/minerals
Nutren 1 (Clintec)	maltodextrin, sucrose, corn syrup	40	38	127	v-340 c-390 s-360	1	lactose- and gluten-free; for normal to mildly impaired digestive function; 24% of fat as MCT; vitamins/minerals
Nutren 1.5 (Clintec)	maltodextrin	60	67.6	169.2	u-410 c-590 v-510	1.5	lactose- and gluten-free; for normal to mildly impaired digestive function; low-residue product; 48% of fat as MCT; vitamins/minerals
Nutren 2 (Clintec)	corn syrup solids, maltodextrin, sucrose	80	106	196	710	2	lactose- and gluten-free; for normal to mildly impaired digestive function; low-residue product; 73% of fat as MCT; vitamins/minerals
Replete Oral (Clintec)	maltodextrin, sucrose	62.5	34	113.2	350	1	lactose- and gluten-free; for increased protein needs; vitamins/minerals
Peptamen (Carnation)	maltodextrin, starch	40	39.2	127.2	270	1	lactose- and gluten-free; 70% of fat as MCT; for impaired digestive function or bowel disorders; for tube feeding only; vitamins/minerals
Citrotein Powder and Liquid (Sandoz)	sugar, hydrolyzed corn starch	41	1.6	122	500	0.67	lactose-free; vitamins/minerals; contains egg white solids as a protein source
Pulmonary/Ventilator Patient Care							
Pulmocare (Ross)	hydrolyzed corn starch, sucrose	62	92	104	475	1.5	lactose-free; vitamins/minerals
Respalor (Mead Johnson)	corn syrup, sugar	75	70	146	580	1.5	lactose-free; vitamins/minerals
Lactose-Free							
Entrition 0.5 (Clintec)	maltodextrin	17.5	17.5	68	120	0.5	tube feeding only; available only in a closed system; vitamins/minerals
Entrition HN Entri-Pak Liquid (Clintec)	maltodextrin	44	41	114	300	1	tube-feeding only; available only in a closed system; for additional protein; vitamins/minerals
Jevity (Ross)	hydrolyzed corn starch	44.3	35	150.8	300	1.06	tube-feeding only; vitamins/minerals; high-fiber
Osmolite (Ross)	hydrolyzed corn starch	37	37	143	300	1.06	tube-feeding only; vitamins/minerals
Osmolite HN (Ross)	hydrolyzed corn starch	44	35	140	300	1.06	tube-feeding only; high-protein; vitamins/minerals
Ensure Plus (Ross)	corn syrup, sucrose	54.2	53	197.1	690	1.5	high-protein; vitamins/minerals
Magnacal (Sherwood)	maltodextrin, sucrose	70	80	250	590	2	high-protein; high-calorie; vitamins/minerals
Isocal HCN (Mead Johnson)	corn syrup	75	102	200	640	2	high-protein; high-calorie; vitamins/minerals
Sustacal (Mead Johnson)	sugar, corn syrup	60.4	23	138	650–690	1	vitamins/minerals

Table 18-5. Nutritional Supplements for the Cancer Patient (continued)

Product (Manufacturer)	Carbohydrate Source	Protein (g/L)	Fat (g/L)	Carbohydrate (g/L)	Osmolarity (mOsm/kg H₂O)	Caloric Density (kcal/ml)	Comments
Lactose-Free (cont.)							
Sustacal Plus Liquid (Mead Johnson)	corn syrup solids, sugar	61	58	190	480	1.52	vitamins/minerals
Lipisorb Powder (Mead Johnson)	corn syrup solids, sucrose	35	48	117	320	1	vitamins/minerals
Vivonex T.E.N. Powder (Sandoz)	unknown	38.2	2.77	205	630	1	elemental formula; requires minimal digestion; vitamins/minerals
Isocal Liquid (Mead Johnson)	maltodextrin	34	44	135	270	1.06	tube feeding only; vitamins/minerals
Isocal HN Liquid (Mead Johnson)	maltodextrin	44	45	123	270	1.06	unflavored; tube feeding only; vitamins/minerals
Ensure With Fiber (Ross)	hydrolyzed corn starch, sucrose	39	37	160	480	1.1	vitamins/minerals
Criticare HN Liquid (Mead Johnson)	maltodextrin, modified corn starch	38	5.3	220	650	1.06	tube-feeding only; vitamins/minerals
Resource (Sandoz)	sugar, hydrolyzed corn starch	37	37	145	430	1.06	gluten-free; vitamins/minerals
Gluten-Free							
Travasorb HN (Clintec)	glucose oligosaccharides	45	13	175	560	1	lactose-free; low-residue; high-protein; elemental formula; requires minimal digestion; vitamins/minerals
Travasorb MCT (Clintec)	corn syrup solids	49.6	33	122.8	250	1	lactose-free; low-residue; high-protein; low-sodium; vitamins/minerals
Isosource (Sandoz)	hydrolyzed corn starch	43	41	170	360	1.2	fiber-free; vitamins/minerals
Isosource HN (Sandoz)	hydrolyzed corn starch	53	41	160	330	1.2	high-protein; vitamins/minerals
Resource Plus (Sandoz)	maltodextrin, sucrose	55	53	200	600	1.5	high-protein; high-calorie; vitamins/minerals
Travasorb STD (Clintec)	glucose oligosaccharides	30	14	190	560	1	lactose-free; low-residue; vitamins/minerals
Special Formulas							
Travasorb Renal Diet Powder (Clintec)	glucose oligosaccharides, sucrose	23	17.7	270.5	590	1.35	electrolyte-free; contains B and C vitamins
Amin-Aid Instant Drink Powder (McGaw)	maltodextrin, sucrose	6.6	15.7	124.3	700	2	for acute and chronic renal failure; high-calorie; limited sodium
Travasorb Hepatic (Clintec)	glucose oligosaccharides, sucrose	29.4	14.7	215.2	600	1.1	for hepatic dysfunction/failure; 50% of protein as BCAA; vitamins/minerals
Hepatic-Aid II Instant Drink Powder (McGaw)	maltodextrin, sucrose	15	12.3	57.3	560	1.2	for chronic liver disease; may contain tartrazine
Glucerna (Ross)	hydrolyzed corn starch, fructose, soy fiber	41	55	93	375	1	for abnormal glucose intolerance; vitamins/minerals

Table 18-5. Nutritional Supplements for the Cancer Patient (continued)

Product (Manufacturer)	Carbohydrate Source	Protein (g/L)	Fat (g/L)	Carbohydrate (g/L)	Osmolarity (mOsm/kg H$_2$O)	Caloric Density (kcal/ml)	Comments
Special Formulas (cont.)							
TraumaCal (Mead Johnson)	corn syrup, sugar	83	69	195	490	1.5	lactose-free; for moderately and severely stressed patients (e.g., multiple trauma, major burns); high-protein; high-calorie; vitamins/minerals
Impact (Sandoz)	hydrolyzed corn starch	56	28	130	375	1	lactose-free; for severe metabolic stress, trauma, and sepsis; vitamins/minerals
Immun-Aid Powder (McGaw)	maltodextrin	18.5	11	60	460	500	for immunocompromised patients; vitamins/minerals
Milk-Based							
Carnation Instant Breakfast + 8 oz. low-fat milk (Carnation)	lactose	14[a]	5	22	545–578	0.7	contains egg white solids as a protein source
Carnation Instant Breakfast + 8 oz. whole milk (Carnation)	lactose, sucrose	14[a]	8	36	671–758	1	contains egg white solids as a protein source

SOURCE: adapted with permission from Liter ME, Corelli RL, Gericke CR, et al. Total quality management in cancer support. *Pharm Pract News* 1996;24:55–64. MCT, medium-chain triglycerides; BCAA, branched-chain amino acids.
[a]Calculations based on 9 oz.

Table 18-6. Specialty Enteral Nutrition Immune-Enhancing Formulas

	Vivonex Plus	Impact	Immun-Aid
Arginine	+	+	+
Glutamine	+	+	+
Omega-3 fatty acids	+	+	−
RNA	−	+	−
BCAA	+	−	+

Recently, enteral products with immune-enhancing substrates that may benefit the immunocompromised cancer patient have been emphasized (Table 18-6). Arginine not only increases the nitrogen content of the formulation with its additional nitrogen but also aids in T-cell activation and is a precursor to nitric oxide, a vasodilating substance. Glutamine has a role in decreasing bacterial translocation across the GI tract. Omega-3 fatty acids are precursors of the even-numbered leukotrienes, prostaglandins, and thromboxanes, which are immunoenhancing and anti-inflammatory. RNA is thought to have a positive effect on immunity and is also present in some formulations (Table 18-6).[70]

Products vary in complexity of the substrate. Blenderized diets, although less costly than commercial preparations, are not sterile and tend to be more viscous, requiring a feeding tube with a large bore. Protein sources in enteral formulations may include milk, meat, or fish, and they are available as intact protein, protein hydrolysates, or crystalline amino acids. The patient's digestive and absorptive abilities need to be considered in the product selection. Hyperosmolar formulations may cause rapid fluid and electrolyte shifts, resulting in severe diarrhea, if they are fed directly into the small bowel. Patients with lactose intolerance may need a lactose-free formula. Patients with reduced absorption surfaces may require an elemental feed or one with decreased fat and low residual. Patients who have disorders that affect pancreatic exocrine function and patients who have problems with amino acid transport may require formulas with hydrolyzed proteins or crystalline amino acids. Gastrectomy patients would best utilize a complex carbohydrate formula to reduce dumping.

Patients who have recently undergone abdominal radiation or who have not been fed via their gut for a few days may benefit from enteral products supplemented with glutamine. Glutamine has been found to decrease bacterial translocation while increasing villous height and number.[71] Prophylactic administration of glutamine in such patients appears to protect the small bowel.[72]

The digestion of fat is more complex. It depends on both bile acids and pancreatic enzymes to emulsify and hydrolyze fat so that absorption can occur. Medium-chain triglycerides in place of fat are indicated in conditions of fat malabsorption. In selecting the most appropriate regimen for the patient, all these factors, as well as product cost, should be considered.

Complications of enteral feedings include nausea, vomiting, diarrhea, constipation, inappropriate hydration status, and pulmonary aspirations, as well as infection from product contamination. Displacement or dislodgement of the enteral tube may cause discomfort. Depending on the site of insertion and type of tube, patients may be at risk for infectious complications. Patients should be monitored at first and followed periodically after they stabilize to ensure that the enteral product has not caused or contributed to these or other problems. Careful attention should be paid when administering enteral nutrition to patients with escalating analgesic needs. Rapid adjustments in narcotic doses can slow GI motility, predisposing these patients to high gastric residuals and aspiration pneumonia.

Although enteral feedings are administered to preserve or rebuild a patient's nutritional state, the psychological effect on the patient can be profound. Patients may refuse life-sustaining support because of inadequate education about nutritional needs or for aesthetic reasons.

Total Parenteral Nutrition

Intravenous hyperalimentation should be used when enteral feedings are not tolerated or are contraindicated. Cancer patients constitute approximately one third of the patients who receive total parenteral nutrition (TPN).[73] TPN can improve immune response and increase body weight.[74] TPN also has been used to suppress gluconeogenesis, although endogenous glucose production rates may not be affected.[67]

Retrospective trials have reported that TPN may improve treatment response, tolerance, and survival. These types of reviews are not recommended for evaluating clinical response and outcomes in the general cancer patient population, however, because intervening improvements in health care, patient management, or selection may change interpretation of data.[73] A review of retrospective studies evaluating TPN use among cancer patients concluded that TPN use decreased surgical complications and operative mortality, but there was no statistical benefit in improved survival or tolerance to toxicity to cancer patients who received chemotherapy or radiation therapy.[73]

Deitel and coworkers[75] observed that when TPN was started preoperatively in cancer patients with resectable cancers and continued postoperatively until enteral diets were resumed, no significant problems were encountered (mortality rate, 0%). However, when TPN was started after life-threatening complications arose, or when it was used in operable, cachectic patients, the mortality rates were 17 and 37.5%, respectively.

Some evidence suggests that specific modifications of widely used TPN formulations may benefit patients with cancer. For example, many current TPN regimens may not provide adequate amounts of branched-chain amino acids to support muscle synthesis in cancer cachexia.[76] TPN solutions enriched with branched-chain amino acids may improve fractional rates of albumin synthesis; however, the clinical significance to cachectic cancer patients is unknown.

Manipulation of TPN amino acid components has been studied with the use of glutamine. Glutamine is a nonessential amino acid that serves as a principal substrate for lymphocytes, macrophages, and intestinal mucosal cells. Although glutamine is a nonessential amino acid, certain conditions (e.g., sepsis, trauma, or malignancies) may make it an essential amino acid.[77] Currently, glutamine is not commonly a component of amino acid solutions. Studies have found that glutamine depletion occurs in cancer patients, which may be caused by glutamine use by the tumor or catabolic effects of antineoplastic treatment. As a result, these patients lose muscle mass because skeletal muscle is the major storage site for glutamine. Glutamine is also required for proper functioning of host tissues; if glutamine is decreased, sepsis and bacterial translocation may occur. Studies involving glutamine supplementation in TPN has shown favorable results, including improved nitrogen balance, alleviation of glutamine skeletal muscle depletion, and decreased bacterial translocation.[78-80]

Research has shown that the addition of glutamine to TPN benefits patients undergoing bone marrow transplantation (BMT). Ziegler et al.[81] studied the effects of glutamine-free and glutamine-enriched TPN on allogeneic BMT patients. Patients received isonitrogenous and isocaloric solutions beginning day one of BMT. Patients who received the glutamine-enriched TPN had improved nitrogen balance, decreased incidence of infection, and decreased length of stay.[82] Scheltinga et al.[82] observed similar results, including decreased fluid accumulation in the patients receiving glutamine-enriched TPN. A study that looked at 29 patients, 14 allogeneic and 15 autologous BMT patients, also reported decreased fluid accumulation with the glutamine-enriched TPN but did not find any significant difference in clinical infections or positive bacterial cultures.[83]

The decision to administer lipids as part of TPN is a clinical decision based on the patient's ability to clear the lipid fraction and the need for a concentrated calorie source, the desire to provide a mixed fuel system or prevent essential fatty acid deficiency, and the patient's hematological status. Lipids should be administered with caution to patients who are thrombocytopenic secondary to antineoplastic treatment. Limited data suggests that lipids may adversely affect platelet function by decreasing platelet aggregation and number in patients who are thrombocytopenic or actively bleeding.[84-86] There is also evidence that lipids have no effect on or increase the adhesiveness of platelets.[87] The mechanism of action in either case is not well understood. The most widely accepted theory for a deleterious effect on platelets is that the phospholipid portion of exogenously administered lipids adheres to and coats the platelet surface, preventing normal aggregation. The clinical significance of alterations in platelet membranes is unclear. No randomized, controlled studies evaluating the effects of lipids on the incidence of bleeding or on bleeding time in thrombocytopenic patients have been done. Some clinicians suggest withholding lipids, particularly when the platelet count reaches a critical level for spontaneous bleeds (e.g., 10,000 platelets/mm^3). The administration of platelets should be carefully considered in actively bleeding thrombocytopenic individuals.

The American College of Physicians evaluated 12 randomized, controlled trials and pooled the results on use of parenteral nutrition in patients who were undergoing chemotherapy and radiotherapy.[88] It concluded that TPN was associated with net harm and that routine use of TPN could not be recommended. The analysis did not show any benefits in survival or response to therapy for the chemotherapy and radiotherapy patients. It does appear that TPN may benefit some subgroups of cancer patients; one such subgroup is BMT patients.[89,90]

PREVENTION

Diet is thought to cause nearly one third of all human cancers in the United States[91] and has long been hypothesized to play an important role in the etiology of cancer. Although many studies have been conducted to assess the relationship between cancer and diet, the results are not consistent. Analysis of the many studies indicates that there are trends with respect to diet and cancer, however.

A known avoidable cause of cancer is tobacco. Smoking causes about 90% of lung cancers and also contributes to cancers of the mouth, esophagus, stomach, kidney, pancreas, bladder, and, possibly, the colon, as well as to leukemia.

Dietary components that have been linked to causing or contributing to the development of cancer include diets high in fat and diets low in fiber, antioxidants, and trace minerals. High fat and alcohol intake has been associated with an increased risk of breast cancer. Associations between fat and breast cancer were found to be specific for postmenopausal, but not premenopausal, women.[92] The mechanism may be related to a neoplastic conversion at the DNA level. Some studies have suggested that animal fat, specifically red meat, may increase the incidence of colon, breast, and prostate cancers. Most consistent has been the relationship between red meat consumption and increased colon cancer risk. Fat alone may not be the culprit; total caloric intake rather than fat intake is reported to be more significant when evaluating the effect of diet on the development of cancer.

The relationship between fiber and colon cancer has been studied.[93] Fiber intake may lower the risk of colon, GI, breast, ovary, and endometrial cancers. The physiological effect of fiber on the GI tract is more commonly known, with its influence on the entire GI tract and its necessity for normal function. Fiber aids in retaining water and increases stool weight, increasing defecation frequency and decreasing GI transit time. The result is increased mobility of possible carcinogens through the GI tract. The association between fiber and breast, ovary, and endometrial cancers may be related to modifications of biological actions of hormones and micronutrient content. Whether any specific fiber, such as oat or wheat bran, is more beneficial than another is still controversial. The National Cancer Institute recommends ingesting 20–30 g/day of any type of fiber.

Antioxidants, such as carotenoids, ascorbic acid, and vitamin E, have been studied in cancer prevention because of their presumptive role against free radicals and reactive oxygen molecules. Free radicals produced by numerous exogenous sources (e.g., pollutants, pesticides, and tobacco smoke) cause cellular damage. Antioxidants trap these free radicals and reactive oxygen molecules to prevent the damage. Three large-scale, randomized trials testing antioxidants in cancer prevention have been completed. The Alpha-Tocopherol Beta Carotene (ATBC) Cancer Prevention Study was conducted in 29,133 Finnish male smokers over six years.[94] The men were supplemented with beta carotene and/or vitamin E. The results showed no protective effect. There was, however, an increased risk of lung cancer shown with beta carotene. The Chinese Cancer Prevention Trial studied 29,584 residents of a community with known high risk for esophageal and gastric cancers and poor diets. Participants received various combinations of retinol, zinc, riboflavin, niacin, vitamin C, molybdenum, beta carotene, vitamin E, and selenium. The subjects who had received beta carotene, vitamin E, and selenium had decreased mortality and gastric cancer–related deaths.[95] The Beta Carotene and Retinol Efficacy Trial (CARET), as can be seen in the above studies[96] (Table 18-7), includes a list of other agents that are under investigation for their chemoprotective effects.[97]

Detecting a protective effect of diet is not a simple matter. Modifications in fat intake generally increase the intake of fiber and vitamins, so a single dietary intervention may affect several components of the diet. We have learned from the above studies that supplementing the diet with antioxidants without diet modification may not be beneficial.

Table 18-7. Promising Cancer Chemoprotective Agents in Phase I Clinical Trials and Preclinical Toxicology Testing

Agent	Toxicology/Phase I	Target
S-Allyl-L-cysteine	Tox	Lung
Curcumin	I	Colon, breast
Fluasterone	Tox	Breast
Genistein	Tox	Breast, prostate, colon
Ibuprofen	I	Colon, bladder
Indole-3-carbinol	I	Breast
Lycopene	I	Prostate
Perillyl alcohol	I	Breast, colon
PEITC	I	Lung
9-cis-Retinoic acid	I	Breast, cervix
Sulindac sulfone	I	Colon, breast
Tea/EGCG	Tox	Colon
Ursodiol	I	Colon
Vitamin D_3 analogues	Tox	Breast, colon
p-XSC	Tox	Breast, colon
NAC + DFMO	Tox	Breast
DFMO + 4-HPR	Tox	Breast
DFMO + Oltipraz	Tox	Bladder, colon
DFMO + Piroxicam	I	Colon, bladder
4-HPR + Oltipraz	Tox	Breast, bladder
NAC + Oltipraz	Tox	Lung

SOURCE: reprinted with permission from Kelloff GJ, Hawk ET, Karp JE, et al. Progress in clinical chemoprevention. *Semin Oncol*; 1997;24:246.
PEITC, phenylethyl isothiocyanate; Tea/EGCG, green tea catechin extract and epigallocatechin gallate; p-XSC, 1,4-phenylenebis-(methylene)selenocyanate; NAC, N-acetyl-L-cysteine; DFMO, 2-difluoromethylornithine; 4-HPR, N-(4-hydroxyphenyl)retinamide.

SUMMARY

Identifying and treating nutritional deficits are extremely important to the comprehensive management of patients with cancer. Nutritional problems may be caused by the tumor or by the various therapies that are used to treat it (i.e., surgery, radiation, or chemotherapy). Because many of these problems are caused by drug therapy, pharmacists are often responsible for distinguishing drug-related causes from other causes. Both pharmacologic and nutritional support interventions are used to manage the anorexia and weight loss associated with advanced cancer. Pharmacists are important members of the nutritional support team. They not only make recommendations regarding the appropriate use of these interventions but also monitor patients receiving nutritional therapies.

REFERENCES

1. DeWys WD, Begg C, Lavin P, et al. Prognostic effect of weight loss prior to chemotherapy in cancer patients. *Am J Med* 1980;69:491–7.
2. Langstein HN, Norton JA. Mechanisms of cancer cachexia. *Hematol Oncol Clin North Am* 1991;5:103–23.
3. Hansell DT, Davies JWL, Burns HJG. The relationship between resting energy expenditure and weight loss in benign and malignant disease. *Ann Surg* 1986;203:240–5.
4. Knox LS, Crosby LO, Flurer ED, et al. Energy expenditure in

malnourished cancer patients. *Ann Surg* 1983;197:152–62.
5. Young VR. Energy metabolism and requirements in the cancer patient. *Cancer Res* 1977;37:2336–47.
6. Moley JF, Morrison SD, Norton JA. Preoperative insulin reverses cachexia and decreases mortality in tumor bearing rats. *J Surg Res* 1987;43:21–8.
7. Mirtallo JM. Nutrition metabolism in health and disease. In: DiPiro JJ, Talbert RL, Hayes PE, et al., editors. *Pharmacotherapy: A Pathophysiological Approach*. 3rd ed. New York: Elsevier; 1997. p. 2711–33.
8. Parnes HL, Fung E, Schiffer CA. Chemotherapy-induced lactose intolerance in adults. *Cancer* 1994;74:1629–33.
9. DeWys WD, Walters K. Abnormalities of taste sensation in cancer patients. *Cancer* 1975;36:1888–96.
10. Souba WW, Copeland EM. Parenteral nutrition and metabolic observations in cancer. *Nutr Clin Pract* 1988;3:183–90.
11. Ballie P, Mullar FK, Pratt AW. Food and water intakes and walker tumor growth in rats with hypothalamic lesions. *Am J Physiol* 1965;209:293–300.
12. Norton JA, Moley JF, Green MU. Parabiotic transfer of cancer anorexia/cachexia in male rats. *Cancer Res* 1985;45:5547–52.
13. Masumo H, Yamasak N, Okuda H. Purification and characterization of a lipolytic factor (toxohormone-L) from cell free fluid of ascites sarcoma 180. *Cancer Res* 1981;41:284–8.
14. Beck SA, Tisdale MJ. Production of lipolytic and proteolytic factors by a murine tumor producing cachexia in the host. *Cancer Res* 1987;47:5919–23.
15. Tisdale MJ, Brennan RA. Metabolic substrate utilization by a tumor cell line which induces cachexia in vivo. *Br J Cancer* 1986;54:601–6.
16. Tisdale MJ, Leung YC. Changes in host liver fatty acid synthetase in tumor-bearing mice. *Cancer Lett* 1988;42:231–5.
17. Gibbs J, Smith GP. The actions of bombesin-like peptides on food intake. *Ann NY Acad Sci* 1988;547:210–6.
18. Krause R, Humphrey C, Von Meyerfeldt M, et al. A central mechanism for anorexia in cancer: a hypothesis. *Cancer Treat Rep* 1981;65(*Suppl* 5):15–23.
19. Ternell M, Moldawer LL, Lonnroth C, et al. Plasma protein synthesis in experimental cancer compared to paraneoplastic conditions, including monokine administration. *Cancer Res* 1987;47:5825–30.
20. Torti M, Dieckman B, Beutler B, et al. A macrophage factor inhibits adipocyte gene expression in an in vitro model of cachexia. *Science* 1985;229:867–9.
21. Kawakami M, Pekala PH, Lane MD, et al. Lipoprotein lipase suppression in 3T3-L1 cells by an endotoxin-induced mediator from exudate cells [abstract]. *Proc Natl Acad Sci USA* 1982;79:912–6.
22. Pekala PH, Kawakami M, Angus CW, et al. Selective inhibition of synthesis of enzymes for de novo fatty acid biosynthesis by an endotoxin-induced mediator from exudate cells. *Proc Natl Acad Sci USA* 1983;80:2743–7.
23. Nathanson L, Hall TC. A spectrum of tumors that produce paraneoplastic syndromes. Lung tumors: how they produce their syndromes. *Ann NY Acad Sci* 1974;230:367–77.
24. Beutler B, Mahoney J, LeTrang N, et al. Purification of cachectin, a lipoprotein lipase-suppressing hormone from endotoxin induced RAW 2647 cells. *J Exp Med* 1985;161:981–95.
25. Beck SA, Tisdale MJ. Production of lipolytic and proteolytic factors by a murine tumor-producing cachexia in the host. *Cancer Res* 1987;47:5919–23.
26. Brennan MF. Uncomplicated starvation versus cancer cachexia. *Cancer Res* 1977;37:2359–64.
27. Owen OE, Morgan AP, Kemp HG, et al. Brain metabolism during fasting. *J Clin Invest* 1967;46:1589–95.
28. Brennen MF. Total parenteral nutrition in the cancer patient. *N Engl J Med* 1981;305:375–82.
29. Popp MB, Kirkemo AK, Morrison SD, et al. Tumor and host carcass during total parenteral nutrition in an anorectic rat-tumor system. *Ann Surg* 1984;199:205–10.
30. Copeland EM, Daly JM, Ota DM, et al. Nutrition, cancer and intravenous hyperalimentation. *Cancer* 1979;43:2108–16.
31. Holroyde CP, Gabuzda TG, Putman RC, et al. Altered glucose metabolism in metastatic carcinoma. *Cancer Res* 1975;35:3710–4.
32. Gold J. Proposed treatment of cancer by inhibition of gluconeogenesis. *Oncology* 1968;22:185–207.
33. Kern KA, Norton JA. Cancer cachexia. *J Parenter Enteral Nutr* 1988;12:286–98.
34. Young VR. Energy metabolism and requirements in the cancer patient. *Cancer Res* 1977;37:2336–47.
35. Holroyde CP, Skutches CL, Boden G, et al. Glucose metabolism in cachectic patients with colorectal cancer. *Cancer Res* 1984;44:5910–3.
36. Lundholm K, Bylund AC, Schersten T. Glucose tolerance in relation to skeletal muscle enzyme activities in cancer patients. *Scand J Clin Lab Invest* 1977;37:267–72.
37. Gold J. Cancer cachexia and gluconeogenesis. *Ann NY Acad Sci* 1974;230:103–10.
38. Burt ME, Lowry SF, Gorschboth CM, et al. Metabolic alterations in a non-cachectic animal tumor system. *Cancer* 1981;47:2138–46.
39. Waterhouse C, Jeanpretre N, Kellson J. Gluconeogenesis from alanine in patients with progressive malignant disease. *Cancer Res* 1979;39:1968–72.
40. Carmichael MI, Clague M, Keir M, et al. Whole body protein turnover, synthesis and breakdown in patients with colorectal carcinoma. *Br J Surg* 1980;67:736–9.
41. Cohn SH, Garenhaus W, Vartsky D, et al. Body composition and dietary intake in neoplastic disease. *Am J Clin Nutr* 1981;34:1997–2004.
42. Reynolds JV, Thom AK, Zhang SM, et al. Arginine, protein calorie malnutrition and cancer. *J Surg Res* 1988;45:513–22.
43. Barbul A. Arginine and immune function. *Nutrition* 1990;6:53–8.
44. Washsman BA. Cancer cachexia: the metabolic alterations. *Nutr Clin Pract* 1988;3:191–7.
45. Waterhouse C, Kemperman JH. Carbohydrate metabolism in subjects with cancer. *Cancer Res* 1971;31:1273–8.
46. Edmonson JH. Fatty acid mobilization and glucose metabolism in patients with cancer. *Cancer* 1966;19:1277–80.
47. Long CL, Schaffel N, Geiger JW, et al. Metabolic response to injury and illness: estimation of energy and protein needs from indirect calorimetry and nitrogen balance. *J Parenter Enteral Nutr* 1979;3:452–6.
48. Jacot E, Defronzo RA, Jequier E, et al. The effect of hyperglycemia, hyperinsulinemia and rate of glucose administration on glucose oxidation and glucose storage. *Metabolism* 1982;31:922–30.

49. Burke JF, Wolfe RR, Mullany CJ, et al. Glucose requirements following burn injury. *Ann Surg* 1979;190:274–85.
50. Fredrix EM, Soetera PB, Wovless EM, et al. Effect of different tumor types on resting energy expenditure. *Cancer Res* 1991;51:6138–41.
51. Bozetti HF, Pagnoni AM, Delvecchio M. Excessive caloric expenditures as a cause of malnutrition in patients with cancer. *Surg Gynecol Obstet* 1980;150:229–34.
52. Parnes HL, Mascioli EA, LaCivita CL, et al. Parenteral nutrition in overweight patients: are IV lipids necessary to prevent EFAD? *J Nutr Biochem* 1994;5:243–7.
53. Burge JC, Gordon A, Choban PS, et al. Efficacy of hypocaloric TPN in hospitalized obese patients: a prospective, double-blind, randomized trial. *J Parenter Enteral Nutr* 1994;18:203–7.
54. Moley JF, Morrison SD, Norton JA. Insulin reversal of cancer cachexia in rats. *Cancer Res* 1985;45:4925–31.
55. Tcheckmedyian NS, Tait N, Moody M, et al. High dose megestrol acetate. *JAMA* 1987;267:1195–8.
56. Aisner J, Tcheckmedyian NS, Tait N, et al. Studies of high-dose megestrol acetate: potential applications in cachexia. *Semin Oncol* 1988;15:68–75.
57. Loprinzi CL, Ellison NM, Schaid DJ, et al. A controlled trial of megestrol acetate in patients with cancer anorexia/cachexia [abstract]. *Proc Am Soc Clin Oncol* 1990;9:321.
58. Tcheckmedyian NS, Hariri L, Sian J, et al. Megestrol acetate in cancer anorexia and weight loss [abstract]. *Proc Am Soc Clin Oncol* 1990;9:336.
59. Kardinal CG, Loprinzi CL, Schaid DJ, et al. A controlled trial of cyproheptadine in cancer patients with anorexia and or cachexia. *Cancer* 1990;65:2657–62.
60. Loprinzi CL, Goldberg RM, Su JQ, et al. Placebo controlled trial of hydrazine sulfate in patients with newly diagnosed non-small cell lung cancer. *J Clin Oncol* 1994;12:1126–9.
61. Piantadosi S. Hazards of small clinical trials. *J Clin Oncol* 1990;8:9–15.
62. Loprinzi CL, Kuross SA, O'Fallon JR, et al. Randomized placebo controlled evaluation of hydrazine sulfate in patients with advanced colorectal cancer. *J Clin Oncol* 1994;12:1121–5.
63. Chlebowski RT, Bulcavage L, Grosvenor M, et al. Hydrazine sulfate in cancer patients with weight loss. *Cancer* 1987;59:406–10.
64. Moertel CG, Schult AJ, Reitemeier RJ. Corticosteroid treatment of preterminal gastrointestinal cancer. *Cancer* 1974;33:1607–9.
65. Shivshanker K, Bennett RW, Hayne TP. Tumor associated gastroparesis: correction with metoclopramide. *Am J Surg* 1983;145:221–5.
66. Curtis EB, Walsh TD. Prescribing practices of a palliative care service. *J Pain Sympt Manage* 1993;8:312–6.
67. Burt ME, Gorschboth CM, Brennan MF. A controlled prospective, randomized trial evaluating the metabolic effects of enteral and parenteral nutrition in the cancer patient. *Cancer* 1982;49:1092–105.
68. Alverdy JC, Aoys E, Moss GS. Total parenteral nutrition promotes bacterial translocation from the gut. *Surgery* 1988;104:185–90.
69. Liter ME, Corelli RL, Gericke CR, et al. Total quality management in cancer support. *Pharm Pract News* 1996;23:21–7.
70. Alexander JW. Immunoenhancement via enteral nutrition. *Arch Surg* 1993;128:1242–5.
71. Klimberg VS, Souba WW, Dolson DJ, et al. Oral glutamine supports crypt cell turnover and accelerates intestinal healing following abdominal radiation. *J Parenter Enteral Nutr* 1989;13(Suppl):11S.
72. Klimberg VS, Souba WW, Dolson DJ, et al. Prophylactic glutamine protects the intestinal mucosa from radiation injury. *Cancer* 1990;66:62–8.
73. Klein S, Sinaes J, Blackburn GL. Total parenteral nutrition and cancer clinical trials. *Cancer* 1986;58:1378–86.
74. Copeland EM, MacFadyen BV Jr, Lanzotti V, et al. Intravenous hyperalimentation as an adjunct to cancer chemotherapy. *Am J Surg* 1975;129:167–73.
75. Deitel M, Vasic V, Alexander M. Specialized nutrition support in the cancer patient: is it worthwhile? *Cancer* 1978;41:2359–63.
76. Tayek JA, Bistrian BR, Hehir DJ, et al. Improved protein kinetics and albumin synthesis by branched chain amino acid-enriched total parenteral nutrition in cancer cachexia. *Cancer* 1986;58:147–57.
77. Souba WW, Herskowitz K, Austgen TR, et al. Glutamine nutrition: theoretical considerations and therapeutic impact. *J Parenter Enteral Nutr* 1990;14(Suppl):237S–42S.
78. Burke D, Alverdy JC, Aoys E, et al. Glutamine supplemented total parenteral nutrition improves gut immune function. *Arch Surg* 1989;124:1396–9.
79. Alverdy JC, Aoys E, Weiss-Carrington P, et al. The effect of glutamine supplemented total parenteral nutrition on gut immune cellularity. *J Surg Res* 1992;52:34–8.
80. Hammarqvist F, Wernermand J, Ali R, et al. Addition of glutamine to total parenteral nutrition after elective abdominal surgery spares free glutamine in muscle, counteracts the fall in muscle protein synthesis, and improves nitrogen balance. *Ann Surg* 1989;209:455–61.
81. Ziegler TR, Young LS, Benfall K, et al. Clinical and metabolic efficacy of glutamine supplemented parenteral nutrition after bone marrow transplant. *Ann Intern Med* 1992;116:821–8.
82. Scheltinga MR, Young LS, Benfall K, et al. Glutamine enriched IV feedings attenuate extracellular fluid expansion after a standard stress. *Ann Surg* 1991;214:385–95.
83. Schloerb PR, Amare M. Total parenteral nutrition with glutamine in bone marrow transplant and other clinical applications. *J Parenter Enteral Nutr* 1993;7:407–13.
84. Kapp JP, Duckert F, Hartman G. Platelet adhesiveness and serum lipids during and after Intralipid infusions. *Nutr Metab* 1971;13:92–9.
85. Aviram M, Deckelbaum RJ. Intralipid infusion into humans reduces in-vitro platelet aggregation and alters platelet lipid composition. *Metabolism* 1989;38:343–7.
86. Thomas MP, Gargett CE, West KR, et al. The effect of Intralipid on platelet function during parenteral nutrition. *Acta Chir Scand Suppl* 1979;494:70–1.
87. Jarnvig I, Naesh O, Hindberg I, et al. Platelet response to intravenous infusion of Intralipid in healthy volunteers. *Am J Clin Nutr* 1990;52:628–31.
88. American College of Physicians. Parenteral nutrition in patients receiving cancer chemotherapy. *Ann Intern Med* 1989;110:734–5.
89. Reed MD, Lazarus HM, Herzig RH, et al. Cyclic parenteral nutrition during bone marrow transplantation in children. *Cancer* 1983;51:1563–70.

90. Schmidt GM, Blume KG, Bross KJ, et al. Parenteral nutrition in bone marrow transplant recipients. *Exp Hematol* 1980;8:506–11.
91. Doll R, Peto R. The cause of cancer: quantitative estimates of avoidable risks of cancer in the United States. *J Natl Cancer Inst* 1981;66:1191–308.
92. Howe GR, Hirohata T, Hisiop GT, et al. Dietary factors and risk of breast cancer: combined analysis of 12 case-control studies. *J Natl Cancer Inst* 1990;82:161–9.
93. Willett WC, Stampfer MJ, Colditz GA, et al. Relation of meat, fat, and fiber intake to the risk of colon cancer in a prospective study among women. *N Engl J Med* 1990;323:1664–72.
94. [Anonymous]. The effect of vitamin E and beta carotene on the incidence of lung cancer and other cancers in male smokers. *N Engl J Med* 1994;330:1029–35.
95. Blot W, Li J, Taylor P, et al. Nutrition intervention trials in Linxian, China: supplementation with specific vitamin/mineral combinations, cancer incidence, disease-specific mortality in the general population. *J Natl Cancer Inst* 1993;85:1483–91.
96. Thornquist MD, Omenn GS, Goodman GL, et al. Statistical design and monitoring of the carotene and retinol efficacy trial. *Controlled Clin Trials* 1993;14:308–23.
97. Kelloff GJ, Hawk ET, Karp JE, et al. Progress in clinical chemoprevention. *Semin Oncol* 1997;24:241–52.

Suggested Readings

Bloch AS. *Nutrition Management of the Cancer Patient.* Rockville, MD: Aspen Publishers; 1991.

Rombeau JL, Caldwell MD, editors. *Enteral and Tube Feedings: Clinical Nutrition*, vol. 1. Philadelphia, PA: WB Saunders; 1990.

Rombeau JL, Caldwell MD, editors. *Parenteral Nutrition: Clinical Nutrition*, vol. 2. Philadelphia, PA: WB Saunders; 1986.

Scalfani LM, Lowry SF. Nutritional support. In: Gorerger JS, editor. *Critical Care of the Cancer Patient.* 2nd ed. Baltimore, MD: Mosby; 1991. p. 283–98.

SELF-STUDY QUESTIONS

1. List five effects of cancer chemotherapy or radiation therapy that may contribute to weight loss.

2. Name four mechanisms by which a tumor may contribute to weight loss.

3. During periods of chronic starvation, normal, nonstressed patients rely on what substrate as the predominant energy source?

4. Why is there increased Cori cycle activity in some cancer patients who have lost weight? Because . . .
    a. the tumor relies on anaerobic utilization of glucose.
    b. the Cori cycle is an energy-consuming process.
    c. aerobic utilization of glucose is increased.
    d. the tumor relies on the oxidation of glucose to lactate as an energy substrate.

5. List four common nutritional indices that may *not* accurately reflect nutritional state in patients with cancer.

6. List the eight elements of a thorough nutritional history and assessment.

7. When are fats a useful calorie source for cancer patients?

8. What two signs of continued protein malnutrition signal that protein allowances should be adjusted?

9. Which of the following statements is true of breast cancer patients who receive high-dose megestrol acetate and experience weight gain?
    a. Weight gain occurs only when their tumor decreases in size.
    b. The weight gain is due to edema.
    c. The weight gain is due to increased body mass.
    d. Appetite does not improve.

10. Total parenteral nutrition decreases complications and operative mortality in cancer patients who undergo surgery.
    a. true
    b. false

11. Glutamine is a substrate for which types of cells?

12. What are the major dietary components that have been linked to an increased risk of developing cancer?

13. Name three appetite stimulants that could benefit patients with poor appetites and mild nausea.

Chapter 19: Oncological Complications

Cynthia L. LaCivita, Pharm.D.
Clinical Coordinator, Department of Pharmacy
Shady Grove Adventist Hospital
Rockville, Maryland
Clinical Assistant Professor
University of Maryland School of Pharmacy
Baltimore, Maryland

Hypercalcemia	342
Calcium Homeostasis	342
Etiology	343
Clinical Presentation	344
Treatment	344
Hydration and Diuretics	344
Calcitonin	345
Glucocorticoids	345
Plicamycin	345
Inorganic Phosphates	345
Prostaglandin Inhibitors	345
Bisphosphonates	346
Etidronate Disodium	346
Pamidronate Disodium	346
Gallium Nitrate	346
Management	346
Superior Vena Cava Syndrome	347
Etiology	347
Clinical Presentation	347
Diagnosis	347
Treatment	347
Small Cell Lung Cancer	347
Non-Small Cell Lung Cancer	348
Non-Hodgkin's Lymphomas	348
Thrombolytic Therapy	348
Supportive Therapy	348
Spinal Cord Compression	348
Etiology	348
Clinical Presentation	349
Diagnosis	349
Treatment	349
Surgery	349
Radiation	350
Tumor Lysis Syndrome	350
Etiology	350
Metabolic Complications	350
Hyperkalemia	351

Hyperuricemia 351
Hyperphosphatemia and Hypocalcemia 351
Prevention of Tumor Lysis Syndrome 352
Malignant Pleural Effusions 352
Etiology 352
Clinical Presentation 352
Diagnosis 352
Treatment 352
Summary 353
References 354
Self-Study Questions 355

Relatively few conditions associated with cancer require immediate therapeutic intervention. However, there is a group of disorders that require immediate recognition and treatment to avoid premature mortality or excessive morbidity. Collectively, these disorders are often referred to as oncological complications or oncological emergencies.

Oncological complications usually are related directly to a tumor mass and may develop rapidly or insidiously. However, they can also be caused or aggravated by antineoplastic therapy. The acuity of the complication and treatment needs are often dictated by the presenting signs and symptoms and the rapidity with which they evolve. The patient's overall prognosis, including information about the underlying malignancy, is important to consider before initiating treatment for the oncological complication. If the complication occurs in the terminal phase of the disease, treating the complication may needlessly prolong life without meaningful improvement in symptoms or the quality of life.

Although initial treatment of the oncological complication may be aimed at treating the acute situation, treatment must also be directed at the underlying malignancy, or the complication is likely to recur. Several oncological complications are of particular interest to pharmacists because they (1) require immediate intervention with drug therapy, (2) may be confused with toxic reactions from drug therapy, or (3) necessitate changes in other drug therapy because of the organ dysfunction they may produce.

This chapter discusses five oncological complications: hypercalcemia, superior vena cava syndrome, spinal cord compression, tumor lysis syndrome, and malignant pleural effusions. The causes, signs, and symptoms of these oncological complications, as well as their treatment and prevention, are reviewed.

After completing this chapter, the reader should be able to:

1. Describe the pathogenesis of hypercalcemia associated with malignancy and identify the presenting signs and symptoms.
2. Describe treatment for hypercalcemia.
3. Discuss medications that can contribute to or cause hypercalcemia.
4. Describe treatment for superior vena cava syndrome.
5. Describe treatment for spinal cord compression.
6. Describe treatment for tumor lysis syndrome.
7. Discuss the possible alternatives for treating malignant pleural effusions.

HYPERCALCEMIA

Hypercalcemia of malignancy can develop over an extended period or present as an acute medical emergency. In the acute situation, this metabolic abnormality may present a more immediate threat to life than the underlying malignancy. A variety of factors can produce or aggravate hypercalcemia.

Calcium Homeostasis

Calcium homeostasis is the delicate balance of the oral intake of calcium, hydration status, bone turnover, and the kidneys' ability to excrete calcium. The normal range for serum calcium is 8.5–10.4 mg/dl.[1] Unbound serum calcium (also known as ionized or free calcium)—the portion of serum calcium that is not bound to plasma proteins—is the only calcium fraction with physiological activity. The normal range of ionized calcium is 4.6–5.2 mg/dl, which constitutes approximately 45% of total serum calcium. Of the remaining serum calcium, 40% is bound to albumin and approximately 15% is bound to organic and inorganic anions.[1]

Low serum albumin (normal range, 3.5–5 g/dl), which is frequently seen in cancer patients, results in a decrease of serum calcium bound to albumin and an increase in the unbound (physiologically active) serum calcium. Unless otherwise specified, serum calcium levels measure the total calcium (bound and unbound). Therefore, in patients with low serum albumin levels (<4.0 g/dl), the total serum calcium level can be within normal limits while the proportion of active, ionized calcium is higher than normal. Interpretation of the serum calcium (Ca) level must therefore be adjusted when a patient has low serum albumin:

Ca corrected for albumin = [(Normal serum albumin − patient's serum albumin) × 0.8 mg/dl] + serum calcium

For each gram per deciliter that albumin is below 3.5 g/dl the serum calcium is increased by approximately 0.8 mg/dl.

Other conditions may require altered interpretation of serum levels of calcium. For example, in a patient with multiple myeloma, serum proteins may interfere with the interpretation of serum calcium. Although fluctuations in serum globulin (e.g., stimulation of humoral immunity) do not normally affect calcium binding significantly, the serum calcium may be abnormally high in a patient with dramatically elevated paraproteins (immunoglobulins produced by a clone of neoplastic cells in conditions such as multiple myeloma). In this situation, the ionized calcium remains normal because of increased binding of calcium to the paraproteins. Other physiological conditions that affect serum calcium include increases in serum pH (e.g., in respiratory alkalosis), which favor protein binding, and increases in serum phosphate, which binds ionized calcium and redeposits it into bone.[1] These would result in a decrease of ionized or physiologically active calcium.

Normally, serum calcium levels are maintained by several hormones, one of which is parathyroid hormone (PTH). PTH works to increase or sustain serum calcium by stimulating bone resorption, intestinal absorption, and renal reabsorption. By a negative feedback mechanism, serum calcium regulates PTH secretion.[2] PTH and serum calcium are therefore inversely related to each other.

Another hormone responsible for regulating serum calcium, calcitonin, is released from the parafollicular cells of the thyroid gland. Calcitonin's major function is to lower serum calcium by promoting renal excretion and inhibiting bone resorption by osteoclasts. The hydroxylated form of vitamin D also regulates calcium absorption from the intestines and stimulates bone resorption.

Etiology

Hypercalcemia can be caused or aggravated by nonmalignant diseases and certain medications (Table 19-1). Primary hyperthyroidism (including benign parathyroid adenomas and parathyroid hyperplasia) is the most common cause of nonmalignant hypercalcemia. Endocrine disorders (e.g., thyrotoxicosis and acute adrenal insufficiency) can also cause hypercalcemia. In addition, the granulomatous diseases (e.g., tuberculosis, sarcoidosis, and berylliosis) and extensive skeletal immobilization have been associated with causing or contributing to hypercalcemia. Thiazide diuretics, calcium supplements, hormone therapy, and vitamins can cause or exacerbate hypercalcemia, especially in persons predisposed to rising serum calcium.

The malignancies most frequently associated with hypercalcemia include breast, lung, and kidney tumors; associated to a lesser degree are cancers of the thyroid, colon, and ovaries and epidermoid tumors of the head, neck, and esophagus.[3] The high incidence of hypercalcemia associated with breast cancer is in part due to the tumor's ability to metastasize to bone. In addition, hormone treatment in breast

Table 19-1. Diseases and Drugs Associated with Hypercalcemia

Endocrine and metabolic diseases
  Primary hyperthyroidism
  Osteopetrosis
  Familial hypercalcemia with hypercalciuria
  Pheochromocytoma
  Infantile hyperphosphatasia

Infectious diseases
  Tuberculosis
  Human immunodeficiency virus (HIV) infection
  Coccidioidomycosis

Renal insufficiency

Cancer

Granulomatous diseases
  Sarcoidosis
  Berylliosis

Diet- or drug-related conditions
  Vitamin D or A intoxication
  Calcium suppplements
  Lithium
  Milk-alkali (Burnett's syndrome)

SOURCE: Warrell RP. Metabolic emergencies. In: DeVita VT, Hellman S, Rosenberg SA, editors. *Cancer: Principles and Practice of Oncology.* 5th ed. Philadelphia, PA: JB Lippincott; 1997. p. 2281.

cancer patients may increase their risk of hypercalcemia. Approximately 10–20% of cancer patients develop some degree of hypercalcemia during the course of their disease.

Tumors that are able to metastasize to bone may cause hypercalcemia by increasing bone turnover. However, bone invasion is not required, nor is it solely responsible, for producing hypercalcemia. Patients with no clinically documented bone metastasis account for up to 20% of the cancer patients who experience hypercalcemia; furthermore, the degree of bone invasion does not correlate well with the clinical severity of or responsiveness to treatment for hypercalcemia. Hypercalcemia also occurs in patients with hematological malignancies, most commonly in patients with multiple myeloma, where the incidence may be as high as 50%.

In patients with bone metastasis, hypercalcemia results from several mechanisms. Originally, it was thought that the hypercalcemia of solid tumors with bone metastasis was caused by release of calcium into the circulation due to local bone destruction. However, tumors such as prostate and small cell lung cancers, which frequently metastasize to bone, are rarely associated with hypercalcemia. It is currently thought that substances produced by the tumor, such as hormones and growth factors, may also destroy bone, a process known as humoral hypercalcemia. Substances produced by squamous cell tumors, and possibly by other neoplasms, stimulate osteoclasts directly or indirectly. Osteoclasts excavate a cavity and cause bone to be resorbed. Osteoclasts may be stimulated by prostaglandins, osteoclast-activating factors, or both.[1,4,5]

Mundy suggests several additional mechanisms for humoral hypercalcemia.[6] Transforming growth factors (TGFs), which are produced by almost all tumors, are suspected of causing humoral hypercalcemia. TGFs are tumor-derived polypeptides that stimulate cell replication. TGFs and polypeptides derived from squamous cells have been known to cause hypercalcemia in rodents. TGFs may increase osteoclastic bone resorption by stimulating the production of an osteoclast precursor and prostaglandin.[6]

Increased prostaglandin production is also thought to cause hypercalcemia. Prostaglandin E_2 does cause bone resorption in vitro. However, prostaglandin inhibitors (such as indomethacin) are rarely successful in reducing serum calcium in patients with hypercalcemia. Although prostaglandin E_2 may play a role in bone resorption, it does not appear to be a major cause of humoral hypercalcemia.

Colony-stimulating factors and leukocyte cytokinin (previously grouped with osteoclast-activating factors) are additional catalysts for stimulating bone resorption.[1,6,7] These factors are implicated as causes of hypercalcemia in hematological malignancies (e.g., multiple myeloma).

Increased metabolism of vitamin D to its hydroxylated form may also be associated with hypercalcemia. In general, patients with humoral hypercalcemia normally have depressed levels of 1,25-dihydroxy(vitamin D_3), the biologically active form of vitamin D. Occasionally, patients have an increased level of this form of vitamin D, which is thought to result from increased metabolism by the tumor.[1]

Humoral hypercalcemia was originally thought to be caused by atopic production of PTH. Recently, a PTH-like hormone has been identified from several different cancers. The sequence of the first 13 amino acids in the PTH-like protein is the same for all the tumors and for endogenous PTH. These amino acids form the biologically active part of PTH, which causes both bone resorption and bone formation.[4] The PTH-like hormone has uncoupled this process and directed its dominant effect at bone resorption.[4,8] Unlike PTH, it does not stimulate 1,25-dihydroxy(vitamin D_3) production.

In general, oral intake of calcium does not contribute to the hypercalcemia of malignancy. However, calcium should be deleted from parenteral sources to avoid contributing to rising serum calcium.

Clinical Presentation

Patients with hypercalcemia may present with a variety of symptoms. Serum calcium concentration does not always correlate with severity of symptoms. Some patients may be asymptomatic with serum levels of 14 mg/dl, whereas others may have noticeable neurological impairment at 13 mg/dl. Patients tend to tolerate slowly rising serum calcium, which gives the body time to acclimate to the metabolic changes. Five organ systems are affected by rising calcium (Table 19-

Table 19-2. Organ System Effects of Hypercalcemia

Gastrointestinal	Genitourinary
Anorexia	Polydipsia
Nausea	Renal calculi
Vomiting	Polyuria
Constipation	Renal failure
Hyporeflexia	
	Central Nervous System
Musculoskeletal	Confusion
Weakness	Lethargy
Bone pain	Coma
Fatigue	
Ataxia	**Cardiac**
	Q-T interval changes
	Arrhythmias

2): the gastrointestinal (GI), central nervous, musculoskeletal, genitourinary, and cardiac organ systems.

Hypercalcemia may worsen because its symptoms contribute to the deterioration of the condition (e.g., progressive dehydration from nausea and vomiting leads to further renal impairment and deteriorating mental status).

Treatment

Ideally, the best treatment for hypercalcemia is ablation of the tumor. When ablation is impossible or unsuccessful and metabolic urgency or emergency has been created by rising serum calcium, treatment should be started immediately. The objectives of treatment are to

- reduce serum calcium,
- prevent further toxicities,
- reverse organ toxicities, and
- provide support to reduce the likelihood of recurrence.

Hydration and Diuretics

The preferred initial therapy is vigorous hydration. Most hypercalcemic patients will be dehydrated and unable to tolerate or maintain adequate oral intake. Rehydration with approximately 3–6 L of normal saline per day, given intravenously, is usually required to replenish intravascular volume and promote calciuria. Although hydration alone is usually not effective in normalizing or controlling hypercalcemia, it is essential to replenish intravascular volume before initiating other therapies. Hydration is also relatively inexpensive.

Sodium and calcium are both excreted via the proximal renal tubule. Renal elimination of calcium can be augmented by concurrently administering a loop diuretic, which prevents reabsorption of calcium in the thick ascending loop of the renal tubule. Caution must be taken not to cause dehydration or other electrolyte abnormalities by forcing diuresis. Serum levels of potassium and magnesium should be monitored frequently and repleted as necessary, because low electrolyte levels can potentiate the deleterious effects of hypercalcemia on cardiac muscle.

Calcitonin

Calcitonin is commercially available as synthetically prepared salmon and human calcitonins. Although these calcitonins differ in amino acid sequence, their pharmacologic activity is the same. Salmon calcitonin is more potent and less expensive than the human variety and has a longer duration of activity. The dosage for salmon calcitonin is in international units (IU). Before salmon calcitonin is administered, a skin test may be advisable, to identify any allergies. The human calcitonin dosage is in milligrams. Because the potency of human and salmon calcitonin differ, the dosages are not interchangeable. Human calcitonin is only approved for the treatment of Paget's disease.

Calcitonin is a safe adjuvant to hydration and diuretics. Calcitonin also may be advantageous for hypercalcemic patients who are unable to tolerate large volumes of fluids because of underlying cardiac or pulmonary disease. It has few serious side effects and promptly lowers serum calcium with the first dose. Calcitonin must be administered parenterally, because it is inactivated in the gut. Subcutaneous administration is the preferred route of delivery, although it has been administered intramuscularly. In the treatment of hypercalcemia, the initial dose of salmon calcitonin is 4 IU/kg administered every 12 hours, to a maximum dose of 8 IU/kg given every 6 hours.

The clinical effects of calcitonin are evident within 2–4 hours after administration, and they last for approximately 8–12 hours. Patients with hypercalcemia usually respond to this therapy for 5–7 days before tolerance develops. Reports that tolerance to calcitonin is delayed by administering glucocorticoids are not supported with reproducible in vivo data.

Glucocorticoids

Glucocorticoids inhibit bone resorption in vitro.[9] They may be useful in treating hypercalcemia, particularly in patients whose tumors are sensitive to the cytolytic effects of glucocorticoids. Multiple myeloma and some of the hematological tumors appear to respond best to this treatment for hypercalcemia. Because responses with glucocorticoids may take as long as 5–10 days, it is not considered first-line therapy for the treatment of severe hypercalcemia or for symptomatic patients.[10] Steroid use is not supported by the data for treating hypercalcemia in solid tumors, with the possible exception of rare responses in breast cancer cases.[11]

Plicamycin

Plicamycin (formerly known as mithramycin), an antineoplastic agent originally used to treat testicular cancer, is considered second- or third-line treatment of hypercalcemia, since newer agents with fewer adverse effects are available. It was observed that patients treated with plicamycin often had dramatic decreases in serum calcium. Plicamycin is thought to exert its hypocalcemic effect by inhibiting DNA-dependent RNA synthesis, causing a decrease in osteoclastic activity. The usual dose recommended for treatment of hypercalcemia is 25 mg/kg as a single dose.[1] Waiting 48–72 hours before administering more plicamycin is advised, so that the patient's response can be fully evaluated and unnecessary toxicity can be avoided.[5] The effects of plicamycin are clinically evident within 24–48 hours, and almost all patients respond. After the initial dose is administered, the hypocalcemic effects may last from several days to 2 weeks.

Because plicamycin is an antineoplastic antibiotic, its side effects must be considered before therapy is begun. Major toxicities include nephrotoxicity, hepatic toxicity, and lytic effects on rapidly dividing cells, such as those in the bone marrow and GI tract. The toxicities are dose-related (the dose used for hypercalcemia is only one-tenth the dose used to treat testicular cancer), and the severity and incidence are greatest in those who receive multiple doses of plicamycin, although organ toxicities may be evident after a single dose.

The manufacturer recommends that plicamycin be diluted in 1 L of 5% dextrose or 0.9% sodium chloride and administered intravenously over 4–6 hours. Because plicamycin is an irritant, care is needed to avoid an extravasation when it is being infused for a prolonged period of time. Others advocate administering plicamycin as a bolus intravenous (IV) injection.[10-13] If nausea and vomiting result from a bolus injection, prolonging administration time or adding antiemetics will reduce or prevent GI toxicity.

Inorganic Phosphates

Administering IV inorganic phosphates decreases serum calcium by

- inhibiting bone resorption;
- forming calcium-phosphate complexes, which are redeposited in bone and other tissues; and
- possibly stimulating bone formation.

This form of therapy is effective in depressing serum calcium rapidly, and the results are dose dependent. Although inorganic phosphates are effective, they are rarely used today because of their severe toxicities, which include hypotension related to rate of administration, renal failure, and extraskeletal calcification in the eye, heart, lung, and muscle.

Prostaglandin Inhibitors

Hypercalcemia may be mediated to a small extent by prostaglandin E_2. However, only a small percentage of patients with hypercalcemia respond to antiprostaglandin therapy. Historically, 25 mg of indomethacin given orally three times per day has been used, although other nonsteroidal anti-inflammatory drugs (NSAIDs) would theoretically be equally effective. NSAIDs should be used with caution when treating elderly patients and in patients with compromised renal function. NSAIDs should be avoided in neutropenic and thrombocytopenic patients, because the drugs' antipyretic activity may mask infection-related fever and because the drugs have negative effects on platelet aggregation.

Bisphosphonates

Bisphosphonates are chemical analogues of the naturally occurring pyrophosphate found in the bone matrix. They have a carbon substituted in place of the oxygen in endogenous pyrophosphate, which makes bisphosphonates resistant to cleavage from phosphatase during the process of bone resorption. They exert their activity by adsorbing to bone surface, inhibiting calcium resorption. A number of bisphosphonate compounds have been used in clinical trials for treating hypercalcemia and osteoporosis. Currently, etidronate disodium, pamidronate disodium, and alendronate sodium are available commercially in the United States. Only etidronate and pamidronate are approved for hypercalcemia. Alendronate is available as an oral formulation for the treatment of postmenopausal osteoporosis. These agents are considered first-line therapy (after rehydration) and should be used concomitantly with saline diuresis in patients with hypercalcemia.

Etidronate Disodium

Patients should receive 7.5 mg/kg of IV etidronate disodium daily over 2 hours for 3 days to load the bone adequately. When hypercalcemia has persisted, infusions have been continued for up to 7 days to return serum calcium to a normal range. It is recommended that a week elapse before re-treatment is considered, to observe the full effect of therapy on serum calcium levels. Bolus infusions should be avoided; bolus infusions in dogs have caused structural renal abnormalities that contribute to renal failure. Oral etidronate has been used in an effort to maintain normal serum calcium if the patient has responded to IV etidronate. Because of the poor bioavailability of oral etidronate, doses of 20 mg/kg per day have been recommended when the formulation is switched from IV to oral for periods up to 90 days. Administering oral etidronate in divided doses increases GI tolerance. Studies have reported that up to 30% of patients may derive benefit from the addition of oral etidronate once they have become normocalcemic.[14,15] Oral etidronate is not effective as initial therapy for hypercalcemia. Dosage reductions are recommended for IV etidronate in patients whose serum creatinine is >2.5 mg/dl, and IV etidronate is contraindicated in those with serum creatinine >5 mg/dl. In general, IV and oral etidronate are well tolerated, without major side effects. Prolonged use of high-dose oral etidronate has been associated with osteomalacia. However, prolonged use is uncommon in patients with advanced malignancies.

Pamidronate Disodium

Pamidronate disodium may be administered at two dose levels. For patients with moderate hypercalcemia (12–13.4 mg/dl), a single dose of 60 or 90 mg of pamidronate disodium should be administered intravenously over 2–4 hours. Patients with severe hypercalcemia (>13.5 mg/dl) should receive a single dose of 90 mg administered over a minimum of 2 hours. The onset of action is usually observed within 24–48 hours, and maximum responses generally occur within 4–7 days. If hypercalcemia recurs, therapy may be repeated 1 week after the initial dose, which is sufficient time to observe the full response to the initial dose. Pamidronate disodium is only available as a parenteral product; GI effects of the oral dose used to treat hypercalcemia were unacceptable. Animal data indicate that pamidronate disodium is approximately 100 times more potent than etidronate disodium. Clinical trials comparing pamidronate disodium to etidronate disodium demonstrated that a single dose of pamidronate disodium was more effective in correcting serum calcium than 3 days of etidronate disodium.[16,17]

Etidronate and pamidronate have similar side effect profiles. Adverse effects associated with bisphosphonate administration include transient fever, a local reaction at the site of infusion, hypomagnesemia, hypokalemia, hypophosphatemia, and hypocalcemia.

Gallium Nitrate

Gallium nitrate was initially developed as an antineoplastic agent and was observed to cause hypocalcemia in patients being treated for lymphoma. Gallium nitrate is incorporated into hydroxyapatite crystals, producing larger and more uniform crystals that are less susceptible to dissolution. The net effect is inhibition of calcium resorption from the bone. Gallium nitrate is indicated for the treatment of symptomatic hypercalcemia that has not responded to hydration and diuretics. Gallium nitrate is administered at 200 mg/m^2 daily for 5 days as a 24-hour IV infusion. A dose of 100 mg/m^2 can be administered for less severe cases. If serum calcium normalizes before the course of gallium nitrate is completed, therapy should be stopped. Responses to treatment are evident within 48 hours and persist for 4 days to 2 weeks.[18] The most common adverse effect associated with gallium nitrate is renal toxicity. The drug's primary route of elimination is renal. Patients who receive gallium nitrate should be well hydrated, with a urine output maintained at or above 2000 ml/day. The manufacturer recommends that patients who are receiving other nephrotoxic agents or who have a serum creatinine level >2.5 mg/dl should not receive gallium nitrate because of the increased risk of nephrotoxicity.

Management

Hypercalcemia is best managed by a combination of hydration, diuretics, and bisphosphonates when the tumor cannot be controlled by antineoplastic therapy. Pamidronate has the advantage of being administered as a single-dose regimen at a potentially lower cost. Gallium nitrate is more expensive than pamidronate but should be considered if the patient does not respond to bisphosphonates. Plicamycin is generally reserved for patients who have not responded to bisphosphonates or gallium nitrate. It is considerably less expensive than calcitonin, bisphosphonate or gallium nitrate; however, its toxicity profile precludes it from being considered as a first-line therapy for the treatment of hypercalcemia.

SUPERIOR VENA CAVA SYNDROME

Superior vena cava syndrome (SVCS) results from decreased venous flow in the superior vena cava due to compression of the vessel wall by an extrinsic mass (i.e., a tumor), tumor invasion, or thrombosis.

Etiology

Malignancy is the most common cause of SVCS.[19] Before antibiotics were developed, infectious causes, such as tuberculous mediastinitis and syphilitic aneurysm, contributed to 40% of SVCS cases.[20,21] The nonmalignant causes of SVCS include benign tumors, pulmonary diseases (e.g., mediastinal emphysema and pneumothorax), trauma, aortic aneurysm, and central venous catheter devices.[22,23] The increased number of reports of SVCS caused by central venous devices is due to the increased use of pacemakers and Swan-Ganz and Hickman catheters.[21,22,24,25] Central venous catheters are frequently placed in cancer patients to administer both chemotherapy and supportive therapies.

The most common malignant causes of SVCS are lung cancer (3%) and lymphoma (8%).[22] All histological types of lung cancer have been associated with SVCS. However, small cell (or oat cell) lung cancer is the bronchiogenic carcinoma most likely to cause SVCS.[26] Roughly 3–20% of SVCS cases are caused by other metastatic malignant diseases, especially metastases from testicular and breast cancers.[27]

Clinical Presentation

Patients with SVCS usually have symptoms related to increased venous pressure. The severity of the signs and symptoms is related to the rate and extent of obstruction.[27] The most common complaint is dyspnea (shortness of breath), followed by facial swelling and head fullness, cough, arm swelling, and chest pain.[26,28] Some of the other, less common symptoms are nasal stuffiness, hoarseness, stridor, dizziness, dysphagia, epistaxis, lethargy, and obtundation.[26,28] Patients may complain that symptoms worsen when they lean forward, stoop, or recline.[22,26,29,30] Symptoms may be mild with slow or incomplete obstruction, or severe and sudden with complete or rapid obstruction. Patients may complain of symptoms being present several weeks before diagnosis.[28] The most common physical findings are dilated thoracic and neck veins. However, other common signs are edema of the face, neck, and upper extremities, as well as tachypnea and cyanosis.[24,26,30]

Diagnosis

For the past several decades, SVCS has been viewed as a medical emergency that needs immediate treatment, often before a histological diagnosis of the underlying disease is made.[21,27,31] However, current literature suggests that SVCS rarely is a true medical emergency.[28,32] SVCS demands immediate attention only when the trachea is obstructed, which can be life threatening.

Histological diagnosis should be attained before treatment in patients who are not in acute distress so that appropriate therapy for the underlying cause can be initiated. This point is especially important if radiation therapy is given, because irradiating the obstruction causes radiation tissue necrosis and makes a histological diagnosis unattainable.[29,32] Although a concern, complications are reduced when skilled clinicians perform these diagnostic and invasive procedures.[33] In the past, there were clinically unsupported concerns that performing invasive procedures on SVCS patients might cause respiratory obstruction, aspiration, or excessive bleeding due to elevated venous pressures.[19,21,31]

Full-blown SVCS is relatively easy to recognize and can be confirmed by a chest X-ray or computed tomography (CT) of the thorax.[29] A small percentage of patients may have normal chest X-rays.[34] Computed tomography is able to provide more details about the involvement of the bronchi and spinal cord and the presence of collateral veins. In addition, the use of magnetic resonance imaging (MRI) has been very effective in the diagnosis of spinal cord compressions and may actually be cost effective.[35] The diagnosis may not be obvious if the onset is insidious and signs are subtle.

The etiology of SVCS can be determined by sputum cytology, bronchoscopy with bronchial biopsies and washings, or biopsy of palpable lymphadenopathy. These methods yield a correct diagnosis in approximately 70% of cases. If these procedures fail to establish a definitive cause, aggressive steps, such as thoracotomy or mediastinoscopy, may be pursued. Phlebography can be used to determine whether the obstruction is vascular and what degree of obstruction exists.

Treatment

Patients with acute, life-threatening obstruction should receive irradiation to the chest. Radiation is the standard palliative therapy for SVCS if it presents as a true medical emergency.[21,31] Radiation treatment is generally administered at 300–400 rads daily for 3 days, followed by 150–200 rads per day, for a total of 3000–6000 rads, depending on the patient's condition and the extent of disease.[19,21,29,31] Subjective response is measured by objective resolution of symptoms; edema, orthopnea, dyspnea, and elevated venous pressure should subside. Although most patients respond to radiation therapy, some of the response may be due to the development of collateral venous circulation.[32] If time permits and the patient is not in imminent danger, therapy should be specific for the disease or neoplasm.

Small Cell Lung Cancer

Combination chemotherapy has been used to treat SVCS caused by small cell lung cancer (SCLC) and has produced favorable responses.[28,35] Most patients with SCLC present with disseminated disease at first. SCLC is an aggressive disease that is sensitive to chemotherapy. Studies have indicated that chemotherapy is as good as radiation for the initial treatment of SVCS in this population.[20,36,37] Prognosis was determined not by the presence of SVCS but rather by adequate disease control, age, and the patient's performance status.[36]

Non-Small Cell Lung Cancer

Patients with non-small cell lung cancer (NSCLC) who have SVCS should receive radiation therapy, particularly if the tumor is unresectable. NSCLC is usually unresponsive to chemotherapy. The best option for survival of NSCLC patients who do not have SVCS is usually surgery and, to a lesser extent, radiation therapy.

Non-Hodgkin's Lymphomas

Non-Hodgkin's lymphomas include several different histological types. Selecting the most appropriate therapy for a patient who presents with SVCS depends on the type of lymphoma and its response to specific treatment modalities. In general, chemotherapy is used alone or in combination with radiation therapy for optimal local and systemic response.

Thrombolytic Therapy

Neither radiation nor chemotherapy would be appropriate therapy if SVCS is caused by occlusion due to a thrombosis. Streptokinase or urokinase may be indicated, particularly if the thrombosis is caused by an indwelling central venous catheter (see chapter 10).

Supportive Therapy

It is important to remember that some of these patients are in considerable discomfort while being evaluated for the cause of SVCS. Procedures should be done as quickly as practical, so that efforts to reduce discomfort are not delayed. While the patient is awaiting a histological diagnosis, general measures, such as elevating the head of the bed and giving oxygen, diuretics, and steroids, may temporarily reduce symptoms. Diuretic therapy should not be so aggressive that cardiac output is decreased and antidiuretic hormone production is stimulated.

SPINAL CORD COMPRESSION

The most common neurological complication of metastatic malignancy is extradural spinal cord compression, with an incidence of approximately 5–10% in patients with advanced cancer.[38,39] Intramedullary spinal cord compression does occur, although rarely.[40] Tumor invasion of the spinal cord can cause mechanical or vascular compromise, which leads or contributes to ischemia, infarction, or hemorrhage.[40,41] Spinal cord compression may be the first sign of a malignancy in up to 35% of cases.[40]

Etiology

Tumors that metastasize to bone (e.g., lung, breast, and prostate tumors; lymphomas; and myelomas) account for most neoplastic spinal cord compressions. Less common malignant causes of spinal cord compression include cancers of the stomach, colon, thyroid, and kidney.[41] Spinal cord compression in men is caused primarily by lung cancer, followed by prostate cancer. Spinal cord compression in women is caused primarily by breast cancer.[39,42] Lung cancer may soon be the most common metastatic cause of spinal cord compression for both sexes, because the incidence of lung cancer among women has risen significantly over the past two decades.

Some tumors are more likely to produce compression in specific areas of the spine. GI tumors have a greater propensity to metastasize to the lumbosacral spine, whereas lung and breast tumors are usually associated with thoracic cord compression.[38] Epidural cord compression should be included in the list of differential diagnoses for cancer patients with back pain.

There are other disease states or syndromes that may cause back pain, with or without neurological dysfunction, and they should be ruled out for patients who have no history of malignancy (Table 19-3). The most common nonmalignant cause of back pain is a herniated or ruptured intervertebral disc. Infectious processes may cause extradural abscesses with or without osteomyelitis. In addition, tuberculosis of the spine (Pott's disease), epidural catheter complications, and rheumatoid arthritis can all present with back pain as the chief complaint.[42,43] Nonmalignant causes of radicular pain, which include

Table 19-3. Causes of Back Pain

Nonmalignant causes[a]
- Herniated or ruptured disc
- Extradural abscess
- Tuberculosis of the spine
- Rheumatoid arthritis
- Cervical spondylosis
- Radiation myelitis
- Epidural catheter-related complications[b]
- Radicular pain
- Pleurisy
- Cholecystitis
- Pancreatitis

Most common malignant causes
- Lung cancer
- Breast cancer
- Prostate cancer

Low-incidence malignant causes
- Stomach cancer
- Colon cancer
- Thyroid cancer
- Kidney cancer

[a]From reference 43.
[b]From reference 44.

pleurisy, cholecystitis, and pancreatitis, should be considered when diagnostic tests are negative for cord compression.[41]

Clinical Presentation

Approximately 75–95% of all patients complain of pain as the first symptom of spinal cord compression, often months before neurological symptoms are apparent.[39,44,45] Pain may be bilateral, local, or radicular. Patients with epidural cord compression may complain of more pain when they lie flat, or pain may be exacerbated by flexing the neck or raising the leg straight. Increased pain in these positions is caused by extending the spinal cord.[43] Radicular pain is caused by trauma to the nerve root, which results from direct tumor compression, collapse of the vertebrae, or infarction.[43] Radicular pain is more commonly associated with cervical or lumbosacral cord compression.[38] Onset of pain may be very gradual, varying from days to years. Pain is generally localized and can be elicited by palpating the spine. Point tenderness usually correlates well with the site of cord compression.[45]

Pain is usually followed by neurological deficits. Progression can be rapid, and paraplegia may develop if the compression goes untreated. Patients may complain first of sensory deficits or muscular weakness. Sensory loss is described as a tingling or numbness of the toes. It is reported that up to 68% of patients experience sensory loss at the time of diagnosis.[39,44] Some patients may not notice any sensory deficits even though a neurological exam reveals mild to moderate losses.[43] Muscular weakness may lead patients to complain of difficulty in climbing stairs or weakness in their knees when they try to walk.[39]

Autonomic dysfunctions are late-occurring symptoms that often have a poor prognosis.[39] Patients may complain of urinary hesitancy, problems in voiding, bowel constipation, or obstipation.[39,42,45]

The patient's status prior to intervention is the best indicator of prognosis. Patients who are ambulatory at the time of recognition and treatment have a more favorable prognosis regardless of treatment modalities. Approximately 60% of surgically treated ambulatory patients remain ambulatory after treatment; only 7% of surgically treated paraplegic patients become ambulatory.[41]

In general, the prognosis is more favorable for patients whose symptoms are progressing slowly or who have distal symptoms than for those with rapidly changing deficits (significant changes in 48–72 hours) or proximal neurological deficits.[38,41] Loss of anal sphincter tone, particularly when it is long lasting, is generally associated with a poor prognosis.[41]

Diagnosis

Spinal cord compression should be suspected in cancer patients with new-onset back pain, particularly in patients with tumors that are associated with a high probability of bone metastasis (Table 19-3). Diagnosis is relatively easy when patients have the classic symptoms, including neurological complaints. If signs or symptoms are more subtle, however, the diagnosis may be delayed, particularly if the patient has a history of chronic back problems.

MRI can be used to diagnose and locate the region of involvement.[46–48] The two advantages of MRI over a myelogram are that it is a noninvasive procedure and is therefore safer and that it allows visualization of the area, which can be useful when selecting and implementing treatment. Because MRI provides greater visualization of the spine than other methods, it is the preferred method of evaluating intramedullary disease, disc space, and degenerative disease. In addition to being effective, the use of MRI may be more cost effective than other diagnostic tools.[35]

Lumbar puncture (LP), which is necessary to perform a myelogram, has been reported to cause rapid neurological deterioration due to the withdrawal of cerebrospinal fluid.[38] LPs are generally not advised. However, if an LP is performed to aid in distinguishing an epidural abscess from metastatic cancer, it should be done in conjunction with myelography.[41] Although myelograms are able to identify the site and extent of the lesion, when a block is observed, the areas above the obstruction need to be evaluated (e.g., with another myelogram) to determine whether there are multiple compression sites.[38,41] Metastatic lesions are almost always extradural.[39] When an epidural block is visualized, other causes, such as abscesses, hematomas, or a herniated disc, should also be considered as a cause of back pain.[39]

Metastases to the cervical spinal cord are less common. However, compression above the C5 vertebra can cause muscle weakness and atrophy and lead to respiratory failure.

Early recognition of the signs and symptoms of spinal cord compression and avoidance of unnecessary delays in diagnosis and treatment may save the patient from paraplegia.

Treatment

Assessing the clinical outcome of treatment—which may include surgery, radiation, or a combination of surgery, radiation, and chemotherapy—is difficult for several reasons. First, outcome is poor, particularly in patients with severe neurological symptoms. Second, good controlled, randomized studies are lacking. Third, the differences in outcome between radiotherapy and surgery do not appear to be significant.[38] Factors that may influence the selection of treatment include symptoms, rate of progression, site of cord compression, and tumor type.

Surgery

Surgery may be used to decompress the spinal cord and debulk the tumor. However, most epidural tumors are located anterior to the spinal cord and often destroy the vertebral bone.

When vertebrae have been weakened by tumor destruction or infiltration, surgical removal can be difficult.[38]

Posterior laminectomy is usually performed to excise the tumor. It is an anatomically awkward procedure that can lead to destabilization at the existing site of stress. Laminectomy would clearly be an appropriate choice for a spinal cord compression caused by a tumor situated posterior or lateral to the spine.[49] Surgical removal of an anterior tumor may not be as successful. In the worst scenario, surgery could contribute to or cause neurological damage, particularly in an unstable spine. Immediate support is often needed to stabilize the spine. Fast-setting acrylic gels, bone graphs, and steel rods have all been used to alleviate instability caused by surgery.

The potential risks and benefits of surgery must be considered in treating patients who are neutropenic, thrombocytopenic, or expected to survive a short time or whose quality of life is poor. The current trend is to treat rapidly progressing symptoms with surgery.

Radiation

Radiation is indicated for patients with slower progressing symptoms or an incomplete block.[41] Radiotherapy is an alternative to surgery for patients who are in poor health and cannot tolerate a surgical procedure. Radiation has better results in radiosensitive tumors, such as lymphoma, myeloma, seminoma, Ewing's sarcoma, and neuroblastoma. However, slightly less radiosensitive tumors (such as breast and prostate tumors) and renal cancer do respond to radiotherapy.

The dose of radiation should be delivered so that the cytolytic response is rapid and maximized. In addition, the total cumulative dose of radiation must be monitored to avoid permanent damage to the spinal cord. There has been some concern in the past, based on animal models, that radiation may increase edema of the spinal cord and therefore worsen neurological symptoms. This danger has not been well substantiated in humans.

Greenberg and colleagues used high doses of radiation (500 rads/day for 13 days) followed by a brief rest period and lower fractionated doses for a total of 3000 rads.[50] In addition, dexamethasone was administered as a 100-mg bolus at the time of diagnosis, continued as an oral dose for 3 days, and then tapered. The results did not differ significantly from results of other studies; approximately 59% of the patients were ambulatory after treatment.

High-dose dexamethasone did appear to alleviate pain. Pain probably was reduced because edema and inflammation were decreased around the site of cord compression, or perhaps because of the cytotoxic effects on the tumor. Lower doses of dexamethasone (16 mg/day) have been used. Titrating the dose of steroids to achieve maximal effects is advised, particularly in patients with worsening symptoms or pain.[45] Patients may complain of a burning or tingling of the perineal area or of retropubic pain with IV administration, which may be confused with worsening of the spinal cord compression.

In conclusion, patients with spinal cord compression need aggressive treatment to reverse new-onset neurological symptoms and to prevent further deterioration. Surgery is used to establish a pathological diagnosis in patients with no history of malignancy, to decompress the spinal cord, and to debulk tumors. Postsurgical radiation is generally recommended to eradicate residual disease. Radiation is also recommended for those who are not surgical candidates. Patients with systemic disease may be considered for chemotherapy specific for their tumor type. Steroids should be used to reduce inflammation and edema and to help control pain.

TUMOR LYSIS SYNDROME

Tumor lysis syndrome (TLS) results from the rapid destruction of neoplastic cells. The rapid lysis of tumor cells releases intracellular contents into the systemic circulation faster than the body can eliminate them. Electrolyte abnormalities associated with TLS are hyperkalemia, hyperuricemia, hyperphosphatemia, and hypocalcemia. Patients who are at risk for TLS are those with large tumor burdens (bulky solid tumors, leukemias, and lymphomas), a high growth fraction, rapid growth rates, and great sensitivity to the lytic effects of cytotoxic therapy.

Etiology

TLS usually results from aggressive cytotoxic therapy that may include both radiation and chemotherapy at a time when tumor burden is the greatest. Although TLS is more common with initial courses of therapy, patients with rapidly growing tumors may experience TLS with subsequent cytotoxic regimens. TLS is most commonly described in patients who have lymphomas (especially Burkitt's lymphoma), acute myelogenous leukemia, or chronic lymphocytic leukemia. Solid tumors rarely produce TLS, although there are case reports of patients with small cell lung cancer, breast cancer, testicular cancer, and medulloblastoma who have experienced TLS.[51]

Metabolic Complications

High concentrations of uric acid and phosphate become insoluble in the urine, and precipitation of these products in the renal tubule can result in renal failure. Subsequent decreased elimination of these cellular by-products can further impair function and worsen the effects of TLS. These electrolyte and metabolic disturbances can result in mental status changes, tetany, neuromuscular problems, renal failure, cardiac arrhythmias, and sudden death. Therefore, efforts to minimize the risk of TLS are warranted, and appropriate measures should be taken before cytotoxic therapy is begun.

Although TLS is the result of cytotoxic reductive therapy, other therapies may potentiate electrolyte abnormalities. Medications that can contribute to electrolyte abnormalities should be reviewed and eliminated if possible (Table 19-4). Drugs

Table 19-4. Therapies Contributing to Electrolyte Abnormalities with Tumor Lysis

Supplements
  Calcium
  Potassium

Nutritional supplements
  Enteral formulas
  Parenteral nutrition

Potassium-sparing diuretics
  Spironolactone
  Triamterene
  Amiloride

Nephrotoxic drugs

that have narrow therapeutic ranges, are nephrotoxic, or rely on the kidneys for elimination must be monitored carefully, and their doses should be adjusted when warranted.

TLS usually occurs within the first 48 hours of treatment. The risk of TLS decreases significantly if the first few days of therapy are tolerated without significant electrolyte abnormalities. Patients with slowly lysing tumors or tumors refractory to treatment are less likely to develop TLS, because slowly lysing neoplastic cells put less demand on organ systems for clearing waste products.

Hyperkalemia

Elevations in serum potassium are seen frequently in TLS and are usually evident within the first 12–48 hours after therapy is begun. Potassium is the major intracellular cation responsible for maintaining osmotic equilibrium between extracellular and intracellular fluid and for establishing the resting membrane potential. Normally, serum potassium is held in a narrow range and most of the cation is intracellular. Excessive extracellular potassium adversely affects the resting membrane potential. The most significant effect of hyperkalemia is cardiac arrhythmias, although neuromuscular abnormalities may occur. Hyperkalemia is considered mild when serum potassium is 5 mEq/L (approximately 5 mmol/L) and electrocardiogram changes are limited to peaking T waves. Hyperkalemia is classified as severe if serum potassium is >8 mEq/L or electrocardiogram changes include more serious abnormalities, such as absent P waves, prolongation of the QRS interval, or ventricular arrhythmias.[52]

Potassium can be removed from the body by administering sodium polystyrene sulfonate (Kayexalate). This cation exchange resin releases sodium in place of other cations. It can be administered orally or rectally as a retention enema. Decreases in serum potassium may be evident within hours of administration of a retention enema. Its effects are not immediate, and so it should not be used to treat acute toxicities.

Calcium can counteract the deleterious effects of hyperkalemia. For severe cardiac toxicities, IV infusions of 10–30 ml of 10% calcium gluconate have been infused over 1–5 minutes. The effects are rapid; however, they do not correct the underlying problem of hyperkalemia.

Hyperuricemia

Hyperuricemia in TLS results from accelerated production of uric acid that surpasses the body's ability to eliminate it. Hyperuricemia secondary to neoplastic disease occurs when there is high cellular turnover or lysis. Uric acid is the final product in the oxidation of purine nucleotides. The oxidation of hypoxanthine and xanthine, precursors of uric acid, depends on xanthine oxidase.

Hyperuricemia is defined as a serum uric acid concentration >7 mg/dl. Higher concentrations exceed the solubility limits in serum and may result in adverse effects. Efforts to maximize solubility and clearance are used to avoid nephrotoxic effects in patients who have hyperuricemia. Nephropathy can result from urate crystals forming in interstitial renal tissue or obstructing the collecting tubules, renal pelvis, or ureters. Nephrolithiasis (i.e., renal deposits of urate crystals) may occur when uric acid excretion is high (>1100 mg/day).

Alkalinizing the urine generally increases solubility. Increases in urine pH favor urate in an ionized state, preventing urate crystals from forming in renal structures. Alkalinization should be done with care because it decreases the solubility of phosphate complexes, placing the patient at risk for renal dysfunction from phosphate precipitation. Patients should be well hydrated to maintain good urine output and maximize solubility.

Allopurinol, a xanthine oxidase inhibitor, can be used to prevent the oxidation of hypoxanthine to xanthine and of xanthine to uric acid. Oral daily doses of 200–400 mg/m^2 are used in patients who are at high risk of TLS. Allopurinol has been reported to cause xanthine nephropathy. It is excreted in the urine, and dose adjustments are necessary in patients with renal dysfunction. Toxicities associated with allopurinol therapy include fever, hepatitis, and erythematous desquamative skin rash. The oxidative metabolism of azathioprine and mercaptopurine by xanthine oxidase is inhibited by allopurinol. This decrease in metabolism can increase their toxic effects. Dose reductions may be necessary when these antineoplastics are given with allopurinol.

Uricosuric agents (e.g., probenecid and sulfinpyrazone) are not recommended, because they promote the renal excretion of uric acid, decrease renal solubility, and increase the risk of renal calculi. Medications that are known to increase serum uric acid, such as thiazide and loop diuretics, need to be monitored closely and discontinued if hyperuricemia becomes a clinical problem.

Hyperphosphatemia and Hypocalcemia

Hyperphosphatemia can result in renal failure and hypocalcemia. Lymphocytic leukemia cells, for example, reportedly contain four times the amount of phosphate found in mature cells, which can result in the substantial release of phosphate when they are lysed during therapy.[53]

In acute hyperphosphatemia, serum levels may exceed the solubility of calcium and phosphate, resulting in precipitation of the calcium-phosphate complex. Acute renal failure can result if precipitation occurs in the renal parenchyma or collecting ducts.

Hyperphosphatemia can be treated with phosphate binders (aluminum hydroxide or aluminum carbonate, 30 ml four times daily). Phosphates should also be eliminated from or reduced in the diet, and careful attention must be given to enteral feedings and parenteral nutrition formulations that may contain phosphate.

Hypocalcemia, a result of the effects of hyperphosphatemia on osteoclasts, causes bone resorption and the formation of calcium-phosphate complexes. Hypocalcemia is normally self correcting if serum phosphate is corrected.

Prevention of Tumor Lysis Syndrome

To reduce the likelihood of TLS, high-risk patients should be well hydrated to maintain good urine output and maximize the serum solubility of the lysis products. Allopurinol should be started, if possible, 24–48 hours before cytotoxic therapy. Alkalinization of the urine may reduce the risk of uric acid crystals in the kidneys and ureters, although the risk of calcium-phosphate precipitation must be considered. Before therapy, medications and feeding products should be reviewed for related drug interactions and potential aggravation of TLS complications. When metabolic disturbances cannot be corrected medically or renal failure develops, hemodialysis or peritoneal dialysis may be necessary.

MALIGNANT PLEURAL EFFUSIONS

During the course of a day, an average of 5–10 L of fluid moves through the pleural space (i.e., the space between the pleura and the lungs), most of which is reabsorbed. Pleural effusions are abnormal fluid collections resulting from changes in capillary permeability or changes in pressure gradients.

Etiology

Nonmalignant causes of pleural effusions include increased hydrostatic pressure secondary to congestive heart failure, decreased oncotic pressure due to decreased serum proteins, and increased negative intrapleural pressure, such as that which occurs with atelectasis.[54]

Malignant pleural effusions occur primarily as a result of impaired capillary permeability or impaired pleural drainage. Increased pleural oncotic pressure caused by tumor involvement of the pleural space can also encourage the development of pleural effusions. Impaired capillary permeability can result from an inflammatory process or altered integrity of the capillary endothelium. Tumor infiltration that results in an obstructive process can impair lymph or venous drainage, hampering pleural drainage.[54,55] Cancer patients may have multiple etiologies for pleural effusions, such as hypoalbuminemia, organ failure, or tumor invasion. Advanced breast and lung cancers, leukemia, and lymphomas are the most common cancers associated with malignant pleural effusions.[56,57]

Clinical Presentation

Symptoms of pleural effusions include cough, chest pain, and dyspnea. Patients often present with confined chest wall expansion, tachypnea, and labored breathing. It is not uncommon for the pleural effusion to be the first symptom of the malignancy.

Diagnosis

Malignant pleural effusions can be detected by chest radiographs or computed tomography. The diagnosis of malignant effusions can be made by cytologic examination, biochemical analysis of the pleural fluid, pleural biopsy, or thoracoscopy. The presence of a bloody effusion is a strong indicator that the underlying pathology is malignant. Malignant effusions are described as an exudate effusion with protein content and specific gravity exceeding, respectively, 3 g/dl and 1.015. The pleural protein/serum protein ratio is >0.5, and the pleural lactate dehydrogenase/serum lactate dehydrogenase ratio is >0.6.[55]

The diagnosis of a malignant pleural effusion is generally associated with a poor prognosis, particularly since this is often a complication of advanced disease. Treating the pleural effusion without correcting the underlying cause will have little effect on survival. In general, treatment of the malignant pleural effusion is palliative and directed at improving the patient's quality of life. Therapy is generally not considered unless the patient is symptomatic and/or has recurrent pleural effusions.

Treatment

Thoracentesis is a temporary measure that provides immediate relief, although fluid reaccumulation is usually rapid. Thoracostomy tubes as a solitary modality are equally ineffective in controlling the effusion.[58] If the underlying pathology is one that will respond to antineoplastic therapy, then patients should receive systemic treatment. For patients who have unresponsive tumors, therapy is palliative and chemical sclerosants are used to close the pleural space. Chemical sclerosants exert their effects by causing an inflammatory or irritative pleurodesis. Candidates for sclerosants are patients who have obtained some relief with thoracentesis and have minimal drainage.

Typically, chemical sclerosants are administered through a chest tube when drainage has decreased to 100 ml/24 hours. The sclerosing agent is diluted to a volume of 50–100 ml, instilled into the chest tube, and clamped. The patient is repositioned every 15 minutes to facilitate drug distribution throughout the pleural space. After 4 hours (range, 2–12 hours), the tube is unclamped and suction is applied to drain the remaining drug and encourage a good seal. Sclerosing is painful, so premedication with analgesics 30 minutes before the procedure is recommended.

A number of drugs have been tried as sclerosing agents. The list includes thiotepa, tetracycline, doxycycline, minocycline, bleomycin, interleukin 2, interferon alfa-2b, mitoxantrone, doxorubicin, cisplatin, cytarabine, and etoposide. Most agents have not been used outside investigational settings because of efficacy, safety, toxicity, and cost concerns. The most commonly used sclerosing agents are talc, bleomycin, and doxycycline (Table 19-5).[59–68]

Talc, although inexpensive, is not available commercially as a sterile product. Sterilization and the administration of general anesthesia to perform thoroscopic talc poudrage adds significantly to the cost of therapy. One comparative trial reported the success rate of pleurodesis to be greater with talc than with bleomycin.[59] However, other studies are needed to confirm this report. Serious adverse effects include adult respiratory distress syndrome and deteriorating respiratory distress of unknown etiology.[69,70]

Bleomycin, an antineoplastic drug, has been administered through a chest tube or thoracentesis catheter. Response rates with a single application are good. Toxicities for the most part are mild and include fever, pain, and nausea.[71] Because bleomycin is an expensive agent, cost should be a consideration.

Agents of the tetracycline family have been used as sclerosing therapy. Production of IV tetracycline ceased in 1991, and the use of minocycline as a sclerosing agent is not widely reported, leaving only doxycycline as an alternative to talc or bleomycin.

When selecting a sclerosing agent, factors such as experience with a particular agent, cost, toxicities, and patient-related variables influence the selection. There is still considerable discussion over which agent clinicians prefer. Comparisons of the agents are difficult because studies are generally small and uncontrolled, so objective measurements of response vary from study to study. Treatment should be aimed at improving the quality of life and should be safe, simple, and economical.

SUMMARY

The oncological complications discussed in this chapter—hypercalcemia, superior vena cava syndrome, spinal cord compression, tumor lysis syndrome, and malignant pleural effusions—may develop suddenly or insidiously and require immediate therapeutic intervention.

Primary hyperthyroidism is the most common cause of nonmalignant hypercalcemia. Other causes of or contributors to hypercalcemia include granulomatous diseases, extensive skeletal immobilization, thiazide diuretics, calcium supplements, hormone therapy, and vitamins. The solid tumors most commonly associated with hypercalcemia are breast, lung, and kidney tumors.

The best treatment for hypercalcemia is ablation of the tumor. Initial therapy should consist of vigorous hydration and diuretics along with careful monitoring of electrolytes. Calcitonin, plicamycin, or bisphosphonates may be necessary to lower serum calcium in patients who do not respond adequately to hydration and diuretics.

The most common cause of superior vena cava syndrome (SVCS) is malignancy, although it may be caused by other, nonmalignant diseases. The leading malignant causes of SVCS are lung cancer, lymphoma, and metastatic disease (most commonly due to breast or testicular cancer). Although symptoms can be severe, a histological diagnosis is recommended before treatment, if possible. Therapy for SVCS depends on its underlying cause and the malignancy's response to chemotherapy, radiation, or surgery.

Extradural spinal cord compression, the most common neurological complication of metastatic malignancy, should be suspected in a cancer patient with back pain. The cancers most commonly associated with this emergency are lung, breast, and prostate cancers, as well as lymphoma and myeloma. The most common complaint is back pain, and onset may be acute or associated with more subtle signs. An MRI should be performed to verify diagnosis, locate the site of cord compression, and determine the extent of the lesion. Treatment is influenced by the presenting symptoms, the rate of tumor progression, the site of cord compression, and the tumor type. Surgery, radiation, and chemotherapy may all be useful in treating this emergency.

Tumor lysis syndrome (TLS) results from neoplastic cells being destroyed faster than the body can eliminate them. TLS usually occurs in patients who have large tumor burdens (e.g., lymphoma, leukemia, or bulky solid tumors) and who are receiving radiation or chemotherapy. Significant tumor lysis can produce hyperkalemia, hyperuricemia, hyperphosphatemia, and hypocalcemia.

Malignant pleural effusions are the result of impaired capillary permeability

Table 19-5. Sclerosing Agents

Schlerosing Agent	Dose Range	Reported Response Rates (%)	References
Talc	3.0–10.5 g	87–100	59–63
Bleomycin	60 units	42–70	59, 60, 64, 65
Doxycycline	500 mg	61–88	66–68

or impaired pleural drainage secondary to hypoalbuminemia, organ failure, or tumor invasion. Symptoms associated with pleural effusions may be the presenting sign of a malignancy. The diagnosis of a malignant pleural effusion has a poor prognosis. If the malignancy does not respond to treatment, therapy for the pleural effusion is palliative.

REFERENCES

1. Levine MM, Kleeman CR. Hypercalcemia: pathophysiology and treatment. *Hosp Pract* 1987;22:93–110.
2. Guyton AC, Itall JE. *Medical Physiology.* 9th ed. Philadelphia, PA: WB Saunders; 1996. Chapter 79, Parathyroid hormone, calcitonin, calcium and phospate metabolism, vitamin D, bone and teeth. p. 985–1002.
3. Mundy GR, Martin TJ. The hypercalcemia of malignancy: pathogenesis and management. *Metabolism* 1982;31:1247–77.
4. Insogna KL, Broadus AE. Hypercalcemia of malignancy. *Annu Rev Med* 1987;38:241–56.
5. Green L, Ringenberg SQ. Current concepts in the management of hypercalcemia of malignancy. *Hosp Formul* 1988; 23:268–87.
6. Mundy GR. The hypercalcemia of malignancy. *Kidney Int* 1987;31:142–55.
7. Broadus AE, Mangin M, Ikeaa K, et al. Humoral hypercalcemia of cancer. *N Engl J Med* 1988;319:556–63.
8. Burtis WJ, Wu TL, Insogna KL, et al. Humoral hypercalcemia of malignancy. *Ann Intern Med* 1988;108:454–7.
9. Raisz LG, Trummel CL, Werner JA, et al. Effect of glucocorticoids on bone resorption in tissue culture. *Endocrinology* 1972;90:961–7.
10. Stewart AF. Therapy of malignancy associated hypercalcemia. *Am J Med* 1983;74:475–80.
11. Percival RC, Yates AJ, Gray RE, et al. Role of glucocorticoids in management of malignant hypercalcemia. *Br Med J* 1984;289:287.
12. Perlia CP, Gubisch NJ, Woller J, et al. Mithramycin treatment of hypercalcemia. *Cancer* 1970;25:389–92.
13. Max M. Acute hypercalcemia crisis. *Heart Lung* 1976;5:624–6.
14. Jacobs TP, Gordon AC, Silverberg SJ, et al. Neoplastic hypercalcemia: physiologic response to intravenous etidronate disodium. *Am J Med* 1987;82(*Suppl* 2A):42–50.
15. Ringenberg QS, Ritsch PS. Efficacy of oral administration of etidronate disodium in maintaining normal serum calcium levels in previously hypercalcemic cancer patients. *Clinical Therapeutics (Excerpta Medica)* 1987;9:318–25.
16. Gucalp R, Ritch P, Wiernik P, et al. Comparative study of pami- dronate disodium and etidronate disodium in the treatment of cancer-related hypercalcemia. *J Clin Oncol* 1992; 10:134–42.
17. Ralston SH, Gallacher SJ, Patel U, et al. Comparison of three intravenous bisphosphonates in cancer associated hypercalcemia. *Lancet* 1989;2:1180.
18. Warrell RP Jr, Skelos A, Alcock NW, et al. Gallium nitrate for acute treatment of cancer-related hypercalcemia:clinicopharmacological and dose response analysis. *Cancer Res* 1986; 46:4208–12.
19. Lokich JJ, Goodman R. Superior vena cava syndrome: clinical management. *JAMA* 1975;231:58–61.
20. Dombernowsky P, Hansen HH. Combination chemotherapy in the management of superior vena cava obstruction in small cell anaplastic carcinoma of the lung. *Acta Med Scand* 1978; 204:513–6.
21. Davenport D, Ferree C, Blake D, et al. Response of superior vena cava syndrome to radiation therapy. *Cancer* 1976; 38:1577–80.
22. Sculier JP, Feld R. Superior vena cava obstruction syndrome: recommendations for management. *Cancer Treat Rev* 1985; 12:209–18.
23. Mahajan V, Strimlan V, Van Ordstrand HS, et al. Benign superior vena cava syndrome. *Chest* 1975;68:32–5.
24. Halery A, Leonoo Y, Levinsohn G, et al. Thrombosis of superior vena cava during total parenteral nutrition managed successfully with low dose streptokinase. *Intensive Care Med* 1988; 14:72–3.
25. Bertrand M, Presant CA, Klein L, et al. Iatrogenic superior vena cava syndrome. *Cancer* 1984;54:376–8.
26. Bell DR, Woods RL, Levi JA. Superior vena cava obstruction: 10-year experience. *Med J. Aust* 1986;145:566–8.
27. Nieto AF, Doty DB. Superior vena cava obstruction: clinical syndrome, etiology, and treatment. *Curr Prob Cancer* 1986; 10:442–84.
28. Sculier JP, Evans WK, Feld R, et al. Superior vena cava obstruction syndrome in small cell lung cancer. *Cancer* 1986; 57:847–51.
29. Frank AR. Superior vena cava syndrome: current management concepts. *Nebr Med J* 1989;74:8–16.
30. Schechler MM. The superior vena cava syndrome. *Am J Med Sci* 1954;227:46–56.
31. Davenport D, Ferree C, Blake D, et al. Radiation therapy in the treatment of superior vena cava obstruction. *Cancer* 1978; 42:2600–3.
32. Ahmann FR. A reassessment of the clinical implications of the superior vena caval syndrome. *J Clin Oncol* 1984;2:961–9.
33. Painter TD, Karpf M. Superior vena cava syndrome: diagnostic procedures. *Am J Med Sci* 1983;285:2–6.
34. Parish JM, Marschke RF, Dines DE, et al. Etiologic considerations in superior vena cava syndrome. *Mayo Clin Proc* 1981;56:407–13.
35. Jordan JE, Donaldson SS, Enzmann DR. Cost effectiveness and outcome assessment of magnetic resonance imaging in diagnosing cord compression. *Cancer* 1995;75:2579–86.
36. Maddox A, Valdivieso M, Lukeman J, et al. Superior vena cava obstruction in small cell bronchogenic carcinoma. *Cancer* 1983;52:2165–72.
37. Kane RC, Cohen MH, Broder LE, et al. Superior vena caval obstruction due to small cell anaplastic lung carcinoma. *JAMA* 1975;16:1717–8.
38. Kanblith PL, Cassady RJ. Central nervous system emergencies. In: DeVita V, Hellman S, Rosenberg SA, editors. *Cancer: Principles and Practice of Oncology.* 2nd ed. New York: JB Lippincott; 1985. p. 1860–5.
39. Neilan BA. Metastatic spinal cord compression. *Am Fam Physician* 1983;27:191–4.
40. Rodriques M, Dinapoli RP. Spinal cord compression with special reference to metastatic epidural tumors. *Mayo Clin Proc* 1980;55:442–8.

41. Bruckman JE, Bloomer WD. Management of spinal cord compression. *Semin Oncol* 1978;5:135–40.
42. Harrison KM, Muss HB, Ball MR, et al. Spinal cord compression in breast cancer. *Cancer* 1985;55:2839–44.
43. Kalia S, Tentinalli JE. Emergency evaluation of the cancer patient. *Ann Emerg Med* 1984;13:723–30.
44. Shoskes DA, Perrin RG. The role of surgical management for symptomatic spinal cord compression in patients with metastatic prostate cancer. *J Urol* 1989;142:337–9.
45. Gilbert RW, Kim JH, Posner JB. Epidural spinal cord compression from metastatic tumor. *Ann Neurol* 1978;3:40–51.
46. Aichner F, Poewe W, Rogalsky W, et al. Magnetic resonance imaging in the diagnosis of spinal cord diseases. *J Neurol Neurosurg Psychiatry* 1985;48:1220.
47. Smoker WRK, Godersky JC, Knutzon RK, et al. The role of MR imaging in evaluating metastatic spinal disease. *AJNR* 1987;8:901.
48. Sarpel S, Sarpel G, Yu E, et al. Early diagnosis of spinal-epidural metastasis by magnetic resonance imaging. *Cancer* 1987;59:1112.
49. Sundaresan N, Galicich JH, Lane JM, et al. Treatment of neoplastic epidural cord compression by vertebral body section and stabilization. *J Neurosurg* 1985;63:676–84.
50. Greenberg HS, Kim JH, Posner JB. Epidural spinal cord compression from metastic tumor: results with a new treatment protocol. *Ann Neurol* 1980;8:361–6.
51. Sparano J, Ramirez M, Wiernik PH, et al. Increasing recognition of corticosteroid induced tumor lysis syndrome in non-Hodgkin's lymphoma. *Cancer* 1990;65:1072–3.
52. Levenski NG. Fluid and electrolytes. In: Wilson JD, Braunward E, Isselbacher KJ, et al., editors. *Harrison's Principles of Internal Medicine*. 12th ed. New York: McGraw-Hill; 1991. p. 278–89.
53. Ettinger D, Harker WG, Gerry HW, et al. Hyperphosphatemia, hypocalcemia, and transient renal failure: results of cytotoxic treatment of acute lymphoblastic leukemia. *JAMA* 1978;239:2472–4.
54. Hausheer FH, Yarbo JW. Diagnosis and treatment of malignant pleural effusion. *Semin Oncol* 1985;12:54.
55. Pass HI. Treatment of malignant pleural and pericardial effusions. In: DeVita VT, Hellman S, Rosenberg SA, editors. *Cancer: Principles and Practice of Oncology*. 4th ed. Philadelphia, PA: JB Lippincott; 1993. p. 2246–61.
56. Pierson DJ. Disorders of the pleura, mediastinum, and diaphragm. In: Wilson JD, Braunwald E, Isselbacher KJ, et al., editors. *Harrison's Principles of Internal Medicine*. New York: McGraw-Hill; 1991. p. 1111–12.
57. Sahn SA. Pleural effusion in lung cancer. *Clin Chest Med* 1993;14:189–200.
58. Schafers SJ, Dresler CM. Update on talc, bleomycin, and the tetracyclines in the treatment of malignant pleural effusions. *Pharmacotherapy* 1995;15:228–35.
59. Hartman DL, Gaither JM, Kesler KA, et al. Comparison of insufflated talc under thoracoscopic guidance with standard tetracycline and bleomycin pleurodesis for control of malignant pleural effusion. *J Thorac Cardiovasc Surg* 1993;105:743–8.
60. Aelony Y, King R, Bouten C. Thoracosopic talc poudrage pleurodesis for chronic recurrent pleural effusions. *Ann Intern Med* 1991;115:778–82.
61. Daniel TM, Tribble CG, Rodgers BM. Thoracoscopy and talc poudrage for pneumothoraces and effusions. *Ann Thorac Surg* 1990;50:186–9.
62. Webb WR, Ozmen V, Moulder PV, et al. Iodized talc pleurodesis for the treatment of pleural effusions. *Thorac Cardiovasc Surg* 1992;103:881–6.
63. Ruckdeschel JC, Moores D, Lee JY, et al. Intrapleural therapy for malignant pleural effusions. *Chest* 1991;100:1528–35.
65. Ostrowksi MJ, Priestman TJ, Houston RF, et al. A randomized trial of intracavitary bleomycin and *Corynebacterium parvum* in the control of malignant pleural effusions. *Radiother Oncol* 1989;14:19–26.
66. Mansson T. Treatment of malignant pleural effusions with doxycycline. *Scand Infect Dis* 1988;53(Suppl):29–34.
67. Robinson LA, Fleming WH, Galbraith TA. Intrapleural doxycycline control of malignant pleural effusions. *Ann Thorac Surg* 1993;55:1115–22.
68. Kitamura S, Sugiyama Y, Izumi T, et al. Intrapleural doxycycline for the control of malignant pleural effusion. *Curr Ther Res* 1981;30:515–21.
69. Rinaldo JE, Owens GR, Rogers RM. Adult respiratory distress syndrome following intraplerual instillation of talc. *Thorac Cardiovasc Surg* 1983;85:523–6.
70. Bouchama A, Chastre J, Gaudichet A, et al. Acute pneumonitis with bilateral pleural effusion after talc pleurodesis. *Chest* 1984;86:795–7.
71. Bitran JD, Brown C, Desser RK, et al. Intracavity bleomycin for the control of malignant effusions. *J Surg Oncol* 1981;16:273–7.

SELF-STUDY QUESTIONS

1. In what four ways does salmon calcitonin differ from human calcitonin?

2. Glucocorticoids are beneficial in treating hypercalcemia secondary to which tumor types?

3. Which statement is true of bisphosphonates, such as etidronate disodium?

   a. They are chemical analogues of the endogenous pyrophosphate found in bone matrix.
   b. When administered orally, they have excellent bioavailability.
   c. They should be given as a bolus infusion to avoid renal toxicities.
   d. They are used in place of hydration and diuretics in patients with hypercalcemia.

4. A patient with a small colorectal tumor is considered at high risk for developing tumor lysis syndrome.

   a. true
   b. false

5. Chemotherapy and radiation have been shown to be equally effective against superior vena cava syndrome secondary to small cell lung cancer.
   a. true
   b. false

6. What is the most likely therapy for superior vena cava syndrome secondary to non-Hodgkin's lymphoma?

7. What four factors may influence treatment selection for spinal cord compression?

8. What three effects does dexamethasone have on spinal cord compression?

9. To avoid hyperuricemia, what should be administered 24–48 hours before cytotoxic therapy?

10. Which treatment is used to counteract the cardiac effects of hyperkalemia?
    a. calcium
    b. plicamycin
    c. steroids
    d. potassium supplements

Chapter 20

Pharmacy Practice Issues in Oncology

Rebecca S. Finley, Pharm.D., M.S.
Chair and Associate Professor
Department of Pharmacy Practice
and Pharmacy Administration
Philadelphia College of Pharmacy
Philadelphia, Pennsylvania

Carol Balmer, Pharm.D.
Associate Professor
University of Colorado School of Pharmacy
Denver, Colorado

Handling of Hazardous Drugs	358
Causes for Concern	358
Occupational and Clinical Research	359
Protective Measures	360
Biological Safety Cabinets	360
Protective Garments	361
Drug Preparation and Manipulation	361
Administration	361
Spills	362
Disposal of Cytotoxics	363
Regulatory Issues	363
Worker Health Evaluation	363
Policies and Procedures	363
Reviewing Medication Orders for Cancer Chemotherapy	364
Professional Training	364
Drug Ordering or Prescribing	364
Order Processing and Delivery	367
Drug Administration	368
Protocol Development	369
Patient Education	369
Drug Information in Oncology	369
Patient-Specific Information	369
Formulary and Guideline Development	370
Patient or Consumer Information	371
Summary	372
References	372
Appendix 20-A	374
Self-Study Questions	390

Providing pharmaceutical care (i.e., assuming responsibility for optimal drug therapy outcomes) for patients with cancer encompasses a diverse spectrum of knowledge and skills. As the previous chapters of this book have shown, optimizing drug therapy outcomes requires a comprehensive understanding of the pathophysiology of the malignant process as well as a clear understanding of how to maximize the therapeutic effects of drugs used to treat cancer and its complications. By integrating this information with basic clinical skills, pharmacists can play an integral role in the care of patients with cancer.

In addition to this knowledge and basic clinical skills, important specialized pharmaceutical and pharmacy practice expertise is crucial to the field of oncology. This expertise includes handling hazardous drugs, reviewing chemotherapy orders to minimize medication-related errors and preventable adverse drug reactions, providing drug information specific to oncology, choosing oncology products for an institution's formulary, and developing clinical guidelines and pathways that include oncology products. Although these issues do not typically involve direct patient care (with the possible exception of drug information), they do constitute a vital part of the quality framework when caring for patients with cancer.

This chapter is designed to clarify some of the areas that pharmacists must be competent in when providing comprehensive pharmaceutical care for patients with cancer.

After completing this chapter, the reader should be able to:

1. Describe the recommended procedures for handling hazardous drugs in order to optimize both worker and environmental protection.
2. List the elements that should be included in each chemotherapy order and describe the process pharmacists should follow when reviewing the order for appropriateness.
3. Outline the elements that should be included in a systematic health-system procedure to prevent medication-related errors involving chemotherapy.
4. Identify topics specific to oncology pharmacy practice that should be included in department policies and procedures.
5. List examples of oncology-specific resources that are helpful in responding to inquiries regarding specific patient care decisions; patient, caregiver, or consumer concerns; and the development of population-based clinical practice guidelines or pathways.

This chapter provides an overview of each of these areas and provides some references and resources that may be helpful in establishing comprehensive pharmacy services that will ultimately improve patient outcomes and enable pharmacists to assume integral roles in oncology practice.

HANDLING OF HAZARDOUS DRUGS

Over the past 20 years, health care workers handling cytotoxic agents have become increasingly concerned about potential hazardous effects. Although the harmful adverse effects these drugs produce in patients receiving therapeutic doses are well recognized, the potential risks to health care workers or other individuals with chronic low-level exposure are not well characterized. Good common sense, however, dictates that exposure to potentially harmful materials should be minimized. Since the early 1980s, several groups have published recommendations to protect both workers and the environment from unnecessary exposure to hazardous drugs in the workplace (Appendix 20-A).[1-5] Although widespread attention to the issue has certainly improved hazardous drug handling in the workplace, problems still exist.[6] Before discussing the essential elements of these recommendations, it may be helpful to review the fundamental causes for concern.

Causes for Concern

It is well known that many anticancer agents are genotoxic—that is, they are capable of causing damage to genetic material. Teratogens, mutagens, and carcinogens are specific types of genotoxins. Teratogens injure the fetus, mutagens alter DNA (which may result in the miscoding of RNA and the synthesis of abnormal proteins), and carcinogens cause neoplasms to form. Some carcinogens are probably teratogens, but mutagens and teratogens are not necessarily carcinogens. Besides the genotoxic potential, other criteria that would classify a drug as potentially hazardous in the workplace would include properties that result in impairment of fertility or evidence of serious organ or other toxicity following either chronic low-level exposure (i.e., small amounts during routine preparation) or acute/accidental exposure (e.g., spillage) to a larger amount.

The potential carcinogenic or mutagenic effects of commonly used cytotoxics have been widely investigated in animal models and in long-term follow-up of patients receiving therapeutic doses. The development of secondary malignancies, including leukemias, lymphomas, and bladder cancer, are well-described late complications of chemotherapy (see chapter 7).[7-9] However, many questions remain unanswered regarding the risk of occupational exposure. The only indisputable method to document occupational exposure would be to determine the amount of drug that has been absorbed by the individual handling it. This, of course, could only be done by measuring drug concentrations in the blood or other body tissues. Such monitoring would require an assay method for each drug that was sensitive enough to be both reliable and reproducible at the very low concentrations that would likely result from exposure due to spills on the skin, inhalation of aerosolized particles, or ingestion during drug manipulation. Furthermore, even if the drug or metabolites were documented, there is not sufficient evidence to define relative risk at varying levels and durations of exposure. At present, no satisfactorily sensitive assay exists for most drugs, and the resources and degree of coordination required to monitor chronic exposure for all persons handling these drugs would likely be impractical.

Occupational and Clinical Research

Environmental studies, however, have attempted to assess toxic exposure both directly (using drug or metabolite assays of urine or blood) and indirectly (using suspected biological markers). The accepted genotoxic risks of these drugs coupled with the information derived from these reports has served as the catalyst for the development and implementation of procedures to minimize worker exposure. Most indirect methods have measured the amount of urine mutagenicity or evidence of chromosomal damage in workers who either prepared or administered cytotoxic drugs, with the assumption that the urine mutagenicity or chromosomal damage was a result of occupational exposure (Table 20-1).[10]

Other reports that are frequently cited to provide indirect evidence of the risks of cytotoxic exposure have implicated the reproductive risks to workers handling these drugs. The results of many of the studies assessing worker exposure are considered inconclusive and controversial because baseline measurements were not performed, confounders such as medications or smoking were not controlled, or control groups were not appropriately selected; nonetheless, such studies have generated considerable concern among pharmacists, nurses, and hospital safety officers. It is also important to remember that most of these studies or reports were completed before the implementation of protective handling procedures, and it is firmly believed that adherence to current recommendations protects individuals handling hazardous drugs in the workplace today.

Widespread concern among personnel handling cytotoxics first began in 1979, when Falck and colleagues[11] reported that the level of mutagenic activity detectable in the urine of nurses handling cytotoxic agents was significantly greater than that of a control group. Shortly afterward, Norppa and colleagues[12] reported an increase in frequency of sister chromatid exchange (SCE) in the lymphocytes of nurses routinely handling cytotoxics. In addition, Waksvik and colleagues[13] found an increased incidence of chromosomal gaps and a slight increase in SCE in nurses preparing and administering cytotoxics. One of the more convincing studies was reported by Anderson and colleagues.[14] That study demonstrated mutagenicity in the urine of pharmacy personnel during periods in which they prepared cytotoxics in horizontal laminar airflow hoods, both when using no protective garments and when wearing gloves or masks. The report also showed that there was no urinary mutagenicity when cytotoxics were prepared in a biological safety cabinet (BSC) by personnel wearing gloves. This comparison of personnel working in horizontal laminar airflow hoods versus BSCs resulted in the universal recommendation of BSCs for cytotoxic preparation.

Concern about the reproductive risk to workers handling cytotoxics has also risen. Several reports in the literature have shown increases in fetal loss and malformation during pregnancy when women received chemotherapy during the first trimester.[15] Other reports have cited normal pregnancies and births following exposure during pregnancy.[15] At least two studies have examined the reproductive risks to female nurses who were pregnant when they worked with antineoplastics. One study reported a significant association between fetal loss (miscarriages) and the degree of occupational exposure during the first trimester.[16] The other study reported an association between the birth of children with malformations and the mother's preparation of chemotherapy while a nurse during the first trimester.[17] Both studies have been heavily criticized because data collection depended largely on worker recall of their exposure as long as 10 years prior to the survey. Although therapeutic exposure to many chemotherapy drugs is known to temporarily or permanently impair spermatogenesis, the risk of occupational exposure has not been assessed.

Other, more direct evidence that documents occupational exposure to cytotoxics also exists. Hirst and colleagues[18] demonstrated absorption through intact skin and detectable concentrations in the urine of nurses handling

Table 20-1. Indirect Methods of Assessing Occupational Exposure to Hazardous Drugs During Routine Manipulations

Biological evidence of drug absorption	
Urinary mutagenesis	Tests rely on the ability of sample to induce specific mutations in bacteria genetically engineered to be deficient in amino acid biosynthesis
Urinary thioethers	Measures glutathione-conjugated metabolites of alkylating agents excreted in the urine
Cytogenetic effects (a measure amount of chromosomal damage)	
Sister chromatid exchange	Symmetrical rearrangement of DNA within a chromosome
Chromosomal aberrations	Gaps, breaks, fragments, translocations
Micronuclei in peripheral blood lymphocytes	Micronuclei form when acentric chromosome fragments or whole chromosomes are not incorporated into the nuclei of daughter cells during division

SOURCE: references 5 and 6.

cyclophosphamide. Similarly, Jagun and colleagues[19] reported that oncology nurses had increased urinary levels of thioethers as a result of exposure to alkylating agents. The effect that absorption has on future health risks of workers is unclear, but absorption of cytotoxic agents through intact skin is a significant finding and could be particularly important in light of reports concerning damage related to duration of exposure. For example, Palmer et al.[20] correlated the degree of chromosome damage in patients receiving chlorambucil (Leukeran) with both the daily dose and the duration of treatment. Other clinical trials have documented cumulative organ system toxicities of many chemotherapy drugs, such as the cardiac toxicity reported with doxorubicin and the pulmonary toxicity associated with bleomycin.

It should be mentioned that in addition to these seemingly positive reports, other investigators have not been able to document similar direct or indirect evidence of cellular modification presumably due to cytotoxic exposure. Wilson and Solimando[21] reported that the urine of health care workers was not mutagenic after they had prepared cytotoxics in a horizontal laminar airflow hood. These results were attributed to strict adherence to aseptic technique while cytotoxics were being prepared. Another negative report by Staiano and colleagues[22] demonstrated the lack of mutagenic activity in the urine of pharmacists while they were preparing cytotoxics in a BSC. Dorr and Alberts[23] studied the extent of percutaneous absorption of daunorubicin (Cerubidine), doxorubicin (Adriamycin), mitoxantrone (Novantrone), vinblastine (Velban), vincristine (Oncovin), and melphalan (Alkeran) through human abdominal skin samples (obtained during reductive abdominoplasty) and found that penetration was negligible using an assay technique with a sensitivity limit that could measure ≤0.001% possible absorption of the exposed amount of drug. Another group of researchers also reported that they could not detect platinum in the urine of 10 pharmacists and nurses who worked with cisplatin (Platinol) and carboplatin (Paraplatin); however, these workers did employ some handling precautions.[24]

Protective Measures

The preceding concerns led to the development of guidelines regarding the handling of hazardous drugs by nationally recognized institutions and organizations. In 1983, guidelines were published by the National Institutes of Health (NIH) and later that year by the National Study Commission on Cytotoxic Exposure.[1,2] These documents were followed by guidelines from the American Society of Health-System Pharmacists (ASHP), the American Medical Association, and the Occupational Safety and Health Administration (OSHA).[3-5] This chapter is not intended to replace the information in these guidelines; rather, the goal is to provide practical information to health care workers so that they may take appropriate precautions to minimize potential risk associated with handling cytotoxic agents.

Biological Safety Cabinets

Several measures can be taken to prevent or minimize exposure to cytotoxics during drug preparation. First, the value of using a biological safety cabinet (BSC) rather than a conventional horizontal laminar airflow hood should be clearly understood. When preparing drugs in the horizontal flow hoods, the worker may be bathed in aerosolization from the product because the direction of airflow blows the aerosolized particles directly on the preparer. In separate reports, Kleinberg and Quinn[25] and Neal and colleagues[26] demonstrated the presence of drugs (1) in the downstream air after sterile ampules and vials had been manipulated in a horizontal laminar airflow hood and (2) in the room air of medication preparation areas, respectively.

Another type of hood frequently used is the vertical laminar airflow hood. The air in this hood flows in vertically from the top of the hood to the work space below, and the contaminated air is not carried directly into the face of the operator. Many of these hoods have no containment capability, and the design allows the air to flow directly into the room environment. The term *vertical laminar airflow hood* in the literature is sometimes confused with the term *BSC*. BSCs have vertical laminar airflow, but they are self-contained units from which the contaminated air does not escape into the environment. Class II BSCs are recommended by published guidelines to be the minimum requirement for preparing cytotoxic agents. Class II BSCs provide high-efficiency particulate air (HEPA)-filtered laminar airflow for product protection, they recirculate a major portion of the contaminated air, and they exhaust only HEPA-filtered air into the work area or to the outside, protecting the environment and the operator. Class II, type A hoods recirculate air, exhausting a small portion of filtered air to the room environment; class II, type B hoods exhaust air to the outside, providing more protection. Most experts prefer type B to type A for preparing cytotoxic agents. Like other hoods used for drug preparation, BSCs should be certified upon installation and recertified every 6 months or whenever they are moved. Inspectors who certify BSCs should be selected carefully by verifying their state-approved credentials.

The exposed surfaces of BSCs should be cleaned and disinfected regularly to ensure proper product protection. For routine cleaning, water with or without a small amount of cleaner should be used. The BSC should be disinfected with 70% alcohol before any aseptic manipulation is begun. The BSC should be decontaminated at least weekly (or whenever there is a spill) with the use of a good cleaning agent that removes chemicals from stainless steel, water, and disposable gauze or towels. BSCs should be reserved only for preparing hazardous materials. More specific information regarding BSCs is available in the ASHP Technical Assistance Bulletin (ASHP TAB) and OSHA guidelines.[3,5]

Nonsterile liquid and powder dosage forms should also be manipulated in a BSC. The same kind of cleaning equipment that is used for sterile products should be used to prepare and dispose of unused drugs and paraphernalia.

Protective Garments

All cytotoxic handling guidelines recommend wearing gloves, and most recommend using powder-free surgical latex gloves of good quality. In a report by Laidlaw and colleagues,[27] glove thickness was found to be a major determinant of breakthrough time. Latex surgical gloves were found to be less permeable than thin polyvinyl chloride gloves. However, gloves of both types were permeated by some drugs, leading some experts to recommend that workers wear double gloves. Double gloving is done by placing the gown cuff over the inner glove and the outer glove over the gown cuff. Personnel should begin each session in the BSC with fresh gloves. It is not necessary to use sterile gloves, but workers should wash their hands before using gloves and immediately after removing them. The outer glove should be replaced if contaminated; otherwise, change both gloves approximately every 30 minutes.

The use of disposable, lint-free, low-permeability protective gowns with long sleeves and closed cuffs is currently recommended by most published guidelines. Gowns should not be worn outside the preparation area and should be changed if overtly contaminated. Questions about the use of nondisposable gowns are usually directly related to the cost of using disposable gowns. There are immediate concerns with the use of nondisposable gowns. Cloth gowns are immediately saturated by the spilling liquid, posing a possibly serious exposure problem. Contaminated cloth gowns also present a laundering problem. They must be handled separately and carefully by workers in the laundry. The use of nondisposable gowns has been debated with only one resolution—that cleaning these gowns is difficult, at best, without contaminating other personnel, articles, and laundering equipment.

Surgical masks and protective glasses are of limited value when cytotoxics are being prepared in a BSC if the cabinet is being operated with the blower on and the view screen located at the recommended access opening. Surgical masks provide no respiratory protection against either powdered or liquid aerosols. Eye protection is important only for working outside the BSC. If workers prepare cytotoxic agents outside a BSC, several other protective articles are required. The reader should consult the ASHP videotape *Safe Handling of Cytotoxic Drugs* for further information.[28]

Drug Preparation and Manipulation

There is no doubt that good aseptic technique as well as the use of protective equipment during preparation and administration plays an important role in reducing exposure to these agents. Because unsatisfactory methods have been used to determine the risk to workers handling these agents, current concern regarding carcinogenic effects can be answered only with long-term epidemiologic studies, which still need to be conducted. Therefore, pharmacists who handle these agents and who are responsible for other employees who handle them should take a proactive approach. They should review the guidelines for safe handling of cytotoxic agents and determine which measures should be used to protect themselves and others working in the area. The importance of good technique to reduce or prevent exposure to these agents should be foremost in workers' minds while they are preparing and administering cytotoxics. Furthermore, all preparers should demonstrate competence in the preparation and handling techniques at least annually. Table 20-2 delineates some important steps in the recommended techniques for preparing and administering hazardous drugs.

Some guidelines recommend that workers handling cytotoxics be periodically rotated to areas that are not associated with hazardous materials. There is clearly no correct scientific response to this recommendation at present. If the staff is large enough to accommodate such an exchange of personnel, the safe answer would be to rotate trained, competent workers in and out of cytotoxic handling areas. Workers must make some personal decisions and be certain that guidelines for safe handling and specific monitoring procedures are developed and adhered to at all times. All personnel involved with the handling of hazardous drugs must be informed of the potential risks as well as the recommended procedures for drug preparation, administration (when applicable), accidental exposure, and clean-up of spills. Workers should remember that, in addition to these measures, good technique in preparing all sterile products is the best method of assuring an aseptic product while reducing operator risk.

As mentioned previously, some reports suggest a possible association between occupational exposure to certain cytotoxic agents during the first trimester of pregnancy and fetal loss or malformation.[16,17] These data suggest the need for concern and caution for women who are pregnant, attempting to conceive, or breast-feeding, because they could potentially be exposed to cytotoxic agents. Policies should be in place that enable such individuals to avoid contact with these drugs by providing them with alternative functions during that period. Because individuals (both male and female) may attempt to conceive for long periods of time, the ASHP TAB recommends that a specific period (e.g., 3 months) be agreed on during which the individual is reassigned.[3] All affected workers may want to seek outside medical advice to assist in making a safe and logical decision, and the institution may want to obtain legal counsel when establishing institutional policies for personnel who handle cytotoxics.

Table 20-2. Important Steps and Techniques in Preparing and Administering Hazardous Drugs

Only individuals specifically trained in the preparation and administration of cytotoxic and hazardous drugs should participate in these activities.

Preparation
1. Hazardous drugs should be prepared in a biological safety cabinet (BSC). If a BSC is not available, consult the American Society of Health-System Pharmacists Technical Assistance Bulletin[3] and Occupational Safety and Health Administration guidelines[5] for recommendations.
2. Powder-free surgical latex or specifically designed chemotherapy gloves and a disposable, lint-free, low-permeability gown should be worn. Protective eyewear is only necessary in situations with potential eye contact (i.e., outside of the glass shield of a BSC).
3. All drug and nondrug items required for preparation should be placed in the BSC before preparation begins.
4. Syringes and intravenous sets with Luer-Lok fittings should be used for preparing and administering hazardous drugs. Syringes should be large enough that they are not completely full when containing the total volume of drug to ensure that the plunger does not separate from the barrel.
5. Contents of ampuls should be gently tapped down from the neck and top portion before the ampul is opened. A sterile gauze pad should be wrapped around the neck when it is opened.
6. When manipulating hazardous drugs in vials, substantial positive or negative pressure within the vial must be avoided. A slight negative pressure within the vial is recommended when withdrawing drug solutions to avoid excessive aerosolization (i.e., blow-back). Venting devices may be used as an alternative.
7. Priming of the intravenous tubing should be done, whenever possible, in the BSC.
8. The outside of bags or bottles should be wiped with moist gauze to remove inadvertent contamination prior to leaving the BSC.
9. All final products should be labeled as hazardous substances and placed in sealable containers (e.g., zip-lock bags) before leaving the preparation area.
10. All waste that came in contact with hazardous drugs should be disposed of according to institutional policies for hazardous drugs.

Administration
1. Syringes and intravenous sets with Luer-Lok fittings should be used when administering hazardous drugs. Whenever possible, nonvented intravenous administration sets should be used.
2. Disposable latex gloves and gowns should be worn during cytotoxic manipulation and administration. Protective eyewear is strongly recommended.
3. If priming cannot be done within a BSC, a hazardous drug solution may be connected to a primary drug-free solution via a Y-site connection, and the tubing of the hazardous drug solution may be primed by retrograde flow of the primary solution into the secondary (hazardous drug) solution tubing. All connections should be taped securely.
4. All waste that came in contact with hazardous drugs should be disposed of according to institutional policies for hazardous drugs.
5. Gloves should be worn when handling urine and other excreta from patients receiving hazardous drugs.

Administration

Recommendations for protective measures to reduce risks to health care workers during administration of cytotoxic agents are also available. Most guidelines agree that workers administering hazardous drugs should use the same protective garments recommended for those who prepare the drugs (i.e., latex surgical gloves and barrier gowns). Although most guidelines recommend safety apparatus that protects the eyes or the entire face, many nurses feel that the wearing of face shields, masks, and protective glasses may cause undue concern to already anxious patients.

Syringes and intravenous (IV) administration sets with Luer-Lok fittings should be used whenever possible. IV administration sets should be primed with special care. The distal tip or needle cover must be removed before priming. The priming can be done into a sterile, alcohol-dampened gauze sponge. Other acceptable techniques for priming include using a closed receptacle (e.g., evacuated container) or backfilling IV sets. Administration sets should not be primed in an open receptacle, and materials should not be allowed to escape into the local environment. Because of the inherent risks associated with priming of IV tubing with a hazardous drug in a patient care and public area, many pharmacy departments attach the IV tubing to the bag or bottle and prime the tubing with a drug-free IV solution prior to admixture of the cytotoxic drug in the BSC. Alternatively, a back-flow closed system method may be used for priming.[3]

Spills

All personnel who handle cytotoxic drugs should be properly trained in the clean-up of spills to avoid unnecessary exposure to themselves, other workers, patients, and the environment.

Many institutions have either purchased or prepared spill kits that contain the necessary equipment for containing and removing spills. Spill kits should be placed in all areas where hazardous drugs are handled—in the pharmacy, in the drug administration areas, and in the storeroom. Workers should be instructed to wear protective garments when cleaning spills. It is also important to assure that housekeeping personnel who may be involved with a clean-up are well informed of the potential risks and appropriate clean-up procedures. The ASHP TAB and videotape and the OSHA guidelines each provide more in-depth information regarding the recommended procedures (Appendix 20-A).[1-3,28]

Disposal of Cytotoxics

Within the clinic, office, or hospital setting, hazardous (noninfectious) drug waste should be placed in leak-proof containers that are distinct from other trash containers and clearly labeled for hazardous waste. This includes items such as gowns, gloves, empty drug containers, and sterile needles and syringes. Contaminated (infectious) needles and syringes that have been used for drug administration should be placed (uncapped) in a sharps container before they are placed in the hazardous waste container. A hazardous waste disposal container should be available in each location where these drugs are prepared or administered. All hazardous wastes collected from these areas should be held in a secure location in labeled, leak-proof containers until terminal disposal. When hazardous drugs are to be administered in the home, patients or caregivers should be provided with containers for disposing of hazardous waste that can then be returned to the clinic or retrieved by a home care or hazardous waste disposal service.

Ultimately, hazardous drug waste should be disposed of separately from other trash in accordance with applicable Environmental Protection Agency, state, and local regulations. The terminal disposal may involve either incineration or burial at a licensed sanitary landfill for toxic wastes. Most institutions use a licensed commercial waste disposal company.

Regulatory Issues

In 1989, OSHA issued a hazard communication standard that states that the identification of hazardous agents and the generation of information about hazardous substances begin with chemical manufacturers or importers. The standard further delineates the responsibility of manufacturers, importers, and distributors to communicate the hazard information and associated protective measures to customers through labels and material safety data sheets (MSDSs). Employers or responsible pharmacists must:

- identify and list the hazardous chemicals used in their work places;
- obtain MSDSs and labels for each hazardous chemical;
- have a written hazardous communication program, including MSDSs and label information for all hazardous chemicals that they use; and
- communicate this hazard information to their employees through labels, MSDSs, and formal training programs.

Drugs regulated by the Food and Drug Administration (FDA) in the nonmanufacturing sector are exempt from the MSDS requirement, and the manufacturer's label and package insert may be used as the MSDS. Information about investigational drugs may be found in the sponsor's clinical brochure, which satisfies the MSDS requirements. If clinical brochures involving hazardous substances are not available, the principal investigator, the manufacturer, or the sponsor of the particular hazardous drug should be contacted.

When developing procedures to educate workers about protection from hazardous material, information about state and local hazardous waste programs and air and water quality control requirements should be included.

Worker Health Evaluation

Currently, no recognizable physiological changes can be detected by routine medical evaluation after a worker has been chronically exposed to low-level concentrations of cytotoxic agents. Tests to determine mutagenicity or chromosomal damage are useful only if conducted under rigidly controlled conditions and should not be considered for routine monitoring procedures, because of their complexity, lack of specificity, and undetermined threshold for positive or meaningful results.[10] At present, no general procedures or techniques are available for monitoring individual workers that would provide useful information regarding harmful exposure. It is generally recommended that a pre-employment health history and physical examination and periodic follow-ups be done at least annually. These exams ordinarily include a complete blood count (including differential), urinalysis, skin evaluation, physical examination of all palpable organs, and other tests as recommended by the local medical staff. Meanwhile, any evidence of a worker's exposure (i.e., overt exposure due to spillage, ingestion, inhalation, or accidental inoculation of chemical carcinogens) should be reported to the appropriate authorities and recorded in the workers' medical records.

Policies and Procedures

Policies and procedures developed to address the proper handling of cytotoxic agents should be based on scientific fact, applicable regulations and guidelines, and sound professional judgement. This point is particularly true of policies for handling hazardous materials because many recommendations are judgmental rather than scientific.

Written institutional policies and procedures should address methods of minimizing workers' exposure to cytotoxic agents. Prospective new employees should be informed about the possible hazards associated with handling cytotoxics.

It is recommended to record in employees' personnel files that they have been so advised. Some institutions have employees sign a statement about the potential risks associated with handling cytotoxics. New employees, current employees, and others (such as volunteers and individuals in training) should have education and training in proper methods to minimize their exposure. This must include pharmacy students who are completing experiential rotations. Recertification should follow periodically for all individuals who continue to work with these agents. This process should assess the worker's competence, and include determination of adherence to departmental or institutional procedures as well as their understanding of potential risks.

Procedure manuals should contain, at a minimum, specific details on worker protection, equipment maintenance, drug preparation, transportation of a formulated drug inside or outside the institution, drug administration, disposal of unused drugs and paraphernalia used in preparation and administration, and spill management. Like all institutional policies, these should be reviewed and updated at regular predetermined intervals. Information to assist in preparing manuals may be obtained from national professional association standards, pharmaceutical manufacturers, governmental regulations, and other knowledgeable personnel. It should be emphasized that safe handling of cytotoxic agents is a health-system-wide concern. Therefore, numerous hospital departments should be involved in preparing manuals, including pharmacy, nursing, medical service, hospital safety officers, hospital legal staff, housekeeping, maintenance, laundry, delivery personnel, and any other departments that have contact with hazardous agents.

REVIEWING MEDICATION ORDERS FOR CANCER CHEMOTHERAPY

Antineoplastic drugs, as a class, are the most toxic drugs distributed through health-system pharmacies. Serious and sometimes life-threatening toxicities are common, even when antineoplastic drugs are administered in conventional doses. Safe dose ranges may be narrow, and patient outcomes of inadvertent overdose can be devastating. Disabling major organ toxicity or death may occur, depending on the toxicity patterns of the drugs involved. A detailed discussion of specific systemic and major organ toxicities can be found in chapters 7 and 8. Perhaps as important as overdose, although less dramatic, are errors of underdosing. Patients may lose their best opportunity for cure or remission because a medication was underprescribed or improperly prepared.

The potential medical and legal implications of chemotherapy dosing errors are also daunting. Several highly publicized chemotherapy dosing errors have illustrated the compelling need for each health system to develop multidisciplinary systems to prevent chemotherapy medication-related errors.[29] Although the details of such guidelines must be customized to accommodate the unique practice situations of each health system, some core precautions apply to most practice settings.

Published analyses of chemotherapy medication errors have highlighted several common weaknesses in drug-use systems that increase the risk of dosing errors with chemotherapy drugs.[30-32] Some of the factors known to contribute to dosing errors include verbal orders; multiple-day drug courses; abbreviations; poor documentation for cited regimens or protocols; errors in references; inadequate interdisciplinary communication; limited education of health care professionals and patients; and the wide variability in chemotherapy doses that may be appropriate for different disease states, drug combinations, and patient situations.

Suggested interventions to minimize errors will be addressed within the following sections: professional training, drug ordering or prescribing, drug order processing and delivery, drug administration, protocol development, and patient education. These policy suggestions have been assimilated from several recent reviews of preventive strategies for chemotherapy dosing errors, as well as from policies in place at the authors' institutions.[30-32] Modifying these areas of risk should result in fewer serious chemotherapy errors, although objective data to prove this hypothesis are not yet available.

Professional Training

Suggestion: All health care practitioners involved in the chemotherapy process should be knowledgeable about the mechanisms of action, doses, schedules, predictable toxicities, and toxicity management of the cytotoxic drugs in use at that institution. The educational process for each discipline must focus on its members' particular responsibilities. Pharmacists, for example, must be trained in safe preparation practices, whereas nurses should be trained in drug administration. Outcome-based certification processes should be implemented to verify competence in required skills for each discipline.

Suggestion: Informational guidelines about conventional and investigational chemotherapy agents must be readily available to all health care practitioners involved in the chemotherapy process. Several useful references for cytotoxic agents are described later in this chapter.

Suggestion: Educational sessions directed specifically at prevention of medication-related errors should be included in the certification process for physicians, pharmacists, and nurses who work with chemotherapy agents. Review and analysis of actual medication-related errors is an effective teaching tool that encourages compliance with institutional guidelines for prevention of chemotherapy medication-related errors.

Drug Ordering or Prescribing

Suggestion: Verbal orders for chemotherapy drugs leave greater potential for misinterpretation or transcription errors than do written orders. Written, signed orders should be required to initiate chemotherapy. Verbal orders may be acceptable to modify an existing order. Ideally, two health care professionals should receive and document verbal orders. Examples of situations in which verbal orders are acceptable might include reducing chemotherapy doses, altering infusion fluids or rates, modifying antiemetics, or reconciling discrepancies in patient height or weight. Specific criteria for acceptance of verbal orders should be specified in the health system's chemotherapy policies.

Suggestion: Orders for cytotoxic agents should be written only by board-certified or -eligible oncologists or hematologists, or by experienced oncology fellows. Chemotherapy orders should not be written by medical residents. Orders written by oncology fellows must be countersigned by a qualified attending physician before the chemotherapy is administered. Some institutions may choose to waive the requirement for countersignature of orders written by oncology fellows once the capability of the fellow has been certified within institution guidelines. In some settings, chemotherapy order writing (under approved protocol) and/or the review function for oncology fellows' orders may be granted to experienced oncology pharmacy practitioners. Specially trained physicians' assistants or nurse clinicians may write chemotherapy orders within approved protocol guidelines. Countersignatures should still be required.

Suggestion: Chemotherapy orders should be written on approved chemotherapy order forms to encourage adherence to a standard order format and to help ensure that information that is essential to safe processing and administration of the drugs is available to pharmacists and nurses who will work with that order (Figure 20-1). Chemotherapy order forms should include specification of the chemotherapy protocol and/or regimen; cycle number; patient age, weight, height, and calculated body surface area; pertinent lab data (including white blood cell count, absolute neutrophil count, platelets, hemoglobin and hematocrit, blood urea nitrogen, serum creatinine, and bilirubin); hydration fluids; and antiemetics for pre- and postchemotherapy administration. The standard format for the chemotherapy drug order should include the generic name of the drug, the dose to be given in dose units (e.g., milligrams) per meter squared, calculated dose, route of administration, frequency, days of administration, and infusion guidelines. An abbreviated order form may be developed for very simple parenteral regimens or for oral chemotherapy regimens. Chemotherapy order forms have been proved to improve the completeness of orders and to decrease pharmacists' time required to clarify orders.[33]

Suggestion: Standardized preprinted order forms or computer order sets should be developed for complicated drug regimens or protocols. All preprinted standardized orders or computer order sets should be exhaustively reviewed by members of each discipline involved to avoid errors that could affect every patient treated with that regimen.

Suggestion: Vocabulary and terminology for chemotherapy ordering should be standardized. This guideline applies to both orders for cytotoxics and for pharmacy and nursing records of the cytotoxic orders. Brand names and abbreviations should not be used as substitutes for generic drug names. Many drug names and abbreviations look alike and could be easily misinterpreted, particularly in handwritten orders. An example is confusion between orders written for "Adria" (Adriamycin, the brand name for doxorubicin), a common chemotherapy drug for treatment of breast cancer patients, and Aredia (pamidronate), a bisphosphonate used to decrease the risk of bone degeneration in patients with breast cancer or multiple myeloma. Abbreviations present a particular problem in oncology because they are widely used to describe complete regimens as well as individual drugs. Examples of abbreviations known to produce confusion are listed in Table 20-3.

Suggestion: Zeros in dose orders or pharmacy records lead to many dosing errors. Trailing zeros follow a decimal point, as in this example: cytarabine 200.0 mg. The decimal point may easily be overlooked or may be lost on carbon or faxed orders.

Table 20-3. Examples of Abbreviations That Increase the Risk of Chemotherapy Errors

Abbreviation	Drug	Risk
CDDP	*c*is-*d*iamino-*d*ichloro*p*latinum (cisplatin)	Suggests four different drugs of a multidrug regimen
MTX	Methotrexate or mitoxantrone	Two generic chemotherapy drugs with similar key letters
MTX and MTC	Methotrexate or mitoxantrone and mitomycin C	Easily confused abbreviations
VCR and VBL	Vincristine and vinblastine	Easily confused abbreviations for very similar drugs with dissimilar doses.
DTIC	*D*iamino-*t*riazo-*i*midazole-*c*arboxamide (dacarbazine)	Suggests four different drugs of a multidrug regimen
Plat or platinum	Cisplatin or carboplatin	Term can refer to any platinum derivative

ANTINEOPLASTIC MEDICATION ORDER FORM

Date					HT. cm
Wbc					WT. Kg
Hct					BSA m^2
PLTS					AGE
CREAT					
BUN					

PATIENT NAME	ALLERGIES	Hx NO.

CHEMOTHERAPY ORDERS

PROTOCOL NO.	COURSE NO.	DOSE MODIFICATION? ☐ NO ☐ YES	☐ INCREASE? ☐ DECREASE? %

DRUG (mg/m^2) ROUTE/ADMINISTRATION GUIDELINES	ACTUAL DOSE	DATES/DAYS TO BE GIVEN	DATE/TIME GIVEN/INITIALS				
1.							
2.							
3.							
4.							
5.							

☐ Antiemetics per Health-System guidelines
☐ Antiemetics as written below.
Reason: ☐ Pt emetic hx ☐ Protocol specfic ☐ Prior ADR ☐ Other

NON-CHEMOTHERAPY ORDERS (E.G., HYDRATION, ANTIEMETICS)	DATE/TIME GIVEN/INITIALS				
1.					
2.					
3.					
4.					

DATE AND TIME ORDER WRITTEN	DAY ONE (1) OF CYCLE TO BE

NURSE(S) SIGNATURE	DOCTOR/NP

Figure 20-1. Example of a chemotherapy order sheet. Wbc, white blood count; Hct, hematocrit; PLTS, platelets; CREAT, serum creatinine; BUN, blood urea nitrogen; HT., height; cm, centimeters; Kg, kilograms; WT., weight; BSA, body surface area; m^2, meters squared; Hx No., history number; Pt emetic hx, patient's emetic history; ADR, adverse drug reaction; NP, nurse practitioner.

A dose intended as 200 mg would then be interpreted as 2000 mg. Both doses are within the broadly acceptable dose ranges for cytarabine, but the second results in a 10-fold overdose. It is just as important that leading zeros be required before decimal points when the chemotherapy dose is less than a whole number to avoid overdosing if the decimal point is lost or overlooked. An example of this kind of error would be an order for dactinomycin .5 mg, which could easily be read as 5 mg. Recording the dose as 0.5 mg minimizes this risk.

Suggestion: Multiple-day bolus and continuous infusion chemotherapy regimens also hold potential for factorial errors. Daily doses must be very clearly distinguished from the total dose per course to avoid the risk of overdosing with each dose portion. The greatest risk is that the total course dose will be given each day. It is generally best to specify the dose each day and the specified days (examples: cisplatin 20 mg/m^2 = 40 mg IV over 1 hour each day on days 1, 2, 3, and 4; or cytarabine 200 mg/m^2 per day = 400 mg in 1 L dextrose 5% in water over 24 hours on days 1–7). Total doses should not be included. An exception is made for continuous infusions to be delivered by pump. These orders should include the total dose to be infused over the time period of the infusion, but they must also note how much drug will be delivered by the pump each day.

Suggestion: Most chemotherapy doses are based on body surface area (BSA), a size parameter estimated from height and weight. To improve dosing accuracy, BSA must be based on measured values rather than estimates by patients. Changes in height and weight are common among cancer patients as a consequence of disease or treatment. For example, spinal compression fractures secondary to bony metastases to the spine can decrease a patient's height by several inches. Weight may be decreased because of chemotherapy or cancer cachexia or increased because of the appetite-stimulating effects of certain hormonal agents. Patients may also under- or overestimate their body size because of lack of knowledge or because of their perceptions of what is acceptable in our society. It is a clinical impression that women patients often underestimate their body weight, whereas males are likely to overestimate their true height.

Suggestion: BSA and doses should be calculated independently by physicians, pharmacists, and nurses. Most adults have BSAs between 1.5 and 2.2 m^2. BSAs outside this range should be rechecked. It is also important that heights and weights that fall outside the normal ranges for that person's age and gender should be verified by remeasurement. An actual error of this type occurred in a university teaching hospital. The height of an adult Hispanic male with newly diagnosed acute myelogenous leukemia was recorded on the order form as 59 inches. This measurement represents 4 feet, 11 inches, which is a possible but improbable height for an adult male in our society. The discrepancy was not noted, and seven days of induction chemotherapy were administered based on a calculated BSA that was 15% lower than the patient's true BSA. The patient required a second cycle of induction chemotherapy to achieve remission, perhaps because of this error. The unusually short height for an adult should have made the pharmacists and/or nurses suspect that the height might be incorrect. In this case, the patient's actual height was 5 feet, 9 inches (69 inches). Heights measured in centimeters can also be a source of error. For example, it is unlikely that most pharmacists in America would recognize a reported height of 185 cm as that of a short, average, or tall patient without translating the figure into feet and inches. Metric height measurements reduce the chance that errors will be detected during routine screening.

Order Processing and Delivery

Suggestion: Chemotherapy orders must be double-checked against the original order at the point of order entry by two pharmacists. Transcribed orders are not acceptable. In the case of a patient's first cycle of a particular regimen, one of these pharmacists should be a pharmacist recognized and approved by the pharmacy as competent in chemotherapy drug dosing and very familiar with the protocols and regimens in use at that institution. Use of fax machines and electronic transfer of orders may permit distant verification of orders in centrally located pharmacies or satellite pharmacies staffed by a single pharmacist.

Suggestion: A systematic verification process should be implemented for chemotherapy order processing. Some institutions include a checklist for order verification as part of the chemotherapy order form. Patient-specific parameters, such as body size, blood counts, and relevant major organ function, should be checked and considered in dosing. A computerized or manual perpetual chemotherapy drug profile should be maintained, and it should be reviewed before any chemotherapy dose is dispensed to screen for unexplained increases or decreases in dose. Each drug dose should be compared with speci-

---

Chemotherapy Checklist

	Intervention Made
❏ Informed Consent	❏
❏ Required Information Completed	❏
❏ BSA Verified	❏
❏ Protocol Review	❏
❏ Dose Confirmation	❏
❏ Inventory Verified	❏
❏ PreMeds/Ancilliary Therapies	❏

Initials _____ Date _____

Figure 20-2. Example of a chemotherapy checklist

fied doses in the chemotherapy regimen or protocol cited on the order and with institutional guidelines for acceptable dose ranges. The need to modify doses based on impaired renal or hepatic function must be considered. Antiemetics appropriate for the emetogenic potential of the chemotherapy regimens (see chapter 9) should be included. A sample checklist is outlined in Figure 20-2.

Suggestion: Chemotherapy must be prepared using safe handling techniques (as outlined earlier in this chapter) and with very careful attention to accuracy. The measured volume and identity of each cytotoxic agent should be checked before the drug is added to infusion fluids. Diluent fluids and volumes should also be confirmed. A very serious error occurred at a large university hospital when a dose of methotrexate was being prepared for intraventricular administration through an Ommaya reservoir (see chapter 10). The order specified 12 mg of methotrexate in a final volume of 5 ml of nonpreserved saline solution. Preparation required 0.5 ml of liquid methotrexate (25 mg/ml), diluted with 4.5 ml of saline solution. An experienced pharmacy technician prepared the dose with 5 ml of methotrexate and no saline solution. The preparation was checked by an experienced pharmacist working a double shift who did not notice the error. The 10-fold overdose (125 mg) of methotrexate was administered into the patient's central nervous system (CNS). Similar doses have been reported in anecdotal literature to cause irreversible neurological toxicity and death. Fortunately, the error was detected soon after the dose was administered. The patient's immediate onset of headache and vomiting prompted the physician to call the oncology pharmacist, who traced the preparation records and questioned the preparer to determine how the drug was prepared. A portion of the methotrexate dose was quickly withdrawn via the Ommaya reservoir, reducing the concentration in the cerebrospinal fluid. Large doses of leucovorin were administered, although leucovorin enters the CNS very poorly. Neurosurgeons placed a drain low in the patient's spine and lavaged his CNS to wash out more methotrexate. With these interventions, the patient recovered completely, without evidence of any neurological damage.

Suggestion: Chemotherapy drugs dispensed in syringes should have labels placed directly on each syringe that include contents and route of drug administration. Syringe labels must include drug concentration to permit nurses administering the drug to double-check dose calculations. IV push drugs requiring more than one syringe to provide the entire dose should be labeled as such. Labeling of route is important for drugs intended for administration by unusual routes, such as intrathecally or into chest tubes for treatment of pleural effusions. It is just as important that drugs intended only for IV use be so labeled. The patient outcome can be devastating when a vesicant drug (such as vincristine) is inadvertently administered into the CNS.[34] An example of appropriate labeling is shown in Figure 20-3.

Suggestion: Careful documentation must be made of the drugs, doses, volumes, and lot numbers of drugs used in chemotherapy preparation. Perpetual manual or computerized profiles aid in this process. In addition to preparation information, these profiles should include notes about the chemotherapy cycle to assist in subsequent dosing. For example, if the patient experiences neutropenic fever requiring dose reduction in the next cycle, this reaction should be noted in the patient's chemotherapy profile. This notation may prevent inadvertent full-dose administration in subsequent cycles.

Suggestion: Chemotherapy should be prepared and administered during specified working hours, usually weekday shifts in hospitals, when adequate qualified staff is available to review orders. Examples of emergency situations that justify off-shift preparation or administration are superior vena cava syndrome caused by small cell lung cancer and, occasionally, institution of treatment for acute leukemia or a rapidly growing lymphoma. Patient or physician convenience or increased hospital stay because of delay in writing orders are not acceptable reasons for failing to observe this safety guideline.

Suggestion: Physicians, pharmacists, and nurses must work together to develop institution-specific dose limits for cytotoxic agents in use within that health system. Dosing guidelines should include the maximum amount permitted in a single dose, in a 24-hour period, over an entire chemotherapy course, and per patient lifetime.[30]

Suggestion: Pharmacists preparing chemotherapy and nurses administering it have the right and responsibility to confirm documentation that supports a selected dose regimen. Only with this knowledge can they adequately fulfill their responsibility to the patient for the outcomes of care. Chemotherapy orders that do not follow institution-approved protocols or established regimens should be accompanied in the patient's chart records with copies of the journal article, protocol, or other supporting references. Whether a physician's order for unsupported dose regimens or doses that exceed established dose limits should be honored may be resolved by a peer-review process established according to institutional guidelines.

Drug Administration[30,35]

Suggestion: Nurses administering chemotherapy drugs should implement a double-check system in which two nurses check

---

Doxorubicin 2 mg/ml
Delivers 50 mg/25 ml
Number of syringes required for patient's dose: 3
Total dose in 3 syringes = 130 mg/65 ml
For INTRAVENOUS use only

Figure 20-3. Example of appropriate chemotherapy labeling

the prepared chemotherapy product against the original orders. At least one of the nurses should be a nurse certified in chemotherapy administration. The verification procedure should be similar to that regularly employed for administration of blood products and should also include confirmation of the patient's identity.

Suggestion: Nurses must independently check the appropriateness of the drugs and doses against the supporting documentation (protocol, standard regimen, journal article, etc.) and calculate the patient's BSA. They must review pertinent laboratory data, dose modifications, need for ancillary medications, and infusion guidelines.

Suggestion: Nurses have the additional responsibility of checking the pharmacy dose calculations to the extent feasible. The syringe or infusion bag should be compared with the original order for accuracy of patient name and identification, route, drug, dose, volume, and infusion time.

Suggestion: Nurses must verify that the patient (or in the case of a child, the parent) understands the procedure and toxicities expected from the chemotherapy drugs and has given consent to the procedure.

Suggestion: Chemotherapy drugs should be administered using safe handling practices. These are detailed earlier in this chapter and in references 3 and 35.

Protocol Development

Suggestion: Concise, consolidated drug information sections should be included in cancer therapy protocols, especially those that study investigational agents, because information on investigational agents may not be readily available in traditional sources. These drug information sections should include pharmacology, pharmacokinetics, known stability and compatibility, storage requirements, vesicant and emetogenic potential, and other toxicities, with an indication of incidence as well as suggestions for prevention or management of toxicity.

Suggestion: Summary schema should be carefully checked for accuracy of dose guidelines and should refer the reader to the specific detailed treatment plan.

Patient Education

Suggestion: One component of the patient care team that may be overlooked in guidelines to prevent chemotherapy medication-related errors is the patient who will be receiving the drugs. The patient should be well educated about the agents he or she is scheduled to receive. Patients and/or family members should know the names of the drugs, doses based on the patient's body size, route of administration, schedule, color of the drugs, and any need for support drugs, such as antiemetics, hydration fluids, antidotes (e.g., leucovorin), or hematopoietic growth factors.

Suggestion: Patients should be encouraged to ask health care professionals about their chemotherapy treatment. It is the patient's right, for example, to question the rationale for choice of the selected regimen, to insist that nurses verify the medication labeling (including the patient's full name) before administering drugs, and to check dose calculations with the nurse or pharmacist if they wish. The patient or family member can then act effectively as an advocate and as the last line of defense against chemotherapy medication-related errors.[30,32]

Many suggestions have been outlined to minimize the potential for chemotherapy medication-related errors. The key to the success of any health-system strategy to prevent errors is effective multidisciplinary communication. Physicians, pharmacists, and nurses must pool the strengths of their individual expertise to honor their mutual commitment to patient safety. Each health system in which chemotherapy agents are administered should develop consensus multidisciplinary practice guidelines designed to prevent chemotherapy errors, educate the health care professionals about these guidelines, monitor the effectiveness of these guidelines using continuous quality improvement parameters, and review the guidelines at least annually. Cancer therapy is a rapidly evolving field. As treatments change, practice guidelines may need to be modified as well. A systematic, multidisciplinary, responsive system should decrease the risk of serious errors with these valuable but dangerous drugs.

DRUG INFORMATION IN ONCOLOGY

Pharmacists working in oncology settings are frequently requested to provide drug information. Like other practice areas this information may be: (1) patient specific—raised by a health care professional and used to make a treatment decision for an individual patient; (2) consumer or patient generated—responding to a question raised by someone other than a health care professional regarding treatment or for adaptation in lay publications or media; or (3) used for the development of population-based tools to optimize drug therapy outcomes in a specific setting (e.g., development of clinical practice guidelines or pathways). Although the standard practices of procuring, evaluating, and interpreting drug information certainly apply to oncology, there are specialized resources that are frequently helpful to oncology pharmacists. In addition, as shown in the previous chapters, the malignancy or its treatment may produce pathological or metabolic changes that may complicate drug therapy and necessitate specialized interpretation of drug information.

Patient-Specific Information

Table 20-4 lists several printed sources of information regarding anticancer drugs and describes the applications for which each reference may be most helpful. In addition to these on-

Table 20-4. Printed Sources of Drug Information for Anticancer Drugs and Related Therapies

Dorr RT and Von Hoff DD, editors. *Cancer Chemotherapy Handbook.* 2nd ed. Norwalk, CT: Appleton & Lange; 1994.

Text contains comprehensive but consise monographs on most commercially available cytotoxics and many immunotherapeutics as well as many monographs on investigational drugs. Monographs contain useful information for pharmacists, including side effects, pharmacokinetics, compatibility/stability information, and administration guidelines.

Perry MC, editor. *The Chemotherapy Sourcebook.* Baltimore, MD: Williams & Wilkins; 1992.

Chapters on chemotherapy principles, special administration techniques, chemotherapy drugs by pharmacologic class, chemotherapy toxicities by organ system, and overview of management of common malignancies. Does not include much pharmaceutical information (compatibilities, stabilities, etc.), but the extensive chapters on toxicities are informative. Unfortunately, many recently marketed drugs are not included.

Chabner BA, Longo DL, editors. *Cancer Chemotherapy and Biotherapy: Principles and Practice.* 2nd ed. Philadelphia, PA: JB Lippincott; 1996.

A basic pharmacology text specifically regarding drugs used in the treatment of cancer, organized by drug class. Reviews are very thorough and include more depth than many of the other references. The reviews do contain information on administration and toxicities. Many tables and figures enhance the presentation.

Pratt WB, Ruddon RW, Ensminger WD, Maybaum J, editors. *The Anticancer Drugs.* 2nd ed. New York: Oxford Univ Pr; 1994.

A basic pharmacology text specifically regarding drugs used in the treatment of cancer, organized by drug class. Reviews are very thorough and include more depth than many of the other references. Figures and tables add insight to the text. Descriptions of side effects are not as thorough as other texts.

DeVita VT, Hellman S, Rosenberg SA, editors. *Biologic Therapy of Cancer.* 2nd ed. Philadelphia, PA: JB Lippincott; 1995.

Most comprehensive text available on biotherapy of cancer. Chapter topics range from principles of immunotherapy to reviews of specific agents to clinical applications in various cancers.

DeVita VT, Hellman S, Rosenberg SA, editors. *Cancer: Principles and Practice of Oncology.* 5th ed. Philadelphia, PA: JB Lippincott; 1997.

Probably the most comprehensive cancer text available. Several chapters deal specifically with chemotherapy and related topics, but the strength of the book is in the extensive reviews of all major cancer types.

---

cology-specific resources, many other general drug information resources (e.g., AHFS DI, USP-DI, MedAxon, and Micromedex) provide much pertinent information. When responding to a patient-specific request, pharmacists must ask the appropriate questions to ascertain the full scope of the issue. For example, if an oncologist questions whether an unusual adverse event was caused by a cytotoxic drug, it may be important to know the type and extent (i.e., the sites of metastases) of the patient's malignancy as well as their other medications and concomitant illnesses. All of this information may help to assess whether the malignant disease itself may either cause the reaction or impair the elimination of the drug and increase its potential for causing the adverse effect.

Formulary and Guideline Development

The collation of information regarding a new anticancer drug for the purpose of formulary review and guideline development can be challenging. Typically, anticancer drugs are initially approved by the FDA for only one indication (e.g., metastatic breast cancer) with one dosing regimen (e.g., 90 mg/m^2 IV every 3 weeks). However, as soon as the drug becomes available, oncologists may begin to prescribe it for several types of cancer, using many different doses and schedules. In addition, the package insert information usually describes the use only as a single agent and, as shown in previous chapters, anticancer drugs are most frequently used in combinations. The challenges for the pharmacist are to:

- verify the appropriateness of the alternative dosages and combinations;
- work with the oncologist to develop guidelines for use that specify adjunctive medications that will minimize side effects;
- compile accurate information for the pharmacy and nursing staffs regarding type and volume of infusates, stability, compatibility, and acute and late toxicities; and
- develop a strategy for follow-up assessment of the new drug's utilization.

When anticancer drugs are used in combination, pharmacists must often refer to the primary literature and make determinations of information that may only be available in abstract form (such as the proceedings of a clinical or scientific meeting). As in all situations in which drug therapy is being used, pharmacists must assume responsibility for critically reviewing available information and working with other clinicians to ensure optimal safety and efficacy for every patient. If information is not readily available, it is quite reasonable to request the prescriber to provide it. Likewise, the manufacturer may also be able to provide helpful information. Several Internet resources of information are listed in Table 20-5. However, pharmacists should always be aware that information posted on the Internet is not always subject to the rigor-

Table 20-5. On-line Sources of Drug Information for Anticancer Drugs and Related Therapies

Description	Internet Address
National Library of Medicince web site: free Medline access	http://www.nlm.nih.gov
WebMedLit: oncology news items from journals and PRNewswire, Medline queries via PubMed	http://www.webmedlit.com/topics/OncoLit.html
National Cancer Institute (NCI) web site: access to PDQ	http://www.nci.nih.gov
Cancer Therapy Evaluations Program (CTEP)	http://ctep.info.nih.gov/
National Cancer Institute	http://cancernet.nci.nih.gov/trials/h_clinic.htm
National Comprehenshive Cancer Network	http://www.fccc.edu/NCCN/NCCN.html

ous peer-review process that they have depended on to ensure the integrity of published information. The reader may not even know the identity of the author of the information. In addition, some of these resources require a subscription fee, whereas others are accessible to everyone.

Because of the positive impact that the rational use of supportive care medications can have on patient outcomes as well as the considerable economic impact that inappropriate use may have, many health systems have developed guidelines for use or algorithms for drugs such as the serotonin receptor antagonist antiemetics, the colony-stimulating factors, epoetin, and broad-spectrum antibiotics and antifungals. The oncology pharmacist can play a pivotal role in reviewing the primary literature and drafting the initial guidelines. The oncology pharmacist should become involved in all aspects of development of disease management tools, including clinical practice guidelines and clinical pathways. Although the principles of development, implementation, and monitoring are the same as those used for other disease states, the sources of information may differ.[36,37] It is also important to be aware of practice standards and guidelines that may be published by oncology organizations, such as the American Society of Clinical Oncology (ASCO), the Oncology Nursing Society (ONS), and the National Association of Comprehensive Cancer Centers (NACCC).

Patient or Consumer Information

Perhaps one of the most challenging aspects of providing oncology-related drug information occurs when inquiries are made by someone other than a health care professional—a patient or family member, for example. They frequently obtain selected pieces of information from the lay press or by word of mouth. In many cases, it may represent hope of cure or a lessening of symptoms. Although it may be easy to discount such information, it is always important to the person asking about it.

The first step is usually to find the source of the information and confirm the content and the patient's interpretation. This step may require a call to a newspaper or television station. In addition to the usual sources of drug information, several other organizations or sources may be helpful (Table 20-6). Following retrieval of information, it is then necessary to put it into a context that the patient can understand. An important aspect of this is providing honest information while

Table 20-6. Other Sources of Drug Information for Anticancer Drugs and Related Therapies

Description	Telephone Number or Internet Address
Cancer Information Line	1-800-4-CANCER
American Association for Cancer Research	http://www.aacr.org
American Society of Clinical Oncology	http://www.asco.org
American Cancer Society	http://www.cancer.org/frames.html
CancerGuide: developed by a cancer patient to inform others how to obtain information	http://cancerguide.org
Cancer News on the Net	http://www.cancernews.com
HospiceHands: hospice information, reference articles	http://hospice-cares.com/welcome.html

Table 20-7. Information Sources for Alternative Cancer Therapies

Agency or Information Source	Contact
National Institutes of Health Office of Alternative Medicine Information Clearinghouse (fax-back system)	1-888-644-6226
Office of Dietary Supplements	1-301-495-1508
National Council Against Health Fraud	1-909-824-4690 http://www.ncahf.org
Consumer Product Safety Commission (Food and Drug Administration)	1-800-638-2772
Cancer Information Line	1-800-4-CANCER

not destroying the patient's sense of hope, so compassion and good communication skills are critical.

In many cases, the new information the patient or their family heard is based on preliminary results of clinical trials involving investigational drugs. It then becomes necessary to explain the status of an investigational drug and establish whether a patient may be eligible for participation in that trial or a similar study. A call to the study site, the sponsor (e.g., the pharmaceutical company or the National Cancer Institute), or the Cancer Information Service (1-800-4-CANCER) may help to clarify this issue. The PDQ database described in Table 20-5 is also a good source of information regarding experimental regimens. A brochure entitled "Clinical Studies: Cancer Research in the Clinic—Who, What, Where and Why" provided by the National Cancer Institute may be useful to patients and their families when contemplating participation in a clinical trial. In understandable terminology, it describes what the patient should expect as a requirement for participation in the trial.

It is particularly challenging to find up-to-date, objective information about alternative cancer therapies. In its broadest sense, this term includes any unproven therapies, such as investigational agents still in phase I and II clinical trials. It is used more commonly, however, to refer to therapies that are not available in hospitals, therapies that have no known preclinical rationale, or therapies that are tested in ways that will not give medically sound answers (see chapter 5). In 1993, an Office of Alternative Medicine (OAM) was established at the National Institutes of Health to evaluate and serve as a clearinghouse for information about alternative medical therapies for treatment of cancer and other disorders. Their contact number and several other resources of drug information on alternative cancer therapies are listed in Table 20-7.

SUMMARY

As you learned in the earlier chapters of this book, pharmacists who collaborate with other health care providers to optimize the therapeutic outcomes for patients with cancer must have a comprehensive knowledge of cancer pathophysiology as well as a clear understanding of the pharmacology of drugs used to treat cancer and related symptoms. In addition to the clinical knowledge and skills, however, specialized pharmaceutical and pharmacy practice knowledge and skills are just as important. These skills include handling and preparing cytotoxic drugs, developing and implementing medication use processes that will ensure the highest degree of patient safety, managing formulary decisions for oncology-related drugs, and providing accurate and timely drug information to other health care providers, patients, and consumers. These activities, which are vital to patient care in oncology, ensure the integrity of the drug use process. These activities are all fundamental to the provision of pharmaceutical care and are clearly the responsibility of every pharmacist working in an oncology setting.

REFERENCES

1. Public Health Service, National Institutes of Health [NIH]. Recommendations for the safe handling of parenteral antineoplastic drugs. NIH Publication No. 83-2621. Washington, DC: U.S. Department of Health and Human Services; 1983.
2. [Anonymous]. Recommendations for handling cytotoxic agents. Providence, RI: National Study Commission on Cytotoxic Exposure; September 1987.
3. American Society of Hospital Pharmacists. ASHP technical assistance bulletin on handling cytotoxic and hazardous drugs. *Am J Hosp Pharm* 1990;47:1033–49.
4. American Medical Association Council on Scientific Affairs. Guidelines for handling parenteral antineoplastics. *JAMA* 1985;253:1590–2.
5. Office of Occupational Medicine, Occupational Safety and Health Administration. Controlling occupational exposure to hazardous drugs. *Am J Health-Syst Pharm* 1996;53:1669–85.
6. Valanis B, Vollmer WM, Labuhn K, et al. Antineoplastic drug handling protection after OSHA guidelines: comparison by profession, handling activity, and work site. *J Occup Med* 1992;34:149–55.

7. Kyle RA, Gertz MA. Second malignancies associated with chemotherapy. In: Perry MC, editor. *The Chemotherapy Sourcebook*. Baltimore, MD: Williams & Wilkins; 1992. p. 689–702.
8. Rosner F. Acute leukemia as a delayed consequence of cancer chemotherapy. *Cancer* 1976;37:1033–6.
9. Sieber SM. Cancer chemotherapeutic agents and carcinogenesis. *Cancer Chemother Rep* 1976;59:915–8.
10. Baker ES, Connor TH. Monitoring occupational exposure to cancer chemotherapy drugs. *Am J Health-Syst Pharm* 1996;53:2713–23.
11. Falck K, Grohn P, Sorsa M, et al. Mutagenicity in urine of nurses handling cytotoxic drugs. *Lancet* 1979;1:1250–1.
12. Norppa H, Sorsa M, Vainio H, et al. Increased sister chromatid exchange frequencies in lymphocytes of nurses handling cytostatic drugs. *Scand J Work Environ Health* 1980;6:299–301.
13. Waksvik H, Klepp O, Brogger A. Chromosome analyses of nurses handling cytostatic agents. *Cancer Treat Rep* 1981;65:607–10.
14. Anderson R, Puckett W, Dana W, et al. Risk of handling injectable antineoplastic agents. *Am J Hosp Pharm* 1982;39:1881–7.
15. Doll DC. Chemotherapy in pregnancy. In Perry MC, editor. *The Chemotherapy Sourcebook*. Baltimore, MD: Williams & Wilkins; 1992. p. 703–9.
16. Hemminki K, Kyyronen P, Lindbohm ML. Spontaneous aberrations and malformations in the offspring of nurses exposed to anesthetic gases, cytotoxic drugs, and other potential hazards in hospitals based on registered information of outcome. *J Epidemiol Comm Health* 1985;39:141–7.
17. Lelevan SH, Lindbohm ML, Hornung RW, et al. A study of occupational exposure to antineoplastic drugs and fetal loss in nurses. *N Engl J Med* 1985;333:1173–8.
18. Hirst M, Tse S, Mills D, et al. Occupational exposure to cyclophosphamide. *Lancet* 1984;1:186–8.
19. Jagun O, Ryan M, Waldron HA. Urinary thioether excretion in nurses handling cytotoxic drugs. *Lancet* 1982;2:443–4.
20. Palmer R, Dore C, Denman A. Chlorambucil-induced chromosome damage to human lymphocytes is dose-dependent and cumulative. *Lancet* 1984;1:246–9.
21. Wilson JP, Solimando DA. Aseptic technique as a safety precaution in the preparation of antineoplastic agents. *Hosp Pharm* 1981;16:575–81.
22. Staiano N, Galleli J, Adamson R, et al. Lack of mutagenic activity in urine from hospital pharmacists admixing antitumor drugs. *Lancet* 1981;1:615–6.
23. Dorr RT, Alberts DS. Topical absorption and inactivation of cytotoxic anticancer agents in vitro. *Cancer* 1992;70:983–7.
24. Venitt S, Crofton-Sleigh C, Hunt J, et al. Monitoring exposure of nursing and pharmacy personnel to cytotoxic drugs: urinary mutation assays and urinary platinum as markers of absorption. *Lancet* 1984;1:74–6.
25. Kleinberg ML, Quinn MJ. Airborne drug levels in a laminar flow hood. *Am J Hosp Pharm* 1981;38:1301–3.
26. Neal A, Wadden R, Chiou W. Exposure of hospital workers to airborne antineoplastic agents. *Am J Hosp Pharm* 1983;40:597–601.
27. Laidlaw J, Connor T, Theiss J, et al. Permeability of latex and polyvinyl chloride gloves to 20 antineoplastic drugs. *Am J Hosp Pharm* 1984;41:2618–23.
28. Safe handling of cytotoxic and hazardous drugs [videotape]. Bethesda, MD: American Society of Hospital Pharmacists; 1990.
29. Roush W. Dana-Farber death sends a warning to research hospitals. *Science* 1995;269:295–6.
30. Cohen MR, Anderson RW, Attilio RM, et al. Preventing medication errors in cancer chemotherapy. *Am J Health-Syst Pharm* 1996;53:737–46.
31. Fischer DS, Alfano S, Knobf MT, et al. Improving the cancer chemotherapy use process. *J Clin Oncol* 1996;14:3148–55.
32. Attilio RM. Caring enough to understand: the road to oncology medication error prevention. *Hosp Pharm* 1996;31:17–26.
33. Thorn DB, Sexton MG, Lemay AP, et al. Effect of a cancer chemotherapy prescription form on prescription completeness. *Am J Hosp Pharm* 1989;46:1802–6.
34. Bain PG, Lantos PL, Djurovic V, et al. Intrathecal vincristine: a fatal chemotherapeutic error with devastating central nervous system effects. *J Neurol* 1991;238:230–4.
35. Oncology Nursing Society. *Cancer Chemotherapy Guidelines and Recommendations for Practice*. Powel LL, editor. Pittsburgh, PA: Oncology Nursing Pr; 1996. p. 6–9.
36. Shane R. Critical pathways. Taking the first step on the critical pathway. *Am J Health-Syst Pharm* 1995;52:1051.
37. [Anonymous]. Using clinical practice guidelines to evaluate care. Volumes 1 & 2. Rockville, MD: U.S. Dept. of Health and Human Services, Public Health Service, Agency for Health Care Policy and Research; 1995.

Appendix 20-A ASHP Technical Assistance Bulletin on Handling Cytotoxic and Hazardous Drugs

In 1985, the "ASHP Technical Assistance Bulletin on Handling Cytotoxic Drugs in Hospitals"[1] summarized published information on handling hazardous drugs, referred to as cytotoxics, as of July 1984. As more information became available on the types of hazardous agents that may represent a health risk to the occupationally exposed population, and as the handling of such substances became routine in hospitals, community pharmacies, home care settings, clinics, and physicians' offices, the need to revise the Technical Assistance Bulletin became apparent.

Early concerns regarding occupational exposure to hazardous agents involved primarily drugs used in cancer therapy. Therefore, the terms "antineoplastics" (drugs used to treat neoplasms) and "chemotherapy" were used in early reports and guidelines. Although any chemical used therapeutically may be referred to as chemotherapy, this term is currently used, both in the medical and lay communities, to mean drug therapy of cancer. In an attempt to be more precise, many professionals adopted the term "cytotoxic" or "cell killer." Not all antineoplastics, however, are cytotoxic, nor are all cytotoxics used exclusively in the treatment of cancer. "Cytotoxic" is often used to refer to any agent that may be genotoxic, oncogenic, mutagenic, teratogenic, or hazardous in any way. As our knowledge of the hazardous nature of many agents grows and as new hazardous agents (e.g., genotoxic biologicals and some biotechnological agents) continue to be developed, cytotoxic is a less appropriate term. In deference to the original Technical Assistance Bulletin, cytotoxic remains in the title of this revision. The remainder of the document, however, will refer exclusively to hazardous drugs or agents, except in very specific instances.

In January 1986, the Federal Occupational Safety and Health Administration (OSHA) released recommendations on safe handling of cytotoxic drugs by health-care personnel.[2] This revised Technical Assistance Bulletin includes information from these recommendations, modified by subsequent discussions with OSHA, and from published reports by the National Institutes of Health,[3] the National Study Commission on Cytotoxic Exposure,[4] and the American Medical Association's (AMA) Council on Scientific Affairs,[5] along with other published information on this issue as of June 1988.

The safe handling of hazardous drugs is an issue that must be addressed in health-care settings and one that may even affect, in a home care environment, persons other than the patient. Inasmuch as possible, the pharmacist should take the lead in establishing policies and procedures to ensure the proper handling of all hazardous drugs in any health-care setting. The recommendations contained in this Technical Assistance Bulletin should be applied to any area where hazardous drugs are handled. Procedures specific to noninstitutional care settings have been included where available.[6-8] Because of the many questions about implementing the recommendations in the original Technical Assistance Bulletin, this revision contains detailed information in those areas of greatest concern. The recommendations contained here should be supplemented with the professional judgments of qualified staff and with newer information as it develops.

Hazardous Drug Dangers

The danger to health-care personnel from handling a hazardous drug stems from a combination of its inherent toxicity and the extent to which workers are exposed to the drug in the course of carrying out their duties. This exposure may be through inadvertent ingestion of the drug on foodstuffs (e.g., workers' lunches), inhalation of drug dusts or droplets, or direct skin contact. Drugs that may represent occupational hazards include any that exhibit the following characteristics:

1. Genotoxicity [i.e., mutagenicity and clastogenicity (see Appendix A) in short-term test systems].
2. Carcinogenicity in animal models, in the patient population, or both, as reported by the International Agency for Research on Cancer (IARC).
3. Teratogenicity or fertility impairment in animal studies or treated patients.
4. Evidence of serious organ or other toxicity at low doses in animal models or treated patients.

The oncogenic and teratogenic effects of therapeutic doses of several antineoplastic agents are well established.[9-13] The mutagenic properties of some cytotoxics, immunosuppressants, antiviral agents, and biological response modifiers have also been documented.[14] The long-term effects (e.g., cancer, impaired fertility, and organ damage) of continued exposure to small amounts of one or more of such drugs remain undetermined.

For example, it is known that long-term use of potent immunosuppressive agents may result in the development of lymphoma. It is not known, however, at what drug level or over what period of time this may occur and how this correlates with possible drug levels achieved through occupational exposure during preparation and administration of hundreds or thousands of injectable and oral doses of these agents.

Studies have attempted to assess indirectly the potential exposure of hospital pharmacists and nurses to some hazardous drugs in several health-care settings including physicians' offices.[15-21] These studies examined the urine mutagenicity or evidence of chromosome damage in subjects who prepared or administered primarily antineoplastic injections. The mutagenicity and chromosome damage that were found were thought to document exposure to and absorption of the drugs that had been handled. An association may exist between carcinogenicity and chromosome breakage or mutagenicity. Therefore, one might conclude that handling hazardous drugs entails some danger to health-care personnel. These studies, although not conclusive, support the postulated occupational risks.

However, several reports make the situation slightly more ominous. Palmer and coworkers[22] measured chromosome damage in 10 patients receiving chlorambucil. They found that the damage was cumulative and was related to both the daily dose and the duration of therapy. Another report[23] described permanent liver damage in three nurses who had worked 6, 8, and 16 years, respectively, on an oncology ward. On the basis of histories, the investigators suggested that the liver injuries may have been related to the intensity and duration of exposure to certain toxic agents. The chlorambucil study involved therapeutic doses of drug, and three cases of liver damage is a small base for drawing any final conclusions. Nevertheless, this information is disturbing in view of the fact that many health-care workers prepare or administer hundreds or even thousands of doses of hazardous drugs during their careers. If low-dose exposure to these agents is cumulative, this exposure should be minimized by strict compliance with safe handling procedures.

The value of chromosome and mutagenicity studies as indicators of the occupational risks of exposure to hazardous drugs has been questioned.[24–28] However, several researchers have employed more direct methods of determining whether or not workers have been exposed to and absorbed hazardous drugs handled in the customary manner. Demonstration that absorption has occurred would be strong support for the imposition of safety measures. (The absorption of hazardous drug is presumed to be a health risk.)

A letter[29] described a study that used the presence of thioethers in the urine as an indicator of exposure to alkylating agents (i.e., certain antineoplastic drugs). The mean urinary thioether concentration (UTC) was higher in a group of 15 oncology nurses after a 5-day rotation than it was when they returned to work after a 3-day leave ($p < 0.01$). There was no difference between the mean pre-exposure UTC and that of a group of 20 nurses who never handled antineoplastic drugs. Twelve of the 15 nurses wore gloves when handling the drugs; none wore any other form of protective apparel. Drug preparation procedures were not reported.

Using gas chromatography, Hirst's group[30] found cyclophosphamide in the urine of two nurses working in a cancer clinic who took no special precautions when handling the drug. They also demonstrated that cyclophosphamide can be absorbed through intact skin. On the other hand, another group of researchers[31] looked for (but could not detect) platinum in the urine of 10 pharmacists and nurses who frequently prepared or administered cisplatin and other platinum-containing antineoplastic agents. However, these subjects employed several protective measures when working with the drugs; this may have influenced the results (and demonstrated the effectiveness of the safety precautions employed). Also, the assay method may not have been sensitive enough.

With a different type of approach, Neal et al.[32] detected fluorouracil in the air of a drug preparation room and nearby office (where the drug was not prepared). A similar study[33] showed that routine drug manipulations in a horizontal laminar airflow hood contaminated the air in an intravenous admixture preparation room. Fluorouracil and cefazolin sodium were the test drugs employed.

Certain antineoplastic drugs have also been implicated in reproductive risks in humans. There have been reports of fetal loss or malformation occurring in pregnancies of women receiving drug therapy for cancer during the first trimester.[34] Two controlled, retrospective Finnish studies[35,36] attempted to examine the relationship between occupational exposure to antineoplastics and reproductive risks in nurses. One study of nurses reported a statistically significant correlation between the birth of children with malformations and the nurses' preparation and administration of antineoplastics more than once a week during the first trimester of pregnancy. At the time of these nurses' exposure, few protective mechanisms were used.

The second study was done in cooperation with the U.S. National Institute for Occupational Safety and Health (NIOSH); it examined only the incidence of fetal loss and did not investigate the condition of live births. The study showed a significant association between fetal loss and occupational exposure to antineoplastic drugs during the first trimester. Both studies are subject to criticism regarding recall bias and determination of exposure data. Concern about exposure of pregnant workers to hazardous drugs, at least in the first trimester, is, however, valid in light of the reproductive risk reported with therapeutic exposure to certain antineoplastics. At therapeutic doses, these drugs have also been shown to suppress testicular function and spermatogenesis.[37–39] While the relationship between occupational exposure to hazardous drugs and testicular dysfunction has not been assessed, this potential complication should be considered in light of the effects on treated patients.

To date, these reports provide the primary evidence that health-care workers exposed to hazardous drugs during the course of their work may be absorbing these drugs and may be at risk for adverse outcomes.

Additional research in this area is needed, but awareness of the problem has led to overall reduction of exposures, either by improved drug handling techniques or through the implementation of safety programs,[40,41] and thus fewer exposed health-care workers are available for study. Definitive knowledge of the occupational dangers of handling hazardous drugs may someday be available through epidemiologic studies of health-care workers.

In theory, correct and perfect preparation and handling techniques will prevent drug particles or droplets from escaping from their containers while they are being manipulated. Our opinion is that near-perfect technique is uncommon; therefore, contamination of the workplace is likely and worker exposure may increase without protective equipment and other safety measures. This is particularly true, we think, in the absence of any structured training and quality-assurance programs covering the proper handling of hazardous drugs. (Such programs are most likely to be found in health-care settings where the preparation of hazardous drugs is centralized.) Beyond problems in technique, however, contamination also will occur from inevitable spills and from the breakage of hazardous drug containers. ASHP believes that the occupational dangers of exposure to hazardous drugs can be summarized as follows:

1. If hazardous drugs are handled in the same way as other less hazardous substances (e.g., potassium chloride solutions and multivitamin tablets), contamination of the work environment is almost certain to occur.

2. The limited data available suggest that this contamination may result in exposure to and absorption of the drugs by health-care personnel and others. The amount of drug absorbed by any one individual on any given day probably is very small, except for instances of excessive exposure.

3. However, if experience with the therapeutic use of hazardous drugs indicates that the damage is cumulative, individuals whose job responsibilities require them to prepare or administer large numbers of hazardous drug doses for long periods of time (e.g., oncology or transplant nurses and pharmacy intravenous service staff) are at greater risk.

4. Considering the above, the use of procedures, equipment, and materials that demonstrably or theoretically reduce exposure to hazardous drugs in the health-care workplace is necessary.

The question remains: What safety precautions should be employed?

Safety Precautions

Ideally, the safety precautions employed to protect health-care workers handling hazardous drugs would be those whose efficacy and cost-effectiveness have been documented. Since these drugs have many different physical and chemical properties, research studies into environmental contamination and safety-garment penetration for all questionable drugs are problematic. However, several studies have attempted to demonstrate the effectiveness of certain recommended interventions. Hoy and Stump[42] concluded that a commercial air-venting device, when used with appropriate technique, effectively reduced the release of drug aerosols during reconstitution of drugs packaged in vials. A study by Anderson et al.[16] provides support for preparing hazardous drugs in a vertical laminar airflow biological safety cabinet (BSC) (NSF Class II;[43] see Appendix B) rather than a horizontal airflow clean air work station.

A more recent air-sampling study,[44] carried out in a hospital pharmacy work area where a Class II BSC was used to prepare cytotoxic drugs, detected no fluorouracil during the study period. The study was limited to one drug and two short study periods; the results indicate that a Class II BSC, in conjunction with stringent aseptic technique and recommended procedures for handling hazardous drugs, may reduce environmental contamination by these drugs.

While common sense suggests that the airflow characteristics of containment cabinets would provide greater worker protection than open airflow workstations, it should also suggest that the front opening of the Class II BSC might present potential for environmental contamination and increased worker exposure to hazardous agents. Indeed, as demonstrated by an industrial hygiene experiment,[45] a Class II BSC may cause occasional leakage toward the operator and into the environment if it is placed in an area of strong air drafts or frequent personnel traffic. The containment characteristics of the Class II BSC are compromised whenever the intake or exhaust grilles are blocked (e.g., by placing equipment or supplies on the front grille or too near the back exhaust) or by too much movement on the part of the operator.

Gloves are a major source of protection, whether the work is performed with or without a Class II BSC. The permeability of various glove materials to selected drugs has been examined.[46–49] By using various methods to determine and quantitate penetration, researchers found that permeability of the glove material varied with the drug, contact time, and glove thickness. None of the glove materials tested was impervious to all drugs, and no material was statistically superior except as related to thickness. A thicker glove material is optimal. In addition, several glove materials showed variation in permeability within a manufacturer's lot. These studies do establish that gloves can provide protection against skin contact with the tested drugs, although the degree of protection has not been substantiated. Protection from skin contact is important since many of the problem drugs are skin irritants or even vesicants and, as Hirst et al.[30] showed, at least one (cyclophosphamide) is absorbed through the skin.

Only one study[50] looked at the permeability of gown materials to drugs. Lab coats and disposable isolation gowns were penetrated immediately and were therefore inappropriate for study. Of the four other gown materials studied, Kaycel and nonporous Tyvek had greater permeability than the coated fabrics (Saranex-laminated Tyvek and polyethylene-coated Tyvek). As with gloves, permeability was drug specific. The investigators concluded that users of garments made of Kaycel and nonporous Tyvek should be aware of the potential of these materials for permeability to certain drugs. An earlier report[51] supports the wearing of gloves and gowns. Additional research is needed in the area of protective garments and equipment. Since substantive data are still lacking, health-care professionals should choose protective measures on the basis of expert recommendations, professional judgment, and common sense as well as scientifically established facts.

Recommended Safe Handling Methods

The balance of this article presents our recommendations for policies, procedures, and safety materials for controlling, preparing, administering, containing, and disposing of hazardous drugs. The recommendations are given in a format that can be used either as a base for establishing safe handling methods or for evaluating existing procedures as part of a quality-assurance program. ASHP believes these recommendations represent a conservative but reasonable approach to the precautions that should be taken.

The recommendations are in the format of evaluation criteria organized into four groups. This format should be useful in establishing a quality-assurance system for all nontherapeutic aspects of hazardous drug use. Each group begins with a broad goal, followed by a set of specific criteria and recommendations for achieving the goal. The four goals reflect the following axioms for handling hazardous drugs:

1. Protect and secure packages of hazardous drugs.
2. Inform and educate all involved personnel about hazardous drugs and train them in the safe handling procedures relevant to their responsibilities.
3. Do not let the drugs escape from containers when they are manipulated (i.e., dissolved, transferred, administered, or discarded).
4. Eliminate the possibility of inadvertent ingestion or inhalation and direct skin or eye contact with the drugs.

The handling of hazardous drugs is a complex issue, and the advice of medical experts, occupational physicians, industrial hygienists, legal counsel, and others should be obtained when organizational policy is being established.

Goal I. Accidental contamination of the health-care environment, resulting in exposure of personnel, patients, visitors, and family members to hazardous substances, is prevented by maintaining the physical integrity and security of packages of hazardous drugs.

1. *Access to all areas where hazardous drugs are stored is limited to specified authorized staff.*
2. *A method should be present for identifying to personnel those drugs that require special precautions (e.g., cytotoxics).*[52] *One way to accomplish this is to apply appropriate warning labels (see Figure 1) to all hazardous drug containers, shelves, and bins where the drug products are stored.*
3. *A method of identifying, for patients and family members,*

those drugs that require special precautions in the home should be in place. This may be accomplished in the health-care setting by providing specific labeling for discharge medications, along with counseling and written instructions. Providers of home care and supplies should develop similar labeling and instructional material for the protection of patients and their families.

4. *Methods for identifying shipping cartons of hazardous drugs should be required from manufacturers and distributors of these drugs.*
5. *Written procedures for handling damaged packages of hazardous drugs should be maintained.* Personnel involved in shipping and receiving hazardous drugs should be trained in these procedures, including the proper use of protective garments and equipment. Damaged shipping cartons of hazardous drugs should be received and opened in an isolated area (e.g., in a laboratory fume hood, if available, not in a BSC used for preparing sterile products). Protective apparel—disposable closed-front gown or coveralls, disposable utility gloves over disposable latex gloves, NIOSH-approved[53] air-purifying half-mask respirator (may be disposable) equipped with a high-efficiency filter, and eye protection—should be worn. Broken containers and contaminated packaging materials should be placed in the designated receptacles as described in this article.
6. *Facilities (e.g., shelves, carts, counters, and trays) for storing hazardous drugs are designed to prevent breakage and to limit contamination in the event of leakage.* Bins, shelves with barriers at the front, or other design features that reduce the chance of drug containers falling to the floor should be used. Hazardous drugs requiring refrigeration should be stored separately from nonhazardous drugs in individual bins designed to prevent breakage and contain leakage.
7. *Methods for transporting hazardous drugs to the health-care setting should be consistent with environmental protection and national or local regulations for transporting hazardous substances.* When hazardous drugs are being transported to the home care setting, appropriate containers (e.g., lined cardboard boxes) and procedures should be used to prevent breakage and contain leakage. Hazardous drug containers should be secured to prevent handling by unauthorized persons. Transportation vehicles should be kept locked at all times.

    For transporting hazardous drugs within the healthcare setting, methods that do not cause breakage of or leakage from drug containers should be used. Conveyances that produce severe mechanical stress on their contents (e.g., pneumatic tubes) must not be used to transport hazardous drugs. The drugs must be securely capped or sealed and properly packaged and protected during transport to reduce further the chance of breakage and spillage in a public area such as a corridor or elevator. Adequate instruction and appropriate containers should be provided to patients for transporting discharge and home care medications that require special precautions.

Goal II. The preparation of hazardous drugs does not result in contamination of the health-care work environment or excessive exposure of personnel, patients, or family members to hazardous drug powders, dusts, liquids, or mists.

1. *Written policies and standard procedures for preparing hazardous drugs are maintained.*
    a. They should include a method for identifying for health-care personnel the particular drugs covered by these policies.
    b. Policies and procedures should be consistent with applicable government regulations, professional practice standards, and the recommendations of pharmaceutical manufacturers, hospital safety officers, and other knowledgeable parties.
    c. Since several departments, such as pharmacy, nursing, transportation, maintenance, housekeeping, and medical staff, will be involved with some aspect of the hazardous drug handling issue, preparation of safe handling policies and procedures must be a collaborative effort. Pharmacy should take the lead in this effort.
    d. All personnel who handle cytotoxic and other hazardous agents should have access to the procedures pertaining to their responsibilities. Deviations from the standard procedures must not be permitted except under defined circumstances.
2. *A method for orienting all involved personnel to the special nature of the hazardous drugs in question and the policies and procedures that govern their handling is present.*
    a. The orientation should include, as appropriate, a discussion of the known and potential hazards of the drugs and explanation of all relevant policies. Training done in association with the orientation should cover all relevant techniques and procedures and the proper use of protective equipment and materials. The contents of the orientation program and attendance should be well documented and sufficient to meet "worker right to know" statutes and regulations.
    b. While implementation of a safety program should reduce the risk of personnel exposure to hazardous drugs, the efficacy of such a program in protecting personnel during preparation or administration of these drugs has yet to be demonstrated. The limitations of such a program should be made known to hazardous drug handlers.
    c. Until the reproductive risks (or lack thereof) associated with handling hazardous drugs within a safety program have been substantiated, staff who are pregnant or breast-feeding should be allowed to avoid contact with these drugs. Policies should be in effect that provide these individuals with alternative tasks

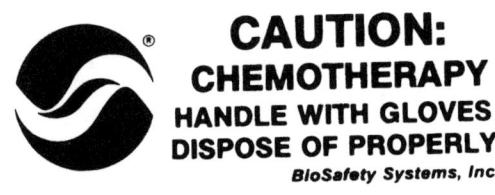

Figure 1. One example of a suitable warning label for cytotoxic and hazardous drugs. Other labels may be used.

or responsibilities if they so desire. In general, these policies should encourage personnel to solicit recommendations from their personal physicians regarding the need for restricted duties. In the case of personnel actively trying to conceive or father a child, a similar policy should be considered, and a specific time period (e.g., 3 months) should be agreed on. Legal counsel should be sought when establishing policies.

    d. Prospective temporary and permanent employees who may be required to work with hazardous drugs should be so notified and should receive adequate information about the policies and procedures pertaining to their use. This notification should be documented during the interview proc-ess and retained as part of the employment record for all employees.

    e. All individuals handling hazardous drugs who do not have employee status (e.g., contract workers, students, residents, medical staff, and volunteers) should be informed through proper channels of the special nature of the drugs. If they choose to handle the hazardous drugs, then they will be expected to comply with established policies and procedures for preparing, administering, and containing hazardous drugs and their associated waste.

3. *A system for verifying and documenting acceptable staff performance of and conformance with established procedures is maintained.*

    a. Methods of determining adherence to departmental safety program policies and procedures should be in place. Proper technique is essential to maintain the sterility of the product being manipulated and to reduce the generation of hazardous drug contaminants. Therefore, after initial training and at regular intervals, the knowledge and competence of personnel preparing and administering these drugs should be evaluated and documented. This evaluation should include written examinations and an observed demonstration of competence in the preparation and simulated administration of practice solutions. The monitoring of staff performance and the control of hazardous drugs usually are best achieved if the storage and preparation of the drugs are centralized within one area or department.

    b. All personnel involved with the transportation, preparation, administration, and disposal of cytotoxic and hazardous substances should continually be updated on new or revised information on safe handling of cytotoxic and hazardous substances. Policies and procedures should be updated accordingly.

4. *Sufficient information is maintained on safe use of the hazardous drugs in the work area.*

    a. The pharmacy should provide access to information on toxicity, treatment of acute exposure (if available), chemical inactivators, solubility, and stability of hazardous drugs (including investigational agents) used in the workplace. This information should be in addition to information required to ensure patient safety during therapy with these drugs and to be in compliance with all applicable laws and regulations. The information must be easily and readily accessible to all employees where these drugs are routinely handled.

    b. Currently, a large number of investigational agents that are potentially hazardous are under clinical study. Staff members should not prepare or administer any investigational agent unless they have received adequate information and instruction about the safe and correct use of the drug. The clinical protocol should include appropriate handling and disposal techniques, if available. When information is limited, pre-clinical data should be used to assess the health risk of the agent.

5. *Appropriate engineering controls should be in place to protect the drug product from microbial contamination and to protect personnel and the environment from the potential hazards of the product.* These engineering controls should be maintained according to applicable regulations and standards.

    a. Class 100 clean air work stations,[54] both horizontal and vertical airflow (with no containment characteristics), are inappropriate engineering controls for handling hazardous drugs because they provide no personnel protection and permit environmental contamination. Although there are no engineering controls designed specifically for the safe handling of hazardous chemicals as sterile products, Class II[43] contained vertical flow BSCs (biohazard cabinets) have been adopted for this use. Biohazard cabinetry is, however, designed for the handling of infectious agents, not hazardous chemicals. Therefore, the limitations of such cabinetry must be understood by purchaser and operator. Manufacturers, vendors, the National Sanitation Foundation (NSF), and some certifying agencies are appropriate sources of information regarding BSCs.

    b. BSCs are available in three classes (Appendix B). Based on design, ease of use, and cost considerations, Class II contained vertical flow biohazard cabinetry is currently recommended for use in preparing sterile doses of hazardous drugs. Class II cabinetry design and performance specifications are defined in NSF Standard 49.[43] BSCs selected for use with hazardous drugs should meet NSF Standard 49 specifications to ensure the maximum protection from these engineering controls. NSF Standard 49 defines four types of Class II cabinetry, depending on the amount of contaminated air that is recirculated through high-efficiency particulate air (HEPA) filters within the cabinet (see Appendix B).

    Selection criteria for Class II cabinetry should include the types and amounts of hazardous drugs prepared, the available location and amount of space, NSF Standard 49, any local requirements for handling hazardous materials and ducting contaminated air, and the cost of the cabinet and related ventilation. Minimum recommendations are a Class II, Type A cabinet (recirculating a major portion of contaminated air through a HEPA filter and back into the cabinet and exhausting a minor portion, through a HEPA filter, to the workroom). In light of the continued development of hazardous drugs having differing physical properties, selection of a Type A cabinet that can be converted to a Type B3 (greater inflow velocity, contaminated ducts and plenums under negative pressure and vented to the outside) may be a prudent investment. There are currently no data to indicate that the use of an auxiliary charcoal filter is more effective in retaining hazardous drugs than the mandatory exhaust HEPA filter of the Type A cabinet.

Type B BSCs are designed to provide more personnel protection than Type A through their greater inflow velocities and required external exhaust of contaminated air. Types B1 (exhausting approximately 70% of the contaminated air to the outside through a HEPA filter) and B2 (exhausting 100% of the contaminated air to the outside through a HEPA filter) require outside exhaust ducts with auxiliary blowers. The Type B2 cabinet is preferred, but unavailability of adequate "makeup" air may eliminate it in favor of the Type B1. All exhaust ducting of any type of BSC must meet applicable codes and ordinances. Ducting into the "dead space" in the ceiling is inappropriate and may be illegal, because it may contaminate ventilation systems and promote contamination of the environment and personnel not directly involved in hazardous drug handling.

In the selection of any BSC, ceiling height should also be considered. Several manufacturers' models have top-load HEPA filters. In workrooms with standard-height ceilings, the filters are difficult to access for certification, which may require that the entire BSC be moved when the filter must be replaced. Because of restrictions of space and cost, the 2-foot wide, Class II, Type A BSC may seem to be the only choice for smaller institutions, outpatient centers, and physician offices. There are, however, many limitations to the smaller cabinet. Because NSF testing facilities are not currently adaptable to 2-foot BSC models, no 2-foot BSC is NSF approved. Selection of a 2-foot cabinet should, therefore, include thorough investigation of cabinet design and knowledge of the reliability of the manufacturer. In all cases, the manufacturer's 2-foot cabinet should not differ extensively from designs used for its NSF-approved larger models.

c. All Class II BSCs have an open front with inward airflow forming a "curtain" or barrier to protect the operator and the environment from contaminants released in the BSC work area. Because BSCs are subject to breaks in their containment properties if there is interference with the inward airflow through the work area access opening, placement of the BSC and operator training are critical. The placement of a BSC in an area with drafts or in close proximity to other airflow devices (e.g., horizontal flow hoods, air conditioners, air vents, fans, and doors) may interfere with the inward airflow through the opening and may release contaminants into the workroom.

The horizontal motion of an operator's arms in the opening may also result in similar workroom contamination. Because smaller BSCs are more sensitive to disruption of the inward airflow barrier, the use of a 2- to 3-foot BSC is associated with a greater risk of releasing contaminants than are larger cabinets and requires that the operator be more carefully trained and monitored. It is critical that all operators know the proper method for preparing hazardous drugs in a BSC and that they understand the limitations of BSCs.

d. Class II BSCs should be certified according to specifications of NSF Standard 49 and Class 100 specifications of Federal Standard 209C.[54] Certification should take place on initial installation, whenever the cabinet is moved or repaired, and every 6 months thereafter. At present, there are no licensing requirements for individuals who certify Class II BSCs. It is, therefore, imperative that the pharmacist responsible for the intravenous preparation area be familiar with the certification requirements for Class II BSCs and the test procedures that should be performed.[55]

All BSCs should be tested for the integrity of the HEPA filter, velocity of the work access airflow and supply airflow, airflow smoke patterns, and integrity of external surfaces of the cabinet and filter housings. Testing of the integrity of the HEPA filter generally ensures that the particulate count in the work area is less than that required to meet Class 100 conditions of Federal Standard 209C.[54] Class II, Type B1 BSCs may be prone to exceed Class 100 particle counts and should have routine particulate testing as part of the certification process. Individuals certifying the BSC should be informed of the hazardous nature of the drugs being prepared in the BSC and should wear appropriate protective apparel (see section 5g).

e. BSCs should be cleaned and disinfected regularly to ensure a proper environment for preparation of sterile products. For routine cleanups of surfaces between decontaminations, water should be used (for injection or irrigation) with or without a small amount of cleaner. If the contamination is soluble only in alcohol, then 70% isopropyl or ethyl alcohol may be used in addition to the cleaner. In general, alcohol is not a good cleaner, only a disinfectant, and its use in a BSC should be limited. The BSC should be disinfected with 70% alcohol before any aseptic manipulation is begun. The excessive use of alcohol should be avoided in BSCs where air is recirculated (i.e., Class II, Type A, B3, and, to a lesser extent, B1) because alcohol vapors may build up in the cabinet.

A lint-free, plastic-backed disposable liner may be used in the BSC to facilitate spill cleanup. Problems with the use of such a liner include introduction of particulates into the work area, "lumping" of a wet liner that causes unsteady placement of drug containers, poor visibility of spills, and creation of additional contaminated disposables. If used, the liner should be changed frequently and whenever it is overtly contaminated.

f. The BSC should be operated with the blower turned on continuously, 24 hours a day, 7 days a week. Hazardous drug aerosols and spills generated in the work area of the BSC routinely accumulate in the deposits of room dust and particles under the work tray. These contaminants are too heavy to be transported to the HEPA filter located at the top of the cabinet. In addition, the plenums in all of the BSCs currently available in the United States become contaminated during use; these plenums cannot be accessed for washing. Turning off the blower may allow contaminated dust to recirculate back into the workroom, especially if other sources of air turbulence, such as horizontal hoods, air intakes, air conditioners, and fans, are located near the BSC. Whether or not the BSC is vented to the outside, the downward airflow velocity is insufficient to move and "trap" room dust, spill debris, and other contaminants on the HEPA filter. If it is necessary to turn off a BSC, first the entire cabinet, including all parts that can be reached, should be thoroughly cleaned with a detergent that will remove surface contamination and then rinsed (see section 5g). Once the BSC is clean, the blower may be turned off and the work access opening of the BSC and the HEPA exhaust area may be covered with impermeable plastic and sealed with tape to prevent any contamination from inadvertently escaping from the BSC. The BSC must be sealed with plastic whenever it is moved or left inoperative for any period of time.

g. The BSC should be decontaminated on a regular basis (ideally at least weekly) and whenever there is a spill or the BSC is moved or serviced, including for certification. While NSF Standard 49 recommends decontamination with formaldehyde to remove biohazard contamination, chemical (drug) contamination is not removed by such treatment. Currently, no single reagent will deactivate all known hazardous drugs; therefore, decontamination of a BSC used for such drugs is limited to removal of contamination from a nondisposable surface (the cabinet) to a disposable surface (e.g., gauze or towels) by use of a good cleaning agent that removes chemicals from stainless steel.

The cleaning agent selected should have a pH approximating that of soap and be appropriate for stainless steel. Cleaners containing chemicals such as quaternary ammonium compounds should be used with caution, because they may be hazardous to humans and their vapors may build up in any BSC where air is recirculated (see section 5e). Similar caution should be used with any pressurized aerosol cleaner; spraying a pressurized aerosol into a BSC may disrupt the protective containment airflow, damage the HEPA filter, and cause an accumulation of the propellant within a BSC where air is recirculated, resulting in a fire and explosion hazard.

During decontamination, the operator should wear a disposable closed-front gown, disposable latex gloves covered by disposable utility gloves, safety glasses or goggles, a hair covering, and a disposable respirator, because the glass shield of the BSC occasionally must be lifted (see 5j). The blower must be left on, and only heavy toweling or gauze should be used in the BSC to prevent it from being "sucked" up the plenum and into the HEPA filter.

Decontamination should be done from top to bottom (areas of lesser contamination to greater) by applying the cleaner, scrubbing, and rinsing thoroughly with distilled or deionized water. All contaminated disposables should be contained in sealable bags for transfer to larger waste containers. The HEPA filter must not become wet during cleaning of the protective covering (e.g., grille front). This covering, therefore, should not be cleaned with spray cleaners while it is in place. Removable parts of the BSC should be cleaned within the containment area of the BSC and should not be removed from the cabinet. The work tray usually can be lifted and placed against the back wall for cleaning of the undersurface of the tray and exposure of the very bottom (or sump) of the BSC.

The drain spillage trough area collects room dust and all spills, so it is the most heavily contaminated area and must be thoroughly cleaned (at least twice with the cleaning agent). The trough provides limited access to the side and back plenums; surfaces should be cleaned as high as possible. BSCs have sharp metal edges, so disposable utility gloves are more durable and appropriate than surgical latex gloves for decontamination. Gloves should be changed immediately if torn. All plenum surfaces must be rinsed well, with frequent changes of water and gauze. If the BSC is equipped with a drainpipe and valve, it may be used to collect rinse water. The collection vessel used must fit well around the drain valve and not allow splashing. Gauze may be used around the connection to prevent aerosol from escaping. The collection vessel must have a tight-fitting cover, and all rinse water (and gauze, if used) must be disposed of as contaminated waste. The outside of the BSC should be wiped down with cleaner to remove any drip or touch contamination.

Cleaner and rinse containers are generally contaminated during the procedure and should remain in the BSC during cleaning or be placed on a plastic-backed, absorbent liner outside the BSC. All bottles must be discarded as contaminated waste after decontamination of the BSC. All protective apparel (e.g., gown, gloves, goggles, and respirator) should be discarded as contaminated waste. Work area surfaces should be disinfected with 70% alcohol before any aseptic operation is begun. With good planning, decontamination of a 4-foot BSC should take about 1 hour.

h. Because of its design and decontamination limitations, the BSC should be considered a contaminated environment and treated as such. The use of the BSC should be restricted to the preparation of sterile dosage forms of hazardous drugs. Access to the BSC should be limited to authorized personnel wearing appropriate protective clothing.

i. If a BSC previously used for biologicals will be adopted for use with hazardous drugs, the BSC should be completely decontaminated of biohazardous agents by use of NSF Standard 49 decontamination techniques. Both HEPA filters should be replaced and the cabinet tested against the *complete* requirements of NSF Standard 49 Appendix B and the particulate limitations of Class 100 conditions of Federal Standard 209C. A BSC used for hazardous drugs that will be recycled for use with hazardous drugs in another section of the institution or in another institution must be surface decontaminated (as described in section 5g), sealed (as in section 5f), and carefully transported to its new location before the filters are replaced (as in section 5j). Once in its new location, the BSC must be recertified.

j. The HEPA filters of the BSC must be replaced whenever they restrict required airflow velocity or if they are overtly contaminated (e.g., by a breach in technique that causes hazardous drug to be introduced onto the clean side of the supply HEPA filter). Personnel and environmental protection must be maintained during replacement of a contaminated HEPA filter. Because replacement of a HEPA filter generally requires breaking the integrity of the containment aspect of the cabinet, this procedure may release contamination from the filter into the pharmacy or intravenous preparation area if carried out in an inappropriate manner.

Before replacement of a HEPA filter contaminated with hazardous drugs, the BSC service agent should be consulted for a mutually acceptable procedure for replacing and subsequently disposing of a contaminated HEPA filter. One procedure would include moving the BSC to a secluded area or using plastic barriers to segregate the contaminated area. Protective clothing and equipment must be used by the servicer. The BSC should be decontaminated before filter replacement (see section 5g). The contaminated filters must be removed, bagged in thick plastic, and prepared for disposal in a hazardous waste dump site or incinerator licensed by the Environmental Protection Agency (EPA).

When arranging for disposal, precise terms should be used to describe the hazard (e.g., "toxic chemicals" or "chemical carcinogens," not "cytotoxic" or "chemotherapy") to ensure that contractors are not inadvertently misled in the classification of the hazard. Disposal of an entire contaminated BSC should be approached in the same manner. The filters should be removed, bagged, and disposed of separately from the BSC. If no available service company will arrange for removal of the filter (or entire BSC) and its ultimate disposal, a licensed hazardous waste contractor should be used. The use of triple layers of thick plastic (e.g., 2-mil low-linear or 4-mil plastic) for initial covering of the filter or cabinet and then the construction of a plywood crate for transport to an EPA-licensed hazardous waste dump site or incinerator is suggested.

6. *Engineering controls should be supplemented with personal protective apparel and other safety materials.* Policies and procedures should be in place to ensure that these materials are used properly and consistently.

   a. Workers should wear powder-free, disposable surgical latex gloves of good quality when preparing hazardous drugs. Selection criteria for gloves should include thickness (especially at the fingertips where stress is the greatest), fit, length, and tactile sensation. While no glove material has been shown to be impervious to all hazardous drugs or to be statistically superior in limiting drug penetration, thickness and time in contact with drug are crucial factors affecting permeability.[47–49]

   The practice of double gloving is supported by research that indicates that many glove materials vary in drug permeability even within lots;[48,49] therefore, double gloving is recommended. This recommendation is based on currently available research findings. Evidence to show that single gloves are sufficiently protective might make this recommendation unnecessary. In general, surgical latex gloves fit better, have appropriate elasticity for double gloving and maintaining the integrity of the glove-gown interface, and have sufficient tactile sensation (even during double gloving) for stringent aseptic procedures.

   b. Powdered gloves increase the particulate level in the filtered air environment of the BSC and leave a powder residue on the surfaces of supplies, final product, and the hands that may absorb contamination generated in the BSC; therefore, powdered gloves should be avoided. The use of sterile gloves is unnecessary during operations involving nonsterile surfaces. Hands must be thoroughly washed and dried before gloves are donned and when a task or batch is completed. If only powdered gloves are available, all powder must be washed off the outside of the outer glove before any operation is begun, and hands should be washed once gloves have been removed.

   c. Two pairs of fresh gloves should be put on when beginning any task or batch. The outer glove should be changed immediately if contaminated. Both gloves should be changed if the outer glove is torn, punctured, or overtly contaminated with drug (as in a spill) and every hour during batch operations. During removal of gloves, care should be taken to avoid touching the inside of the glove or the skin with the contaminated glove fingers. To limit transfer of contamination from the BSC into the work area, outer gloves should be removed after each batch and should be placed in "zipper"-closure plastic bags or other sealable containers for disposal.

   d. The worker should wear a protective disposable gown made of lint-free, low-permeability fabric with a solid front, long sleeves, and tight-fitting elastic or knit cuffs when preparing hazardous drugs. Washable garments are immediately penetrated by liquids and therefore provide little, if any, protection. In addition, washable garments require laundering and thus potentially expose other personnel to contamination.

   e. When double gloving, one glove should be placed under the gown cuff and one over. The glove-gown interface should be such that no skin on the arm or wrist is exposed. Gloves and gowns should not be worn outside the immediate preparation area. On completion of each task or batch, the worker should, while wearing outer gloves, wipe all final products with gauze. The outer gloves should then be removed and placed, along with the gauze, in a sealable container (e.g., a zipper-closure plastic bag) within the BSC. All waste bags in the BSC should be sealed and removed for disposal. The gown should be removed and placed in a sealable container before removal of the inner gloves. The inner gloves should be removed last and placed in the container with the gown.

- f. Workers who are not protected by the containment environment of a BSC should use respiratory protection when handling hazardous drugs. Respiratory protection should be an adjunct to and not a substitute for engineering controls.
- g. Surgical masks of all types provide no respiratory protection against powdered or liquid aerosols of hazardous drugs.
- h. In situations where workers may be exposed to potential eye contact with hazardous drugs, an appropriate plastic face shield or splash goggles should be worn. Eyewash fountains should be available in areas where hazardous drugs are routinely handled. Inexpensive alternatives include an intravenous bag of 0.9% sodium chloride solution (normal saline) or irrigation bottle of water or saline with appropriate tubing.

7. *Proper manipulative technique to maintain the sterility of injectable drugs and to prevent generation of hazardous drug contaminants is used consistently.*
   - a. Proper manipulative technique must be taught to all workers who will be required to prepare hazardous drugs.[56] Preparers should demonstrate competence in these techniques once training has been completed and at least annually thereafter.
   - b. Systems to ensure that these techniques are adhered to should exist, along with systems to ensure patient safety by providing that drugs are properly selected, calculated, measured, and delivered.
   - c. The work area should be designed to provide easy access to those items necessary to prepare, label, and transport final products; contain all related waste; and avoid inadvertent contamination of the work area.
   - d. Maintenance of proper technique requires an organized approach to the preparation of sterile doses of hazardous drugs in a BSC. All drug and nondrug items required for completing a dose or batch and for containing the waste should be assembled and placed in the BSC; care should be taken not to overload the BSC work area. All calculations and any label preparation should be completed at this time. Appropriate gowning, hand washing and gloving (or glove changing), and glove washing should be completed before any manipulations are begun. Unnecessary moving in and out of the BSC should be avoided during aseptic manipulations.
   - e. Syringes and intravenous sets with Luer-lock type fittings should be used for preparing and administering hazardous drug solutions, since they are less prone to accidental separation than friction fittings. Care must be taken to ensure that all connections are secure. Syringes should be large enough so that they are not full when containing the total drug dose. This is to ensure that the plunger does not separate from the syringe barrel. Doses should be dispensed in several syringes when this problem arises.
   - f. The contents of an ampul should be gently tapped down from the neck and top portion of the ampul before it is opened. The ampul should be wiped with alcohol before being opened. A sterile gauze pad should be wrapped around the neck of the ampul when it is opened.
   - g. Substantial positive or negative deviations from atmospheric pressure within drug vials and syringes should be avoided.
   - h. For additional worker protection, equipment such as venting devices with 0.2-μm hydrophobic filters and 5-μm filter needles or "straws" may be used. It is critical that the worker be proficient with these devices before using them with hazardous drugs. Improper use of these devices may result in increased, rather than decreased, risk of exposure.
   - i. Final products should be dispensed in ready-to-administer form. If possible, intravenous administration sets should be attached to the bag or bottle in the BSC and primed with plain fluid before the hazardous drug is added. However, if total volume is a concern, intravenous sets may be primed with diluted drug solution, which is discarded into an appropriate container within the BSC. Potential disadvantages to this approach include difficulty in selecting the appropriate administration set when several methods of administering hazardous drugs exist, potential contamination of the outside of the intravenous set, and the risk of the intravenous set becoming dislodged from the bag or bottle during transport.
   - j. The outside of bags or bottles and intravenous sets (if used) should be wiped with moist gauze to remove any inadvertent contamination. Entry ports should be wiped with sterile, alcohol-dampened gauze pads and covered with appropriate seals or caps.
   - k. Final products should be placed in sealable containers (e.g., zipper-closure plastic bags) to reduce the risk of exposing ancillary personnel or contaminating the environment. Containers should be designed such that damage incurred during storage or transport is immediately visible and any leakage is fully contained. For offsite transport, appropriate storage conditions (e.g., refrigerated, padded, and locked carriers) should also be used.
   - l. Excess drug should be returned to the drug vial whenever possible or discarded into a closed container (empty sterile vial). Placing excess drug in any type of open container, even while working in the BSC, is inappropriate. Discarding excess drug into the drainage trough of the BSC is also inappropriate. These practices unnecessarily increase the risk of exposure to large amounts of hazardous drug.
   - m. All contaminated materials should be placed in leak-proof, puncture-resistant containers within the contained environment of the BSC and then placed in larger containers outside the BSC for disposal. To minimize aerosolization, needles should be discarded in puncture-resistant containers without being clipped.

8. *Procedures for the preparation and dispensing of noninjectable dosage forms of hazardous drugs are established and followed.*
   a. Although noninjectable dosage forms of hazardous drugs contain varying proportions of drug to nondrug (nonhazardous) components, there is potential for personnel exposure and environmental contamination with the hazardous components. Procedures should be developed to avoid the release of aerosolized powder or liquid into the environment during manipulation of these drugs.
   b. Drugs designated as hazardous should be labeled or otherwise identified as such to prevent their improper handling.
   c. Tablet and capsule forms of these drugs should not be placed in automated counting machines, which subject them to stress and may introduce powdered contaminants into the work area.
   d. During *routine handling* of hazardous drugs and contaminated equipment, workers should wear one pair of gloves of good quality and thickness.
   e. The counting and pouring of hazardous drugs should be done carefully, and clean equipment dedicated for use with these drugs should be used. Contaminated equipment should be cleaned initially with water-saturated gauze and then further cleaned with detergent and rinsed. The gauze and rinse should be disposed of as contaminated waste.
   f. During *compounding* of hazardous drugs (e.g., crushing, dissolving, and preparing an ointment), workers should wear low-permeability gowns and double gloves. Compounding should take place in a protective area such as a disposable glove box. If compounding must be done in the open, an area away from drafts and traffic must be selected, and the worker should use appropriate respiratory protection.
   g. When hazardous drug tablets in unit-of-use packaging are being crushed, the package should be placed in a small sealable plastic bag and crushed with a spoon or pestle; caution should be used not to break the plastic bag.
   h. Disposal of unused or unusable oral or topical dosage forms of hazardous drugs should be performed in the same manner as for hazardous injectable dosage forms and waste.
9. *Personnel know the procedures to be followed in case of accidental skin or eye contact with hazardous drugs.*
   a. Each health-care setting should have an established first aid protocol for treating cases of direct contact with hazardous drugs, many of which are irritating or caustic and can cause tissue destruction. Medical care providers in each setting should be contacted for input into this protocol. The protocol should include immediate treatment measures and should specify the type and location of medical followup and work-injury reporting. Copies of the protocol, highlighting emergency measures, should be posted wherever hazardous drugs are routinely handled.
   b. Hazardous drug work areas should have a sink (preferably with an eyewash fountain) and appropriate first aid equipment to treat accidental skin or eye contact according to the protocol.
   c. In settings where hazardous drug handlers are offsite (e.g., home use), protocols must be part of orientation programs, and copies of the procedures should be immediately accessible to handlers, along with appropriate first aid equipment and emergency phone numbers to call for followup and reporting.
10. *All hazardous drugs are labeled with a warning label stating the need for special handling.*
    a. A distinctive warning label with an appropriate CAUTION statement should be attached to all hazardous drug materials, consistent with state laws and regulations. This would include, for example, syringes, intravenous containers, containers of unit-dose tablets and liquids, prescription vials and bottles, waste containers, and patient specimens that contain hazardous drugs.
    b. The hazardous drugs discussed in this Technical Assistance Bulletin are chemical hazards and *not* infectious hazards. Because the term "biohazard" refers to an infectious hazard, the use of this term or the biohazard symbol (in any variation) on the label of drugs that are chemical hazards is inappropriate and may be misleading to staff and contract workers who are familiar with the biohazard symbol. An example of a suitable label is shown in Figure 1.
    c. All staff and contract workers should be informed about the meaning of the label and the special handling procedures that have been established.
    d. In settings where patients or their families will be responsible for manipulating these drugs, they should be made aware of the need for special handling and the reasons behind it.

Goal III. Procedures for administering hazardous drugs prevent the accidental exposure of patients and staff and contamination of the work environment.

1. *A method for informing and training health-care professionals in these procedures is maintained.*
   a. Only individuals trained to administer hazardous drugs should be allowed to perform this function. Training programs should contain information on the therapeutic and adverse effects of these drugs and the potential, long-term health risk to personnel handling them. Each individual's knowledge and technique should be evaluated before administration of these drugs. This should be done by written examination and direct observation of the individual's performance.
2. *Standard procedures for the safe administration of hazardous drugs are established and followed.* These procedures ensure the safety of both the patient and health-care personnel.
   a. Intravenous administration sets (e.g., vented, nonvented, and minidrip) and infusion devices appropriate for use with the final product should be selected.
   b. Syringes and intravenous sets with Luer-lock fittings should be used whenever possible.
   c. Preparation of the final product for administration should take place in a clean, uncluttered area separate from other activities and excessive traffic. A plastic-

backed absorbent liner should be used to cover the work area to absorb accidental spills. A single pair of disposable latex gloves and a disposable gown should be worn. The glove and gown cuffs should be worn in a manner that produces a tight fit (e.g., loose glove tucked under gown cuff; tight glove fitted over gown cuff). Hands must be thoroughly washed before gloves are donned.

Administration sets should be attached with care (if not attached during drug preparation). Administration sets and devices should be monitored for leakage.

d. Priming of intravenous sets should not allow any drug to be released into the environment. Hazardous drug solutions may be "piggybacked" into primary intravenous solutions and primed by retrograde flow of the primary solution into the secondary tubing. All Y-site connections should be taped securely. Alternatively, the intravenous set may be primed with plain solution before the hazardous drug solution bag or bottle is connected. Some intravenous sets can be primed so that the fluid enters the medication port of the intravenous bag. The priming fluid may also be discarded into a sealable plastic bag containing absorbent material if care is taken not to contaminate the sterile needle tip. Likewise, a sterile gauze pad should be placed close to the sterile needle tip when air is expelled from a syringe. The syringe plunger should first be drawn back to withdraw liquid from the needle before air is expelled. Care should be taken not to contaminate the sterile needle with gauze fibers or microorganisms.

e. Intravenous containers designed with venting tubes should not be used. If such containers must be used, gauze should be placed over the tube when the container is inverted to catch any hazardous drug solution trapped in the tube. If containers with solid stoppers are used, any vacuum present should be eliminated before the container is attached to a primary intravenous or to a manifold. If a series of bags or bottles is used to deliver the drug, the intravenous set should be discarded with each container because removing the spike from the container is associated with a greater risk of environmental contamination than priming an intravenous set. (Use of secondary sets for administration of hazardous drugs reduces the cost of this recommendation and the risk of priming.)

f. A plastic-backed absorbent liner should be placed under the intravenous tubing during administration to absorb any leakage and prevent the solution from spilling onto the patient's skin. The use of sterile gauze around any "push" sites will reduce the likelihood of releasing drug into the environment.

g. The use of eye protection (safety glasses or goggles) during work with hazardous drugs, especially vesicants, should be considered. Work at your waist level, if possible; avoid working above the head or reaching up for connections or ports.

h. All contaminated gauze, syringes, intravenous sets, bags, bottles, etc., should be placed in sealable plastic bags and placed in a puncture-resistant container for removal from the patient-care area.

i. Gloves should be discarded after each use and immediately if contaminated. Gowns should be discarded on leaving the patient-care area and immediately if contaminated. Hands must be washed thoroughly after hazardous drugs are handled.

j. Gloves should be worn when urine and other excreta from patients receiving hazardous drugs are being handled. Skin contact and splattering should be avoided during disposal. While it may be useful to post a list of drugs that are excreted in urine and feces and the length of time after drug administration during which precautions are necessary, an alternative is to select a standard duration (e.g., 48 hours) that covers most of the drugs and is more easily remembered.

k. Disposable linen or protective pads should be used for incontinent or vomiting patients. Nondisposable linen contaminated with hazard-ous drug should be handled with gloves and treated similarly to that for linen contaminated with infectious material. One procedure is to place the linen in specially marked water-soluble laundry bags. These bags (with the contents) should be prewashed; then the linens should be added to other laundry for an additional wash. Items contaminated with hazardous drugs should not be autoclaved unless they are also contaminated with infectious material.

3. *Appropriate apparel and materials needed to protect staff and patients from exposure and to protect the work environment from contamination are readily available.* Supplies of disposable gloves and gowns, safety glasses, disposable plastic-backed absorbent liners, gauze pads, hazardous waste disposal bags, hazardous drug warning

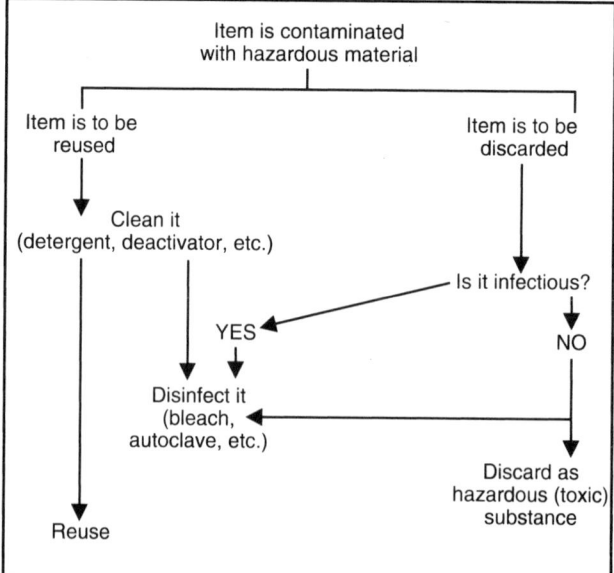

Figure 2. Proposed flow chart for handling chemical hazards versus biohazards. Disinfection of a disposable item contaminated with both infectious and hazardous material may not be necessary, depending on the degree of infectious hazard (e.g., human immunodeficiency virus verses *Escherichia coli*) and depending on the method of disposal (e.g., burial versus incineration).

labels, and puncture-resistant containers for disposal of needles and ampuls should be conveniently located for all areas where hazardous drugs are handled. Assembling a "hazardous drug preparation and administration kit" is one way to furnish nursing and medical personnel with the materials needed to reduce the risk of preparing and administering a hazardous drug.

4. *Personnel know the procedures to be followed in case of accidental skin or eye contact with hazardous drugs. (See Goal II9.)*

Goal IV. The health-care setting, its staff, patients, contract workers, visitors, and the outside environment are not exposed to or contaminated with hazardous drug waste materials produced in the course of using these drugs. (See Figure 2 for proposed flow chart for handling contaminated items.)

1. *Written policies and procedures governing the identification, containment, collection, segregation, and disposal of hazardous drug waste materials are established and maintained.* All health-care workers who handle hazardous drugs or waste must be oriented to and must follow these procedures.
2. *Throughout institutional health-care facilities and in alternative health-care settings, hazardous drug waste materials are identified, contained, and segregated from all other trash.*
   a. Hazardous drug waste should be placed in specially marked (specifically labeled CAUTION: HAZARDOUS CHEMICAL WASTE) thick plastic bags or leakproof containers. These receptacles should be kept in all areas where the drugs are commonly used. All and only hazardous drug waste should be placed in them. Receptacles used for glass fragments, needles, and syringes should be puncture resistant. Hazardous drug waste should not be mixed with any other waste. Waste containers should be handled with uncontaminated gloves.
   b. Health-care personnel providing care in a patient's home should have with them all the equipment and supplies necessary to contain properly any hazardous drug waste that is generated during the visit. Contaminated needles and syringes, intravenous containers, intravenous sets, and any broken ampuls should be placed in leakproof, puncture-resistant containers. Gloves, gowns, drug vials, etc., should be sealed in specially labeled (CAUTION: HAZARDOUS CHEMICAL WASTE) thick plastic bags or leakproof containers. All waste should be removed from the patient's home and transported to a designated area. Additional precautions should be taken during transport, including temporary storage in a spill-resistant container and ensuring that the vehicle is locked at all times. Hazardous waste should be securely stored at a designated area until it is picked up for appropriate disposal. Patients or their caregivers should be instructed on methods for the proper handling of excreta from patients receiving hazardous drugs.
   c. Unless restricted by state or local regulations, hazardous drug waste may be further divided into trace and bulk-contaminated waste, if desired, to reduce costs of disposal. As defined by the EPA, bulk-contaminated materials are solutions or containers whose contents weigh more than 3% of the capacity of the container.[57,58] For example, empty intravenous containers and intravenous administration sets usually are considered trace waste; half-empty vials of hazardous drugs and unused final doses in syringes or intravenous containers are considered bulk-contaminated waste. If trace and bulk-contaminated waste are handled separately, bulk-contaminated waste should be segregated into more secure receptacles for containment and disposal as toxic waste. While this may allow for less expensive overall disposal of hazardous waste, it also requires close monitoring of the containment and segregation process to prevent the accidental discarding of a bulk-contaminated container into a trace-waste receptacle.
   d. All hazardous waste collected from drug preparation and patient-care areas should be held in a secure place in labeled, leakproof drums or cartons (as required by state or local regulation or disposal contractor) until disposal. This waste should be disposed of as hazardous or toxic waste in an EPA-permitted, state-licensed hazardous waste incinerator. Transport to an offsite incinerator should be done by a contractor licensed to handle and transport hazardous waste. (While licenses are generally required to transport infectious waste as well as hazardous waste, these are different classes of contractors and may not be interchanged. Verification of possession and type of license should be documented before a contractor is engaged.)
   e. If access to an appropriately licensed incinerator is not available, transport to and burial in an EPA-licensed hazardous waste dump site is an acceptable alternative. While there are concerns that destruction of carcinogens by incineration may be incomplete, newer technologies and stringent licensing criteria have improved this disposal method. (Again, the existence and type of license should be verified before use of a contract incinerator.)
   f. Chemical deactivation of hazardous drugs should be undertaken only by individuals who are thoroughly familiar with the chemicals and the procedures required to complete such a task. The IARC recently published a monograph describing methods for chemical destruction of some cytotoxic (antineoplastic) drugs in the laboratory setting.[59] The chemicals and equipment described, however, are not generally found in the clinical setting, and many of the deactivating chemicals are toxic and hazardous. Most procedures require the use of a chemical fume hood. The procedures are generally difficult, and the deactivation is not always complete. Serious consideration should be given to the negative aspects of chemical deactivation before one commits to such a course of action.
3. *Materials to clean up spills of hazardous drugs are readily available and personnel are trained in their proper use.* A standard cleanup protocol is established and followed.

a. "Spill kits" containing all materials needed to clean up spills of hazardous drugs should be assembled or purchased. These kits should be readily available in all areas where hazardous drugs are routinely handled. If hazardous drugs are being prepared or administered in a nonroutine area (home setting or unusual patient-care area), a spill kit should be obtained by the drug handler. The kit should include two pairs of disposable gloves (one outer pair of utility gloves and one inner latex pair); low permeability, disposable protective garments (coveralls or gown and shoe covers); safety glasses or splash goggles; respirator; absorbent, plastic-backed sheets or spill pads; disposable toweling; at least two sealable thick plastic hazardous waste disposal bags (prelabeled with an appropriate warning label); a disposable scoop for collecting glass fragments; and a puncture-resistant container for glass fragments.

b. All individuals who routinely handle hazardous drugs must be trained in proper spill management and cleanup procedures. Spills and breakages must be cleaned up immediately according to the following procedures. If the spill is not located in a confined space, the spill area should be identified and other people should be prevented from approaching and spreading the contamination. Wearing protective apparel from the spill kit, workers should remove any broken glass fragments and place them in the puncture-resistant container. Liquids should be absorbed with a spill pad; powder should be removed with damp disposable gauze pads or soft toweling. The hazardous material should be completely removed and the area rinsed with water and then cleaned with detergent. The spill cleanup should proceed progressively from areas of lesser to greater contamination. The detergent should be thoroughly rinsed and removed. All contaminated materials should be placed in the disposal bags provided and sealed and transported to a designated containment receptacle.

c. Spills occurring in the BSC should be cleaned up immediately; a spill kit should be used if the volume exceeds 150 ml or the contents of one drug vial or ampul. If there is broken glass, utility gloves should be worn to remove it and place it in the puncture-resistant container located in the BSC. The BSC, including the drain spillage trough, should be thoroughly cleaned. If the spill is not easily and thoroughly contained, the BSC should be decontaminated after cleanup. If the spill contaminates the HEPA filter, use of the BSC should be suspended until the cabinet has been decontaminated and the HEPA filter replaced. (See Goal II 5j.)

d. If hazardous drugs are routinely prepared or administered in carpeted areas, special equipment is necessary to remove the spill. Absorbent powder should be substituted for pads or sheets and left in place on the spill for the time recommended by the manufacturer. The powder should then be picked up with a small vacuum unit reserved for hazardous drug cleanup. The carpet should then be cleaned according to usual procedures. The vacuum bag should be removed and discarded or cleaned, and the exterior of the vacuum cleaner should be washed with detergent and rinsed before being covered and stored. The contaminated powder should be discarded into a sealable plastic bag and segregated with other contaminated waste materials. Alternatively, inexpensive wet or dry vacuum units may be purchased for this express use and used with appropriate cleaners. All such units are contaminated, once used, and must be cleaned, stored, and ultimately discarded appropriately (i.e., like BSCs).

e. The circumstances and handling of spills should be documented. Health-care personnel exposed during spill management should also complete an incident report or exposure form.

4. *Hazardous drug waste is disposed of in accordance with all applicable state, federal, and local regulations for the handling of hazardous and toxic waste.*

a. Regulatory agencies such as the EPA and state solid and hazardous waste agencies and local air and water quality control boards must be consulted regarding the classification and appropriate disposal of drugs that are defined as hazardous or toxic chemicals. EPA categorizes several of the antineoplastic agents (including cyclophosphamide and daunorubicin) as toxic wastes, while many states are more stringent and include as carcinogens certain cytotoxic drugs (azathioprine) and hormonal preparations (diethylstilbestrol and conjugated estrogens). EPA also allows exemptions from toxic waste regulations for "small quantity generators,"[57] whereas certain states do not. It is critical to research these regulations when disposal procedures are being established.

Other Hazardous Drug Issues

The handling of hazardous drugs, some of which are defined by the EPA as toxic chemicals, has implications that go beyond the health-care setting. Disposal of hazardous materials and toxic chemicals continues to be a controversial issue of which the disposal of hazardous drugs is but a small part. The EPA currently issues permits for both burial and incineration of hazardous waste. Some such facilities may purport to possess permits to handle these types of hazardous agents when, in fact, they do not meet the requirements or are only in the initial stages of obtaining permits. It is imperative that health-care facilities verify the license or permit status of any contractor used to remove or dispose of infectious or hazardous waste. In addition, many hazardous drugs are excreted unchanged or as equally toxic metabolites. The amount of hazardous drug transferred to the environment (primarily through the water supply) from this source may exceed that resulting from the hospital trash pathway. No good methods for reducing this source of contamination are currently known.

Definitive risks of handling these drugs may never be fully determined without epidemiologic data from a national registry of handlers of hazardous drugs (and chemicals). There is no method available for routine monitoring of personnel for evidence of hazardous drug exposure. Tests for the presence of mutagens or chromosomal damage are not drug specific and are of value only in controlled studies. Chemical analysis of urine for the presence of hazardous drugs at the sensitivity level needed to detect occupational exposure is limited to a few drugs and is not yet commercially available.

This document is designed to identify areas of risk in the handling of hazardous drugs and to provide recommendations for reducing that risk. A safety program should be coupled with a strong quality-assurance program that periodically evaluates and verifies staff adherence to and performance of the established safe handling policies and procedures. Until some type of external monitoring of exposure levels from handling hazardous drugs is commercially available, development of and compliance with a safety program remain the most logical means for minimizing occupational risk.

References

1. American Society of Hospital Pharmacists. ASHP technical assistance bulletin on handling cytotoxic drugs in hospitals. *Am J Hosp Pharm.* 1985; 42:131–7.
2. Yodaiken R. Safe handling of cytotoxic drugs by health care personnel. Washington, DC: Occupational Safety and Health Administration; 1986 Jan 29. (Instructional publication 8-1.1).
3. U.S. Public Health Service, National Institutes of Health. Recommendations for the safe handling of parenteral antineoplastic drugs. Washington, DC:U.S. Department of Health and Human Services; 1983. (NIH publication 83-2621).
4. Recommendations for handling cytotoxic agents. Providence, RI: National Study Commission on Cytotoxic Exposure; 1987 Sep.
5. AMA Council on Scientific Affairs. Guidelines for handling parenteral antineoplastics. *JAMA.* 1985; 253:1590–2.
6. Scott SA. Antineoplastic drug information and handling guidelines for office-based physicians. *Am J Hosp Pharm.* 1984; 41:2402–3.
7. Barstow J. Safe handling of cytotoxic agents in the home. *Home Healthc Nurse.* 1986; 3:46–7.
8. Barry LK, Booher RB. Promoting the responsible handling of antineoplastic agents in the community. *Oncol Nurs Forum.* 1985; 12:40–6.
9. Berk PD, Goldberg JD, Silverstein MN, et al. Increased incidence of leukemia in polycythemia vera associated with chlorambucil therapy. *N Engl J Med.* 1981; 304:441–7.
10. Penn I. Occurrence of cancer in immune deficiencies. *Cancer.* 1974; 34:858–66.
11. Schafer AI. Teratogenic effects of antileukemic therapy. *Arch Intern Med.* 1981; 141:514–5.
12. Stephens JD, Golbus MS, Miller TR, et al. Multiple congenital abnormalities in a fetus exposed to 5-fluorouracil during the first trimester. *Am J Obstet Gynecol.* 1980; 137:747–9.
13. IARC monographs on the evaluation of the carcinogenic risk of chemicals to humans. Geneva, Switzerland: World Health Organization; 1981.
14. Benedict WF, Baker MS, Haroun L, et al. Mutagenicity of cancer chemotherapeutic agents in the *Salmonella*/microsome test. *Cancer Res.* 1977; 37:2209–13.
15. Falck K, Grohn P, Sorsa M, et al. Mutagenicity in urine of nurses handling cytostatic drugs. *Lancet.* 1979; 1:1250–1.
16. Anderson RW, Puckett WH, Dana WJ, et al. Risk of handling injectable antineoplastic agents. *Am J Hosp Pharm.* 1982; 39:1881–7.
17. Norppa H, Sorsa M, Vainio H, et al. Increased sister chromatid exchange frequencies in lymphocytes of nurses handling cytostatic drugs. *Scand J Work Environ Health.* 1980; 6:299–301.
18. Waksvik H, Klepp O, Brogger A. Chromosome analyses of nurses handling cytostatic agents. *Cancer Treat Rep.* 1981; 65:607–10.
19. Nikula E, Kiviniitty K, Leisti J, et al. Chromosome aberrations in lymphocytes of nurses handling cytostatic agents. *Scand J Work Environ Health.* 1984; 10:71–4.
20. Chrysostomou A, Morley AA, Sehadri R. Mutation frequency in nurses and pharmacists working with cytotoxic drugs. *Aust N Z J Med.* 1984; 14:831–4.
21. Rogers B, Emmett EA. Handling antineoplastic agents: urine mutagenicity in nurses. *Image J Nurs Sch.* 1987; 19:108–13.
22. Palmer RG, Dore CJ, Denman AM. Chlorambucil-induced chromosome damage to human lymphocytes is dose-dependent and cumulative. *Lancet.* 1984; 1:246–9.
23. Sotaniemi EA, Sutinen S, Arranto AJ, et al. Liver damage in nurses handling cytostatic agents. *Acta Med Scand.* 1983; 214:181–9.
24. How real is the hazard? *Lancet.* 1984; 1:203.
25. Tuffnell PG, Gannon MT, Dong A, et al. Limitations of urinary mutagen assays for monitoring occupational exposure to antineoplastic drugs. *Am J Hosp Pharm.* 1986; 43:344–8.
26. Cloak MM, Connor TH, Stevens KR, et al. Occupational exposure of nursing personnel to antineoplastic agents. *Oncol Nurs Forum.* 1985; 12:33–9.
27. Connor TH, Anderson RW. Demonstrating mutagenicity testing using the Ames test. *Am J Hosp Pharm.* 1985; 42:783–4.
28. Connor TH, Theiss JC, Anderson RW, et al. Re-evaluation of urine mutagenicity of pharmacy personnel exposed to antineoplastic agents. *Am J Hosp Pharm.* 1986; 43:1236–9.
29. Jagun O, Ryan M, Waldrom HA. Urinary thioether excretion in nurses handling cytotoxic drugs. *Lancet.* 1982; 2:443–4.
30. Hirst M, Tse S, Mills DG, et al. Occupational exposure to cyclophosphamide. *Lancet.* 1984; 1:186–8.
31. Venitt S, Crofton-Sleigh C, Hunt J, et al. Monitoring exposure of nursing and pharmacy personnel to cytotoxic drugs: urinary mutation assays and urinary platinum as markers of absorption. *Lancet.* 1984; 1:74–6.
32. Neal A deW, Wadden RA, Chiou WL. Exposure of hospital workers to airborne antineoplastic agents. *Am J Hosp Pharm.* 1983; 40:597–601.
33. Kleinberg ML, Quinn MJ. Airborne drug levels in a laminar flow hood. *Am J Hosp Pharm.* 1981; 38:1301–3.
34. Gililland J, Weinstein L. The effects of chemotherapeutic agents on the developing fetus. *Obstet Gynecol Surv.* 1983; 38:6–13.
35. Hemminki K, Kyyronen P, Lindbohm ML. Spontaneous abortions and malformations in the offspring of nurses exposed to anesthetic gases, cytostatic drugs and other potential hazards in hospitals, based on registered information of outcome. *J Epidemiol Community Health.* 1985; 39:141–7.
36. Selevan SH, Lindbohm ML, Hornung RW, et al. A study of occupational exposure to antineoplastic drugs and fetal loss in nurses. *N Engl J Med.* 1985; 333:1173–8.

37. Richter P, Calamera JC, Morgenfeld MC, et al. Effect of chlorambucil on spermatogenesis in the human with malignant lymphoma. *Cancer.* 1970; 25:1026–30.
38. Maguire LC. Fertility and cancer therapy. *Postgrad Med.* 1979; 65:293–5.
39. Sherins JJ, DeVita VT Jr. Effect of drug treatment for lymphoma on male reproductive capacity. *Ann Intern Med.* 1973; 79:216–20.
40. Gregoire RE, Segal R, Hale KM. Handling antineoplastic-drug admixtures at cancer centers: practices and pharmacist attitudes. *Am J Hosp Pharm.* 1987; 44:1090–5.
41. Cohen IA, Newland SJ, Kirking DM. Injectable-antineoplastic-drug practices in Michigan hospitals. *Am J Hosp Pharm.* 1987; 44:1096–105.
42. Hoy RH, Stump LM. Effect of an air-venting filter device on aerosol production from vials. *Am J Hosp Pharm.* 1984; 41:324–6.
43. National Sanitation Foundation Standard: Class II (laminar flow) Biohazard Cabinetry. Standard 49. Ann Arbor, MI: National Sanitation Foundation; 1987 Jun.
44. McDiarmid MA, Egan T, Furio M, et al. Sampling for airborne fluorouracil in a hospital drug preparation area. *Am J Hosp Pharm.* 1986; 43:1942–5.
45. Clark RP, Goff MR. The potassium iodide method for determining protection factors in open-fronted microbiological safety cabinets. *J Appl Biol.* 1981; 51:461–73.
46. Connor TH, Laidlaw JL, Theiss JC, et al. Permeability of latex and polyvinyl chloride gloves to carmustine. *Am J Hosp Pharm.* 1984; 41:676–9.
47. Laidlaw JL, Connor TH, Theiss JC, et al. Permeability of latex and polyvinyl chloride gloves to 20 antineoplastic drugs. *Am J Hosp Pharm.* 1984; 41:2618–23.
48. Slevin ML, Ang LM, Johnston A, et al. The efficiency of protective gloves used in the handling of cytotoxic drugs. *Cancer Chemother Pharmacol.* 1984; 12:151–3.
49. Stoikes ME, Carlson JD, Farris FF, et al. Permeability of latex and polyvinyl chloride gloves to fluorouracil and methotrexate. *Am J Hosp Pharm.* 1987; 44:1341–6.
50. Laidlaw JL, Connor TH, Theiss JC, et al. Permeability of four disposable protective-clothing materials to seven antineoplastic drugs. *Am J Hosp Pharm.* 1985; 42:2449–54.
51. Falck K, Sorsa M, Vainio H. Use of the bacterial fluctuation test to detect mutagenicity in urine of nurses handling cytostatic drugs. *Mutat Res.* 1981; 85:236–7.
52. Myers CE. Preparing a list of cytotoxic agents. *Am J Hosp Pharm.* 1987; 44:1296, 1298. Questions and Answers.
53. National Institute of Occupational Safety and Health. Respirator decision logic. Washington, DC: U.S. Department of Health and Human Services; 1987. (DHHS, NIOSH publication 87-108).
54. Commissioner, Federal Supply Service, General Serv-ices Administration. Federal Standard 209C. Clean room and work station requirements, controlled environments. Washington, DC: U.S. Government Printing Office; 1988.
55. Bryan D, Marback MA. Laminar-airflow equipment certification: what the pharmacist needs to know. *Am J Hosp Pharm.* 1984; 41:1343–9.
56. Wilson JP, Solimando DA. Aseptic technique as a safety precaution in the preparation of antineoplastic agents. *Hosp Pharm.* 1981; 15:575–81.
57. F40 CFR 261.5.
58. Vaccari PL, Tonat K, DeChristoforo R, et al. Disposal of antineoplastic wastes at the National Institutes of Health. *Am J Hosp Pharm.* 1984; 41:87–93.
59. Castegnaro M, Adams J, Armour MA, et al., eds. Laboratory decontamination and destruction of carcinogens in laboratory wastes: some antineoplastic agents. International Agency for Research on Cancer Scientific Publication 73. Fair Lawn, NJ: Oxford University Press; 1985.

Appendix A—Glossary

Biohazard: An infectious agent presenting a real or potential risk to humans and the environment.

Carcinogen: Any cancer-producing substance.

Chemotherapy: The treatment of disease by chemical means; first applied to use of chemicals that affect the causative organism unfavorably but do not harm the patient; currently used to describe drug (chemical) therapy of neoplastic diseases (cancer).

Clastogenic: Giving rise to or inducing disruption or breakage, as of chromosomes.

Contamination: The deposition of potentially dangerous material where it is not desired, particularly where its presence may be harmful or constitute a hazard.

Cytotoxic: Possessing a specific destructive action on certain cells; used commonly in referring to antineoplastic drugs that selectively kill dividing cells.

Decontamination: Removal, neutralization, or destruction of a toxic (harmful) agent.

Exposure: The condition of being subjected to something, as to chemicals, that may have a harmful effect. Acute exposure is exposure of short duration, usually exposure of heavy intensity; chronic exposure is long-term exposure, either continuous or intermittent, usually referring to exposure of low intensity.

Genotoxic: Damaging to DNA; pertaining to agents (radiation or chemical substances) known to damage DNA, thereby causing mutations or cancer.

Hazardous: Dangerous; risky; representing a health risk.

Mutagen: Chemical or physical agent that induces or increases genetic mutations by causing changes in DNA.

Plenum: Space within a biohazard cabinet where air flows; plenums may either be under positive (greater than atmospheric pressure) or negative pressure, depending on whether the air is "blown" or "sucked" through the space.

Respirator: A National Institute of Occupational Safety and Health (NIOSH) approved, air-purifying half-mask respirator equipped with a high-efficiency filter; may be disposable (discarded after the end of its recommended period of use).

Trough: Drain spillage trough; an area below the biological safety cabinet's work surface, provided to retain spillage from the work area.

Utility gloves: Heavy, disposable gloves, similar to household latex gloves.

Appendix B—Classification of Biohazard Cabinetry (Biological Safety Cabinets)[43]

Class I: A ventilated cabinet for personnel and environmental protection, with an unrecirculated inward airflow away from the operator.
Note: The cabinet exhaust air is treated to protect the environment before it is discharged to the outside atmos-phere. This cabinet is suitable for work with low- and moderate-risk biological agents when no product protection is required.

Class II: A ventilated cabinet for personnel, product, and environmental protection, having an open front with inward airflow for personnel protection, high-efficiency particulate air (HEPA) filtered laminar airflow for product protection, and HEPA-filtered exhausted air for environmental protection.
Note: When toxic chemicals or radionuclides are used as adjuncts to biological studies or pharmaceutical work, Class II cabinets designed and constructed for this purpose should be used.

- *Type A (formerly designated Type 1)*: Cabinets that (1) maintain minimum calculated average inflow velocity of 75 feet per minute (fpm) through the work area access opening; (2) have HEPA-filtered downflow air from a common plenum (i.e., plenum from which a portion of the air is exhausted from the cabinet and the remainder is supplied to the work area); (3) may exhaust HEPA-filtered air back into the laboratory; and (4) may have positive-pressure-contaminated ducts and plenums. Type A cabinets are suitable for work with low- to moderate-risk biological agents in the absence of volatile toxic chemicals and volatile radionuclides.
- *Type B1 (formerly designated Type 2)*: Cabinets that (1) maintain a minimum (calculated or measured) average inflow velocity of 100 fpm through the work area access opening; (2) have HEPA-filtered downflow air composed largely of uncontaminated recirculated inflow air; (3) exhaust most of the contaminated downflow air through a dedicated duct exhausted to the atmosphere after it passes through a HEPA filter; and (4) have all biologically contaminated ducts and plenums under negative pressure or surrounded by negative-pressure ducts and plenums. Type B1 cabinets are suitable for work with low- to moderate-risk biological agents. They may also be used with biological agents treated with minute quantities of toxic chemicals and trace amounts of radionuclides required as an adjunct to microbiological studies if work is done in the directly exhausted portion of the cabinet or if the chemicals or radionuclides will not interfere with the work when recirculated in the downflow air.
- *Type B2 (sometimes referred to as "total exhaust")*: Cabinets that (1) maintain a minimum (calculated or measured) average inflow velocity of 100 fpm through the work area access opening; (2) have HEPA-filtered downflow air drawn from the laboratory or the outside air (i.e., downflow air is not recirculated from the cabinet exhaust air); (3) exhaust all inflow and down-flow air to the atmosphere after filtration through a HEPA filter without recirculation in the cabinet or return to the laboratory room air; and (4) have all contaminated ducts and plenums under negative pressure or surrounded by directly exhausted (nonrecirc-ulated through the work area) negative-pressure ducts and plenums. Type B2 cabinets are suitable for work with low- to moderate-risk biological agents. They may also be used with biological agents treated with toxic chemicals and radionuclides required as an adjunct to microbiological studies.
- *Type B3 (sometimes referred to as "convertible cabinets")*: Cabinets that (1) maintain a minimum (calculated or measured) average inflow velocity of 100 fpm through the work access opening; (2) have HEPA-filtered downflow air that is a portion of the mixed downflow and inflow air from a common exhaust plenum; (3) discharge all exhaust air to the outdoor atmosphere after HEPA filtration; and (4) have all biologically contaminated ducts and plenums under negative pressure or surrounded by negative-pressure ducts and plenums. Type B3 cabinets are suitable for work with low- to moderate-risk biological agents treated with minute quantities of toxic chemicals and trace quantities of radionuclides that will not interfere with the work if recirculated in the downflow air.
- *Other Types*: Other cabinets may be considered Class II if they meet these requirements for performance, durability, reliability, safety, operational integrity, and cleanability.

Class III: A totally enclosed, ventilated cabinet of gas-tight construction. Operations in the cabinet are conducted through attached rubber gloves. The cabinet is maintained under negative air pressure of at least 0.5 inch (12.7 mm) water gauge (wg). Supply air is drawn into the cabinet through HEPA filters. The exhaust air is treated by double HEPA filtration or by HEPA filtration and incineration.

Revised by ASHP's Clinical Affairs Department in collaboration with Luci A. Power, M.S., Senior Consultant, Power Enterprises, San Francisco, CA. Reviewed by the officers of the ASHP Special Interest Group (SIG) on Oncology Pharmacy Practice and approved by the ASHP Council on Professional Affairs, September 20, 1989. Approved by the ASHP Board of Directors, November 15–16, 1989. Supersedes a previous version approved by the Board of Directors on November 14, 1984.

Copyright © 1990, American Society of Hospital Pharmacists, Inc. All rights reserved.

The bibliographic citation for this document is as follows: American Society of Hospital Pharmacists. ASHP technical assistance bulletin on handling cytotoxic and hazardous drugs. *Am J Hosp Pharm.* 1990; 47:1033–49.

This Technical Assistance Bulletin was reviewed in 1996 by the Council on Professional Affairs and by the Board of Directors and was found to still be appropriate.

SELF-STUDY QUESTIONS

1. List at least four research methodologies that have been used to assess exposure to cytotoxics in the workplace and briefly describe the limitations of each strategy.

2. Measurement of urinary thioethers assesses the:
   a. ability of substances in the urine to induce bacterial mutations.
   b. glutathione-conjugated metabolites of alkylating agents.
   c. sister chromatid exchange.
   d. all of the above.
   e. none of the above.

3. In the study done by Anderson and colleagues, mutagenicity was demonstrated in the urine of pharmacy personnel when they prepared cytotoxics in:
   a. horizontal laminar flow hoods when using no protective garments.
   b. horizontal laminar flow hoods while wearing gloves or masks.
   c. biological safety cabinets when using gloves.
   d. both a and b.
   e. all of the above.

4. Explain the difference between class II, type A and class II, type B biological safety cabinets.

5. Surgical masks should always be worn when preparing cytotoxic drugs, whether or not a biological safety cabinet is being used.
   a. true
   b. false

6. Because there is minimal risk of cytotoxic exposure when a biological safety cabinet and recommended garments are properly used, the ASHP Technical Assistance Bulletin states that it is reasonable for women to continue their usual cytotoxic preparation activities during the first trimester of pregnancy.
   a. true
   b. false

7. Describe the health evaluation monitoring procedures that are recommended for workers who prepare or administer cytotoxic drugs.

8. List nine common factors associated with the prescribing of cancer chemotherapy that have been implicated in contributing to medication errors.

9. List the standard elements that should be included in every chemotherapy order.

10. The following order is faxed to the oncology pharmacy. Discuss potential problems associated with the following order: Adria 40.0 mg days 1–3. BSA = 1.7 m^2

11. To avoid contamination of chemotherapy and unnecessary worker exposure, chemotherapy prepared in syringes should be sealed in a plastic bag, and the label should always be attached to the bag.
    a. true
    b. false

12. Describe the order verification process that the pharmacist should follow prior to filling chemotherapy orders.

13. A chemotherapy order is received by the pharmacy at 10 p.m. with doses that far exceed the usual dose range for a new cytotoxic agent. The medical resident on call insists that the order is correct and demands that it be prepared. What processes could prevent this situation and how should the evening pharmacist respond?

14. You have been asked to develop a print library for the new oncology satellite pharmacy. List four textbooks that you would purchase and explain why you chose these books.

15. A patient who is receiving chemotherapy at your clinic confides that she is taking many different "vitamin supplements" recommended by a nutritional therapist and asks what you think of them. After examining the labels you find that you are not familiar with some of these alternative therapies. Where can you obtain more information about these substances?

16. A patient approaches you in the clinic and asks about a new "miracle drug" for bladder cancer that they heard about last evening on the television news. He knows that his disease is not controlled by his current therapy and wants to know how to get this new medication. Unfortunately, you were working late again and missed the news. How should you respond?

Appendix I—The Mammalian Cell Cycle

Tumors grow because the cells they contain are undergoing division. Like other mammalian cells, malignant cell division proceeds through a series of sequential phases and results in two daughter cells. When normal cells divide, these daughter cells are almost always identical. Malignant cells are far more likely to experience genetic aberrations. Uncontrolled tumor growth or expansion occurs because the homeostatic control mechanisms that maintain the appropriate number of cells in normal tissues are defective. Understanding the cell cycle and biological events that occur during each phase are key to understanding the interaction of cytotoxic drugs and tumor cells.

A complete cycle, from one mitosis to the next, is called the *generation time*. The generation time is different for all tumors, ranging from hours to days. In fact, the generation time may even differ between cells within a single tumor mass or between the cells of a primary tumor and its metastases. The transition from one phase of the cell cycle to the next is controlled by cellular proteins. After mitosis, each daughter cell enters the G_1 (or postmitotic) phase (Figure A-1) and remains in the G_1 phase until it receives some stimulus to enter the S (or DNA synthesis) phase. It is believed that the enzymes necessary for DNA synthesis are produced during the G_1 phase and that once a cell is stimulated to proceed to the S phase it is committed to proceed through the division process. Until that point, the cell could reversibly leave the dividing process, reverting to the resting (G_0) phase.

DNA synthesis occurs during the S phase. The DNA coils unwind, separating the two strands and exposing the nucleotide bases that were once paired. Each DNA strand serves as a template, allowing enzymes (DNA polymerases) to match free nucleotides in the nucleus with the exposed nucleotide bases along the sugar-phosphate backbone of each strand of DNA. When the DNA replication is complete, the new DNA molecule coils up.

The premitotic G_2 phase is a short phase during which RNA and specialized proteins are produced. When new pro-

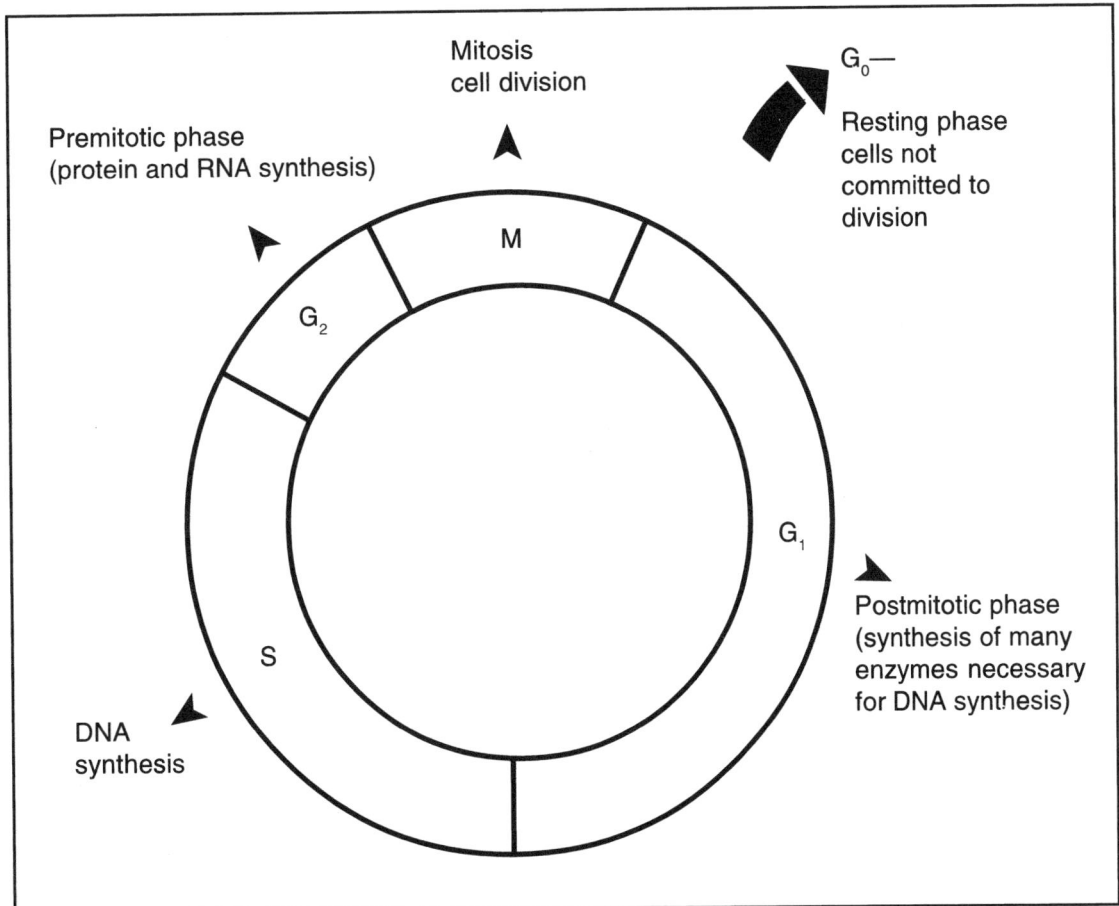

Figure A-1. The cell cycle

SOURCE: Erlichman C. The pharmacology of anticancer drugs. In: Tannock IF, Hill RP, editors. *The Basic Science of Oncology*. New York: Pergamon; 1987. p. 292–307; and Fox M. Drug resistance and DNA repair. In: Fox BW, Fox M, editors. *Antitumor Drug Resistance*. Berlin: Springer-Verlag, 1984. p. 335–69.

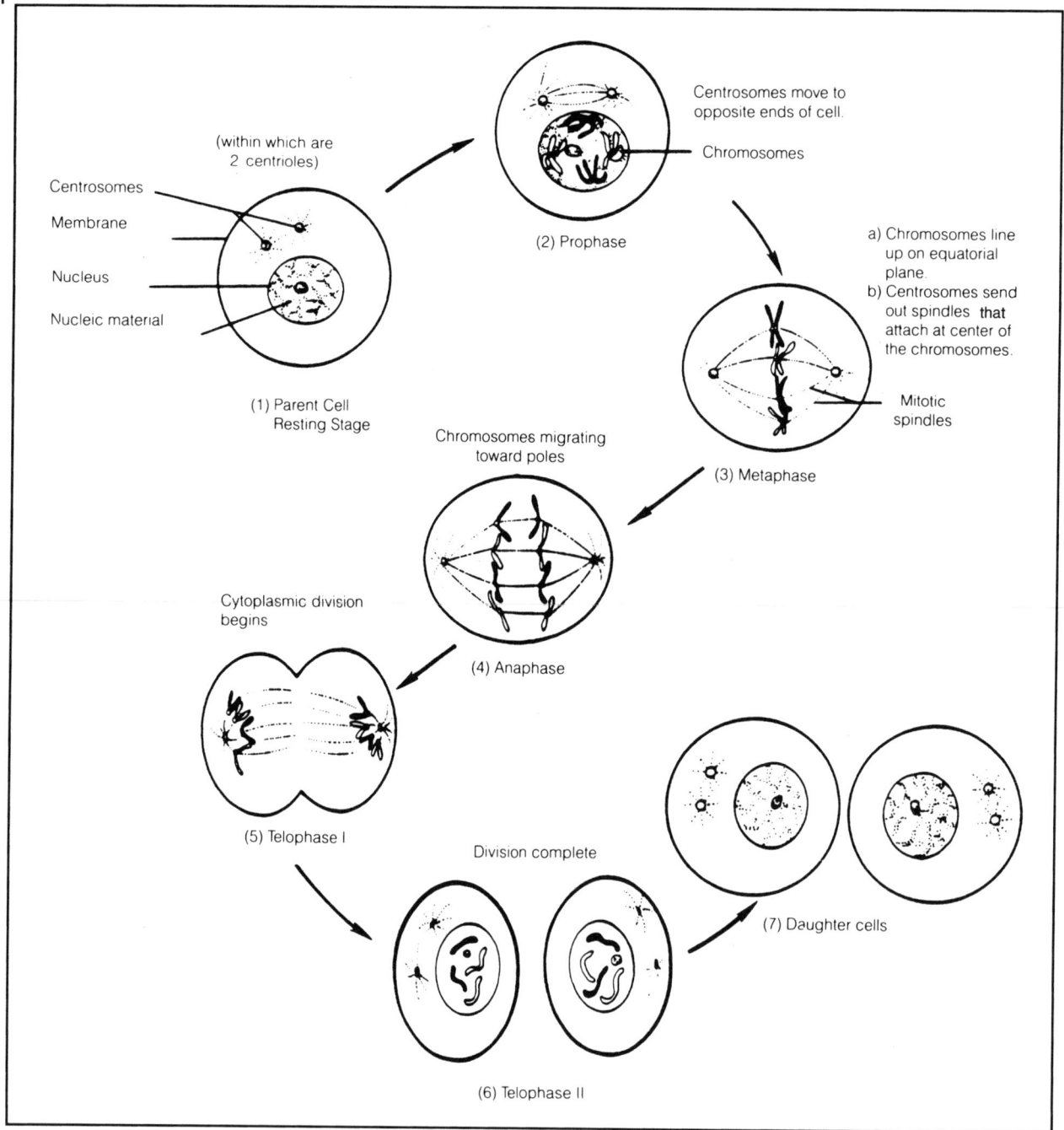

Figure A-2. Mitosis (cell division)

teins or enzymes are needed, DNA begins to unravel at the point that bears the code for the necessary enzyme. The exposed nucleotides are acted on by RNA polymerase II to pair free nucleotides with the backbone, forming messenger RNA (mRNA), which then passes through holes in the nuclear membrane and migrates to the ribosome. The ribosome moves along the mRNA, and transfer RNA delivers and attaches amino acids to assemble the new protein.

The mitosis phase of the cell cycle can be divided into four phases: prophase, metaphase, anaphase, and telophase (which has two parts, parts I and II) (Figure A-2). Each cell has two centrosomes (within which are two centrioles) that lie close to each other in the cytoplasm between mitotic divisions. The first event of mitosis (prophase) is the movement of these centrosomes away from each other to opposite ends of the cell. Small fibers called protein microtubules (spindles) grow between the centrioles during prophase, pushing the centrioles apart. Simultaneously, chromatin is transformed into chromosomes, each containing a pair of chromatids. Metaphase begins with the disappearance of the nuclear membrane and continues with the chromosomes lining up between the centrioles. Anaphase follows, as the chromatids are pulled toward the centrioles by the microtubules. During the final phase of mitosis, telophase, the nuclear membrane forms around each set of chromosomes, causing division. After mitosis, the cells can die, return to the cell cycle at the G_1 phase, or enter the G_0 phase. Most normal human cells exist predominantly in the G_0 phase. Cancer cells in the G_0 phase are not generally susceptible to the toxic effects of chemotherapy, because the lethal activity of most cytotoxics depends on the cell attempting to proceed to the next step in the division process. For example, if an alkylating agent binds to DNA, the cell typically will not suffer lethal damage until its DNA is unable to separate during the S phase of the cell cycle.

Cells in the G_0 phase retain the capacity to begin dividing again following an appropriate stimulus (e.g., a growth factor or nutrient). Before a cell (malignant or normal) can re-enter the dividing process from the G_0 phase, three things must occur: (1) one or more growth factors must interact with receptors on the cell's surface; (2) the growth factor–receptor complex must signal the cell's nucleus; and (3) this signal must activate genes in the nucleus that stimulate production of cellular proteins that regulate the other proteins necessary for the remainder of the cell division process.

Two terms are used to describe cellular division activity: *growth fraction* is the percentage of dividing cells in a tumor mass, and the *mitotic index* is the percentage of cells in mitosis at any given time. These terms are important because tumors with a large growth fraction or a high mitotic index (i.e., many cells dividing) are more likely to be susceptible to chemotherapy. The proportion of cells that are actively dividing at any time is measured by incubating tumor cells with ^{3}H-thymidine for a short period of time (labeling index or thymidine labeling index). Because ^{3}H-thymidine is either incorporated into DNA during synthesis or rapidly broken down, an autoradiographic scan can be used to assess the proportion of cells that are synthesizing DNA (i.e., are in their S phase). Cells may also be studied using flow cytometry, which sorts cells by the amount of DNA in the nucleus and estimates the cell-phase distribution (proportion of cells in each phase), growth fraction, and kinetic properties.

Cytotoxic agents are commonly grouped by the phase of the cell cycle in which they are active (see Figure 3-4, page 37). Some agents are reported to be most active during a particular phase of the cycle (cell cycle specific), whereas others appear to act relatively independently of a specific phase (cell cycle nonspecific). These classifications should not be considered absolute, because the precise mechanism or mechanisms of each agent are not known and others act by more than one mechanism. The mechanisms of action of some of the most widely used cytotoxic drugs are explained in chapters 3 and 4.

Appendix II—Common Toxicity Criteria

	Toxicity	Grade 0	Grade 1	Grade 2	Grade 3	Grade 4
Blood/Bone Marrow	WBC	≥4.0	3.0–3.9	2.0–2.9	1.0–1.9	<1.0
	PLT	WNL	75.0–normal	50.0–74.9	25.0–49.9	<25.0
	Hb	WNL	10.0–normal	8.0–10.0	6.5–7.9	<6.5
	Granulocytes/Bands	≥2.0	1.5–1.9	1.0–1.4	0.5–0.9	<0.5
	Lymphocytes	≥2.0	1.5–1.9	1.0–1.4	0.5–0.9	<0.5
	Hemorrhage—clinical	none	mild, no transfusion	gross, 1–2 units transfusion per episode	gross, 3–4 units transfusion per episode	massive, >4 units transfusion per episode
	Infection	none	mild	moderate	severe	life-threatening
Gastrointestinal	Nausea	none	able to eat reasonable intake	intake significantly decreased but can eat	no significant intake	—
	Vomiting	none	1 episode in 24 hr	2–5 episodes in 24 hr	6–10 episodes in 24 hr	>10 episodes in 24 hr, or requiring parenteral support
	Diarrhea	none	increase of 2–3 stools/day over pre-Rx	increase of 4–6 stools/day, or nocturnal stools, or moderate cramping	increase of 7–9 stools/day, or incontinence, or severe cramping	increase of ≥10 stools/day, or grossly bloody diarrhea, or need for parenteral support
	Stomatitis	none	painless ulcers, erythema, or mild soreness	painful erythema, edema, or ulcers, but can eat	painful erythema, edema, or ulcers, and cannot eat	requires parenteral or enteral support
Liver	Bilirubin	WNL	—	<1.5 × N	1.5–3.0 × N	>3.0 × N
	Transaminase (SGOT, SGPT)	WNL	≤2.5 × N	2.6–5.0 × N	5.1–20.0 × N	>20.0 × N
	Alk Phos or 5′-nucleotidase	WNL	≤2.5 × N	2.6–5.0 × N	5.1–20.0 × N	>20.0 × N
	Liver—clinical	no change from baseline	—	—	precoma	hepatic coma
Kidney, Bladder	Creatinine	WNL	<1.5 × N	1.5–3.0 × N	3.1–6.0 × N	>6.0 × N
	Proteinuria	no change	1+ or <0.3 g% or <3 g/L	2–3+ or 0.3–1.0 g% or 3–10 g/L	4+ or >1.0 g% or >10 g/L	nephrotic syndrome
	Hematuria	neg	micro only	gross, no clots	gross + clots	requires transfusion
	Alopecia	no loss	mild hair loss	pronounced or total hair loss	—	—
	Pulmonary	none or no change	asymptomatic, with abnormality in PFTs	dypsnea on significant exertion	dypsnea at normal level of activity	dypsnea at rest
Heart	Cardiac dysrhythmias	none	asymptomatic, transient, requiring no therapy	recurrent or persistent, no therapy required	requires treatment	requires monitoring, or hypotension, or ventricular tachycardia, or fibrillation
	Cardiac function	none	asymptomatic, decline of resting ejection fraction by <20% of baseline value	asymptomatic, decline of resting ejection fraction by >20% of baseline value	mild CHF, responsive to therapy	severe or refractory CHF
	Cardiac—ischemia	none	nonspecific T wave flattening	asymptomatic, ST and T wave changes suggesting ischemia	angina without evidence for infarction	acute myocardial infarction
	Cardiac—pericardial	none	asymptomatic effusion, no intervention required	pericarditis (rub, chest pain, ECG changes)	symptomatic effusion, drainage required	tamponade, drainage urgently required

Appendix II—Common Toxicity Criteria (continued)

	Toxicity	Grade 0	Grade 1	Grade 2	Grade 3	Grade 4
Blood Pressure	Hypertension	none or no change	asymptomatic, transient increase by >20 mmHg (D) or to >150/100 if previously WNL; no treatment required	recurrent or persistent increase by >20 mmHg (D) or to >150/100 if previously WNL; no treatment required	requires therapy	hypertensive crisis
	Hypotension	none or no change	changes requiring no therapy (including transient orthostatic hypotension)	requires fluid replacement or other therapy but not hospitalization	requires therapy and hospitalization; resolves within 48 hr of stopping the agent	requires therapy and hospitalization for >48 hr after stopping the agent
Neurological	Neuro—sensory	none or no change	mild paresthesias, loss of deep tendon reflexes	mild or moderate objective sensory loss; moderate paresthesias	severe objective sensory loss or paresthesias that interfere with function	—
	Neuro—motor	none or no change	subjective weakness; no objective findings	mild objective weakness without significant impairment of function	objective weakness with impairment of function	paralysis
	Neuro—cortical	none	mild somnolence or agitation	moderate somnolence or agitation	severe somnolence, agitation, confusion, disorientation, or hallucinations	coma, seizures, toxic psychosis
	Neuro—cerebellar	none	slight incoordination, dysdiadochokinesis	intention tremor, dysmetria, slurred speech, nystagmus	locomotor ataxia	cerebellar necrosis
	Neuro—mood	no change	mild anxiety or depression	moderate anxiety or depression	severe anxiety or depression	suicidal ideation
	Neuro—headache	none	mild	moderate or severe but transient	unrelenting and severe	—
	Neuro—constipation	none or no change	mild	moderate	severe	ileus >96 hr
	Neuro—hearing	none or no change	asymptomatic, hearing loss on audiometry only	tinnitus	hearing loss interfering with function but correctable with hearing aid	deafness not correctable
	Neuro—vision	none or no change	—	—	symptomatic subtotal loss of vision	blindness
	Skin	none or no change	scattered macular or papular eruption or erythema that is asymptomatic	scattered macular or papular eruption or erythema with pruritus or other associated symptoms	generalized symptomatic macular, papular, or vesicular eruption	exfoliative dermatitis or ulcerating dermatitis
	Allergy	none	transient rash, drug fever <38°C (100.4°F)	urticaria, drug fever = 38°C (100.4°F), mild bronchospasm	serum sickness, bronchospasm, requires parenteral meds	anaphylaxis
	Fever in absence of infection	none	37.1–38.0°C 98.7–100.4°F	38.1–40.0°C 100.5–104.0°F	>40.0°C >104.0°F for <24 hr	>40.0°C (104.0°F) for >24 hr or fever accompanied by hypotension
	Local	none	pain	pain and swelling, with inflammation or phlebitis	ulceration	plastic surgery indicated
	Weight gain/loss	<5.0%	5.0–9.9%	10.0–19.9%	≤20.0%	—

Appendix II—Common Toxicity Criteria (continued)

	Toxicity	Grade 0	Grade 1	Grade 2	Grade 3	Grade 4
Metabolic	Hyperglycemia	<116	116–160	161–250	251–500	>500 or ketoacidosis
	Hypoglycemia	>64	55–64	40–54	30–39	<30
	Amylase	WNL	$<1.5 \times N$	$1.5–2.0 \times N$	$2.1–5.0 \times N$	$>5.1 \times N$
	Hypercalcemia	<10.6	10.6–11.5	11.6–12.5	12.6–13.5	≥13.5
	Hypocalcemia	>8.4	8.4–7.8	7.7–7.0	6.9–6.1	≤6.0
	Hypomagnesemia	>1.4	1.4–1.2	1.1–0.9	0.8–0.6	≤0.5
Coagulation	Fibrinogen	WNL	$0.99–0.75 \times N$	$0.74–0.50 \times N$	$0.49–0.25 \times N$	$≤0.24 \times N$
	Prothrombin time	WNL	$1.01–1.25 \times N$	$1.26–1.50 \times N$	$1.51–2.00 \times N$	$>2.00 \times N$
	Partial thromboplastin time	WNL	$1.01–1.66 \times N$	$1.67–2.33 \times N$	$2.34–3.00 \times N$	$>3.00 \times N$

SOURCE: developed by the National Cancer Institute. WBC, white blood cell count; PLT, platelet count; WNL, within normal limits; Hb, hemoglobin; Rx, treatment; N, normal; SGOT, serum glutamic-oxaloacetic transaminase; SGPT, serum glutamic-pyruvate transaminase; Alk Phos, alkaline phosphatase; PFTs, pulmonary function tests; CHF, congestive heart failure; ECG, electrocardiogram.

Appendix III—Karnofsky Performance Status Scale

Description	Karnofsky Scale
Normal; no complaints; no evidence of disease	100
Able to carry on normal activity; minor signs or symptoms of disease	90
Normal activity with effort; some signs or symptoms of disease	80
Cares for self; unable to carry on normal activity or to do active work	70
Requires occasional assistance but is able to care for most of own needs	60
Requires considerable assistance and frequent medical care	50
Disabled; requires special care and assistance	40
Severely disabled; hospitalization indicated although death is not imminent	30
Very sick: hospitalization necessary; active supportive treatment necessary	20
Moribund; fatal processes progressing rapidly	10
Dead	0

SOURCE: Karnofsky DA, Abelmann WH, Craver LF, et al. The use of the nitrogen mustards in the palliative treatment of carcinoma. *Cancer* 1948;1:634–56.

Answers to Self-Study Questions

Chapter 1

1. Proliferation of normal cells is controlled by feedback mechanisms that halt proliferation when there are sufficient cells to meet the physiological needs of the individual. In contrast, genetic changes in malignant cells result in loss of these feedback mechanisms and uncontrolled proliferation. Malignant cells continue to divide, often invading and destroying adjacent normal tissues. They can also break away from the primary tumor mass and establish metastases in distant tissues or organ. Uncontrolled proliferation will eventually result in death.

2. Malignant cells are undifferentiated and have lost the physiological function of the tissue of origin. In addition, these cells may exhibit gross changes in morphology, as well as alterations in their cellular membranes, and have chromosomal abnormalities that result in protein and enzyme content that is significantly different from their normal counterparts. Collectively, these differences influence the cells' sensitivity to chemotherapy and radiation.

3. b
4. tumor suppressor genes
5. d
6. b
7. They do not metastasize or destroy adjacent normal tissues. It is frequently the metastases of malignant tumors that invade and destroy vital organs, such as the liver, brain, or lungs. Pain and symptoms caused by either benign or malignant tumors may result from growth of the tumor mass and compression of surrounding tissues.
8. sun exposure, alcohol ingestion, cigarette smoking, and high-fat, low-fiber diet
9. a
10. lung (in the smoker and in the spouses of smokers due to passive smoking), mouth, lip, pharynx, esophagus, bladder
11. breast, ovarian
12. Epstein-Barr virus: Burkitt's lymphoma in African children

    Epstein-Barr virus: nasopharyngeal carcinoma

    hepatitis B and human papillomavirus: hepatocellular carcinoma and cervical cancers

    HTLV-1 virus: adult T-cell leukemia

    Infection of cells with these viruses is believed to lead to genetic mutations that ultimately contribute to the malignant transformation.
13. sarcomas, leukemias, lymphomas
14. clinician breast examination, mammography, pelvic examination with Pap smear. In addition, she should be instructed to perform monthly breast self-examination.
15. digital rectal exam, prostate-specific antigen test, stool guaiac, sigmoidoscopy
16. A cancer screening initiative should be both sensitive (resulting in true positives) and specific (resulting in true negatives) enough that if applied to either the general or a high-risk population it will result in a measurable decrease in morbidity and mortality of the target cancer. In addition, the screening test or procedure must be acceptable to the target population. That is, it should not be excessively painful, discomforting, or inconvenient. The test or procedure should present little or no risk (i.e., it is unlikely that an asymptomatic individual will be harmed). Finally, the process (including the test and its interpretation) should be economically justifiable to society.
17. colon, breast, lung
18. lung
19. b

Chapter 2

1. c. The tumor doubled in number of cells twice (from 4 to 8 cells, then 8 to 16). Two doublings in one year is a doubling time of 6 months (12 months divided by 2 doublings).

2. a

3. The curve should show an early phase of exponential growth (steep curve) that occurs early in the life of a tumor mass when the growth fraction is high. Gradually tumor growth slows and the curve levels off to a plateau phase as the percentage of cells actively dividing decreases (the tumor may be outgrowing its food and blood supply) and more cells are dying.

4. a. True. It takes about 30 doublings to reach a tumor that is 1 cm in diameter, which is the lower limit of size for clinical detection. Only a few more doublings are required to reach a 1–2 kg mass, which is incompatible with life.

5. b. Cells can shed from a tumor at any point in the tumor's life. Whether or not these shed cells result in metastases depends on "seed and soil"—does the cell reach a tissue that provides the growth conditions it needs? Answer *c* is not correct, because most hematological malignancies grow quickly (short doubling time that may be measured in hours, days, or weeks) compared with most solid tumors (doubling time in weeks or months, sometimes years).

6. b. False. Some cancers in some stages of growth are not known to be curable. This is true for most solid tumors diagnosed as metastatic disease, for example.

7. c. Chemotherapy may be given to relieve symptoms if the side effects of the chemotherapy are not more troublesome than the symptoms.

8. a. In general, the more there is to gain, the greater the risk that is acceptable.

9. a. The best way to cure most solid tumors is to surgically remove the tumor while it is still contained in the tissue of origin.

10. c. Although some radiation is given by interstitial techniques (from within the tumor mass), most is given by external beam (from outside the body). Surgery and radiation are the best treatment modalities for managing localized tumors. Fractionating the dose of radiation therapy refers to giving the dose in many small doses to decrease toxicity to normal tissue. Radiation doses are measured in grays or centigrays.

11. d

12. Some nononcological uses of oncology drugs include treatment of rheumatoid arthritis, ectopic pregnancy, plantar warts, steroid-dependent asthma, lupus nephritis, hepatitis, psoriasis.

13. adjuvant chemotherapy

14. Patients may receive adjuvant chemotherapy when they are already cured by surgery or radiation therapy because the patient population for adjuvant treatment is the patients who are free of *visible disease* but at high *statistical* risk of recurrence. Decisions are made on population statistics because there is no way at present to select with complete accuracy the patients who have already been truly cured and those with residual micrometastases. Use of prognostic indicators helps in patient selection and can suggest that an individual is at high or low risk of recurrence, but no indicator or panel of indicators is 100% accurate.

15. The clearest examples of cancers for which adjuvant therapy increases the number of patients cured of cancer are breast cancer and colorectal cancer. Other less well-established cancers are melanoma, ovarian cancer, and osteogenic sarcoma.

16. b. A partial response requires a decrease in tumor size by ≥50%.

17. c. Stable disease is defined as an increase or decrease of <25%. To be officially defined as progression, tumor size must increase by ≥25% compared with, previous measurements.

18. breast and prostate cancers

19. b

20. Response rate (also called objective response rate) is the combined percentage of complete and partial responses.

21. c. To make a significant impact on cancer outcomes, chemotherapy regimens must increase overall survival. Regimen C increases overall survival by the greatest length of time (6 months), although it has the lowest response rate.

Chapter 3

1. Alkylating agents: cyclophosphamide, ifosfamide, melphalan, chlorambucil, mechlorethamine, thiotepa

   (1) The template or DNA strand being replicated may be misread or mispaired during DNA synthesis; (2) cross-linking may prevent the DNA strands from unwinding, which could hinder replication; and (3) the alkylating agents may produce either single- or double-strand breaks in the DNA. Any of these processes could inhibit DNA, RNA, or protein synthesis.

2. b. Alkylating agents are cell cycle nonspecific (i.e., they can exert their effect during any phase of the cell cycle) and, as a class, they are significantly myelosuppressive.

3. e. Ifosfamide/cyclophosphamide hemorrhagic cystitis is dose-related but not influenced by urinary pH and can be effectively prevented by administering mesna before and after drug administration. Once hemorrhagic cystitis has occurred, mesna will not alleviate it. On a milligram-to-milligram basis, the risk is equal with these two drugs; however, the conventional dose of ifosfamide is higher (to produce equivalent alkylating activity) than the conventional dose of cyclophosphamide. Thus, hemorrhagic cystitis is more common following ifosfamide.

4. e. In addition to each of these mechanisms, the anthracyclines, like doxorubicin, also catalyze the production of oxygen free radicals that may damage cell membranes. It is likely that a combination of all these effects ultimately leads to the death of the cell.

5. b. Dexrazoxane is a strong iron chelator that removes iron from the anthracycline (e.g., doxorubicin) complex and reduces the generation of oxygen free radicals. In some clinical trials, myelosuppression was slightly more severe when dexrazoxane was given with an anthracycline.

6. *reduced*. Bleomycin is excreted primarily unchanged in the urine, and increases in the serum half-life secondary to decreased glomerular filtration have been associated with an increased risk of pulmonary toxicity.

7. b. False. Bleomycin pulmonary toxicity is related to the total cumulative dose.

8. e. All of the above can cause severe tissue damage if extravasated during administration.

9. Topoisomerases are enzymes that facilitate the unwinding, separation, and orderly rejoining of complementary DNA strands during DNA synthesis and transcription. Topoisomerase I relaxes the supercoiled, double-stranded DNA above and below the site that is unwinding, which allows the cleaving and resealing of the strand. Topoisomerase II facilitates double-strand breaks by relaxing and swiveling the supercoiled helix during DNA synthesis and resealing. Topoisomerase II may also contribute to the separation of the two daughter cells at the end of mitosis.

10. b. In patients receiving transplant regimens of 4 mg/kg per day for 4 days, AUCs were significantly higher in patients developing hepatic veno-occlusive disease than those not experiencing hepatic effects.

11. e. All of these mechanisms are believed to contribute to the activity of cisplatin and carboplatin.

12. c. Clinical responses have been correlated to adduct formation in both tumors cells and peripheral blood leukocytes of patients receiving cisplatin therapy.

13. c. thrombocytopenia

14. The most frequent mechanism of resistance to anthracyclines is increased drug efflux due to amplification of the gene for P-glycoprotein, a multidrug cell transporter.

15. b. Both the parent drug and the metabolites are excreted in the bile, necessitating dosage reductions in patients with biliary obstruction. Doxorubicin may cause cardiomyopathy leading to congestive heart failure and may be contraindicated in patients with significant underlying cardiac disease. Dose reduction would only decrease the likelihood of clinical response and place the patient at increased risk of further cardiac deterioration.

Chapter 4

1. In tumor cells, there is a higher concentration of the larger polyglutamated methotrextate molecules, which have more difficulty exiting the tumor cells than the nonglutamated methotrexate molecules. The resulting higher intracellular concentration of polyglutamated methotrexate is more difficult to displace with leucovorin administration.

2. Three mechanisms that slow methotrexate elimination include: (1) drugs that impair methotrexate elimination, such as ibuprofen, ketoprofen, aspirin, and penicillin; (2) renal dysfunction; and (3) fluid accumulations, such as pleural effusions or ascites.

3. b. False. The answer is false because gemcitabine is retained intracellularly significantly longer than cytarabine. This is one explanation for gemcitabine's broader in vitro activity.

4. d. Patients receiving high-dose cytarabine can experience a severe conjunctivitis that is prevented by the administration of corticosteroid eye drops throughout treatment. High-dose cytarabine is also quite emetogenic.

5. c. The pneumonitis is usually reversible and resolves spontaneously over several weeks with or without steroid therapy.

6. b. About 30% of patients have transient elevations in transaminases. The rise in transaminases typically occurs early in therapy, peaks by cycle 2, and returns to baseline by the end of therapy.

7. In contrast to high-dose methotrexate treatment, in which leucovorin therapy rescues normal cells from

the lethal effects of methotrexate, administration of leucovorin with fluorouracil increases the binding of the fluorouracil metabolite FdUMP to the reduced folate and its catalyzing enzyme thymidylate synthase. This increased binding increases the inhibition of DNA synthesis by fluorouracil.

8. c. If fluorouracil is given by continuous infusion over several days, mucosal damage manifesting as stomatitis and diarrhea is usually the dose-limiting toxicity. If fluoruracil is given by weekly or monthly bolus injections, the predominant toxicity is myelosuppression.

9. b. Paclitaxel exhibits nonlinear pharmacokinetics, and the duration of paclitaxel above a critical plasma concentration appears to influence neutropenia more than the peak serum concentration. Because hepatic extraction and biliary secretion account for most elimination, renal dysfunction does not appear to influence toxicity. Premedication with corticosteroids helps prevent hypersensitivity reactions.

10. d. The fluid retention caused by docetaxel does not appear to be related to cardiac, renal, endocrine, hepatic, or pulmonary disease. The only recognized predisposing factor is cumulative dose. Treatment with corticosteroids with each cycle appears to delay the onset of this manifestation.

11. c

12. a. Early diarrhea is believed to be a cholinergic effect that can be managed with atropine. Late diarrhea can be very serious and result in life-threatening dehydration and electrolyte imbalances. Aggressive therapy with loperamide is recommended for late diarrhea, and fluid and electrolyte therapy should be initiated whenever clinically warranted. Subsequent doses of irinotecan should be reduced.

13. a

14. b. The other agents can all be safely administered by rapid bolus injection.

15. b

16. The taxanes, like paclitaxel, promote microtubule assembly and bind to the stabilized microtubules once they have been formed. The net effect is arrest of the mitotic cellular division. In contrast, the vinca alkaloids inhibit assembly of the microtubules, arresting cells during metaphase of mitosis.

Chapter 5

1. d
2. b
3. a
4. a
5. c
6. d
7. b
8. d
9. c
10. a
11. c
12. b
13. a
14. b
15. d
16. a
17. d
18. b
19. a
20. d
21. c
22. a
23. c
24. bystander effect
25. b

Chapter 6

1. Both toxic and therapeutic effects of chemotherapy have a steep dose-response curve. If the dose is reduced to avoid a toxic effect, then the therapeutic efficacy may be compromised. If the dose-related toxicity is intolerable or life-threatening, then dose reductions may be necessary unless another strategy (e.g., use of chemoprotectant or rescue drug) are available to manage the toxic effects.

2. Small cell lung cancer is most likely to be sensitive to chemotherapy. Most chemotherapy drugs are capable of killing only dividing cells, so the tumor is most susceptible to chemotherapy when it is growing rapidly.

3. d
4. c
5. first-order. The absolute number of cells that are killed by a chemotherapy regimen is proportional to the dose administered.

6. Cells within the mass are heterogenous and not equally susceptible to cytotoxic effects. In addition, the cells may not have equal access to oxygen or nutrients necessary to sustain growth, and the drug molecules may not be able to penetrate the tumor mass and affect all cells.
7. d
8. (1) Cells lack necessary drug-activating enzyme(s); (2) cells overproduce enzymes responsible for drug destruction; (3) cells have faulty transport mechanisms that prevent drug entry into the cell; (4) efflux of the drug from the cell is so rapid that the cytotoxic effect cannot be realized; or (5) cells may be able to repair cytotoxic damage to DNA.
9. mutations, gene amplifications
10. b
11. e
12. b
13. It has a short half-life and is only active during the S phase of the cell cycle. Administration by prolonged infusion allows many more leukemia cells to come into contact with the drug during their S phase.
14. activation
15. Within a tumor there may be thousands of tumor cells clones, each with its own pattern of drug sensitivity. By administering multiple drugs, there is a greater chance of eradicating more cells or clones. In addition, more than one drug may attack a cancer cell simultaneously, and multiple drug-induced biochemical lesions may have an increased likelihood of inflicting mortal injury to the cell.
16. b
17. c
18. The disadvantages of combination chemotherapy include: (1) they have multiple toxicities; (2) it is often necessary to reduce doses for individual drugs and potentially compromise their effectiveness; (3) they are complicated to administer; and (4) they are expensive.
19. The principles for developing combination therapies include: (1) each drug has demonstrated single-agent activity in the tumor type; (2) drugs have minimal overlapping toxicities; and (3) drugs have different mechanisms of action.
20. Three strategies that minimize dose-related neutropenia while maintaining chemotherapy effectiveness include: (1) modestly reducing the dose of myelosuppressive drugs; (2) administering filgrastim or sargramostim; and (3) administering non-myelosuppressive antineoplastic agents between cycles of myelosuppressive drugs.
21. b. False. The decision whether to use chemotherapy should not be based on age but rather on the patient's organ function and baseline performance status.
22. Whenever possible, corticosteroids should be avoided because they impair cell-mediated immunity. Several studies have shown that patients are less likely to respond to chemotherapy if their cell-mediated immunity is impaired. If the reaction is severe or life threatening, the benefit of steroids may outweigh this risk.

Chapter 7

1. b
2. c
3. cytarabine, fluorouracil, docetaxel, doxorubicin, or methotrexate
4. b
5. d
6. c
7. b
8. a
9. c
10. b
11. a
12. d
13. The advantages of ice pack use are that it decreases hair loss by producing vasoconstriction in scalp vessels and decreasing drug circulation to the scalp and that it is inexpensive. The disadvantages are that ice pack use is uncomfortable and cumbersome and that there is a risk of creating a tumor sanctuary.
14. d
15. c
16. b
17. a
18. b
19. c
20. Although chemotherapy can produce sterility in males, mature sperm are resistant to the effects of cytotoxic drugs. Because of this resistance, sperm counts usually do not drop until 2–3 months after chemotherapy begins. Because this patient started treatment just 3 weeks ago, it is likely that his sperm count is still unaf-

fected. If he and his girlfriend do not wish to risk pregnancy, it is essential that they use an effective form of birth control.

Chapter 8

1. b
2. d. Risk of anthracycline-induced cardiac toxicity is greater in females than males.
3. Dexrazoxane is a metal chelator. Iron is required to produce the free radicals that are believed to be responsible for the classic form of anthracycline-induced cardiac muscle damage. Dexrazoxane is believed to chelate the iron, making it unavailable for formation of free radicals and thereby preventing the development of cardiac muscle damage.
4. a. True. Anthracycline-induced cardiac damage is associated with high peak levels of anthracyclines in cardiac tissue. Interventions that decrease the peak levels decrease the risk of cardiac damage without compromising antitumor effects.
5. c
6. b
7. d
8. a. Providing a high concentration of chloride ions helps keep cisplatin in its nonaquated and less nephrotoxic form. Magnesium supplementation replaces magnesium lost as a result of cisplatin-induced renal defects.
9. d
10. b. False. It is likely that the glomerular filtration rate decreases with each cisplatin cycle, but this is not always reflected by changes in the serum creatinine.
11. a
12. c. Urine alkalinization increases the solubility of methotrexate in the urine and decreases the risk of precipitation. Leucovorin does not affect the risk or incidence of methotrexate-induced renal damage.
13. Carboxypeptidase G2 is an enzyme that cleaves methotrexate into inactive components. It serves as an alternate route of elimination of methotrexate in patients who cannot clear methotrexate renally.
14. c. Chronic low-dose administration of methotrexate increases the risk of liver damage, but renal damage is linked with high-dose administration and concomitant administration of other agents that can reduce methotrexate clearance, such as cisplatin and nonsteroidal anti-inflammatory drugs.
15. b
16. Conventional doses of parenteral cyclophosphamide have only a low risk of producing bladder damage. Oral hydration is usually an adequate intervention. Patients should be counseled to drink at least 2 L of fluid the day of cyclophosphamide administration and for 1–2 days following treatment. At least two large glasses of fluid should be consumed before bedtime to ensure that the patient will need to awaken during the night to void.
17. Hydration flushes acrolein, the bladder-toxic metabolite of cyclophosphamide and ifosfamide, from the bladder, decreasing its contact time with the bladder wall. Mesna is a sulfhydryl donor that complexes with acrolein, making a nontoxic complex that can then be eliminated in the urine.
18. d. Recommended mesna dosing for ifosfamide short infusion is a dose equal to 20% of the ifosfamide dose before ifosfamide and every 4 hours for two additional doses.
19. b
20. d. Vigorous fluid administration (hyperhydration regimens) and/or mesna can decrease the risk of bladder damage secondary to high-dose cyclophosphamide.
21. b. Long-term methotrexate therapy produces gradual onset of liver fibrosis or cirrhosis. It is most common with low oral daily doses.
22. a
23. a
24. c. Fluorouracil and levamisole both have low risks of liver damage as single agents. This risk is not increased by combination of fluorouracil and leucovorin, but about 40% of patients receiving the combination of fluorouracil and levamisole have increases in liver function tests (LFTs).
25. d. Hepatic toxicity is a rare and unpredictable side effect of tamoxifen. Routine monitoring of LFTs is not useful or recommended.
26. Most antineoplastic drugs that cause pulmonary damage produce a similar clinical picture. Characteristic symptoms are shortness of breath, often with nonproductive cough, weakness, and fatigue. Chest X-rays show a reticulonodular pattern. Pulmonary function test results are nonspecific but may show abnormal carbon monoxide diffusing capacity.
27. b. False. Corticosteroids are rapidly effective in management of the retinoic acid syndrome, the characteristic pulmonary toxicity caused by tretinoin.

28. a
29. d
30. Interleukin 2 causes a capillary leak syndrome that results in fluid retention, causing fluid accumulation in the lungs and interfering with air exchange.
31. b
32. a. Risk of neurological toxicity from HDAC is increased in the elderly and greatly increased in patients with impaired renal function.
33. a. Vincristine, cisplatin, and paclitaxel characteristically produce peripheral neuropathies with numbness and tingling in the extremities.
34. c
35. a

Chapter 9

1. d
2. b
3. d
4. b
5. e
6. c
7. b
8. d
9. c
10. a
11. d
12. a
13. c
14. d
15. d
16. e
17. a
18. d
19. b
20. e
21. a
22. a
23. a
24. a
25. b
26. b
27. b
28. a
29. b
30. a

Chapter 10

1. twice
2. phlebitis, embolization, extravasation, enhanced toxicity due to higher serum concentrations
3. (1) The purpose and duration of the injection—some sites are inappropriate for vesicant injections or prolonged infusions.

    (2) The type of venous access device that will be used.

    (3) The physical condition and level of activity of the patient.
4. a
5. Irritant drugs produce local pain, erythema and swelling around the site of injection. Vesicants may cause the same type of local symptoms initially but then go on to cause tissue damage that may be quite severe. Local hypersensitivity reactions may occur even if the drug is not extravasated and cause erythema or a rash along the vein track.
6. c
7. vascular disease; elevated venous pressure; previous radiation therapy to the site; injection at the antecubital fossa, wrist, or dorsum of the hand; recent venipuncture in the same vein
8. dull ache in the shoulder, arm or neck; supraclavicular fullness or swelling; venous distension in the neck or chest; and arm swelling
9. b. False. Locking the catheter with heparinized saline may help to prevent the formation of clots at the tip of the catheter or within the lumen but will not prevent the formation of thrombi around the lumen. Heparin "locked" within the catheter lumen would not come in contact with the circulating blood.
10. Staphylococcal epidermidis
11. c. Once the clot has formed, heparin will not dissolve it. Heparin is only effective in preventing clot formation.
12. signs of infection surrounding the exit site or tunnel (e.g., pain, erythema, or swelling) and/or blood cultures that are positive for the same organism drawn from a peripheral vein and the access device

13. The infusion rate is generally preset—the only way to alter it is to change the concentration of drug in the device; and they have no alarms or warning features.
14. Only a small volume of drug can be stored in the device reservoir; the infusion rate must be low; they require a surgical procedure for placement; and they are more expensive unless used for long periods of time.
15. ovarian cancer, melanoma, mesotheliomas, and gastrointestinal cancers
16. bacterial and chemical peritonitis, abdominal pain, bleeding, bowel perforation, ileus, and fluid leakage
17. cytarabine, methotrexate, and thiotepa
18. b. False. Studies have demonstrated that when administered via the Ommaya reservoir, methotrexate distributes throughout the CSF. In addition, the device may also be used for withdrawing CSF for cytologic, biochemical, and bacteriological testing.
19. performance status, size of tumor, presence of extrahepatic disease, extent of prior chemotherapy and radiation therapy

Chapter 11

1. c
2. a
3. e
4. d
5. a
6. e
7. b
8. a
9. d
10. b
11. c
12. e

Chapter 12

1. c
2. b
3. c
4. b
5. d
6. d
7. b
8. c
9. a
10. b
11. a
12. a
13. c
14. b
15. a
16. b

Chapter 13

1. b
2. d
3. c
4. a
5. b
6. d
7. c
8. b
9. a
10. d
11. c
12. b
13. e
14. a
15. c
16. a
17. c
18. b
19. d
20. a
21. a
22. c
23. d
24. a
25. a
26. d
27. b
28. a
29. a

30. b
31. d
32. a
33. d
34. c
35. b
36. e
37. a
38. d
39. b
40. c

Chapter 14

1. a
2. b
3. b
4. In autologous BMT, bone marrow is collected from the patient prior to transplantation, whereas in allogeneic BMT, bone marrow is harvested from another individual (such as a sibling).
5. Chemotherapy doses used in the BMT setting are significantly higher than standard doses. As a result, a number of serious nonhematological toxicities may be observed in this patient population.
6. d
7. d
8. b
9. b
10. a
11. c
12. a
13. Cyclosporine inhibits the activation of T cells by interleukin 2; T cells are the primary initiators of GVHD. Cyclosporine is one of the most effective single agents in the prevention of GVHD.
14. b
15. Hypomagnesemia, hyperkalemia, hypotension, tremors, hirsutism, and renal insufficiency. More serious side effects include serious neurotoxicity and liver toxicity.
16. c
17. b
18. d
19. a
20. Patients with GVHD require prolonged immunosuppressive therapy for as long as they have active disease. Because of this prolonged immunosuppression, they remain at risk for severe opportunistic infections.

Chapter 15

1. 1000 and 100
2. by damaging the mucosa that lines the gastrointestinal and respiratory tracts
3. antipseudomonal penicillin, cephalosporin
4. a
5. how promptly the therapy is begun after symptoms appear
6. amphotericin B
7. Fungal infections are life threatening and often difficult to diagnose.
8. acyclovir
9. intravenous immune globulin
10. Bathe and shampoo daily with a germicidal soap and refuse contact with people who have not washed their hands with a germicidal soap.

Chapter 16

1. d
2. e
3. b
4. e
5. c
6. c
7. b
8. a
9. a
10. b
11. e
12. a
13. c
14. c
15. b
16. a

17. b
18. d
19. a

Chapter 17

1. a
2. Symptoms include pain, nausea, anorexia, depression, anxiety, sleep disorders, and dyspnea.
3. fatigue, weight loss, anorexia, or insomnia
4. dysphoric mood, feeling of hopelessness, guilt, worthlessness, or suicidal thoughts
5. b
6. b
7. poor concentration, poor memory, irritability, dizziness, fatigue, insomnia, nightmares, headache, panic attacks, or tremors
8. a
9. a
10. a
11. b
12. b
13. haloperidol
14. Dyssomnia is a primary disorder that results as a disturbance of quantity, quality, or timing of nocturnal sleep.
15. a
16. disturbances of nighttime sleep, medications, metabolic disorders (such as hypercalcemia), or disturbances of the sleep-wake cycle
17. b
18. a
19. See Table 17-5.
20. b
21. opiates, benzodiazepines, and antihistamines; not tested: theophylline, respiratory stimulants, and prostaglandins

Chapter 18

1. nausea and vomiting, taste alterations, mucositis, xerostomia, and malabsorption
2. obstruction of gastrointestinal or biliary tract, secretion of humoral factors, development of fistulas leading to protein loss, and difficulty chewing or swallowing because of tumor mass
3. fat
4. a
5. lymphocyte counts, anergy panels, albumin, and anthropometric measurements
6. height; estimate of ideal body weight; actual weight; weight before illness; measurements of triceps skin fold and mid-upper-arm circumference; serum albumin; prealbumin or transferrin; and record of current oral intake
7. when patients have hyperglycemia or are fluid restricted
8. decreased serum proteins and negative nitrogen balance
9. c
10. a
11. lymphocytes, macrophages, and mucosal cells
12. fat, total calories, and low fiber
13. dexamethasone, delta-tetrahydrocannabinol, and metoclopramide

Chapter 19

1. They differ in amino acid sequencing. Salmon calcitonin is more potent and has a longer duration of activity. Doses are not interchangeable.
2. multiple myeloma and some of the hematological tumors
3. a
4. b
5. a
6. chemotherapy alone or combined with radiation
7. presenting symptoms, rate of progression, site of cord compression, and tumor type
8. It decreases edema and inflammation, alleviates pain, and is cytotoxic to some tumors.
9. allopurinol
10. a

Chapter 20

1. Measurement of urine mutagenicity and urine thioethers, assessment of chromosomal damage, studies of fetal loss, and measurement of serum or urine concentrations of cytotoxics. When assessing urine mutagenicity or chromosomal damage, it is only an assumption that the effect is a result of cytotoxic exposure. It is known that other drugs as well as environ-

mental and lifestyle factors may also produce these types of effects. Also, in many published studies, there were no baseline assessments done prior to the worker's exposure. Studies examining the rate of fetal loss or malformation during pregnancy have relied on worker recall of their exposure during the first trimester. In some cases this recall has been as long as 10 years after the fact and the reliability of the exposure estimation has been questioned. Finally, because of the small amount of drug absorbed through accidental exposure (e.g., through aerosolization or percutaneous absorption), very sensitive assays would be necessary and workers need to be screened for multiple drugs that they presumably would be manipulating.

2. b
3. d
4. Type A hoods recirculate air, exhausting a small portion of filtered air to the room environment, and type B exhaust air to the outside.
5. b. False. Surgical masks are of limited value because they provide no respiratory protection against either powdered or liquid aerosols. Furthermore, if the view screen of the cabinet is properly placed and the cabinet is in good working condition, there should be no appreciable risk of contamination of the room air.
6. b. False. Because of the possible association of fetal loss or malformations and cytotoxic exposure, most published guidelines and recommendations (including the ASHP TAB) state that such workers should be reassigned during these periods.
7. No general procedures or techniques are currently available that would provide useful information regarding hazardous drug exposure. It is recommended that pre-employment health history and physical be completed with annual follow-ups. Any evidence of a worker's exposure (e.g., documentation of a spill) should be reported to appropriate authorities and documented in the worker's medical records.
8. Verbal orders, multiple-day drug orders, abbreviations, poor documentation for cited regimens or protocols, errors in references, inadequate interdisciplinary communication, limited education of health care professionals and patients, and the wide variability of chemotherapy doses commonly used have been implicated in contributing to medication-related errors.
9. Every chemotherapy order should include specification of the chemotherapy regimen or protocol; cycle number; patient age, weight, height, and calculated body surface area (BSA); white blood cell count; platelet count; hemoglobin and hematocrit; hydration fluids and antiemetics (if appropriate); generic name of the drug; dose to be given in standard units (e.g., milligrams) per meter squared; calculated total dose (dose/m^2 × BSA); frequency; days to be administered; and infusion guidelines (for parenteral drugs).

10. Drugs should always be ordered using generic names, never trade names, abbreviations, or synonyms. Presumably, the prescriber was referring to doxorubicin (tradename Adriamycin). Trailing zeros are also dangerous, especially when the orders are faxed or when carbon copy orders are used. Poor quality or artifacts can cause the loss of the decimal point, and the dose could be interpreted as 400 mg. The order is also confusing because it is not clear if the 40 mg is to be administered each day or divided between multiple days. The use of a range (e.g., 1–3 days) rather than explicitly listing the days the drug should be administered may also be misinterpreted. For example, this order could be interpreted in several ways: (1) 40 mg should be administered each day on days 1, 2, and 3; (2) 40 mg should be divided and one third of it given on each of days 1, 2, and 3; (3) 40 mg should be administered on days 1 and 3; or (4) 40 mg should be divided and half administered on days 1 and 2. Finally, the indication of the BSA could also lead one to believe that the intended dose was actually 40 mg/m^2. A more appropriate order would read: doxorubicin 40 mg/m^2 = 68 mg daily on days 1, 2, and 3. BSA = 1.7 m^2.

11. b. False. The label should always be placed directly on the syringe. If multiple syringes are required for a single dose, each syringe should be labeled.

12. Recalculate the patient's BSA and the total dose, compare with previous chemotherapy orders for this patient and question any unexpected changes, compare the dose and schedule with the standard chemotherapy regimen or protocol, assess any need to modify doses based on blood counts or renal or hepatic function, ensure that hydration fluids and antiemetics are appropriately prescribed for the chemotherapy regimen, and ensure that there is adequate drug inventory to complete the patient's course of therapy.

13. Institutional policies should require that all chemotherapy orders be written by oncologists whose credentials have been reviewed by appropriate authorities. Medical residents, non-oncologists, nurse practitioners, and physician assistants should not be permitted to order chemotherapy. The pharmacist should be empowered to request published literature substantiating doses outside the usual dose ranges and once again, written policies should reinforce this practice. If the chemotherapy is an emergency it would be reasonable for the pharmacist to consult with an oncologist

that evening via telephone. The order should not be filled until the issue has been resolved to the satisfaction of the pharmacist.

14. Any of the texts listed in Table 20-4 would be appropriate for your collection. At least one of these should provide in-depth information regarding chemotherapy drugs, including their pharmacology, adverse effects, dosing, and pharmaceutical issues (e.g., compatibility, stability, etc). *The Cancer Chemotherapy Handbook* by Dorr and Von Hoff is probably the most appropriate for this purpose. If specialty oncology services will be supported by your pharmacy, you will probably also want to include texts that deal with areas such as pediatric or gynecological oncology.

15. The Office of Alternative Medicines or the Office of Dietary Supplements at the National Institutes of Health may provide helpful information. In addition, the FDA Consumer Product Safety Commission, the National Council Against Health Fraud, and the Cancer Information Line may also be consulted.

16. Because this drug may represent a last hope for the patient, it is important that he understands that you take his request very seriously. First, you must find the source of the information and determine which drug the patient described. A call to the television station may help. If this is an investigational drug, contacting the National Cancer Institute or the manufacturer (if known) may provide useful information. If not, a call to the source of the news story (probably a medical school or hospital) is warranted. Information you should request would include basic pharmacologic information, the status of the drug's availability (investigational versus marketed), and, if the drug is investigational, ascertain whether there are ongoing clinical trials that the patient may be eligible to participate in.

Glossary

Absolute granulocyte count—the white blood cell concentration multiplied by the fraction of segmented neutrophils or neutrophils.

Adjuvant analgesic drug—a drug that is not a primary analgesic but that research has shown to have independent or additive analgesic properties.

Adjuvant therapy—systemically administered therapy with cytotoxic drugs, hormones, or biological response modifiers to kill micrometastases after the primary tumor mass has been eliminated or destroyed.

Alkylation—the substitution of an alkyl group for a hydrogen atom in an organic compound, such as DNA.

Alopecia—hair loss.

Amenorrhea—absence of menses.

Amnestic agents—drugs that induce memory loss; given to reduce anxiety about chemotherapy.

Anaphylaxis—hypersensitive reaction of bronchospasm and hypotension.

Angiogenesis—development of new blood vessels.

Anorexia—loss of appetite, especially as a result of disease.

Anticancer—*see* **Cytotoxic**.

Antigenic modulation—the loss of an antigen from the tumor cell surface.

Antineoplastic—*see* **Cytotoxic**.

Antitumor—*see* **Cytotoxic**.

Ataxia—impaired ability to coordinate movement.

Azoospermia—few or no sperm.

Benign tumor—a nonmalignant tumor.

Biological response modification—all anticancer treatment approaches that attempt to influence the patient's immune response to a tumor.

Biological safety cabinet—a self-contained cabinet with vertical laminar airflow for preparing hazardous agents (such as cytotoxics) from which the contaminated air does not escape into the environment.

Biomodulation—an agent, which need not be cytotoxic in itself, that is administered to increase either the antitumor effects or the selectivity for tumor cells of an active antineoplastic agent.

Blast cell—an abnormal, immature blood cell; an immature blood cell precursor.

Blast crisis—transformation from the chronic or accelerated phases of chronic myelogenous leukemia to acute leukemia, characterized by excessive leukemic blast cells in the blood and bone marrow.

Bone marrow aspirate—a sample of bone marrow fluid obtained by inserting a large-bore needle into bone tissue.

Bone marrow biopsy—a procedure in which a large-bore needle is inserted into bone, usually the posterior iliac crest, and a core of bone tissue is removed.

Bone marrow suppression—*see* **Myelosuppression**.

Breakthrough pain—intermittent exacerbations of pain that occur spontaneously or in relation to specific activity.

B symptoms—designated as "B symptoms" by the Ann Arbor Staging Classification System for lymphomas; constitutional symptoms, such as fever, weight loss, and night sweats, present in stage B lymphomas (e.g., stage III_B).

Butterfly—stainless steel scalp vein needle.

Calcitonin—a hormone that inhibits bone resorption, lowers serum calcium, and promotes renal excretion.

Cancer—a malignant, uncontrolled cellular growth with local tissue invasion or systemic spread of the disease or both.

Cancer cachexia—the syndrome of diminished appetite, fatigue, anemia, muscle wasting, organ atrophy, weight loss, and decreased performance status that accompanies cancer.

Carcinogen—a type of genotoxin that causes neoplasm formation.

Carcinoma—malignant tumor arising from epithelial tissue.

Cardiomyopathy—breakdown of heart muscle.

Castration—sterilization; removal of the ovaries or testicles.

Cell half-life—average time it takes for half of a cell population to die.

Cell turnover—the rate at which cells are depleted and replaced.

Chemoprotectant—an agent that protects normal tissue from the toxic damage of antineoplastic agents or radiation.

Chemosensitization—administering chemotherapy within a few days of radiation therapy to enhance the therapeutic effects of radiation.

Cholestasis—obstruction of the bile ducts.

Circadian timing—the biological rhythms of organisms during the 24-hour day.

Central nervous system (CNS) prophylaxis—chemotherapy or radiotherapy administered to eradicate clinically undetectable central nervous system leukemia.

Colony-stimulating factors—hormone-like substances that regulate growth, differentiation, and function of blood cells.

Complementary inhibition—a combination chemotherapy strategy in which one agent that inhibits a pathway contributing to DNA synthesis is combined with a drug that reacts directly with the DNA.

Complete response—also complete remission. Loss of evidence of measurable tumor as a result of cancer therapy. It is not necessarily synonymous with cure, because tumor cells may remain in collections too small to be detected clinically.

Concurrent inhibition—a combination chemotherapy strategy in which two or more parallel pathways leading to synthesis of DNA are interfered with at the same time.

Consolidation—chemotherapy administered after successful remission induction therapy in acute leukemia to further reduce any residual leukemic cells.

Cross-resistance—resistance that develops in a tumor mass to more than one agent simultaneously.

Cytokines—protein molecules that are produced by host macrophages and lymphocytes in response to noxious stimuli.

Cytotoxic—causing death to cells.

Disease progression—increase of a tumor mass by >25%, appearance of new lesions, or tumor-induced death.

Dose intensity—*see* Dose rate.

Dose limiting—a degree of toxicity that limits dosing or scheduling of anticancer therapy.

Dose rate—amount of drug given per unit of time.

Doubling time—the time it takes a tumor mass to double in size.

Dysarthria—impaired ability to coordinate muscles that control speech.

Dysdiadochokinesia—impaired ability to perform rapidly alternating movements.

Dysmetria—impaired position sense.

Dyspnea—shortness of breath.

Emesis—coordinated action of the gastrointestinal tract, respiratory muscles, and abdominal muscles to forcefully expel gastrointestinal contents.

Engraftment—the process in which the transplanted bone marrow cells begin producing new blood cells.

Epidural—situated within the spinal canal, on or outside the dura mater (the tough membrane surrounding the spinal cord).

Equianalgesic—having equal controlling effect; morphine sulfate, 10 mg intramuscularly is generally used for opioid analgesic comparisons.

Erythrocytes—red blood cells.

Extravasation—drug escape from the blood vessel.

First-order kinetics—each drug dose kills the same percentage of drug-sensitive cells regardless of the number of cells present.

Generation time—a complete cell cycle from one mitosis to the next.

Genotoxic—toxic to genetic material.

Germinal cells—reproductive cells of the gonads.

Gompertzian growth curve—rapid, logarithmic initial growth of tumors, followed by a plateau. The Gompertzian growth curve (Figure 2-3) demonstrates the theoretical pattern of tumor growth.

Granulocytes—one type of white blood cell.

Granulocytopenic—neutropenic or leukopenic; absolute granulocyte count <5000/mm^3.

Growth fraction—the percentage of actively dividing cells.

Hematological malignancies—cancers of the blood and lymphatic systems.

Hematological toxicities—toxicities of the blood system.

Hepatic veno-occlusive disease—a liver disorder caused by obstruction of blood flow in small hepatic veins.

Hepatomegaly—enlargement of the liver.

Hepatotoxic—toxic to the liver.

Humoral immunity—the process and function of antibody production. The humoral immunity system marks the foreign cells for destruction by the cellular immunity system.

Hybrid combination—a combination chemotherapy regimen that uses half the scheduled number of doses of two different effective combinations over the time usually occupied by a single cycle.

Hybridoma technology—a process that fuses two cells: one a cell that is stimulated to produce antibodies against a specific antigen, and the other a myeloma plasma cell. This process produces pure quantities of monoclonal antibodies.

Immunoconjugate—a monoclonal antibody coupled with a toxic compound.

Immunomodulating—*see* **Biological response modification**.

Immunotherapy—*see* **Biological response modification**.

Induction—chemotherapy administered to induce complete remission in acute leukemia treatment.

Infertility—inability to produce children.

Intensification—consolidation chemotherapy administered in significantly higher doses than those used in remission induction.

Intercalation—insertion of a drug molecule between two strands of DNA.

Interferon—a protein with antiviral, immune-modulating, and antitumor activity.

Interleukin—a protein produced by lymphocytes that has biological effects on either itself or other cells.

Leukemia—malignancy of the blood cells.

Lymphadenopathy—enlargement of a lymph node.

Lymphoma—malignancy of the lymphatic system.

Maintenance—low doses of chemotherapy administered over the long term to maintain remission.

Malignancy—*see* **Cancer**.

McGill Pain Questionnaire—clinical method of reporting patient pain.

Metabolic modulation—*see* **Biomodulation**.

Metastasis—a clone of the original tumor that develops elsewhere in the body.

Mitotic index—percentage of cells in a tumor mass that are in the mitosis phase at any given time.

Mixed opioid agonist/antagonist—a compound that has an affinity for two or more types of opioid receptors and blocks opioid effects on one receptor type while producing opioid effects on a second receptor type.

Monoclonal—cells arising from a single cell.

Monoclonal antibodies—pure clones of immunoglobulin that react with a specific antigen.

Mucositis—inflammation or toxic damage of the mucous membranes of the gastrointestinal tract.

Multipronged attacks on biochemical pathways—a chemotherapy strategy of multiple insults, combining drugs with different mechanisms of action to attack the tumor from several biochemical directions.

Mutagen—a type of genotoxin that alters DNA.

Myelosuppression—suppression of bone marrow activity, resulting in reduced number of platelets, red cells, and white cells.

Nadir of the white blood cell count—lowest concentration of white blood cells in the peripheral blood after chemotherapy.

Nausea—an awareness of the urge to vomit; an autonomic process associated with pallor, flushing, and tachycardia.

Neoadjuvant therapy—treatment given before surgery to debulk tumors and eradicate micrometastases.

Neoplasm—*see* **Cancer**.

Nephrotoxic—toxic to the kidneys.

Neuropathic pain—pain that results from a disturbance of function or pathological change in a nerve.

Neutropenia—the presence of abnormally low numbers of neutrophils in the circulating blood. (Depending on the institution, the range is <500–1000 cells/mm^3.)

Nociceptive—the process of pain transmission; usually relating to a receptive neuron for painful sensations.

Oncogenes—carcinogen-activated genes that act as transforming genes, causing uncontrolled proliferation of cells and other malignant characteristics.

Opioid agonist—any morphine-like compound that produces bodily effects, including pain relief, sedation, constipation, and respiratory depression.

Opioid partial agonist—a compound that has an affinity for and stimulates physiological activity at the same cell receptors as opioid agonists but that produces only a partial (i.e., submaximal) bodily response.

Pain—an unpleasant sensory and emotional experience associated with actual or potential tissue damage or described in terms of such damage.

Palliative therapy—therapy administered to relieve symptoms.

Paraneoplastic syndromes—remote effects of malignancy; signs or symptoms that are produced by a tumor at a distant site.

Paraproteins—immunoglobulins produced by a clone of neoplastic cells in conditions such as multiple myeloma.

Parathyroid hormone—hormone that regulates serum calcium and stimulates bone resorption, intestinal absorption, and renal reabsorption.

Paresthesia—subjective sensation, experienced as numbness, tingling, or pins-and-needles sensation.

Partial response—decrease of measurable tumor by 50% with no new cancer or tumor progression.

Patient-controlled analgesia (PCA)—self-administration of analgesics by a patient instructed in doing so; usually refers to self-dosing with an intravenous opioid administered by means of a programmable pump.

Peristalsis—the worm-like movement by which tubular organs, provided with longitudinal and circular muscle fibers, propel their contents.

Physical dependence—physiological adaptation of the body to the presence of opioid such that sudden discontinuation of the opioid or administration of an opioid antagonist causes a characteristic withdrawal syndrome.

Pleiotropic drug resistance (multidrug resistance)—resistance of some tumor cell clones to more than one drug.

Prerenal azotemia—elevated blood urea nitrogen concentration resulting from something other than primary renal disease.

Psychological dependence (addiction)—pattern of compulsive drug use characterized by a continued craving for an opioid, the need to use the opioid for effects other than pain relief, and continued use of the opioid despite self-harm.

Radiation recall—hypersensitivity reactions caused by chemotherapy following radiation.

Radiosensitization—*see* **Chemosensitization**.

Recombinant DNA technology—the use of genetic engineering techniques to clone individual genes and produce large quantities of highly purified products in cell culture.

Resistance—the ability of a tumor cell to withstand the effects of a drug that should be lethal.

Retching—spasmodic, abortive movements of the diaphragm and the thoracic and abdominal muscles.

Retinoic acid syndrome—acute complex of fever, respiratory distress, weight gain, edema, effusions, and hypotension caused by tretinoin therapy.

Sanctuary site—sites in the body (such as the central nervous system or testes) where residual cancer cells can survive because chemotherapy agents do not distribute well there.

Sarcoma—malignant tumor of the connective tissue.

Secondary malignancies—cancer that arises after treatment and possibly cure of the primary cancer.

Sequential blockade—a combination of chemotherapy strategy in which two or more drugs block a single critical metabolic pathway at different sites, eliminating this pathway from the tumor cell's metabolism.

Solid tumors—cancers of nonhematological origin that arise from solid tissue (such as breast, lung, prostate, and colon cancers).

Somatic mutation theory—a theory, proposed by Goldie and Coldman, that mutational changes result in varying patterns of drug resistance within a tumor mass.

Spermatogenesis—production of sperm.

Splenomegaly—enlargement of the spleen.

Stable disease—measurable tumor that is neither responding nor progressing.

Synergy—the ability of drug combinations to produce a greater response rate or survival time than is possible with each drug used alone at its optimum dose.

Teratogen—a type of genotoxin that injures a fetus.

Thrombocytopenia—low platelet count.

Tolerance—a physiological result of chronic opioid use; it means that a larger dose of opioid is required to maintain the same level of analgesia.

Transforming growth factors—tumor-derived polypeptides that stimulate cell replication.

Tumor—*see* **Cancer**.

Tumor antigens—chemical compounds on the surface of tumor cells that tell the immune system that the cells do not belong in the body.

Tumor burden—quantity of cancer cells. (Cancers with large tumor burdens include lymphoma, leukemia, and some solid tumors.)

Tumor heterogeneity—existence of multiple variant tumor cell subpopulations within a single tumor mass.

Tumor lysis syndrome (TLS)—a condition that results from the rapid destruction of neoplastic cells. The rapid lysis of tumor cells releases intracellular contents into the systemic circulation faster than the body can eliminate them.

Tumor markers—substances secreted by or associated with particular tumor types.

Tumor priming—a chemotherapy strategy that recruits resting cells into active growth to maximize tumor cell kill.

Visual Analog Scale—clinical method of reporting patient pain.

Volume depletion—inadequate fluid in circulating blood volume.

Vomiting—the mechanical expulsion of gastric contents by coordinated respiratory and abdominal muscles.

White blood cell count (WBC) and the differential—the number of white blood cells and the percentage of each type of white blood cell.

Xerostomia—dry mouth.

Index

A

Absolute neutrophil count (ANC) 270
Acute GVHD 256
    GVHD prophylaxis 257
Acute leukemias 233
    acute lymphocytic leukemia 236
    acute myelogenous leukemia 234
    clinically detectable disease 234
    colony-stimulating factors (CSFs) 239
    complications 238
    consolidation 234
    induction 234
    intensification 234
    maintenance therapy 234
    postremission therapy 234
    prognosis 238
    treatment-related toxicities 238
Acute lymphocytic leukemia (ALL) 236, 254
    diagnosis and classification 236
    treatment 237
Acute myelogenous leukemia (AML) 112, 234, 254, 270, 350
    complications 236
    diagnosis and classification 234
    prognosis 236
    treatment 235
    treatment-related toxicities 236
Adjuvant analgesic drugs 296
Adjuvant drugs 304-5
    anticonvulsants 304
    antidepressants 304
    bone pain adjuvants 304
    corticosteroids 304
    nerve blocks 305
Adjuvant therapy 27-8
Adult T-cell leukemia 6
AJCC classification 204
Alkylating agents 37, 112
    busulfan 40
    chlorambucil 40
    cyclophosphamide 39
    mechlorethamine 39
    melphalan 40
    resistance 38
    thiotepa 40
    toxicities 38
Allogeneic bone marrow transplantation 279
Alloimmunization 104
Alopecia 109-10
Alternative cancer therapies 77
    complementary therapy 77
    integrative therapy 77
    unproven or unorthodox therapies 77
Altretamine 42
American Urologic Association (AUA) 221
Anastrozole 217
Anemia 105

Ann Arbor staging classification system 244
Anorexia 324-5
Anthracyclines 43, 122
    daunorubicin 43
    dexrazoxane 44
    doxorubicin 43
    doxorubicin and daunorubicin 44
    idarubicin 43
    liposomal products 44
    resistance 44
Antibody 24
Antiemetic agents 155
    5-HT$_3$ receptor antagonists 153
    adverse effects 156
    benzodiazepines 153, 155
    butyrophenones 153, 155
    cannabinoids 153, 155
    corticosteroids 153, 155
    cost 157
    designing an antiemetic regimen 157
    dosing and administration 156
    metoclopramide 153
    phenothiazines 153, 155
    serotonin antagonists 155
Antiemetic therapy 152
Antimicrobial resistance 274
    vancomycin-resistant enterococci (VRE) 274
Antineoplastic drug resistance 84
    colon cancer 84
    intrinsic resistance 84
    melanoma 84
    multidrug resistance (MDR) 85
    non-small cell lung cancer 84
    pleiotropic drug resistance 85
    renal cancer 84
Antithymocyte globulin (ATG) 258
Anxiety 313, 314
    management of anxiety 314
ASHP Technical Assistance Bulletin on Handling Cytotoxic and Hazardous Drugs 374
Asparaginase 61, 101, 104, 110, 132, 237-8
Ataxia telangiectasia (Louis-Bar sydrome) 6
Azathioprine 6, 260

B

Bacillus Calmette-Guérin (BCG) vaccine 70-1
Back pain 348
Basal energy expenditure (BEE) 328
Benign prostatic hypertrophy (BPH) 220
Benign tumors 4
Bicalutamide 133
Biochemistry 34
    DNA 36
    RNA 36
    specificity of cancer chemotherapy 36
Biological agents 28

Biological safety cabinet (BSC) 359-60, 389
Biological therapy 24, 68
Bisphosphonates 346
Bladder cancer 6, 40, 358
Bladder toxicity 129
Bleomycin 45, 90, 101, 107, 109, 113, 134, 160, 245, 353
Bloom's syndrome 6
Body surface area (BSA) 91-2
    adults 92
    children 91
Bone marrow transplantation (BMT) 130, 218, 246, 252, 255
    allogeneic BMT 252
    autologous BMT 253
    graft-versus-host disease (GVHD) 256
    hepatic veno-occlusive disease 256
    human leukocyte antigens (HLAs) 252
    peripheral stem cell transplantation 253
    syngeneic BMT 252
Brain tumors 42
BRCA1 gene 213
BRCA2 gene 213
Breast cancer 6, 10, 56, 59-60, 347
    anatomy 212
    clinical presentation 213
    diagnosis 214
    etiology 212
    pathology 213
    pathophysiology 212
    prevention 218
    prognosis 214
    screening 214
    staging 214
    treatment 215
Burkitt's lymphoma 6, 350
Busulfan 40, 107, 130, 134, 240
    hepatic veno-occlusive disease 40

C

Cachectin 327
Calcitonin 345
Calcium homeostasis 342
Camptothecins 60
    irinotecan 60-1
    topotecan 60-1
Cancer cachexia 324, 330
Cancer chemotherapy 271, 364
Cancer diagnosis 7
Cancer pain 291, 293, 301
    acute pain 292
    addiction 301
    causes 291
    chronic pain 292
    contributing factors 291
    management 292
    patient assessment 293
    physical dependence 301
    prevalence 291
    reassessment 295

    tolerance 301
Cancer prevention 4
    aflatoxin 4
    dietary factors 4
    environmental factors 4
    lifestyle factors 4
    medical drugs 4
    occupational factors 4
    reproductive history 4
Cancer screening 8
Cancer statistics 9
Capillary leak syndrome 126
Carboplatin 41
    Calvert formula 42
Carcinoma in situ 213
Carcinoma of the colon or rectum 61
Cardiac toxicity 122
    anthracyclines 122
    cyclophosphamide 125
    fluorouracil 125
    ifosfamide 125
    mechanism of toxicity 123
    prevention 124
    risk factors 123
    taxanes 126
    treatment 124
Central venous access 178
    catheter-related infections 182
    intravascular thrombosis and occlusion of catheter 181
    percutaneous (nontunneled) central venous access 178
    peripherally inserted central venous catheters 179
    totally implantable intravascular devices 180
    tunneled central venous catheters 179
Central venous catheters 347
Cervical cancer 6
Chemoprotective agents 337
Chemotherapy 21-2, 94, 174
    intravenous administration 175
    oral administration 174
Chemotherapy errors 365
Chlorambucil 40, 112, 241-2, 360
Chronic leukemias 239
    chronic lymphocytic leukemia 241-2
    chronic myelogenous leukemia 239-40
Chronic lymphocytic leukemia 55, 57, 241-2, 255, 350
    clinical presentation 241
    complications 242
    diagnosis and classification 241
    prognosis 242
    treatment 241
    treatment-related toxicities 242
Chronic myelogenous leukemia 239-40
    accelerated phase 240
    blast crisis 240
    chronic phase 239
    clinical presentation 239
    complications 240
    diagnosis and classification 239
    Philadelphia chromosome 239
    prognosis 240
    treatment 239
    treatment-related toxicities 240

Cisplatin 41, 89, 101, 104, 139-40, 152, 164, 200-1, 326, 353
  toxicities 41
Cladribine 57, 137
Colon 56
Colony-stimulating factors (CSFs) 238, 344
Colorectal cancer 10, 203
  clinical presentation 204
  diagnosis 204
  etiology 203
  pathophysiology 204
  prognosis 206
  screening 204
  staging 204
  treatment 205
Combination chemotherapy 86-7, 89
Common ALL antigen 237
Confusion 314-5
  management of confusion 315
Constipation 165
  pathophysiology and etiology 165
  prevention and treatment 165
  risk factors 165
Cori cycle 327
Cryotherapy, 223
Cyclophosphamide 6, 39, 86, 89, 107, 112, 125, 130, 151, 200, 237, 246, 257, 260, 328
  hemorrhagic cystitis 39
  mesna 40
Cyclosporine 257, 260
Cytarabine 54-5, 107, 131, 136, 140, 160, 235, 238, 353
Cytomegalovirus 278

D

Dacarbazine 42, 90, 107, 109, 113, 133, 245
Dactinomycin 46, 107, 109, 160
Daunorubicin 122, 124, 160, 235, 237-8, 360
Depression 311-2
  management of depression 312
  medications 311
  symptoms 311
Dermatological reactions 106
  alopecia 109
  busulfan 106
  dactinomycin 106
  drug reactions 106
  fluorouracil 106
  hydroxyurea 106
  nonchemotherapy drug reactions 109
  photosensitivity reactions 109
  radiation and chemotherapy reactions 109
  recombinant cytokine reactions 109
  thiotepa 106
Dexamethasone 237-8
Dexrazoxane 125
Diarrhea 163
  octreotide 164
  pathophysiology and etiology 163
  prevention and treatment 164
  risk factors 163

Diet 5
  breast cancer 6
  colon cancer 5
  esophageal cancer 6
  gastric cancer 6
  larynx neoplasms 6
  liver cancer 6
  oropharynx cancer 6
Diethylstilbestrol (DES) 24, 225
Digital rectal exam (DRE) 220-1
Dihydrotestosterone (DHT) 219
Docetaxel 60, 107, 110, 126, 133, 139
Doxorubicin 89-90, 107, 109, 113, 122, 124, 126, 159, 237-8, 245-6, 353, 360
Doxycycline 353
Drug administration 368
Drug information 369
  formulary and guideline development 370
  patient or consumer information 371
  patient-specific information 369
Ductal carcinoma in situ (DCIS) 213
Dukes' staging system 204
Dyspnea 316-7
  management of dyspnea 317

E

Embryonal rhabdomyosarcoma 46
Endocrine therapy 22
Endometrial carcinoma 6
Enteral nutrition 331
  immune-enhancing formulas 335
Environmental factors 4
  acute leukemia 4
  bladder cancer 4
  mesothelioma 4
Environmental studies 359
Epipodophyllotoxins 58
  etoposide 58
  teniposide 58
Epoetin alfa 105-6
Epstein-Barr Virus 6, 279
Erythropoietin 105
Estrogen receptors 214
Estrogens 6, 104, 255
Etidronate disodium 346
Etoposide 58, 107, 200, 238, 353
Evaluation of response 25
  complete response or remission (CR) 25-6
  disease progression (treatment failure) 25
  duration of response 27
  duration of survival 25
  partial response (PR) 25
  response rate 26
  stable disease 25
Ewing's sarcoma 46
Extravasation 192-3

F

Fanconi's anemia 6
Female fertility 115
Floxuridine 56-7
Fludarabine 55, 104, 137, 242
Fluorouracil 56-7, 87-8, 93, 107, 109, 140, 152, 159, 162-4, 205
Fluorouracil and levamisole 132
Flutamide 133
Fungal infections 276

G

Gallium nitrate 346
Gemcitabine 55-6, 135
Gene therapies 24
Gene therapy of cancer 76
Genetic factors 6
    BRCA1 gene 6
    breast cancer 6
    colon cancer 6
    stomach cancer 6
Genetic mutations 3
Gleason grading system 219
Gluconeogenesis 328
Gompertzian growth curve 18
Gompertzian tumor growth curve 17
Gonadal dysfunction and infertility 113
    prevention of gonadal damage 115
Gonadotropin-releasing hormone (GnRH) 223, 225
Graft-versus-host disease (GVHD) 256
    acute GVHD 256
    chronic GVHD 259
    grading of GVHD 257
    GVHD prophylaxis 259
Granulocyte colony-stimulating factor (G-CSF) 102, 281
Granulocyte-macrophage colony-stimulating factor (GM-CSF) 102, 162, 281
Granulocytopenia 270-2

H

Harris-Benedict equation 328
Hazardous drugs 358, 362
Hazardous drugs, handling of
    disposal of cytotoxics 363
Head and neck cancers 56
Hematological malignancies 58, 254
Hematological toxicity 100, 104
    anemia 105
    myelosuppression 100
    neutropenia 101
    neutropenic fever 102
    thrombocytopenia 103
Hematopoietic colony-stimulating factors (CSFs) 103
Hematopoietic growth factors 71, 93, 101, 105, 281
    filgrastim and sargramostim 93
    oprelvekin 93
Hemorrhagic cystitis 129-30

Hepatic arterial infusions 187, 206
Hepatic toxicity 131
    asparaginase 132
    cytarabine 131
    fluorouracil and levamisole 132
    interferon alfa 133
    interleukin 2 133
    mercaptopurine 131
    methotrexate 132
Hepatic veno-occlusive disease 133
Hepatitis B virus 6
HER2/neu gene 214
Herpes simplex virus (HSV) 162, 278
High-dose cytarabine (HDAC) 135-7, 235, 238
High-efficiency particulate air (HEPA) filter 360
Hodgkin's disease (HD) 6, 42, 113, 242-3, 245, 255, 278
Hodgkin's lymphomas 52
Hormonal agents 22
Hormonal therapy 22
Hormones 28
Hospice care 317
Human leukocyte antigens (HLAs) 104, 252
Human papillomavirus 6
Human T-cell leukemia virus type 1 (HTLV-1) 6
Hydroxyurea 62, 107, 160, 240
Hypercalcemia 342-3
    calcium homeostasis 342
    clinical presentation 344
    etiology 343
    management 346
    treatment 344
Hyperkalemia 351
Hyperphosphatemia 351
Hypersensitivity reactions 110-1
Hyperuricemia 351
Hypocalcemia 351

I

Idarubicin 122, 124, 235
Ifosfamide 39, 86, 107, 125, 130, 136, 200
Immune system 24, 68
    antibody-dependent cell-mediated cytotoxicity 70
    cytotoxic T lymphocytes 69
    interferon gamma 69
    lymphocyte 69
    natural killer (NK) cells 69
    tumor-associated antigens (TAAs) 70
    tumor necrosis factors 69
Immunotherapies 70
    active interventions 70
    Bacillus Calmette-Guérin (BCG) vaccine 70
    passive immunity 70
Infections 270-1
    granulocytopenia 270
Infectious and related complications 260
    hematopoietic growth factors in BMT 262
    interstitial pneumonitis 261
Inorganic phosphates 345
Insomnia 316

Insulin resistance 328
Interferon alfa (INF-α) 68, 133, 138, 206, 240, 246
Interferon alfa-2b 353
Interferon β2 327
Interferon gamma (INF-γ) 327
Interferons 24, 71
   alpha 71
   antitumor mechanisms 72
   clinical applications 72
   interferon alpha-2b 71
   interferon alpha-2a 71
   pharmacokinetics 72
   toxicity 73
Interleukin 1 327
Interleukin 2 (aldesleukin, IL-2) 126, 129, 133, 138, 328, 353
Interleukin 6 327
Interleukins 24, 71, 73
   antitumor mechanisms 73
   clinical applications 74
   pharmacokinetics 73
   toxicity 74
Intra-arterial administration 187
   hepatic arterial infusions 187
   regional limb perfusion 187
Intramuscular administration 184
Intraperitoneal chemotherapy 184, 194
Intrathecal (IT) injections 185
Intravenous (IV) administration of chemotherapy 175
   central venous access and administration 178
   peripheral venous access and administration 175
Intravenous infusion devices 182
   ambulatory infusion devices 182
Irinotecan 61, 163

K

Karnofsky performance status criteria 94
Keratinocyte growth factor (KGF) 162

L

Letrozole 217
Leucovorin 53, 55, 57, 88, 205
Leucovorin rescue 101
Leukemia 6, 55
Leukemias 233, 358
   acute leukemias 233
   chronic leukemias 233
   etiology 233
   pathophysiology 233
Levamisole 205
Liarozole 226
Lifestyle-related factors 4
   breast cancer 4
   leukemias 4
   lung cancer 4
   passive smoking 4
   radiation exposure 4
   radon 4
   thyroid cancer 4
Liposomal doxorubicin and daunorubicin 125

Local and regional chemotherapy administration 184
   intra-arterial administration 186
   intraperitoneal administration 184
   intrathecal and intraventricular administration 185
   intravesical administration 186
Lumpectomy 215
Lung and head and neck tumors 41
Lung and testicular cancers 58
Lung cancer 9, 58-9, 198, 348
   clinical presentation 198
   diagnosis 199
   etiology 198
   non-small cell lung cancer (NSCLC) 198, 200
   pathophysiology 198
   prognosis 202
   screening 198
   small cell lung cancer (SCLC) 198, 202
   staging 199
   treatment 200
Luteinizing hormone (LH) 223
Luteinizing hormone–releasing hormone (LHRH) 223, 225
Lymphocytic leukemia 61
Lymphomas 6, 42, 58, 242, 358
   Ann Arbor staging classification system 244
   bone marrow transplantation 246
   classification 244
   clinical presentation 242
   complications 246
   diagnosis 244
   Hodgkin's disease 242, 245
   non-Hodgkin's lymphoma 242, 246
   treatment 245
   treatment-related toxicities 246

M

Male fertility 113
Malignant pleural effusions 352
   clinical presentation 352
   diagnosis 352
   etiology 352
   treatment 352
Malignant tumors 4
Malnutrition 324
   cancer cachexia 324
   causes of anorexia and cachexia 324
   mechanical problems 325
   prevention 336
   resting energy expenditure (REE) 324
Mammography 214
Mastectomy 215
McGill pain questionnaire 294
Mechlorethamine 6, 39, 90, 112-3, 151, 153, 160, 245
Medication orders 364
Melanomas 42
Melphalan 40, 112, 360
Mercaptopurine 57, 131, 133, 160
Mesna 129-30
Metastases 16
Metastasis 18-9
Methotrexate 52-4, 87-8, 101, 107, 109, 129, 132, 137, 152, 159-60, 238, 257-8

folic acid 52
leucovorin rescue 53
Metoclopramide (Reglan) 155
Minocycline 353
Mitomycin 46, 104, 129, 160
Mitoxantrone 45, 107, 125, 235, 353, 360
Monoclonal antibodies 75
antitumor mechanisms 75
clinical applications 75
toxicity 76
Monthly breast self-examination 214
Mucositis 158, 160, 258, 325
Multidrug resistance (MDR) 85-6
Multiple myeloma 255
Muromonab-CD3 259
Mutagenic effects 358
Myelogenous leukemias 57
Myelosuppression 100, 102

N

Nasopharyngeal carcinoma 6
Nausea and vomiting 149-50, 153, 325
5-HT$_3$ receptor antagonist 152
acetylcholine 150
acute nausea and vomiting 150
anticipatory nausea and vomiting 150
antiemetic agents 153
antiemetic therapy 152
chemoreceptor trigger zone 149-50
chemotherapy-induced 150
corticosteroids 152
cyclophosphamide 152
delayed nausea and vomiting 150
dopamine 150
histamine 150
pathophysiology and etiology 149
risk factors 151
serotonin 150
Southwest Oncology Group (SWOG) toxicity criteria 153
vomiting center 149
Nephrotoxicity 126, 129
Neurological toxicity 136-7
antimetabolites 137
cisplatin 139
cytarabine 136
high-dose cytarabine (HDAC) 136
ifosfamide 136
interferon alfa 138
interleukin 2 138
methotrexate 137
paclitaxel and docetaxel 139
vinca alkaloids 138
Neutropenia 93, 101-2
absolute neutrophil count (ANC) 101
colony-stimulating factors (CSFs) 102
Nilutamide 133
Nitrosoureas
carmustine 40
lomustine 40, 112
streptozocin 40
Non-Hodgkin's lymphoma (NHL) 57, 113, 242-3, 246, 255, 278, 348
Non-small cell lung cancer (NSCLC) 58, 198-9, 201, 348
Nonopioid analgesics 297
Normal hematopoiesis 232
B and T lymphocytes 232
Nosocomial organisms 279
Nucleic acid synthesis 34
DNA 34-5
RNA 34-5
Nutritional supplements 333

O

Occupational Safety and Health Administration (OSHA) 360
Ocular toxicity 140
Ommaya reservoir 238
Oncogenes 2
Oncogenes/Proto-oncogenes 3
ABL 3
BRCA1 3
BRCA2 3
c-myc 3
erb-B 3
N-myc 3
p53 3
ras 3
RASK 3
RB 3
WT1 3
Opioid analgesics 298, 300
Opioids 290
Oprelvekin (interleukin 11) 104
Oral complications 158
analgesics 161
antifungal agents 162
antiviral agents 162
local protective agents 161
mucositis 158
oral cryotherapy 161
oral hygiene 160
other agents 162
pathophysiology and etiology 159
prevention and treatment 160
risk factors 159
Oral contraceptives 6
Orthoclone OKT3 259
Osteogenic sarcomas 52
leucovorin rescue 52
Ototoxicity 139
Ovarian cancer 42, 59, 61
Ovarian carcinoma 41

P

p53 **gene 214**
Paclitaxel 104, 107, 110, 126, 139, 160
Pain intensity scales 294
Pain management 290-1
cancer pain 291
Palliative care 310
Pamidronate 218, 346

Pancreatic cancer 56
Paraneoplastic 199
Paraneoplastic syndromes 9
   autoimmune hemolytic anemia 9
   chronic adrenocortical insufficiency (Addison's disease) 9
   Cushing's syndrome 9
   dermatomyositis and polymyositis 9
   disseminated intravascular coagulation 9
   hypercalcemia 9
   myasthenic syndrome 9
   sensory neuropathies 9
   Sweet's disease 9
   syndrome of inappropriate secretion of antidiuretic hormone (SIADH) 9
   thrombophlebitis 9
Passive smoking 198
Patient education 369
Pediatric leukemias 57-8
Pediatric tumors 255
Pentostatin 57, 137
Peripheral blood progenitor cell transplantation 253
Peripheral stem cell transplantation (PSCT) 253
Peripheral venous administration 175
   extravasation 177
   venous sclerosis and thrombosis 178
Philadelphia chromosome 240
Platinum analogues 41
   carboplatin 41
   cisplatin 41
Plicamycin 345-6
Policies and procedures 363
Porfimer (Photofrin II) 109
Prednisone 90, 113, 153, 237-8, 242, 245-6
Procarbazine 42, 90, 113, 153, 160, 245, 260
Progesterone receptors 214
Prostaglandin E_2 344-5
Prostate cancer 10, 219, 224
   anatomy 219
   clinical presentation 220
   diagnosis 220
   etiology 219
   pathophysiology 219
   prevention 226
   prognosis 221
   screening 220
   staging 221
   treatment 222
Prostate-specific antigen (PSA) 219-22
Proto-oncogenes 2
Protocol development 369
Psoralens plus ultraviolet A radiation (PUVA) therapy 260
Psycho-oncology 311
   anxiety 313
   depression 311
Psychosocial assessment 294
Pulmonary toxicity 133-4
   bleomycin 134
   busulfan 134
   cytarabine 135
   gemcitabine 135
   interleukin 2 136
   tretinoin 136

Q

Quality of life 27

R

Radiation 21-2, 215
   palliative radiation therapy 21
   total body irradiation 21
Radiation therapy 20, 94, 205, 218, 271
Radiosensitizers 22
Regional or localized administration of chemotherapy 25
Regulatory issues 363
Renal toxicity 126
   cisplatin 126
   interleukin 2 129
   methotrexate 129
   mitomycin 129
Resting energy expenditure (REE) 324
Rhabdomyosarcoma 46

S

Safe handling of cytotoxic drugs 361
Sarcomas 42
Sclerosing agents 352-3
Secondary malignancies 111, 358
   chemotherapy 112
   radiation therapy 111
Selective aromatase inhibitors 217
Selective estrogen receptor modulators (SERMs) 217
Sister chromatid exchange (SCE) 359
Skin 10
Skin reactions 107
Sleep disorders 316
   dyssomnias 316
   insomnia 316
   management of sleep disorders 316
   parasomnias 316
Small cell lung cancer (SCLC) 199-200, 202, 347
Solid tumors 28, 255
Southwest Oncology Group (SWOG) toxicity criteria 153
Spill kits 363
Spinal cord compression 348
   clinical presentation 349
   diagnosis 349
   etiology 348
   treatment 349
Stomatitis 158
Stomatotoxicity 159
Subcutaneous administration 184
Superior vena cava syndrome (SVCS) 347
   clinical presentation 347
   diagnosis 347
   etiology 347
   treatment 347
Surgery 19, 22, 218
   diagnosis 20
   prevention 20

reconstruction 20
relief of symptoms 20
staging 20
Syndrome of inappropriate secretion of antidiuretic hormone (SIADH) 199
Syndromes 199

T

Tacrolimus 258
Tamoxifen 6, 24, 104, 133, 216-7
Taste alterations 325
Taxanes 59
   docetaxel 60
   paclitaxel 59
Teniposide 58, 238
Teratogens 358
Testicular cancer 58
Testosterone 219
Tetracycline 353
Thalidomide 260
Thioguanine 57, 133, 160
Thiotepa 40, 107, 112, 353
Thoracentesis 352
Thrombocytopenia 93, 101, 103-4
   platelet transfusions 104
   thrombopoietic growth factors 104
Thrombolytic therapy 348
TNM staging system 199, 205, 214, 222
Tobacco smoking 198
Topoisomerase enzymes 36
Topotecan 61
Total parenteral nutrition (TPN) 335
Toxicities 27
Transforming growth factor beta (TGF-β) 162
Transforming growth factors (TGFs) 212, 344
Transrectal ultrasound (TRUS) 221
Tretinoin 133, 235
Tumor burden 83
Tumor cell proliferation 3
Tumor growth 17
Tumor growth kinetics 16, 82
Tumor lysis syndrome 350, 352
   etiology 350
   metabolic complications 350
   prevention 352
Tumor markers 9
   α-fetoprotein (AFP) 9
   calcitonin 9
   cancer antigen 125 (CA-125) 9
   carcinoembryonic antigen (CEA) 9
   human chorionic gonadotropin (HCG) 9
   immunoglobulins 9
   prostatic acid phosphatase (PAP) 9

Tumor necrosis factor (TNF) 327
Tumor nomenclature 6
   blood cells 7
   connective 6-7
   epithelial 6-7
   lymph tissue 7
   lymph vessels 7
   mesothelium 7
   nerve 7
   neuroectoderm 7
   synovia 7
Tumor size 83
Tumor suppressor genes 3
   BCRA1 genes 3
   retinoblastoma susceptibility (RB) gene 3
   p53 gene 3
Tumor vaccines 24, 76
Tumor vascularization 83
Tumor-associated antigens (TAAs) 68
Tumors 56
Type II topoisomerase inhibitors 112

U

United States Agency for Health Care Policy and Research 293
Urinary urea nitrogen (UUN) 327

V

Vancomycin-resistant enterococci (VRE) 274
Varicella-zoster virus 278
Vertical laminar airflow hood 360
Vinblastine 58, 90, 107, 109, 113, 138, 165, 245, 360
Vinca alkaloids 58, 140, 160
   vinblastine 58
   vincristine 58
   vinorelbine 58
Vincristine 58, 90, 101, 107, 113, 138, 153, 165, 237-8, 245-6, 360
Vinorelbine 58, 138, 165
Viral infections 278
Visual Analog Scale (VAS) 294

W

Wilms' tumor 46
World Health Organization three-step analgesic ladder 296

X

Xeroderma pigmentosum 6
Xerostomia 162, 325-6